CAMBRIDGE TEXTBOOK OF
Neuroscience for Psychiatrists

"Burgeoning neuroscience research and numerous advancements in psychopharmacology have made it a challenge for a busy clinician to remain current in their knowledge base. *Neuroscience for Psychiatrists* provides a pithy and succinct overview of a wide array of neuroscience topics relevant to a practicing clinician, ranging from neurotransmission, functional neuroanatomy and genetics to a discussion of neuroplasticity. This comprehensive text, written by the leading experts in the field, is intuitively organized and richly illustrated. It distils complex subject matter into information that is easy to digest and remember. I would wholeheartedly recommend this book to psychiatrists, residents in training or any other advanced neuroscience enthusiasts."

Vladimir Maletic, MD, MS
Clinical Professor of Psychiatry and Behavioral Science
University of South Carolina School of Medicine, USA

"Improving the treatment for our patients is based on a better understanding of neuroscience. The foundation of evidence-based, rational, prescribing is built upon solid neuroscience knowledge. As this textbook clearly provides both, it is a must for any psychiatrist who pursues to upgrade the treatment she/he provides to their patients."

Joseph Zohar
Professor (Emeritus) of Psychiatry, Tel Aviv University, Israel
Chair, Neuroscience-based Nomenclature (NbN)
President, the International College of Neuropsychopharmacology (CINP)

"*The Cambridge Textbook of Neuroscience for Psychiatrists* is truly a unique compendium of the neurobiological and clinical bases of Psychiatry. It is a self-standing masterpiece for anyone interested understanding and deepening their knowledge of psychiatric disorders without having to search various sources. It represents an up-to-date, comprehensive, and scholarly representation of our current knowledge of Neuroscience relevant to Psychiatry. Furthermore, it is superbly illustrated thereby facilitating a rapid grasp of the fundamental principles and concepts described in the text. The editors realized a *tour de force* in gathering these outstanding contributions from such a group of experts in their own field."

Pierre Blier, MD, PhD
Professor, Departments of Psychiatry and
Cellular & Molecular Medicine
University of Ottawa, Canada

"The editors have succeeded in developing an impressive textbook of neuroscience that speaks directly to psychiatrists. Chapters on basic and translational neuroscience use language that is accessible to clinicians. Moreover, there are illustrations on nearly page to guide the reader through the most complex concepts in neuroscience. Although speaking directly to psychiatrists, the authors manage to present complex concepts in areas that include receptor pharmacology, genetics, neural circuits, and connectivity. Other chapters discuss the underlying neuroscience of basic functions such as sleep, appetite, motivation, cognitive functions and social behaviours. This text is perfectly suited for neuroscience courses for psychiatry training programs and it will also be valued by clinicians who are eager to understand the underlying neuroscience of psychiatric disorders and their treatments."

Stephen R. Marder, MD
Distinguished Professor of Psychiatry
Semel Institute for Neuroscience at UCLA
Director, VA Desert Pacific Mental Illness Research, Education, and Clinical Center

CAMBRIDGE TEXTBOOK OF
Neuroscience for Psychiatrists

Edited by

Mary-Ellen Lynall
University of Cambridge

Peter B. Jones
University of Cambridge

Stephen M. Stahl
University of California, San Diego

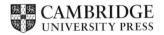

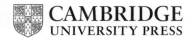

Shaftesbury Road, Cambridge CB2 8EA, United Kingdom

One Liberty Plaza, 20th Floor, New York, NY 10006, USA

477 Williamstown Road, Port Melbourne, VIC 3207, Australia

314–321, 3rd Floor, Plot 3, Splendor Forum, Jasola District Centre, New Delhi – 110025, India

103 Penang Road, #05–06/07, Visioncrest Commercial, Singapore 238467

Cambridge University Press is part of Cambridge University Press & Assessment,
a department of the University of Cambridge.

We share the University's mission to contribute to society through the pursuit of
education, learning and research at the highest international levels of excellence.

www.cambridge.org
Information on this title: www.cambridge.org/9781911623113

DOI: 10.1017/9781911623137

First published 2024

Printed in the United Kingdom by TJ Books Limited, Padstow Cornwall

A catalogue record for this publication is available from the British Library.

A Cataloging-in-Publication data record for this book is available from the Library of Congress.

ISBN 978-1-911-62311-3 Paperback

Cambridge University Press & Assessment has no responsibility for the persistence
or accuracy of URLs for external or third-party internet websites referred to in this
publication and does not guarantee that any content on such websites is, or will remain,
accurate or appropriate.

Every effort has been made in preparing this book to provide accurate and up-to-date information that
is in accord with accepted standards and practice at the time of publication. Although case histories
are drawn from actual cases, every effort has been made to disguise the identities of the individuals
involved. Nevertheless, the authors, editors, and publishers can make no warranties that the information
contained herein is totally free from error, not least because clinical standards are constantly changing
through research and regulation. The authors, editors, and publishers therefore disclaim all liability for
direct or consequential damages resulting from the use of material contained in this book. Readers are
strongly advised to pay careful attention to information provided by the manufacturer of any drugs or
equipment that they plan to use.

Contents

For lecturers and instructors interested in using this text on their course, please email collegesales@cambridge.org and lecturers@cambridge.org for further information, including lecture slides

Laith Alexander
Institute of Psychiatry, Psychology and Neuroscience, King's College London, London, UK
and
South London and the Maudsley NHS Foundation Trust, London, UK

Manny Bagary
Department of Neuropsychiatry Birmingham and Solihull Mental Health NHS Foundation Trust, Birmingham, UK

David Baldwin
Clinical and Experimental Sciences, Faculty of Medicine, University of Southampton, Southampton, UK

Roger Barker
Department of Clinical Neurosciences,
Cambridge Centre for Brain Repair, University of Cambridge, Cambridge, UK

Simon Baron-Cohen
Autism Research Centre, Department of Psychiatry, University of Cambridge, Cambridge, UK

Waiel A. Bashari
Metabolic Research Laboratories, Wellcome–MRC Institute of Metabolic Science, University of Cambridge, Cambridge, UK
and
National Institute for Health Research Cambridge Biomedical Research Centre, Addenbrooke's Hospital, Cambridge Biomedical Campus, Cambridge, UK

Richard Bethlehem
Department of Psychology, University of Cambridge, Cambridge, UK

Markus Boeckle
Department of Psychology, University of Cambridge, UK,
Department of Transitory Psychiatry, Karl Landsteiner University of Health Sciences, Austria
and
University Hospital Tulln, Austria

Ed Bullmore
Department of Psychiatry, University of Cambridge, Cambridge, UK

Chloe Campbell
Research Department of Clinical, Educational and Health Psychology, University College London, London, UK

Rudolf N. Cardinal
Department of Psychiatry, University of Cambridge, Cambridge, UK,
Liaison Psychiatry Service, Cambridgeshire and Peterborough NHS Foundation Trust, Cambridge, UK
and
Cambridge University Hospitals NHS Foundation Trust, Cambridge, UK

Hannah F. Clarke
Department of Physiology, Development and Neuroscience, University of Cambridge, Cambridge, UK

Nicola S. Clayton
Department of Psychology, University of Cambridge, UK

Bru Cormand
Department of Genetics, Microbiology and Statistics, University of Barcelona, Barcelona, Catalonia, Spain,

Institute of Biomedicine of the University of Barcelona, Barcelona, Catalonia, Spain,
Center for Biomedical Network Research on Rare Diseases, Instituto de Salud Carlos III, Spain
and
Sant Joan de Déu Research Institute (IR-SJD), Esplugues de Llobregat, Catalonia, Spain

Herbert E. Covington III
Empire State University School of Social and Behavioral Sciences,
Saratoga Springs, NY, USA

Colm Cunningham
School of Biochemistry and Immunology and Trinity College Institute of Neuroscience,
Trinity College, Dublin, Ireland

Jeffrey W. Dalley
Department of Psychology, University of Cambridge, Cambridge, UK
and
Department of Psychiatry, Herschel Smith Building for Brain and Mind Sciences,
University of Cambridge, Cambridge, UK

Marisa Casanova Dias
National Centre for Mental Health, MRC Centre for Neuropsychiatric Genetics and Genomics,
Cardiff University, Cardiff, UK

I. Sadaf Farooqi
Wellcome-MRC Institute of Metabolic Science, Addenbrooke's Hospital, Cambridge, UK

Emilio Fernandez-Egea
Department of Psychiatry, University of Cambridge, Cambridge, UK
and
Cambridgeshire and Peterborough NHS Foundation Trust, Cambridge, UK

Naomi A. Fineberg
Department of Clinical, Pharmaceutical and Biological Science, University of Hertfordshire, Hatfield, UK
and
Hertfordshire Partnership University NHS Foundation Trust

Paul C. Fletcher
Department of Psychiatry, University of Cambridge, Cambridge, UK

Peter Fonagy
Research Department of Clinical, Educational and Health Psychology, University College London, London, UK

Andre Felix Gentil
Department of Neurosurgery, Hospital Israelita Albert Einstein, Universidade de São Paulo,
São Paulo, Brazil

Claire M. Gillan
School of Psychology and Global Brain Health Institute,
Trinity College Dublin, Ireland

Glenda Gillies
Division of Brain Sciences, Imperial College London, London, UK

Ian M. Goodyer
Department of Psychiatry, University of Cambridge, Cambridge, UK

Mark Gurnell
Metabolic Research Laboratories, Wellcome–MRC Institute of Metabolic Science, University of Cambridge and National Institute for Health Research Cambridge Biomedical Research Centre, Addenbrooke's Hospital, Cambridge Biomedical Campus, Cambridge, UK

Jeremy Hall
Neurosciences & Mental Health Innovation Institute, Hadyn Ellis Building, Cardiff University, Cardiff, UK

Catherine Harmer
Psychopharmacology and Emotion Research Laboratory (PERL), Department of Psychiatry, University of Oxford, Oxford, UK

Alexandra Hayes
Neuropsychopharmacology Unit, Division of Psychiatry, Department of Brain Sciences, Imperial College London, London, UK

Joe Herbert
John van Geest Centre for Brain Repair, Department of Clinical Neurosciences, University of Cambridge, Cambridge, UK

Louise M. Howard
Section of Women's Mental Health, Institute of Psychiatry, Psychology and Neuroscience, King's College London, London, UK

Nathan Huneke
Clinical and Experimental Sciences, Faculty of Medicine, University of Southampton, Southampton, UK
and
Southern Health NHS Foundation Trust, Southampton, UK

Masud Husain
Nuffield Department of Clinical Neurosciences and Department of Experimental Psychology, University of Oxford and John Radcliffe Hospital, Oxford, UK

Bethan Impey
Clinical and Experimental Sciences, Faculty of Medicine, University of Southampton, Southampton, UK

Ian Jones
National Centre for Mental Health, MRC Centre for Neuropsychiatric Genetics and Genomics, Cardiff University, Cardiff, UK

Peter B. Jones
Department of Psychiatry, University of Cambridge, Cambridge, UK
and
Cambridgeshire and Peterborough NHS Foundation Trust, Cambridge, UK

Eileen M. Joyce
Department of Clinical and Movement Neurosciences, UCL Queen Square Institute of Neurology, London, UK
and
The National Hospital for Neurology and Neurosurgery, London, UK

Alexander Kaltenboeck
Psychopharmacology and Emotion Research Laboratory (PERL), Department of Psychiatry,
University of Oxford, Oxford, UK

Kimberley Kendall
Centre for Neuropsychiatric Genetics and Genomics, Cardiff University School of Medicine, Cardiff, UK

George Kirov
MRC Centre for Neuropsychiatric Genetics & Genomics, Cardiff University School of Medicine, Cardiff, UK

Meng-Chuan Lai
Centre for Addiction and Mental Health and The Hospital for Sick Children, Department of Psychiatry,
University of Toronto, Toronto, Canada
and
Autism Research Centre, Department of Psychiatry, University of Cambridge, Cambridge, UK

Matthew A. Lambon Ralph
MRC Cognition and Brain Sciences Unit, University of Cambridge, Cambridge, UK

Rebecca P. Lawson
Department of Psychology, University of Cambridge, Cambridge, UK

Michael C. Lee
University Division of Anaesthesia, University of Cambridge, Cambridge, UK

Victoria Leong
Psychology, School of Social Sciences, Nanyang Technological University, Singapore
and
Department of Paediatrics, University of Cambridge, Cambridge Biomedical Campus, Cambridge, UK

Anne Lingford-Hughes
Neuropsychopharmacology Unit, Division of Psychiatry, Department of Brain Sciences, Imperial College London,
London, UK

Anne Lingford-Hughes
Division of Psychiatry, Dept of Brain Sciences, Imperial College London, London, UK

Patrick Luyten
Research Department of Clinical, Educational and Health Psychology, University College London, London, UK
and
Faculty of Psychology and Educational Sciences, KU Leuven, Belgium

Mary-Ellen Lynall
Department of Psychiatry, University of Cambridge, Cambridge, UK
and
Cambridgeshire and Peterborough NHS Foundation Trust, Cambridge, UK

James MacFarlane
Metabolic Research Laboratories, Wellcome–MRC Institute of Metabolic Science, University of Cambridge , Cambridge, UK
and
National Institute for Health Research Cambridge Biomedical Research Centre, Addenbrooke's Hospital, Cambridge
Biomedical Campus, Cambridge, UK

Ruaidhrí McCormack
Department of Liaison and Neuropsychiatry, Addenbrooke's Hospital, Cambridge, UK
and
Peterborough NHS Foundation Trust, Cambridge, UK

Klaus A. Miczek
Departments of Psychology, Neuroscience, and Psychiatry, Tufts University, Medford and Boston, MA, USA

Amy L. Milton
Department of Psychology, University of Cambridge, Cambridge, UK

Marina Mitjans
Department of Genetics, Microbiology and Statistics, University of Barcelona, Barcelona, Catalonia, Spain,
Institute of Biomedicine of the University of Barcelona, Barcelona, Catalonia, Spain,
Center for Biomedical Network Research on Mental Health, Instituto de Salud Carlos III, Spain
and
Sant Joan de Déu Research Institute (IR-SJD), Esplugues de Llobregat, Catalonia, Spain

John D. Mollon
Department of Psychology, University of Cambridge, Cambridge, UK

Sarah E. Morgan
Department of Psychiatry, University of Cambridge, Cambridge, UK

Alexander G. Murley
Department of Clinical Neurosciences, University of Cambridge, Cambridge, UK

Camilla L. Nord
MRC Cognition and Brain Sciences Unit, University of Cambridge, Cambridge, UK

Mark A. Oldham
University of Rochester Medical Center, University of Rochester, New York, USA

Emanuele F. Osimo
Department of Psychiatry, University of Cambridge, Cambridge, UK,
Cambridgeshire and Peterborough NHS Foundation Trust, Cambridge, UK
and
Faculty of Medicine, Imperial College London, London, UK

Guilherme Carvalhal Ribas
Hospital Israelita Albert Einstein, Universidade de São Paulo, São Paulo, Brzil

Eduardo Carvalhal Ribas
Hospital Israelita Albert Einstein, Universidade de São Paulo, São Paulo, Brazil

Trevor W. Robbins
Department of Psychology and the Behavioural and Clinical Neuroscience Institute,
University of Cambridge, Cambridge, UK

Angela C. Roberts
Department of Physiology, Development and Neuroscience, University of Cambridge, Cambridge, UK

Hugh Robinson
Department of Physiology, Development and Neuroscience, University of Cambridge, Cambridge, UK

Jonathan Roiser
Institute of Cognitive Neuroscience, University College London, London, UK

James B. Rowe
Department of Clinical Neurosciences, University of Cambridge, Cambridge, UK

Barbara J. Sahakian
Department of Psychiatry and the Behavioural and Clinical Neuroscience Institute,
University of Cambridge, Cambridge, UK

Sophie Scharner
Department for Psychosomatic Medicine, Charité – Universitätsmedizin Berlin, Berlin, Germany
and
Child and Adolescent Psychiatry, Massachusetts General Hospital, Boston, USA

Wolfram Schultz
Department of Physiology, Development and Neuroscience, University of Cambridge, Cambridge, UK

Kirsten Scott
Department of Clinical Neurosciences,
Cambridge Centre for Brain Repair, University of Cambridge, Cambridge, UK

Jakob Seidlitz
Department of Psychology, University of Cambridge, Cambridge, UK

Russell Senanayake
Metabolic Research Laboratories, Wellcome–MRC Institute of Metabolic Science, University of Cambridge and
National Institute for Health Research Cambridge Biomedical Research Centre, Addenbrooke's Hospital,
Cambridge Biomedical Campus, Cambridge, UK

Pascal Sienaert
Academic Center for ECT and Neuromodulation (AcCENT), University Psychiatric Center,
KU Leuven (Catholic University of Leuven), Belgium

Jon S. Simons
Department of Psychology, University of Cambridge, Cambridge, UK

Ewan St John Smith
Department of Pharmacology, University of Cambridge, Cambridge, UK

Stephen M. Stahl
University of California, San Diego, CA, USA

Ute Stead
Insomnia and Behavioural Sleep Medicine Clinic, Royal London Hospital for Integrated Medicine,
University College London, London, UK
and
London Hospitals NHS Foundation Trust, London, UK

Andreas Stengel
Department for Psychosomatic Medicine, Charité – Universitätsmedizin Berlin, Berlin, Germany
and
Department of Psychosomatic Medicine and Psychotherapy, University Hospital Tübingen, Tübingen, Germany

Lane Strathearn
Department of Pediatrics, University of Iowa, Iowa City, Iowa, USA

Jack F. G. Underwood
Neurosciences and Mental Health Innovation Institute, Cardiff University, Cardiff, UK

Vincent Valton
Institute of Cognitive Neuroscience, University College London, London, UK
and
National Institute of Health Research,
University College London Hospitals Biomedical Research Centre, London, UK

Merel van der Meulen
Metabolic Research Laboratories, Wellcome–MRC Institute of Metabolic Science, University of Cambridge and
National Institute for Health Research Cambridge Biomedical Research Centre, Addenbrooke's Hospital,
Cambridge Biomedical Campus, Cambridge, UK

Anne-Laura van Harmelen
Department of Education and Child Studies, Faculty of Social Sciences, Leiden University, Leiden, The Netherlands

Eric Vermetten
Department of Psychiatry, Leiden University Medical Center, Leiden, The Netherlands

James Walters
Centre for Neuropsychiatric Genetics and Genomics, Cardiff University, Cardiff, UK

Paul O. Wilkinson
Department of Psychiatry, University of Cambridge, Cambridge, UK

Mai Wong
Department of Liaison Psychiatry, Addenbrooke's Hospital, Cambridgeshire and Peterborough NHS Foundation
Trust, Cambridge, UK

Nefize Yalin
Centre for Affective Disorders, Department of Psychological Medicine, Division of Academic Psychiatry, Institute of
Psychiatry, Psychology and Neuroscience, King's College London, London, UK

Allan H. Young
Centre for Affective Disorders, Department of Psychological Medicine, Division of Academic Psychiatry, Institute of
Psychiatry, Psychology and Neuroscience, King's College London, London, UK

Shahid H. Zaman
Department of Psychiatry, University of Cambridge, Cambridge, UK
and
Cambridgeshire and Peterborough NHS Foundation Trust, Cambridge, UK

Introduction

In the past 100 years there has been a revolution in our understanding of the brain. So far, this has done little to disrupt mainstream psychiatric practice. That is set to change. New neuroscience-based treatments are emerging, while evidence from neuroscience and genetics is calling into question traditional diagnostic boundaries. Psychiatrists of the future will need to integrate their understanding of brain imaging, molecular diagnostics, psychological factors and social context to provide neuroscience-informed care plans.

In recognition of the changes to come, and the need to train the next generation of psychiatrists in modern neuroscience, the Gatsby Foundation, Wellcome and the UK Royal College of Psychiatrists brought together a board of experts under the brilliant direction of Professors Wendy Burn and Mike Travis. Their brief was to develop and implement a new neuroscience curriculum for psychiatrists in training preparing for the Membership of the Royal College of Psychiatrists (MRCPsych) professional examination. The Cambridge Textbook of Neuroscience for Psychiatrists accompanies that new curriculum and should serve as a 'one-stop shop' for what any psychiatrist needs to know about the brain.

Understanding the brain and mind requires a vast array of techniques and conceptual approaches. In this book, we have brought together basic neuroscientists, geneticists, psychologists, psychiatrists, neurologists, neurosurgeons and endocrinologists to bring you the cutting edge of translational neuroscience, focused on addressing the material most relevant to current or future psychiatric practice. Much of the material draws on the lectures prepared for undergraduate and clinical teaching by the faculty of Cambridge Neuroscience and their collaborators beyond the university. We thank them all for their generous contributions.

The book opens with chapters on the basic neuroscience of cells and synapses; the array of methods used in neuroscience; and the neuroanatomy most relevant to psychiatrists. We move on to consider the brain circuits and modulators which underlie functions relevant to psychiatry such as stress responses, motivation, sleep and empathy. We outline the basics of neural development and developmental models of psychiatric disorders. Finally, we consider the neuroscience of each of the major psychiatric diagnoses. We recommend moving back and forth between these sections as you build your knowledge, using the cross-references provided. For example, if you are interested in the neuroscience of obsessive–compulsive disorder (OCD), you might start with the section on OCD, go back to read the section on the neural circuitry of habits, recap the neuroanatomy of the striatum and frontal lobes, then move on to read the section on the neuroscience of brain stimulation.

Despite the vast neuroscientific literature, we are only beginning to understand the neuroscience of psychiatric symptoms, syndromes and treatments. We've tried to reflect this in the textbook, showcasing what is known, but also highlighting aspects of psychiatry that are less well understood, and key outstanding questions in each area.

Our chapters align with the neuroscience syllabus generated under the Gatsby–Wellcome–RCPsych Neuroscience Project described above, and link to the curriculum from the USA National Neuroscience Curriculum Initiative (NNCI). Throughout the book, QR codes link out to relevant online resources from the NNCI. We are grateful to David Ross and Mike Travis at NNCI for discussions during the production of this book and for providing the hard links allowing us to integrate with their fantastic resources. We are also hugely indebted to our brilliant team of peer reviewers, mainly psychiatry trainees, whose incisive feedback was instrumental to the development of these chapters, honing their accessibility and clinical relevance. We are grateful to Dr Gareth Cuttle at the Royal College of Psychiatrists for coordinating this process.

We are keen that this book and its future editions are as useful as possible to those practising clinically, or researching questions of clinical relevance. We would be grateful for your feedback and suggestions, which you can submit as issues on our GitHub repository at **https://github .com/maryellenlynall/neuroscience_for_psychiatrists**.

Introduction

If something comes up in clinical practise and you find yourself wondering, 'What's the neuroscience of that?', but find that it is not covered in this book, we'd like to know!

Editing this book has been a privilege and a pleasure, in large part because of the fantastic team at Cambridge University Press, including Jessica Papworth, Saskia Pronk, Olivia Boult, Anna Whiting and Catherine Barnes, as well as expert copy-editing by Zoë Lewin.

We hope that this book proves a helpful accompaniment to your study and practice, and that you find the material as insightful and thought-provoking as we do.

Mary-Ellen Lynall
Peter B. Jones
Stephen M. Stahl
March 2023

1

Cells

1.1 Neurons

Hugh Robinson

OVERVIEW

Cells are the fundamental units of tissues in multicellular organisms. Animal cells are sealed sacs constructed of extremely thin ($\approx$5 nm) lipid bilayer plasma membranes, spanning across which are various membrane proteins. Crucially, the membrane separates an intracellular biochemical compartment, the cytoplasm, from the extracellular environment. This separation enables gradients, or differences in concentration, of ions and small molecules to be maintained across the membrane, and acts to contain the cytoplasmic proteins and enzymes involved in metabolism, as well as organelles, or intracellular membrane compartments. Particularly importantly for the nervous system, the membrane is also an excellent electrical insulator: it is energetically very unfavourable for charged entities like free ions and electrons to jettison their interactions with polar water molecules in order to cross through the uncharged, non-polar hydrocarbon interior of the lipid bilayer membrane, and so transporting them across the membrane is normally very difficult. This high resistance allows an electrical potential difference to be maintained across the membrane – the membrane potential. An electrical potential difference is equivalent to a difference in the 'concentration' of unbalanced charges between the two sides of the membrane.

Cells come in a myriad of different types and shapes, with specialised adaptations and purposes. In the brain, neurons are the cells which carry out the rapid electrical signalling underlying sensation, reflexes, decisions and motor action. Neurons are supported by another large population of cells, called glial cells, or glia (which are roughly as numerous as neurons, $\approx 10^{10}$ in the human brain). Glial cells associate intimately with neurons, wrapping around them and providing energy support, transporting and recycling the signalling molecules released by neurons (transmitters) at neuron-to-neuron connections, or synapses. Glia are less studied than neurons, but much new research is shedding light on diverse and important roles of these cells in brain physiology and pathology.

Neurons are highly diverse in shape, but generally have (1) a cell body – a relatively large-diameter compartment of the cell containing the cell nucleus; (2) many dendrites, fine branching elongations, which are covered with synaptic connections from other neurons; and (3) an axon, a tubular elongation of the membrane, which conducts electrical signals to the output synaptic connections of the neuron and may be very long and branched. The axon usually arises from the cell body (in some cases, though, from a dendrite). The structure of the neuron enables the collection of large numbers of synaptic inputs from many different presynaptic neurons, processing of this information, and then dispatching an output, expressing some kind of computation or decision based on the input, to many other neurons. For example, a typical brain neuron might receive on the order of 10,000 input synaptic connections from other cells, and send its output through axonal branches to a similar number of downstream neurons. This extraordinarily high connectivity of individual cells to others in a network, and the ability to modify the strength of these connections in response to patterns of electrical activity, explains the complexity of input–output relations of the brain, and its ability to learn associations between inputs and to store vast amounts of information.

The human brain (Figure 1.1.1) is distinctive in having a particularly large outer mantle or cerebrum, with the 'neocortex', a surface layer some 2–3 mm in thickness, overlying phylogenetically older 'allocortex'. The cerebral cortex is most elaborately folded in humans, giving a total area of something like a quarter of a square metre. The neocortex, which is crucially important for many of the higher cognitive functions of the brain, has a stereotypical structure throughout, albeit with some variation from area to area, with six layers distinguished according to the type and density of neuron cell bodies present, and the arrangements of axons.

There are many different types of neuron in the neocortex. These are distinguished, for instance, by:

- whether they make only nearby, local axonal connections or long-range connections
- their inhibitory or excitatory function
- morphology
- expression of particular peptides (somatostatin, cholecystokinin) or calcium-binding proteins (parvalbumin, calbindin)
- secreted neurotransmitters (commonly glutamate in excitatory cells and gamma-aminobutyric acid (GABA) in inhibitory cells, but also including others such as acetylcholine, dopamine, serotonin, glycine)
- other features.

Estimates of the number of different types of cortical neuron vary, and even definitions of 'type', but up to 50 or more neuronal cell types have been identified from single-cell gene expression patterns.

In the next section, we consider the universal features of how neurons operate as biophysical machines, to carry out their function of electrical and chemical processing of information.

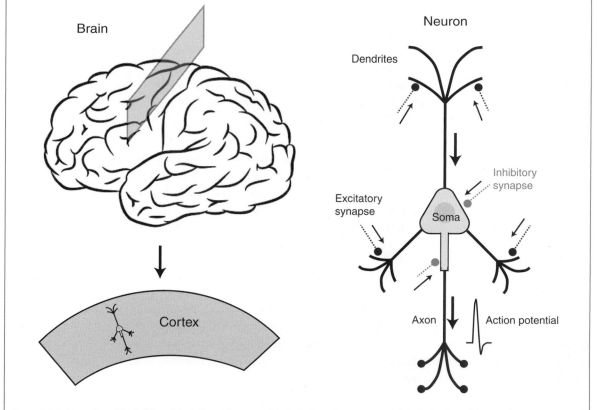

Figure 1.1.1 The cortex of the brain contains billions of neurons. A typical neuron has a soma, or cell body, fine branching membrane extensions called dendrites, and an axon. Information flows in the form of electrical activity arriving from other neurons in the network, to synapses on the dendrites, then electrical current flow to the soma and axon, where an action potential is generated, carrying information down the axon, which forms synapses on other cells. The mapping of the spatiotemporal pattern of synaptic inputs to the timing of the output axonal action potentials defines the information processing function of the neuron.

| **1.2** | **The Physiology of Neurons, Synapses and Receptors** | **Hugh Robinson** |

1.2.1 Ionic Gradients, Ion Channels and the Resting Potential

When a neuron is not electrically active (see Section 1.2.2 below), the plasma membrane potential difference returns to the resting potential: typically −60 mV to −70 mV, meaning the potential inside the cell relative to that outside the cell. The resting potential arises because of the difference in concentration of the major membrane-permeating ions on either side of the plasma membrane: potassium, sodium and chloride (Table 1.2.1).

These gradients arise from the action of the sodium pump, an active (energy-consuming) membrane transporter which pumps three Na^+ ions out of the cell, and two K^+ ions into the cell for each adenosine triphosphate (ATP) molecule hydrolysed. Transporting ions and neurotransmitters across the membrane probably accounts for a large fraction (by some estimates, as much as 75%) of the brain's energy consumption.

In the membranes of neurons are a diverse collection of ion channels: proteins spanning the membrane, each of which contains a pore allowing a continuous pathway for diffusion of ions from one side to the other (Figure 1.2.1). Movement of ions is passive, not linked to ATP consumption, but simply due to diffusion of the charged ions according to the combined effect of their concentration gradient and the influence of the electrical field, if any, within the membrane, on them. The ease with which ions can traverse the pore, and so how much ionic current the pore can conduct, is referred to as its permeability. Typically, the pore is subject to 'gating': conformational changes of the channel protein which open or close the pore. As a result of the precise architecture and charges of amino acid sidechains within the pore formed by the protein channel, many types of ion channel are **selective**, favouring the passage of a particular kind of ion: cations or anions, or specifically potassium, sodium or calcium. The overall ionic permeability and selectivity of a region of neuronal membrane results from the summed effects of all open ion channels. A neuron, depending on its size, may have hundreds or even thousands of ion channels of particular types. Because gating of these channels may itself be controlled by the membrane potential, or by binding of ligands such as neurotransmitters to receptor sites on the channel, ionic permeability and selectivity of the neuronal membrane can be dynamic – changing in time, sometimes very rapidly.

To understand why the combination of ionic gradients and ionic selectivity leads to a resting potential, let us analyse what happens when a cell membrane containing ion channels selective to a particular ion, say K^+, separates a high $[K^+]$ inside from a low $[K^+]$ outside, as in actual neurons. Imagine that only K^+ is allowed to flow

Table 1.2.1 Typical ion concentrations and equilibrium (Nernst) potentials (E_{ion}) for a mammalian neuron

Outside	Inside	Ratio out:in	E_{ion} at 37 °C
$[K^+]_o$ = 5 mM	$[K^+]_i$ = 100 mM	1:20	−80 mV
$[Na^+]_o$ = 150 mM	$[Na^+]_i$ = 15 mM	10:1	62 mV
$[Ca^{2+}]_o$ = 2 mM	$[Ca^{2+}]_i$ = 0.2 μM	10,000:1	123 mV
$[Cl^-]_o$ = 150 mM	$[Cl^-]_i$ = 13 mM	11.5:1	−65 mV

Note that $[Ca^{2+}]_i$ in particular will fluctuate greatly in physiological conditions. The Nernst potential of an ion is the membrane potential difference at which the electrical and chemical (concentration driven) influences on the flux of that ion across the membrane are in balance. There is no net flux of that ion across the membrane when it is at electrochemical equilibrium across the membrane (see text).

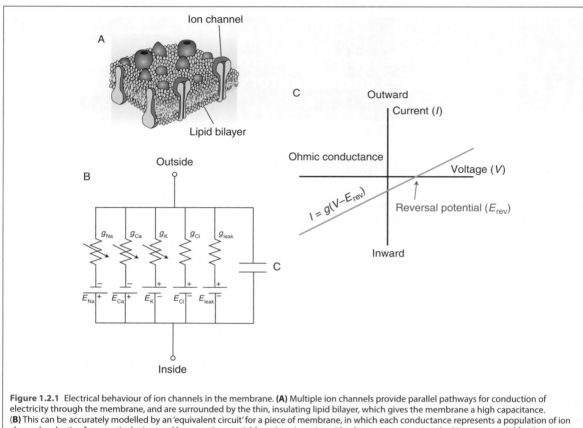

Figure 1.2.1 Electrical behaviour of ion channels in the membrane. **(A)** Multiple ion channels provide parallel pathways for conduction of electricity through the membrane, and are surrounded by the thin, insulating lipid bilayer, which gives the membrane a high capacitance. **(B)** This can be accurately modelled by an 'equivalent circuit' for a piece of membrane, in which each conductance represents a population of ion channels selective for a particular ion, and has a static or variable resistor in series with a battery representing the Nernst potential for that ion. Some conductances are not selective to just one ion, but have a mixed selectivity (e.g. g_{leak}). **(C)** The current through a particular population of ion channels is characterised by its current–voltage relationship. An ohmic conductance, shown here, conducts a current which is a simple linear function of the membrane potential (or voltage), and which is zero at its reversal potential. For a conductance perfectly selective to one ion, the reversal potential is equal to the Nernst potential for that ion.

across the membrane (very crudely, a reasonable model of a resting neuronal membrane). As it flows **down its concentration gradient**, from inside to outside, this leaves a net negative charge inside, that is, it creates a negative (hyperpolarised) membrane potential, because of the loss of positive ions within the cell. This counteracts the outward flux (flow) of the positively charged K^+ ions. Net flux continues until a potential difference is achieved where the concentration drive is balanced by the counteracting electrical force. One can calculate this potential for a given concentration difference, using the **Nernst equation**:

$$E_K = \frac{RT}{zF} \ln \frac{\left[K^+ \right]_o}{\left[K^+ \right]_i}$$

where E_K is the equilibrium potential for potassium, R and F are constants (fixed numbers), T is the temperature in

Kelvin, z is the number of unitary charges of the ion (+1 for potassium), and $[K^+]_i$ and $[K^+]_o$ are the concentrations of potassium inside and outside the cell, respectively. This is exactly true only for a purely K^+-selective membrane. Roughly speaking, though, it serves as an explanation of the resting potential. At rest, the membrane is *predominantly* K^+ permeable. With 150 mM inside and 5.5 mM outside, E_K is about −90 mV at 37 °C. The resting potential therefore is predicted to be −90 mV. However, inward leakage of some Na^+, through a much smaller Na^+ permeability, and balanced by an equal and opposite movement of K^+, means that zero net flux of charge (and therefore a stationary membrane potential) is actually reached at a somewhat more depolarised (more positive) potential, commonly around −70 mV to −65 mV.

The membrane potential **changes** as a result of the flow of electrical current in the form of ions. Considering a patch of membrane at one particular location in a neuron, positive charge, for example, might arrive at the internal face of the membrane either by flowing through the cytoplasm from a neighbouring region of the neuron which is at a higher potential (propagation of depolarisation), or through specialised ion-channel molecules – pore structures allowing flow of ions across the membrane. Positive charge building up on the inside of the membrane makes the membrane potential difference more positive – it is said to **depolarise** the membrane. Loss of net positive charge, either through loss of positive ions or gain of negative ions, causes the membrane potential difference (inside relative to outside) to become more negative – the membrane is said to **hyperpolarise.**

The way in which membrane potential changes in time is heavily influenced by the **electrical capacitance** of the membrane. Capacitance is the storage of charge at an insulating gap between two conductors at different potentials. Positive charge on one side is attracted to negative charge on the other. The amount of charge stored (Q) is proportional to the voltage difference V across the capacitor: $Q = CV$, where the constant of proportionality C is the capacitance (unit C/V = Farad). For a capacitor composed of two conducting plates, the capacitance scales with the area of the plates and inversely with the distance between them.

Applying a voltage across a capacitor stores charge on the capacitor. When the potential difference between the plates is reduced, the charge flows away – the capacitor discharges. In neurons, lipid bilayer membranes represent exceedingly thin insulating gaps between two conducting phases (intra- and extracellular), and therefore have a high capacitance (typically 1 μF/cm^2).

The consequence of this high capacitance is that capacitative current flows when the membrane potential changes. The rate of flow of charge, in other words the current I, is the capacitance times the rate of change of voltage across the capacitor:

$$I = C \frac{dV}{dt}.$$

Depolarisation entails positive charge moving onto the cytoplasmic 'plate' of the membrane capacitor, and off of the external 'plate'. It is transmembrane and intracellular ionic currents which provide this charge: the capacitative current in a patch of membrane is equal and opposite in sign to the ionic and intracellular currents (resulting

from flux from neighbouring regions of the cell having a different membrane potential). It can also be seen from this that, as a current flows, it takes time to change the membrane potential by a given amount: it changes with a finite dV/dt. If the membrane conductance g (the summed conductance of all open ion channels in the membrane) is constant, the membrane potential changes in an exponential manner, relaxing towards a new steady value, with a time constant $\tau = C / g$, which characterises the timescale with which the neuron responds (in the sense of changing its membrane potential) to an input, in the form of a step change in an input current. For a cortical neuron at rest, this time constant might typically be 20–50 ms.

1.2.2 Voltage-Dependent Gating of Ion Channels and Action Potentials

Neurons signal over long distances via fast transient changes in their membrane potential, briefly reaching positive values (usually +20 mV to +60 mV). This rapid pulse of positivity is referred to as an **action potential**, and usually has a characteristic trajectory in time for a given type of neuron, typically lasting a millisecond or two. It is therefore often thought of as a digital pulse, an all-or-nothing event, whose occurrence reflects a decisive signalling switch. Neurons send long-range signals around the brain and through the body, because the action potential **propagates** along axons, with speeds of 0.1–100 m/s. Even the stimulation of a sequence of a few action potentials in one neuron in the brain can influence sensory discrimination.

How does the action potential happen? Work by Hodgkin and Huxley on squid giant axons in the early 1950s used experimental control of the membrane potential (voltage-clamp) and manipulation of ionic gradients to reveal that two populations of **voltage-gated** ion channels, sodium (Na_V) and potassium (K_V), in the membrane open in quick succession. First, triggered by a depolarisation, the Na_V channels open, making the overall membrane conductance strongly selective for Na$^+$, and so the membrane potential swings rapidly towards the sodium equilibrium potential, E_{Na}, ($\approx$+60 mV), as sodium ions enter. After only a brief delay, however, the depolarised membrane potential triggers opening of the K_V channels, and the membrane potential is pulled back towards the resting potential, as K$^+$ ions leave the cell. Overall, a small amount of sodium has entered the cell, and a small amount of potassium has left, slightly dissipating the ionic gradients, which are restored by the subsequent ATP-consuming action of the sodium pump.

The requirement for a certain amount of depolarisation to be exceeded (threshold) in order to trigger the stereotypical sequence of sodium–potassium permeability is referred to as excitability. If depolarisation is not sufficient to reach threshold, it subsides after the input is switched off. If threshold is reached, however, a full-blown action potential is excited.

Action potentials propagate along axons, as mentioned above, in the following way. Consider one location on the axon where an action potential is currently under way. The positive charge entering the cell at this excited location, while the membrane potential there is undergoing the upstroke of the action potential, results in a positive current flowing forward within the cytoplasm of the axon, a little further along. This depolarises the next section of axon membrane, causing it to reach its threshold, and undergo an action potential, and so on. Propagation is not instant, but depends on the time required to charge up the membrane capacitance at each location to threshold, which takes longer the more capacitance there is (see the discussion of the time constant above).

In some axons, especially those adapted for long-range and relatively fast signalling, this time delay for the local depolarisation to threshold is reduced by *myelin*, which consists of multiple layers of membrane wrapped around the axon by so-called Schwann cells, greatly reducing its membrane capacitance by increasing the gap between intracellular and extracellular compartments. However, the thick myelin sheath must be interrupted every milimetre or so, at so-called nodes of Ranvier, where the voltage-gated ion channels are concentrated, and can operate. Runaway depolarisation driven by sodium influx occurs at each node, depolarising the next low-capacitance internode region relatively quickly. The savings in energetic cost (total transmembrane flux of sodium and potassium which must ultimately be pumped back using ATP) and the benefit of much higher conduction speeds make the investment of constructing the myelin sheath worthwhile. However, for short-range information processing in local cortical networks, a very high and complex connectivity is needed, while speed of conduction is less important, and so unmyelinated (and

hence potentially much thinner) axons are used. The high lipid content of the thick myelin sheaths give a white appearance to brain tissue in which long-range axons are bundled together ('white matter'), while areas dedicated to information processing by complex local circuits have a much lower myelin content and appear grey.

1.2.3 Synapses

Synapses are specialised signalling junctions between two neurons where their membranes are separated by only 15–20 nm – the gap is referred to as the synaptic cleft – and action potentials in one neuron, the 'presynaptic' neuron, produce release of transmitter chemicals, or neurotransmitters, into the synaptic cleft via fusion of transmitter-containing presynaptic vesicles with the plasma membrane. The neurotransmitters then bind to clusters of ion-channel receptors on the other side of the gap, on the 'postsynaptic' neuron, which in turn open and conduct ionic current briefly (Figure 1.2.2). The postsynaptic neuron may itself be excited to fire action potentials depending on the spatial and temporal patterns of activation of multiple synapses onto it, and the consequent flow of current. For example, a large pyramidal neuron in the cortex may have up to 100,000 synapses. In this way, a neuron makes decisions, or computes its output as a pattern of action potentials in time.

A fundamental mechanism of plasticity in neuronal circuits – their ability to change their operation with time and through this to implement learning and memory – is the modifiability of the amplitude of the synaptic current with activity. These changes occur at both short and long timescales, and are assisted by the elaborate biochemical signalling networks at the postsynaptic site (often confined within a small evagination of membrane called a dendritic spine). See Section 2.1 for more on synaptic physiology.

1.2.4 Neurotransmitter Receptors

Neurotransmitters may be excitatory, with an action that depolarises, or excites, postsynaptic neurons; or inhibitory, resisting depolarisation, or even hyperpolarising, and so inhibiting postsynaptic neurons. Glutamate is widely used in the brain as an excitatory neurotransmitter, and GABA as an inhibitory neurotransmitter (although there are many other neurotransmitters – see above). For example, glutamate receptors

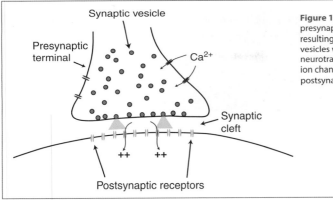

Figure 1.2.2 An excitatory synapse. An action potential arriving at a presynaptic terminal opens voltage-gated calcium channels, and the resulting calcium influx triggers fusion of neurotransmitter-containing vesicles with the plasma membrane facing the synaptic cleft. The neurotransmitter diffuses across the cleft and opens postsynaptic ion channels, allowing influx of cations and depolarising the postsynaptic membrane.

include cation-selective ion channels which have a mixed selectivity for Na^+ and K^+ ions. This means that their opening pulls the membrane potential towards a value in between E_K and E_{Na}, to around 0 mV. This depolarising effect may trigger action potentials in the postsynaptic neuron. Some glutamate receptors are also permeable to calcium, in addition to sodium and potassium, and the calcium entry which they can mediate may serve as a downstream intracellular messenger in the postsynaptic cell. Specialised glutamate receptors called *N*-methyl-D-aspartate (NMDA) receptors both are calcium permeable and experience a block by magnesium ions at hyperpolarised potentials, which is relieved by depolarisation. This block allows the NMDA receptor to act like a switch, gating plastic changes

at the postsynaptic site signalled by calcium influx, but requiring **simultaneous** presynaptic excitation (release of glutamate) and postsynaptic depolarisation (relief of magnesium block) to be effective – a so-called 'Hebbian' mechanism.

In contrast, many types of GABA receptor are chloride channels. Inhibitory neurons release GABA, which increases the chloride permeability of the postsynaptic membrane, pulling the postsynaptic neuron's membrane potential towards E_{Cl}, which is usually close to the resting potential. If this coincides with release of glutamate from a presynaptic excitatory neuron, this has the effect of reducing the amount of depolarisation that would have occurred without the inhibitory input. See Section 2.3 for more on specific neurotransmitter systems.

1.3 Modelling Single Neurons and Their Combinations in Circuits

Hugh Robinson

The principles of electrical current flow in neurons are well understood, from studying the 'equivalent circuits' constructed from resistors and capacitors which represent the corresponding properties of the membrane and cytoplasm, and the differential equations describing the dynamics of the opening probabilities of Na_V and K_V channels as voltage changes. These can give quantitatively accurate predictions of the overall behaviour of the membrane potential, including action potential firing, both single and repetitive, during stimulation – famously in the Hodgkin–Huxley model. For a neuron of complicated morphology (the usual case!), accurate modelling might require hundreds of individual subcompartments, each with its own complement of ion channels and particular membrane characteristics, linked via intracellular resistors to its neighbouring compartments. Modern computational power makes it easy to calculate numerical solutions of these large systems of differential equations for highly complicated neuronal morphologies and for multiple neurons connected by synaptic connections – neural circuits.

This has led to the field of *computational neuroscience*, the endeavour to understand and predict the function of neurons and neuronal circuits by modelling (see also Section 3.4). Efforts are still in their infancy, but aspire to the extraordinary effectiveness and biophysical meaningfulness of the Hodgkin–Huxley model. Many challenges remain, though – our lack of knowledge of the detailed parameters such as the densities and gating properties of particular kinds of ion channel in real neurons, and the ways in which these are adjusted through biochemical signalling such as phosphorylation of ion channels during activity, as well as the still-inadequate experimental characterisation of the massively parallel patterns of activity in biological neuronal networks which computational neuroscience tries to explain. However, the situation is changing rapidly, with new techniques of microscopy for live imaging and genetic approaches.

1.4 Glia

Hugh Robinson

No survey of brain cells would be complete without considering glial cells, or glia. These are non-neuronal, non-electrically active cells, which nevertheless make vital contributions to the function of neurons in the brain. Located throughout the brain, intermingled with and in close proximity to neurons, in similar numbers, they can be divided into several major types, with specific roles.

Astrocytes, the most numerous glial cell type, wrap tightly around blood capillaries to help maintain the blood–brain barrier – regulating transport of substances from the blood into the extracellular space around neurons. Astrocytes are also believed to supply energy to active neurons in the form of lactate, which can be converted into pyruvate and fed into the tricarboxylic acid cycle to produce ATP in neurons. Astrocytes take up and process neurotransmitters released at the synapse, in particular glutamate, thus shaping the strength and timing of synaptic transmission and influencing synaptic plasticity. This is achieved through a very close physical association of astrocytic cell processes with synaptic sites, leading to the concept of the 'tripartite synapse'

(presynaptic neuron–postsynaptic neuron–astrocyte). Astrocytes also rapidly absorb potassium released during neuronal activity, counteracting the lingering depolarisation of neurons produced by extracellular potassium.

Another abundant type of glial cell is the oligodendrocyte, which is responsible for myelination in the central nervous system, principally in the white matter, by wrapping its membrane around axonal processes of neurons. The same role is carried out in the peripheral nervous system by Schwann cells (as described in **Section 1.2.2** above), which are also classed as glial cells. Microglia, yet another glial cell type, are in fact brain-specific macrophages, with an immune function. These are able to move and proliferate within the brain, in response to disease and damage, and to attack and phagocytose foreign or infected cells. Glia also play important roles in neuronal development, guiding the migration of developing neurons and, unlike most neurons, they can continue to undergo mitosis in the adult brain. Glial progenitor cells are the cells of origin of the most prevalent forms of primary brain cancers, the gliomas.

FURTHER READING FOR CHAPTER 1

Hille, B. *Ion Channels of Excitable Membranes*, 3rd ed. Sinauer, 2001.

Hodgkin AL, Huxley AF. A quantitative description of membrane current and its application to conduction and excitation in nerve. *J Physiol* 1952; **117**: 500–544.

Johnston D, Miao-Sin Wu S. *Foundations of Cellular Neurophysiology*. MIT Press, 1994.

Sterratt D, Graham B, Gillies A, Willshaw D. *Principles of Computational Modelling in Neuroscience*. Cambridge University Press, 2011.

National Neuroscience Curriculum Initiative online resources

Synaptic Plasticity: The Role of Learning and Unlearning in Addiction and Beyond

Alejandro Ramirez and Melissa R. Arbuckle

Modern Microglia: Novel Targets in Psychiatric Neuroscience

Jennifer B. Dwyer and David A. Ross

This "stuff" is really cool: Jenny Dwyer, *"Microglia"*

This "stuff" is really cool: Alan Lewis, *"Your Brain In A Dish"* on induced pluripotent stem cells

2

Neurotransmitters and Receptors

Emanuele F. Osimo and
Stephen M. Stahl

2.1 The Chemical Synapse

OVERVIEW

As described in Chapter 1, the generation and propagation of electrical signals in the brain (neurotransmission) happens at specialised sites of the neuron called synapses. Electrical signals which exceed a given threshold can be propagated to nearby neurons nearly instantaneously, and bidirectionally, at electrical synapses.

In this Section 2.1, we focus on chemical synapses: these are slower, as they require an electrical signal to be transduced into the physical movement and fusion of synaptic vesicles, which contain specialised neurotransmitters, in a synaptic cleft. Chemical synapses are monodirectional and allow for much finer regulation of signal transduction. A neurotransmitter is described as excitatory if it increases the likelihood of depolarisation in the postsynaptic neuron, and inhibitory if it decreases it. Chemical signals from one synapse can contact and modulate multiple postsynaptic neurons, and multiple synapses – from more than one presynaptic neuron – can converge on one postsynaptic neuron, allowing for finer control – as well as for amplification – of signals. In the following three sections we will then explore various families of neurotransmitters, as well as the different classes of receptors that can transduce their signals.

2.1.1 Introduction to the Chemical Synapse

Chemical synapses mediate complex transmission in the central nervous system. Differently from electrical synapses, they are classically monodirectional, meaning that there is a presynaptic neuron relaying a message to a postsynaptic one; recently, there has been appreciation that some chemical signalling is retrograde, from postsynaptic to presynaptic, but we will confine our discussion here to classical neurotransmission from presynaptic to postsynaptic, as current knowledge indicates that retrograde transmission plays a less significant role.

Chemical synapses may function to amplify the signal, meaning that the synaptic discharge of neurotransmitter from one neuron can affect many postsynaptic neurons. Each receptor has the ability to activate a metabolic chain of events, as we will see later. Chemical synapses can allow for signals that are richer in quality than electrical synapses: excitatory and inhibitory chemical signals from different neurotransmitters can act on the same receiving neuron on separate receptors, and different receptors can respond to the same chemical signal with graded responses. Chemical ionotropic receptors can be specific for various ions, such as Na^+, K^+, Ca^{2+}, or Cl^-; and they can respond by opening or closing to a neurotransmitter. For example, if a sodium-channel receptor responds to a ligand by opening, it will depolarise the postsynaptic neuron, while if the ligand causes the channel to close further, it will hyperpolarise the neuron; a ligand can have opposite effects if it triggers a channel that is permeable to cations. Metabotropic receptors can activate complex biochemical pathways, both excitatory and inhibitory.

The chemical synapse also has much more diversity in time-specificity than the electrical synapse: metabotropic receptors and ionotropic receptors have different activation kinetics. This complex synaptic physiology allows for the fine modulation of interneuronal communication in the central nervous system, and is an important mechanism underlying higher brain function and disease pathophysiology. Furthermore, most (if not all) psychiatric treatments affect, directly or indirectly, several neurotransmitter pathways.

2.1.2 Ion Channels and Calcium Flux in Relation to Synaptic Physiology

In chemical synapses (Figure 2.1.1), the presynaptic neuron is not in continuity with the postsynaptic neuron, thus forming a gap, called a synaptic cleft. The presynaptic neuron stores one or more neurotransmitters in vesicles – pockets of liquid enclosed by membranes – separating their contents from the cytoplasm. The vesicles are organised in pools (a storage pool and an active pool) and are lined with neurotransmitter transporters, which are usually specific for one, or a few, related neurotransmitters. The cleft is lined with receptors, both postsynaptic receptors that respond to neurotransmitter release, and presynaptic receptors that can exert feedback control of neurotransmission. As seen in more detail below, to terminate the signal quickly, the presynaptic membrane hosts neurotransmitter transporters, which can 're-capture' the neurotransmitter from the cleft; the cleft may also contain enzymes that terminate neurotransmission by destroying the transmitter, such as cholinesterase and monoamine oxidase. The presynaptic membrane, especially the active zone (the site of neurotransmitter release) is lined with voltage-gated ion channels. When the presynaptic neuron is depolarised, these voltage-gated channels open and allow calcium to enter. A high concentration of calcium near the active zone causes vesicles containing neurotransmitter to fuse with the presynaptic membrane and release their contents into the synaptic cleft (a process called exocytosis). The neurotransmitter then binds to both the postsynaptic receptors (effectors), and to presynaptic ones (feedback modulators, which contribute to terminating the discharge).

2.1.3 Transmitter Synthesis

Two sets of substances act as neurotransmitters: small-molecule neurotransmitters, which were discovered first and are the most common targets of existing psychotropic drugs, and neuropeptides (short chains of amino acids, which will be covered in the next section). The main small molecule transmitters are:

- monoamines (including dopamine, adrenaline, noradrenaline and serotonin)
- acetylcholine
- amino acids (including glutamate and gamma-aminobutyric acid (GABA))
- purines (e.g. adenosine triphosphate).

Figure 2.1.2 shows that monoamines are grouped together as they all share a common precursor, the

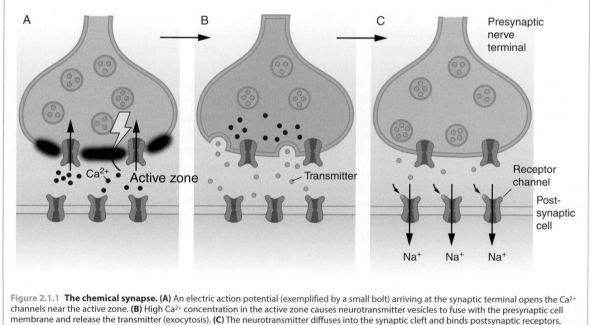

Figure 2.1.1 The chemical synapse. (A) An electric action potential (exemplified by a small bolt) arriving at the synaptic terminal opens the Ca^{2+} channels near the active zone. **(B)** High Ca^{2+} concentration in the active zone causes neurotransmitter vesicles to fuse with the presynaptic cell membrane and release the transmitter (exocytosis). **(C)** The neurotransmitter diffuses into the synaptic cleft and binds postsynaptic receptors. Neurotransmitters can cause ion channels to open or close, affecting postsynaptic cell membrane potential.

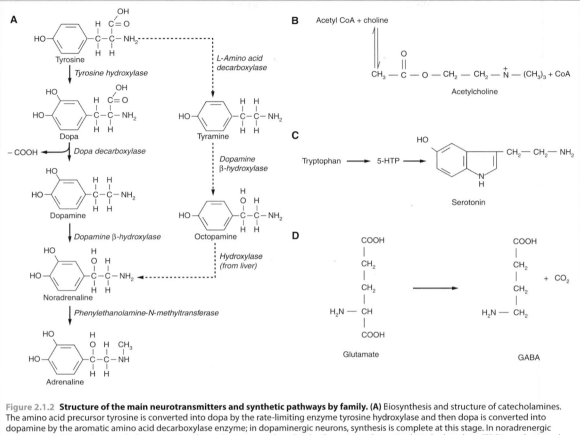

Figure 2.1.2 **Structure of the main neurotransmitters and synthetic pathways by family. (A)** Biosynthesis and structure of catecholamines. The amino acid precursor tyrosine is converted into dopa by the rate-limiting enzyme tyrosine hydroxylase and then dopa is converted into dopamine by the aromatic amino acid decarboxylase enzyme; in dopaminergic neurons, synthesis is complete at this stage. In noradrenergic neurons, an additional step includes converting dopamine into noradrenaline by the enzyme dopamine beta-hydroxylase. **(B)** Biosynthesis and structure of acetylcholine. Acetylcholine is synthesised from the precursor choline by the enzyme choline acetyl transferase. **(C)** Biosynthesis and structure of serotonin. Serotonin, also known as 5-hydroxytryptamine (5-HT), is synthesised from the amino acid tryptophan by the rate-limiting enzyme tryptophan hydroxylase, first converting tryptophan into 5-hydroxytryptophan (5-HTP). Next, aromatic amino acid decarboxylase converts 5-HTP into 5-HT, i.e. serotonin. **(D)** Biosynthesis and structure of GABA. Gamma-aminobutyric acid (GABA) is formed from the amino acid glutamate by the glutamic acid decarboxylase enzyme.

amino acid phenylalanine, which is converted either into tyrosine or into a so-called trace amine called beta-phenethylamine.

Tyrosine can be converted either into dopa by tyrosine hydroxylase, or into the trace amine tyramine and then into another trace amine, octopamine (Figure 2.1.2). Tyrosine hydroxylase is the rate-limiting enzyme (i.e. the bottleneck) for the synthesis of the monoamine neurotransmitters dopamine, noradrenaline and adrenaline and is present in specific cell types, namely dopaminergic and noradrenergic neurons. In dopaminergic neurons, the synthetic pathway terminates with the production of dopamine, while in sympathetic terminals dopamine is further converted into noradrenaline. In the adrenal

TRACE AMINES

Trace amines remain poorly characterised; in the past they were considered simply to be intermediaries of actual neurotransmitters, because they are found in low (i.e. trace) concentrations and not stored in synaptic vesicles. Recently, however, receptors for trace amines (called trace amine associated receptors (TAARs)) were discovered, and new drugs acting as TAAR agonists are in clinical testing; these appear to show early signs of efficacy in schizophrenia, and have opened a new chapter of research into the pathophysiology and potential treatments for serious mental illness.

medulla and certain areas of the central nervous system, some noradrenaline is further converted into adrenaline. Acetylcholine derives from the common Krebs cycle metabolite acetyl coenzyme A (CoA) combined with choline. Serotonin derives from the amino acid tryptophan. Glutamate is an amino acid that also acts as an excitatory neurotransmitter; GABA derives from the decarboxylation of glutamate (Figure 2.1.2).

2.1.4 Transmitter Storage, Release and Reuptake

Neurotransmitters are synthesised in the cytosol, then concentrated into presynaptic vesicles by specific transporters (Figure 2.1.3). Vesicular monoamine transporters (VMATs) transport all monoamines (VMAT2 is the primary VMAT in the brain; VMAT1 is mainly expressed in the peripheral nervous system and in neuroendocrine cells), while other transmitters have specific transporters. Once the transmitter is released into the synaptic cleft, it must be removed quickly to avoid toxic effects, which is the task of two sets of proteins:

- Transporters such as the dopamine (DAT), noradrenaline (NET) or serotonin (SERT) transporters bring the chemical back into the presynaptic neuron, thus allowing recycling.
- Transmitters can also rapidly be degraded by specific enzymes such as monoamine oxidase (MAO) for monoamines or by acetylcholinesterase (AChE) for acetylcholine.

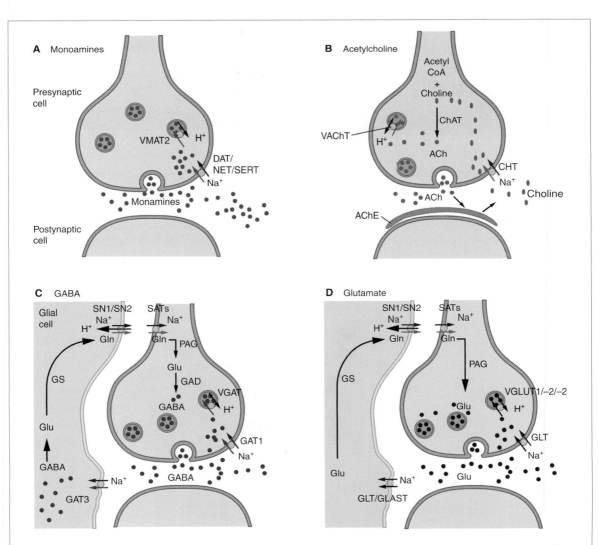

Figure 2.1.3 Transmitter storage, release and reuptake. Transmitters are released by exocytosis, then the signal is terminated by specific proteins at the nerve terminal or in nearby glial cells. **(A)** Monoamines: vesicular monoamine transporter 2 (VMAT2) transports neurotransmitters from the cytoplasm into storage in synaptic vesicles; dopamine transporter (DAT) transports dopamine from the synapse into the presynaptic neuron; noradrenaline (norepinephrine) transporter (NET) transports noradrenaline from the synapse into the presynaptic neuron; serotonin transporter (SERT) transports serotonin from the synapse into the presynaptic neuron. **(B)** Acetylcholine: vesicular acetylcholine transporter (VAChT) transports acetylcholine (ACh) from the cytoplasm into synaptic vesicles; choline acetyltransferase (ChAT) synthesises ACh from the precursor choline; acetylcholinesterase (AChE) inactivates ACh, converting it back into choline. **(C)** Gamma-aminobutyric acid (GABA) and **(D)** glutamate are both neurotransmitters; system A transporters (SATs) and system N (SN1/SN2) transporters are additional transport pumps for amino acids such as glutamate; GABA transporter (GAT) pumps GABA from the synapse into the presynaptic neuron; glutamine synthetase (GS) converts glutamate (Glu) into glutamine (Gln) in glial cells as part of the recycling process to return Glu into the presynaptic neuron, where phosphate-activated glutaminase (PAG) coverts Gln into Glu, and glutamate decarboxylase (GAD) converts Glu into the neurotransmitter GABA; vesicular GABA transporter (VGAT) stores GABA from the cytoplasm in the synaptic vesicles; glutamate transporter (GLT) and glutamate aspartate transporter (GLAST) are additional reuptake pumps for synaptic glutamate into the cytoplasm of either glial cells or presynaptic glutamate nerve terminals; vesicular glutamate transporter (VGLUT) pumps glutamate from the cytoplasm into synaptic vesicles.

<table>
<tr><td>**2.2**</td><td>**Classification of Receptors: Metabotropic and Ionotropic Receptors**</td><td>Emanuele F. Osimo and Stephen M. Stahl</td></tr>
</table>

Chemical neurotransmitters have two main ways of exerting an effect on postsynaptic neurons: by binding to ionotropic or to metabotropic receptors (Figure 2.2.1). Both receptor types are ligand-gated, meaning that they open in response to a chemical binding to them (as opposed to voltage-gated). Ionotropic receptors are membrane channels: ligand binding causes a change in flow of ions through the channel. Metabotropic receptors do not have channels. For metabotropic receptors, binding of the transmitter (the 'first messenger') leads to

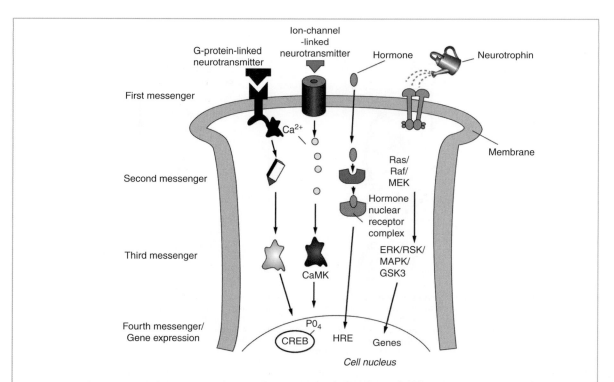

Figure 2.2.1 Different types of neuron receptors and signal transduction cascades. The figure shows four of the most important signal transduction cascades in the brain. These include G-protein-linked systems (metabotropic receptors), ion-channel-linked systems (ionotropic receptors), hormone-linked systems (see Section 6.1) and neurotrophin-linked systems (for growth factors that induce neuron growth/survival, again not described in this section). Each cascade is activated by a specific ligand, which activates a downstream second, and therefore third and fourth, messenger. These are all different and allow for pleiotropy (diversity) in synaptic function. Neurotransmitters activate both G-protein-linked and ion-channel-linked receptors, and both systems activate genes in the nucleus by phosphorylating (adding a phosphoryl group) a nuclear protein called cAMP response-element-binding protein (CREB). Metabotropic receptors act by increasing levels of cyclic adenosine monophosphate (cAMP), while ionotropic receptors increase calcium levels and this in turn activates a protein called calcium/calmodulin-dependent protein kinase (CaMK). Certain hormones, including oestrogens, enter the neuron, combine with a receptor which allows them to enter the nucleus, and there form a hormone response element (HRE) able to affect gene expression. Finally, neuronal growth factors (neurotrophins) activate several G-proteins such as Ras and some kinases (that add phosphate) such as Raf and MEK (mitogen-activated protein kinase). These in turn can activate other downstream proteins such as extracellular signal-regulated kinase (ERK), ribosomal S6 kinase (RSK), mitogen-activated protein kinase (MAPK) or glycogen synthase kinase (GSK), all kinases that affect gene expression.

a conformational change of the receptor itself, which is then able to couple with a specific G protein and activate an enzyme such as adenylate cyclase, which will then synthesise the 'second messenger', such as cyclic AMP (cAMP). cAMP can in turn activate specific protein kinases (PKs) that can then phosphorylate other enzymes and generate a signalling cascade. Each neurotransmitter can activate different receptors, causing the production of different downstream second, third and subsequent chemical messengers within the postsynaptic neuron.

Ion-channel-linked receptors can have antagonistic effects to those of G-protein coupled receptors: binding of a transmitter leads to opening of the channel, calcium ion influx (second messenger) and subsequent activation of enzymes such as calcineurin, a phosphatase (third messenger). Phosphatases remove a phosphate group from proteins and can counteract the actions of cAMP-activated PKs.

2.3	**Neuronal Receptors and Drug Targets**	Emanuele F. Osimo and Stephen M. Stahl

There are different types of neurotransmitter receptors on neuronal surfaces. These are molecules specialised in transforming a chemical signal (neurotransmitter) into a metabolic signal (downstream activation of protein kinases, phosphatases, and/or nuclear effects on DNA accessibility or synthesis) in the target cell. A slightly different but parallel concept is that of drug target. In the central nervous system, very often the two concepts overlap, as over half of psychotropic drug targets are neurotransmitter receptors (Figures 2.3.1B, 2.3.1D and 2.3.1E). Other important drug targets are neurotransmitter transporters

(Figure 2.3.1A) and other enzymes (Figure 2.3.1C), such as neurotransmitter-metabolising enzymes.

2.3.1 Agonistic Spectrum of Chemicals

Both neurotransmitters and psychotropic drugs can activate brain receptors. As such, both can be further classified based on the effects they have on their molecular target (receptor). A full agonist is a transmitter that fully opens a ionotropic receptor (Figure 2.3.2), or that fully activates a G-protein-coupled metabotropic receptor

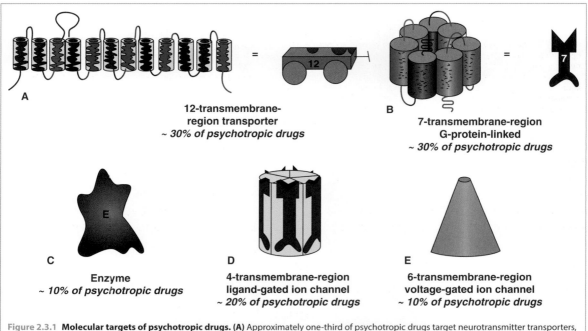

A 12-transmembrane-region transporter
~ 30% of psychotropic drugs

B 7-transmembrane-region G-protein-linked
~ 30% of psychotropic drugs

C Enzyme
~ 10% of psychotropic drugs

D 4-transmembrane-region ligand-gated ion channel
~ 20% of psychotropic drugs

E 6-transmembrane-region voltage-gated ion channel
~ 10% of psychotropic drugs

Figure 2.3.1 **Molecular targets of psychotropic drugs. (A)** Approximately one-third of psychotropic drugs target neurotransmitter transporters, for example selective serotonin reuptake inhibitors (SSRIs, such as citalopram and fluoxetine). **(B)** Another third of drugs target G-protein-linked receptors, for example dopamine D2 receptor antagonists such as haloperidol. **(C)** Approximately 10% of drugs, such as cholinesterase inhibitors (e.g. rivastigmine), target enzymes. **(D)** and **(E)** Other drugs target ion channels, including benzodiazepine receptor agonists (such as diazepam), which act as positive allosteric modulators, enhancing the action of gamma-aminobutyric acid (GABA) at GABA-A receptors.

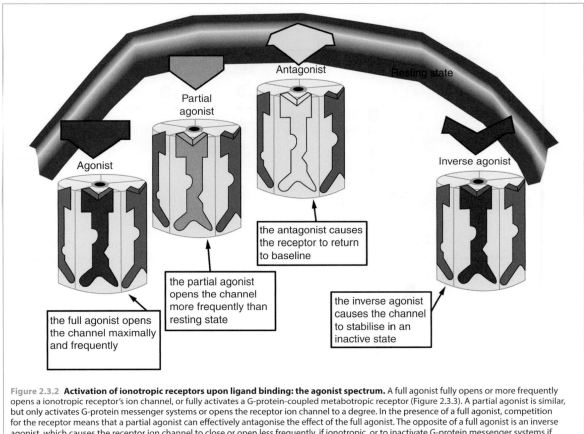

Figure 2.3.2 Activation of ionotropic receptors upon ligand binding: the agonist spectrum. A full agonist fully opens or more frequently opens a ionotropic receptor's ion channel, or fully activates a G-protein-coupled metabotropic receptor (Figure 2.3.3). A partial agonist is similar, but only activates G-protein messenger systems or opens the receptor ion channel to a degree. In the presence of a full agonist, competition for the receptor means that a partial agonist can effectively antagonise the effect of the full agonist. The opposite of a full agonist is an inverse agonist, which causes the receptor ion channel to close or open less frequently, if ionotropic, or to inactivate G-protein messenger systems if metabotropic. A true or silent antagonist is a ligand that is inactive at the receptor in itself, and functions only in the presence of an agonist or partial agonist by competing for binding and reducing their actions.

(Figure 2.3.3). A partial agonist is similar, but only activates or opens the receptor to a degree. In the presence of a full agonist, competition for the receptor means that a partial agonist can effectively antagonise the effect of the full agonist. The opposite of a full agonist is an inverse agonist, which causes the receptor to close if ionotropic, or to inactivate if metabotropic. A true or silent antagonist is a ligand that is inactive at the receptor in itself, and functions only in the presence of an agonist or partial agonist by competing for binding and reducing their action (Figure 2.3.3).

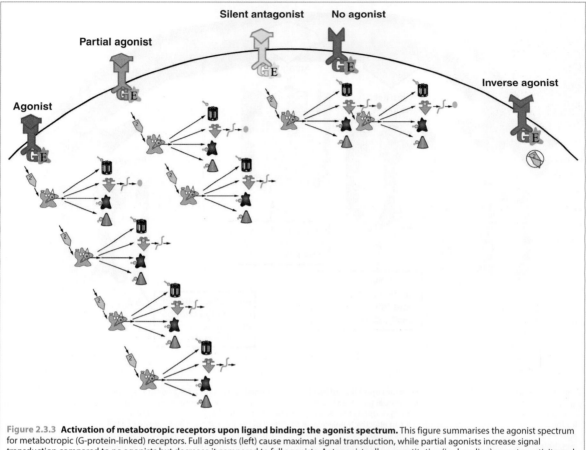

Figure 2.3.3 Activation of metabotropic receptors upon ligand binding: the agonist spectrum. This figure summarises the agonist spectrum for metabotropic (G-protein-linked) receptors. Full agonists (left) cause maximal signal transduction, while partial agonists increase signal transduction compared to no agonists but decrease it compared to full agonists. Antagonists allow constitutive (i.e. baseline) receptor activity and thus, in the absence of an agonist, have no effect themselves. In the presence of an agonist, antagonists lead to reduced signal transduction by competing with the agonist. Inverse agonists (right) reduce signal transduction beyond physiological levels.

<table>
<tr><td>**2.4**</td><td># Basic Pharmacology of Specific Neurotransmitter Pathways</td><td>Emanuele F. Osimo and Stephen M. Stahl</td></tr>
</table>

Many substances act as transmitters in the central nervous system. We will focus on those small molecules which have been most implicated in neuropsychiatric conditions, namely serotonin, dopamine, gamma-aminobutyric acid (GABA), noradrenaline, acetylcholine and glutamate; for further reading, see [1] and [2].

2.4.1 Basic Pharmacology of Serotonin

Most serotonergic neurons in the central nervous system originate in the raphe nucleus or midline regions of the pons and brainstem. Serotonin (5-hydroxytryptamine, 5-HT) has more than 10 receptors in the central nervous system (Figure 2.4.1), most of which are metabotropic and inhibitory. Serotonin dysfunction is closely linked with mood disorders and anxiety: carriers of the short allele of the *SERT* gene, a genetic variant that reduces the expression of *SERT*, are more sensitive to stress-induced activation of the amygdala [3], more prone to anxiety-like temperaments [4] and to depressive recurrence in the context of environmental adversity [5]. Furthermore, all available medications with antidepressant effects have a significant effect on the monoamine system, and most specifically a stimulating effect on serotonergic function. Selective serotonin reuptake inhibitors, such as fluoxetine and citalopram, are believed to work by inhibiting SERT, thus increasing serotonergic function in the brain. Other medications with antidepressant effects, for instance tricyclics (TCAs, such as amitriptyline and imipramine) and serotonin–noradrenaline reuptake inhibitors (SNRIs, such as venlafaxine), are also believed to inhibit SERT (and NET), therefore increasing serotonin signalling.

NbN: NEUROSCIENCE BASED NOMENCLATURE

Neuroscience Based Nomenclature (https://nbn2r.com) is an international effort aimed at using modes of action (such as agonist, antagonist, modulator) and molecular targets (called pharmacological domains, such as serotonergic or noradrenergic pathway) to classify all psychoactive medication. This contrasts with current descriptors, which are based on indication (antidepressants, antipsychotics, etc.) or chemical structure (e.g. benzodiazepines). NbN aligns to nomenclature in other branches of medicine (e.g. calcium-channel blockers, proton pump inhibitors, etc.).

In NbN there are currently 10 described pharmacological domains – (1) acetylcholine, (2) dopamine, (3) GABA, (4) glutamate, (5) histamine, (6) melatonin, (7) noradrenaline, (8) opioid, (9) orexin and (10) serotonin; and nine modes of action – (1) enzyme inhibitor, (2) enzyme modulator, (3) ion-channel blocker, (4) neurotransmitter releaser, (5) positive allosteric modulator, (6) receptor agonist, (7) receptor antagonist, (8) receptor partial agonist and (9) reuptake inhibitor.

Examples of NbN nomenclature are defining citalopram as a serotonin reuptake inhibitor (SSRI) instead of an antidepressant, and calling haloperidol a dopamine (D2) receptor antagonist instead of an antipsychotic.

Critics of NbN find this approach too simplistic, as it usually only captures the main modes of action of a medication; an example could be clozapine, which is classed as a dopamine D2, serotonin 5-HT2 and noradrenaline alpha-2 receptor antagonist. Clozapine also has high affinity for other receptors, including histaminergic, muscarinic and alpha-1 receptors; however, NbN only mentions drug targets that current knowledge considers most relevant for desired effects (and might overlook receptors responsible for side effects).

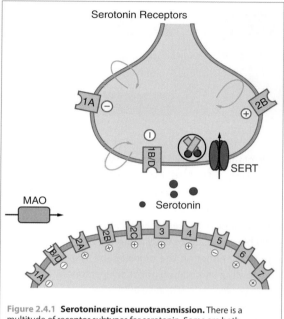

Figure 2.4.1 **Serotoninergic neurotransmission.** There is a multitude of receptor subtypes for serotonin. Some are both presynaptic and postsynaptic (1A, 1B/D and 2B), and many others are only postsynaptic (2A, 2C, 3, 4, 5, 6 and 7). This plethora of receptors allows for many differing functions in different brain circuits, and also allows serotonin to both stimulate and inhibit the neuron.

Older drugs such as the MAO inhibitors (MAOIs, e.g. phenelzine, tranylcypromine) decrease degradation of all monoamines in the synaptic cleft, thereby also increasing synaptic availability of serotonin. The antidepressant and anxiolytic effects of these medications appear to be mediated both by the activation of serotonergic postsynaptic receptors, and by the activation of presynaptic soma-dendritic autoreceptors such as 5-HT1A.

5-HT2A modulation, as well as having effects on mood, has been linked with psychosis: its activation (such as by lysergic acid (LSD)) can lead to hallucinations, and many current drugs used for psychosis, such as clozapine and quetiapine, have an inverse agonist action on 5-HT2A (as well as affecting the dopaminergic pathways, as we will see later). It has been postulated that 5-HT2A modulation might also be related to the mood-stabilising properties of some drugs used for psychosis.

Activation of 5-HT3 (the only ionotropic receptor) is linked both with nausea (note that ondansetron, a 5-HT3 blocker, is an antiemetic) and with depression (the noradrenaline, serotonin antagonist mirtazapine is a 5-HT3 receptor antagonist).

2.4.2 Basic Pharmacology of Dopamine

There are two main families of dopamine receptors, called D1 and D2. The D1 family in humans (Figure 2.4.2) includes D1 and D5 receptors, and is characterised by coupling of the receptors to stimulatory G proteins that activate adenylyl cyclase, tending to activate the postsynaptic neuron. The D2 family includes D2, D3 and D4, and these receptors are coupled to G inhibitory proteins that reduce adenylyl cyclase activity, tending to inhibit the postsynaptic neuron. D1 receptors are mainly found in the striatum, cerebral cortex and hippocampus; D2 receptors are most densely found in the striatum, but also in the cortex, amygdala and hippocampus.

Parkinsonism is characterised by reduced levels of dopamine in the basal ganglia, due to the death of neurons originating from the substantia nigra; pharmacological treatment of these conditions is based on attempts to restore dopamine levels by administering levodopa (precursor of dopamine) or dopamine agonists (such as bromocriptine).

Dopamine dysfunction has also been linked with psychotic disorders using a diverse range of techniques: brain imaging studies have shown that – in patients with psychosis – dopamine synthesis is increased; dopamine is more sensitive to release in the face of stress; there are higher levels of endogenous synaptic dopamine when patients are psychotic; and there is a modest elevation in striatal D2/3 receptor density independent of the effects of drugs used for psychosis. Furthermore, at clinical doses, most if not all currently licensed drugs used for psychosis block striatal D2 receptors (for further reading, see [6] and Sections 9.9 and 9.10).

In addition to psychosis, D1 and D2 agonism can exert positive effects on mood. Dopamine is also closely linked to brain reward pathways: dopamine is involved in learning (Section 5.7), pleasure (Section 5.13) and addiction (Section 9.3). Dopamine pathway manipulation is a core feature of most drugs of addiction (Section 2.7), and the effects on dopamine signalling may be a major causal factor in the development of addiction.

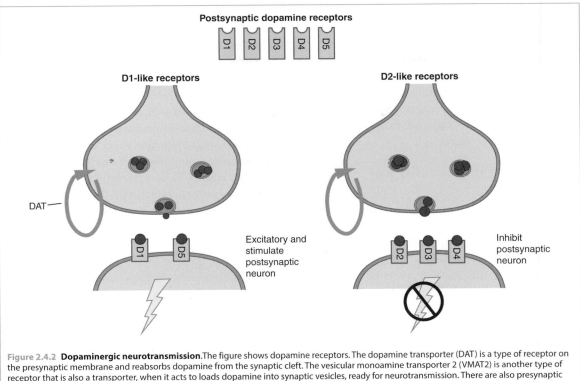

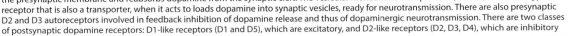

Figure 2.4.2 **Dopaminergic neurotransmission.**The figure shows dopamine receptors. The dopamine transporter (DAT) is a type of receptor on the presynaptic membrane and reabsorbs dopamine from the synaptic cleft. The vesicular monoamine transporter 2 (VMAT2) is another type of receptor that is also a transporter, when it acts to loads dopamine into synaptic vesicles, ready for neurotransmission. There are also presynaptic D2 and D3 autoreceptors involved in feedback inhibition of dopamine release and thus of dopaminergic neurotransmission. There are two classes of postsynaptic dopamine receptors: D1-like receptors (D1 and D5), which are excitatory, and D2-like receptors (D2, D3, D4), which are inhibitory

2.4.3 Basic Pharmacology of GABA

Gamma-aminobutyric acid (GABA) is the main inhibitory neurotransmitter in the central nervous system and is typically secreted by local interneurons. It has a crucial function in maintaining the overall balance between excitation and inhibition in the central nervous system, and is implicated in conditions of reduced inhibition such as epilepsy and anxiety, or of excessive inhibition such as narcolepsy. There are two main GABA receptors, GABA-A and GABA-B (Figure 2.4.3). GABA-A receptors are ionotropic and hyperpolarising (selective for chloride anions) and are the main target of benzodiazepines (such as diazepam). Benzodiazepines amplify the effect of GABA ('positive allosteric modulation'): they bind to the GABA-A receptor, increasing its affinity for GABA, thereby increasing its likelihood of being open, and leading to more hyperpolarisation. Barbiturates such as phenobarbital exert a similar effect to benzodiazepines, but increase both affinity for GABA and the channel opening time, with an associated risk

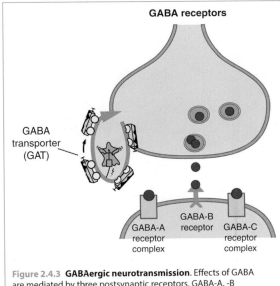

Figure 2.4.3 **GABAergic neurotransmission**. Effects of GABA are mediated by three postsynaptic receptors, GABA-A, -B and -C. GABA-A and -C are ion channels, and are inhibitory (chloride ion channels). GABA-A receptors play a critical role in mediating inhibitory neurotransmission and are the targets of benzodiazepines. GABA-B receptors are metabotropic.

of causing excessive central nervous system depression. Benzodiazepines are sedative and have powerful anti-anxiety, as well as good anticonvulsant and muscle relaxant, properties; however, they can cause pharmacological tolerance and dependence. GABA-B receptors are metabotropic inhibitory receptors and act both by increasing K+ depolarising currents and by decreasing cAMP generation. GABA-B agonists such as baclofen can be used to treat narcolepsy.

2.4.4 Basic Pharmacology of Noradrenaline

Most central noradrenergic neurons are located in the locus coeruleus or reticular formation, but project diffusely to most other regions of the central nervous system. Noradrenaline has several receptors, all metabotropic (Figure 2.4.4). In line with its alerting and arousing behavioural effects, noradrenaline usually exerts an excitatory role on neurons. This can be achieved directly, through alpha-1 and beta-1 receptors, or indirectly, by inhibition of local inhibitory circuits. Alpha-2 receptors

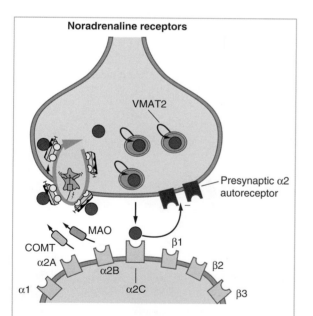

Figure 2.4.4 Noradrenergic neurotransmission. The figure shows noradrenaline (NA) receptors and other regulators of NA transmission. The noradrenaline transporter (NET) reabsorbs NA into the presynaptic neuron. The vesicular monoamine transporter 2 (VMAT2) loads NA into synaptic vesicles, ready for neurotransmission. Presynaptic alpha-2 (α2) receptors contribute to regulating NA transmission by feedback inhibition.

are inhibitory and can exert presynaptic feedback inhibition on noradrenaline release.

SNRIs (e.g. venlafaxine), noradrenaline reuptake inhibitors (NRIs, e.g. reboxetine and atomoxetine) and TCAs such as imipramine all inhibit the NET, thus increasing noradrenaline levels. MAOIs give rise to similar effects by decreasing the degradation of noradrenaline. Other substances can boost noradrenaline levels by reversing NET, thus pumping noradrenaline into the synaptic cleft (amphetamines and methylphenidate). SNRIs, some NRIs, TCAs and MAOIs have powerful antidepressant and anti-anxiety effects; atomoxetine, methylphenidate and amphetamines (with specific indications for prescribing) have been shown to be effective in the treatment of attention deficit hyperactivity disorder (ADHD).

Alpha-2 receptors, mainly present as inhibitory autoreceptors (i.e. on the presynaptic terminal), are hyperpolarising (thus causing a reduction in noradrenaline release). Alpha-2 agonism (such as with clonidine) is anti-hypertensive and has been used in ADHD; alpha-2 antagonism (such as with trazodone) has been shown to have an antidepressant action.

2.3.5 Basic Pharmacology of Acetylcholine

As well as a crucial neurotransmitter in the brain, acetylcholine is also responsible for synaptic transmission at all neuromuscular junctions. Figure 2.4.5 shows that acetylcholine has two sets of receptors: nicotinic (which are ion channels, and mostly peripheral) and muscarinic (which are G-protein-coupled receptors). Most cholinergic receptors in the brain are muscarinic, and most of them cause slow excitation, often mediated by M1 receptors. M1 receptors are unusual as they produce excitation by decreasing membrane K+ permeability. Conversely, M2 receptors produce slow inhibition by opening K+ channels.

Complete blockage of nicotinic receptors causes paralysis and is used in anaesthesia (e.g. pancuronium); tobacco smoke exerts some of its addictive effects through nicotinic receptor stimulation.

In the central nervous system, acetylcholine mediates many cognitive functions, including alertness and memory, and cholinesterase inhibitors such as rivastigmine, which boost acetylcholine levels in the brain, are used in the treatment of some types of dementia.

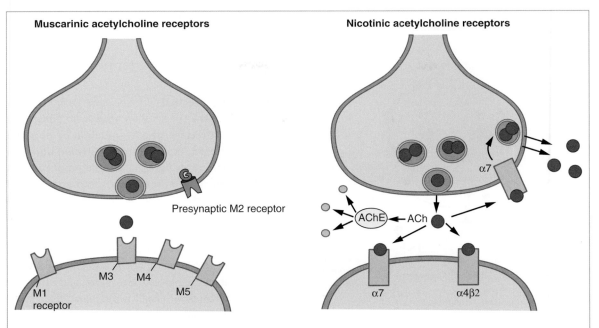

Figure 2.4.5 Acetylcholinergic neurotransmission. The panels show muscarinic and nicotinic acetylcholine (ACh) receptors. Muscarinic receptors are G-protein-coupled; M1 receptors are postsynaptic and important for regulating memory; M2 receptors are both pre- and postsynaptic. Nicotinic ACh receptors are excitatory ionotropic channels. There are multiple subtypes classified by the subunits that they contain. Shown are two of the most important, alpha-7 (α7) (both pre- and postsynaptic, involved in regulation of neurotransmission and cognitive function respectively) and alpha-4, beta-2 (α4β2), which regulate dopamine release in the nucleus accumbens. Acetylcholinesterase (AChE) inactivates ACh, converting it back into choline.

2.4.6 Basic Pharmacology of Glutamate

Glutamate is the main excitatory neurotransmitter in the brain. After its release in the synapse, glutamate is cleared by transporters in surrounding glial cells. Most glutamate receptors are excitatory, and glutamate has been found to have a profound excitatory action on all neurons. Glutamate has both ionotropic and metabotropic receptors. The main receptors are ionotropic and can be further subdivided into three groups: AMPA, NMDA and kainate (Figure 2.4.6). AMPA receptors are present on all neurons, and most are permeable to sodium and potassium cations. NMDA receptors are also ubiquitous, and all are permeable to sodium, potassium and calcium cations; they are tightly regulated, and require both glycine binding and postsynaptic membrane depolarisation to open. However, at normal ambient levels of glycine this site is saturated, and receptor opening is regulated by depolarisation, which causes the expulsion of a magnesium cation, blocking the channel's pore. This mechanism ensures that NMDA receptors are only activated

when there is intense activation of the synapse, or even of many neighbouring synapses; this is the mechanism underlying long-term potentiation, one of the molecular bases of memory formation (Section 5.14). On the other hand, excessive glutamate concentrations, and the consequent powerful calcium influx caused by the activation of NMDA receptors, can also mediate glutamate excitotoxicity, a phenomenon where neurons die, and that has been postulated to be involved in brain damage following strokes and epileptic seizures. Kainate receptors are expressed mostly in the hippocampus, cerebellum and spinal cord, and are similar in function to AMPA receptors. Glutamate also has three classes of metabotropic receptors: type I receptors are postsynaptic and excitatory, while types II and III are inhibitory presynaptic receptors.

Glutamatergic synapses are the most numerous in the human brain; as well as a crucial role in all brain activity, including all motor, sensitive and cognitive functions, glutamatergic dysfunction is likely to be involved in most neuropsychiatric conditions. Glutamate excitatory activity is balanced against GABA's inhibitory activity, and an

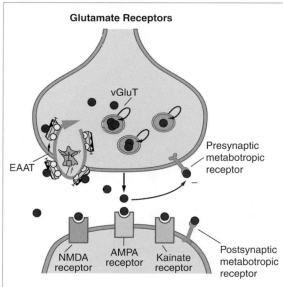

Glutamate Receptors

Figure 2.4.6 **Glutamatergic neurotransmission**. The figure shows glutamate receptors and other regulators of glutamate transmission. The excitatory amino acid transporter (EAAT) reabsorbs glutamate into the presynaptic neuron, thus clearing the synapse. The vesicular transporter for glutamate (vGluT) loads glutamate into synaptic vesicles, ready for neurotransmission. Most glutamate receptors are ionotropic, and are classified as *N*-methyl-D-aspartate (NMDA), alpha-amino-3-hydroxy-5-methyl-4-isoxazole-propionic acid (AMPA) and ersona receptors, all named after specific agonists. Metabotropic receptors are involved pre- and postsynaptically in the regulation of glutamate transmission.

equilibrium must be reached. Epilepsy is due to abnormal discharge of cerebral neurons, and as such some forms are thought to be linked to a relative glutamatergic excess. Most existing antiepileptic medications act either by reducing excitatory signalling, usually glutamatergic transmission (e.g. phenytoin, carbamazepine, lamotrigine, gabapentin, pregabalin), or by enhancing inhibitory signalling, usually GABAergic transmission (such as with diazepam).

Glutamatergic pathways are also affected by medications for dementia (e.g. the NMDA receptor antagonist memantine), and by chemicals used for recreational purposes (such as ethanol, which among other targets is a GABA-A agonist and an NMDA antagonist). Phencyclidine and ketamine, both NMDA receptor antagonists, are drugs of abuse, which can cause psychotic symptoms, both positive and negative; among other findings, these have raised the possibility that glutamatergic function may be crucial in the pathophysiology of psychotic disorders, and

glutamatergic medications are being trialled in patients with schizophrenia.

Conclusions and Outstanding Questions

In conclusion, in Sections 2.1 to 2.4, we have reviewed the function of the chemical synapse, from transmitter synthesis to its release, and degradation or reuptake. We have explored the differences between the main families of neurotransmitters, including monoamines (such as dopamine, adrenaline, noradrenaline and serotonin), acetylcholine and other transmitters, as well as the basic pharmacology of each class. We described the main receptor classes: ionotropic (ligand binding causes a change in flow of ions through the channel) and metabotropic (binding of the transmitter leads to a conformational change of the receptor, and activation of a molecular cascade). Finally, we explored the agonist spectrum for neurotransmitter receptors, and some of the implications for clinical pharmacology.

Outstanding Questions

- Medications in psychiatry are increasingly designed with a specific receptor, and agonist spectrum, in mind. This is the case, for example, for aripiprazole, which was released in 2002 following the specific quest for a dopamine D2 receptor partial agonist. This process tends to minimise side effects from off-target drug effects. Will this targeted approach continue? Will it lead to new, better, more targeted medications? Or does this approach risk developing 'me-too' drugs, similar in profile to current medications rather than having a mechanism of action that can help patients who don't respond to current treatments?

- Most existing medications for psychosis target dopamine receptors, while most existing medications for depression favour serotonergic or monoaminergic activation. Since the mid-2000s we have experienced a great flourishing of complex disorder genomics, which has highlighted the role of other neurotransmitters in disease pathogenesis (e.g. glutamate and calcium channels) – will this lead to the design of drugs aimed at different targets? (See Section 2.6.)

- Most drug targets, as well as catabolic pathways, are genetically encoded. Will the pharmacogenomics boom lead to more personalised treatments, which consider each patient's likely responsivity and expected drug metabolism?

REFERENCES

1. Kandel ER, Schwartz JH, Jessell TM, Siegelbaum SA, Hudspeth AJ. *Principles of Neural Science*, 5th ed. McGraw-Hill, Health Professions Division, 2013.

2. Katzung BG, Masters SB, Trevor AJ. *Basic and Clinical Pharmacology*, 12th ed. McGraw Hill Medical, 2012.

3. Hariri AR, Mattay VS, Tessitore A et al. Serotonin transporter genetic variation and the response of the human amygdala. *Science* 2002; 297(5580): 400–403.

4. Lesch K-P, Bengel D, Heils A et al. Association of anxiety-related traits with a polymorphism in the serotonin transporter gene regulatory region. *Science* 1996; 274(5292): 1527–1531.

5. Caspi A, Sugden K, Moffitt TE et al. Influence of life stress on depression: moderation by a polymorphism in the 5-HTT gene. *Science* 2003; 301(5631): 386–389.

6. Howes OD, Kapur S. The dopamine hypothesis of schizophrenia: version III – the final common pathway. *Schizophr Bull* 2009; 35(3): 549–562.

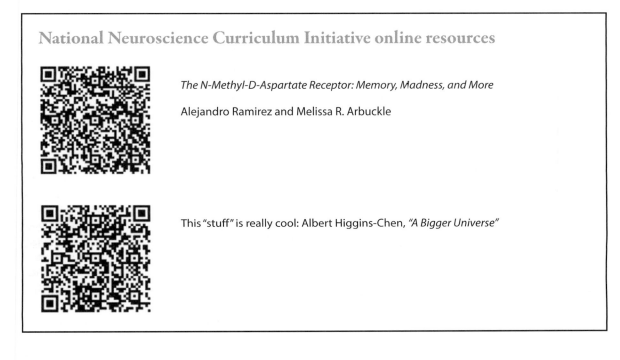

National Neuroscience Curriculum Initiative online resources

The N-Methyl-D-Aspartate Receptor: Memory, Madness, and More

Alejandro Ramirez and Melissa R. Arbuckle

This "stuff" is really cool: Albert Higgins-Chen, *"A Bigger Universe"*

<table>
<tr><td>**2.5**</td><td>**Neuropeptides**</td><td>I. Sadaf Farooqi</td></tr>
</table>

OVERVIEW

The complexity of neuronal signalling is mediated by neurotransmitters (glutamate, gamma-aminobutyric acid), neuromodulators (e.g. serotonin, dopamine, acetylcholine discussed in Section 2.4) and neuropeptides, which are the focus of this section. In contrast to rapid-acting neurotransmitters, which affect the excitability of target neurons by depolarisation or hyperpolarisation (lasting seconds to minutes), neuropeptides exert prolonged actions (lasting hours to days) by changing gene expression and synaptogenesis to mediate a diverse range of physiological and behavioural responses. There are over a hundred different neuropeptides that mediate, for example, eating behaviour, social behaviour, learning, memory, reproduction and analgesia. Most neurons release classical neurotransmitters or amino acid transmitters as well as neuropeptides. A small minority of neurons release only neuropeptides, including the magnocellular neurons in the hypothalamus, which release peptides such as oxytocin and arginine vasopressin directly into the bloodstream.

Neuropeptides are derived from larger precursor molecules called pre-propeptides, made up of a chain of amino acids that are processed first to pro-neuropeptides, which are stored as a reservoir and can have some biological activity. When needed, these pro-neuropeptides are selectively cleaved and then spliced together by specific enzymes to synthesise several smaller neuropeptides. Processing of pre-propeptides is often tissue specific, which allows for the generation of multiple peptides that can have overlapping functions in different brain regions and tissues. Pre-propeptides are synthesised predominantly by neurons (but also by glial cells and non-neuronal cells), then packaged into large dense core vesicles, discrete organelles that reside in the soma (cell body) and act as vehicles to transport neuropeptides down to axon terminals where they are stored prior to release. During this process, enzymatic cleavage of the pre-propeptides occurs within the vesicles (Figure 2.5.1). Smaller secretory vesicles containing neuropeptides are then held or stored at the presynaptic membrane until neuronal stimulation triggers their fusion with the plasma membrane (this

is termed regulated secretion). Neuropeptides then diffuse from the point of release to bind to and signal via receptors, most commonly G-protein-coupled receptors (GPCRs) expressed on the cell surface of other neuronal cells. The absence of mechanisms for the reuptake of neuropeptides, in contrast to neurotransmitters, allows for persistent levels to be maintained at the synapse.

Many neuropeptides play a key role in maintaining homeostasis, whereby neural circuits in the brain respond to and integrate peripheral hormonal, metabolic and sensory inputs, compare those inputs to basic 'set-points' or parameters and then change autonomic, neuroendocrine and behavioural outputs to maintain these set-points (homeostasis).

2.5.1 Opioid Peptides: Enkephalins, Endorphins and Dynorphins

In times of stress and injury, the release of endogenous opioids is an adaptive mechanism, which allows us to ignore pain to focus on productive behaviours that will help us to escape potentially harmful situations.

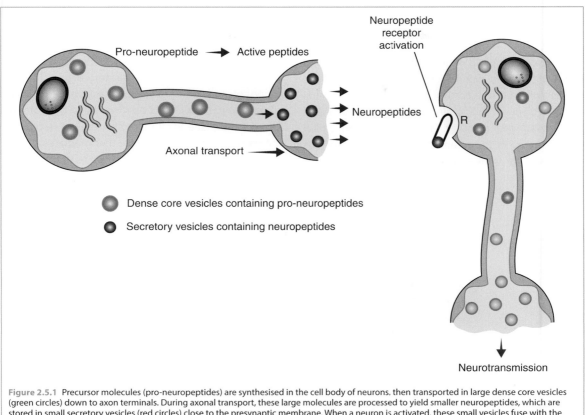

Figure 2.5.1 Precursor molecules (pro-neuropeptides) are synthesised in the cell body of neurons, then transported in large dense core vesicles (green circles) down to axon terminals. During axonal transport, these large molecules are processed to yield smaller neuropeptides, which are stored in small secretory vesicles (red circles) close to the presynaptic membrane. When a neuron is activated, these small vesicles fuse with the presynaptic membrane and release their contents (neuropeptides) into the synaptic cleft. Once released, neuropeptides bind to receptors (often G-protein-coupled receptors (GPCRs)) on adjacent neurons to mediate their effects.

The endogenous opioid system consists of three families of opioid neuropeptides: beta-endorphin, enkephalins and dynorphins. These neuropeptides modulate analgesia, motor coordination, learning, memory, gastrointestinal motility and the reproductive system. Opioids act by signalling through the mu (MOR), delta (DOR) and kappa (KOR) opioid receptors (Table 2.5.1), and the recently identified nociceptin receptor (NOPR), all of which are GPCRs [1]. NOPR has minimal affinity for the endogenous opioid peptides; it is activated by nociceptin, an anti-analgesic which has a significantly higher affinity for NOPR than for the other opioid receptors.

There are three endogenous opioid precursors – proenkephalin, prodynorphin and proopiomelanocortin (POMC). Proenkephalin is the precursor of leucine (Leu)- and methionine (Met)-enkephalins and several other peptides which act at the delta- and mu-opioid receptors expressed in the striatum, the ventromedial nucleus of the

Table 2.5.1 Endogenous opioids act on mu (μ), delta (δ) and kappa (κ) opioid receptors (relative potencies shown as +, ++, +++)

Selectivity of endogenous opioids for opioid receptor subtypes			
	μ	δ	κ
Endogenous peptide			
Beta-endorphin	+++	+++	+++
Leu-enkephalin	+	+++	−
Met-enkephalin	++	+++	−
Dynorphin	++	+	+++

hypothalamus and the dentate gyrus of the hippocampus. Prodynorphin can be cleaved to produce Leu-enkephalin, and several Leu-enkephalin-containing peptides, including dynorphin A, dynorphin B, and alpha- and beta-neoendorphin. Levels of prodynorphin messenger RNA are particularly concentrated in the magnocellular cells of the hypothalamus and in the hippocampal formation, where they signal via kappa receptors. POMC can be cleaved to produce beta-lipoprotein and beta-endorphin, which is a potent agonist at mu, delta and kappa opioid receptors (Table 2.5.1).

Several non-opioid neuropeptides are also derived from POMC. These include adrencorticotropic hormone (ACTH), which drives cortisol synthesis by the adrenal gland (see Section 6.1.1); also, the peptides alpha- and beta-melanocyte stimulating hormone (MSH), which are expressed in the pituitary gland, arcuate nucleus of the hypothalamus and the nucleus tractus solitarius in the brainstem, and play a role in appetite regulation

(Figure 2.5.2). Recent studies into the different pathways by which these receptors signal have paved the way for new analgesics that seek to harness the beneficial analgesic effects of opioids without some of the adverse effects such as constipation and respiratory depression. The actions of exogenous opioids on these neural pathways contribute to their effects on reward and the potential for addiction (see Sections 2.7 and 9.3). Establishing the particular receptor subtype that mediates a beneficial or adverse effect should inform the design of safer treatments.

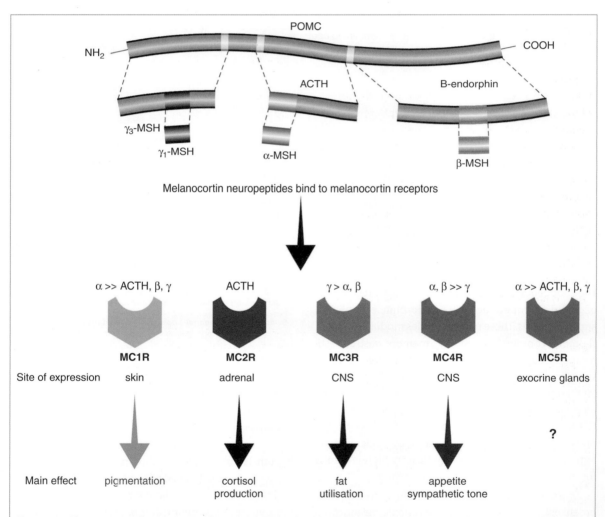

Figure 2.5.2 The precursor molecule proopiomelanocortin (POMC) is cleaved to yield multiple peptides, including beta-endorphin. This acts on opioid receptors and alpha (α)/beta (β)/gamma (γ)-melanocyte stimulating hormone (MSH), which in turn act on the melanocortin receptors to mediate different physiological effects as shown [1–5].

2.5.2 Anorectic (Appetite-Reducing) and Orexigenic (Appetite-Stimulating) Neuropeptides

Many psychiatric and neurodevelopmental disorders affect the regulation of appetite. Moreover, many drugs used in the treatment of psychiatric disease, such as antipsychotic agents, can affect appetite and drive weight gain. These observations speak to the considerable overlap between the neural circuits that regulate appetite and weight and the circuits that regulate complex thoughts and behaviours. The function of these overlapping neural circuits is governed by a shared repertoire of neuropeptides and neurotransmitters including serotonin and dopamine.

Body weight is governed by a complex system whereby peripheral hormonal signals exert their effects in the brain to modulate eating behaviour by changing levels of the POMC-derived melanocortin peptides and other neuropeptides [3]. For example, the endocannabinoids act on cannabinoid-1 (CB1) receptors to affect appetite and mood. Exogenous compounds can affect appetite by engaging these neural circuits. POMC-expressing neurons are activated by nicotine, providing a mechanism for the widely observed appetite-suppressing effect of tobacco consumption. Cannabis causes the 'munchies' by activating CB1 receptors, enhancing the release of the POMC-derived neuropeptide beta-endorphin but not alpha-MSH, which would normally suppress appetite. There is also some evidence that ethanol drives hunger via activation of neurons in the hypothalamus which express the appetite-stimulating neuropeptide agouti related peptide (AGRP).

Eating a meal and/or the presence of nutrients in the intestinal lumen triggers the release of neuropeptides including cholecystokinin from the stomach, glucagon-like peptide 1 and gastric inhibitory polypeptide from the entero-endocrine cells of the small intestine and peptide YY and oxyntomodulin from the large intestine. Their release together with neural signals from the vagus nerve and the enteric nervous system affect fullness after a meal. Ghrelin is the only known orexigenic hormone, which increases food intake when administered to volunteers. Ghrelin exists in two main forms, the inactive, non-acylated form, and the active, acylated

form, converted by the enzyme ghrelin O-acyltransferase (GOAT). Genetic knockout of the GOAT enzyme that activates ghrelin *in vivo* has been demonstrated to reduce hedonic feeding behaviour in mice and GOAT inhibitors are currently in clinical trials. In addition, these peripherally expressed neuropeptides are also expressed in the brain, where they seem to have direct effects on hunger, satiety and reward (see Section 5.1 for more on appetite).

2.5.3 Neuropeptides Involved in Sleep and Arousal

Although the purpose of sleep is the subject of much debate, it clearly has a restorative effect on the brain, enhances the consolidation of memory and is regulated by homeostatic and circadian factors (see Section 5.2). Key neuropeptides involved in arousal/promoting the awake state are orexin A (hypocretin-1) and orexin B (hypocretin-2) which are produced by neurons in the lateral and posterior hypothalamus and project to multiple brain regions to mediate effects on sleep, feeding, reward, emotion and motivated behaviours by signalling through orexin type 1 and 2 receptors (OX1Rs and OX2Rs, respectively). Orexin A activates both OX1Rs and OX2Rs with approximately equal potency, while orexin B preferentially activates OX2Rs. The contribution of these receptors to different phenotypes is only partially understood. OX1Rs are selectively expressed in the locus coeruleus and cingulate cortex, while OX2Rs are selectively expressed in the tuberomammillary nucleus, hypothalamic paraventricular nucleus and nucleus accumbens. Both receptors are expressed in the lateral hypothalamus, medial prefrontal cortex, hippocampus, central nucleus of the amygdala, bed nucleus of the stria terminalis, dorsal raphe, ventral tegmental area and nucleus of the solitary tract [4].

Impaired orexin signalling due to mutations in the *OX2R* gene causes narcolepsy in dogs and is a rare cause of narcolepsy in people. More frequently, an autoimmune process that causes destruction of orexinergic neurons in the lateral hypothalamus causes the condition known as type 1 narcolepsy, a severe chronic neurological sleep disorder characterised by excessive daytime sleepiness, cataplexy (sudden loss of muscle tone), fragmented night-time sleep with episodes of sleep paralysis and hallucinations. Low cerebrospinal fluid levels of orexin are found in these patients. There is increasing interest in the potential utility of selective OX1R antagonists, selective OX2R antagonists and dual OX1/2R antagonists for the treatment of sleep disorders, anxiety and addiction, with some drugs now in clinical use and others in clinical trials [4]. Examples include seltorexant, a selective antagonist of the OX2R that can attenuate depressive symptoms.

2.5.4 Neuropeptides and Social Interactions: Oxytocin and Arginine Vasopressin

As the ability to form social attachments can be considered an adaptive behaviour that favours survival, food-seeking and mating, some authors have hypothesised that reward mechanisms exist to promote such adaptive behaviours. Thus, we seek social attachments and interactions to increase the release of neuropeptides that can result in sensations of pleasure, which in turn motivates us to continue to seek such attachments. One neuropeptide that has received a lot of attention for its role in social interaction and bonding is oxytocin (see Section 8.3 for more on oxytocin and attachment).

Magnocellular oxytocin neurons in the supraoptic nucleus and paraventricular nucleus of the hypothalamus project to the posterior pituitary, from where oxytocin is released into the systemic circulation to control uterine contractions and milk ejection during parturition and lactation. Oxytocin is also released in abundance from the large dendrites of magnocellular neurons. Oxytocin receptors are present in many brain areas including the amygdala, nucleus accumbens and dorsal vagal complex, which mediate the effects of oxytocin on social behaviours, such as maternal care and pair bonding, the attenuation of fear, the stress response and eating [5]. Several human studies have shown that intranasal oxytocin administration can improve social functioning in children with autism.

2.5.5 Targeting Neuropeptide Receptors for Therapy

Many commonly prescribed medicines for psychiatric diseases target a particular type of receptor that mediates the effects of noradrenaline, dopamine and serotonin and a variety of neuropeptides. These are the previously mentioned GPCRs (G-protein-coupled receptors), which are the largest family of cell surface proteins involved in signalling. Classically, upon neuropeptide binding, GPCRs located at the cell surface interact with guanine nucleotide-binding (G) proteins to direct signalling and gene transcription (switching on). This response is attenuated within minutes by molecules called beta-arrestins, which prevent overstimulation and can themselves directly/indirectly mediate signalling through other pathways. Many drugs currently in use act as balanced agonists, signalling with comparable efficacy through multiple pathways (e.g. stimulating both G-protein-dependent and beta-arrestin pathways downstream of GPCR engagement). However, there is considerable interest in the development of 'biased agonists', which preferentially activate signalling through either G-protein-dependent or G-protein-independent beta-arrestin-mediated pathways, an approach that could amplify favourable signals while reducing signals that contribute to adverse effects. For example, experiments in mice have shown that morphine's effects on respiratory depression and constipation are mediated by the beta-arrestin-2 signalling pathway. This work has informed the development of a small-molecule mu-opioid receptor agonist, which stimulates nearly undetectable levels of beta-arrestin compared to morphine and as such is predicted to have the analgaesic effects of morphine without its adverse effects of respiratory depression and constipation. This approach may be generalizable to other GPCRs and could pave the way for a new generation of drugs that target neuropeptide receptors with greater specificity.

Additionally, large-scale genetic studies are revealing that there is substantial variation in the genes that encode GPCRs. Some of these common genetic variants preferentially impair or even enhance signalling via one pathway more than others, which can explain susceptibility to neurobehavioural and physiological traits including weight gain. These genetic variants may also affect the response to drugs that target these receptors in apparently healthy people. For example, by combining genetic predictions with experiments in cells, Hauser et al. showed that specific variants in the gene for the mu-opioid receptor could affect therapeutic responses to morphine and naloxone in cells in vitro. They hypothesised that this might predict clinical responses to these drugs, which may in turn influence tolerance and the risk of dependence [6].

Conclusions

In summary, we are only really beginning to understand how neuropeptides exert a complex array of effects in the brain to direct and modulate human physiology and behaviour. One of the major challenges has been our inability to measure small peptides (many assays for oxytocin for example are unreliable) but recent technological advances are changing this. The use of positron emission tomography ligands for specific neuropeptide receptors has provided insights into the brain regions where neuropeptides exert their effects and molecular studies are providing new insights into the precise mechanisms by which they signal and how they may be targeted for therapeutic benefit.

REFERENCES

1. Corder G, Castro DC, Bruchas MR, Scherrer G. Endogenous and exogenous opioids in pain. *Annu Rev Neurosci.* 2018;41:453–473. doi: 10.1146/annurev-neuro-080317-061522. Epub 2018 May 31. PMID: 29852083

2. Koob GF, Volkow ND. Neurobiology of addiction: a neurocircuitry analysis. *Lancet Psychiatry.* 2016;3(8):760–773. doi: 10.1016/S2215-0366(16)00104-8. PMID: 27475769

3. Heisler LK, Lam DD. An appetite for life: brain regulation of hunger and satiety. *Curr Opin Pharmacol.* 2017;37:100–106. doi: 10.1016/j.coph.2017.09.002. Epub 2017 Nov 5. PMID: 29107871

4. Han Y, Yuan K, Zheng Y, Lu L. Orexin receptor antagonists as emerging treatments for psychiatric disorders. *Neurosci Bull.* 2019 Nov 28. doi: 10.1007/s12264-019-00447-9. PMID: 31782044

5. Horta M, Kaylor K, Feifel D, Ebner NC. Chronic oxytocin administration as a tool for investigation and treatment: a cross-disciplinary systematic review. *Neurosci Biobehav Rev.* 2019;108:1–23. doi: 10.1016/j.neubiorev.2019.10.012. PMID: 31647964

6. Hauser AS, Chavali S, Masuho I et al. Pharmacogenomics of GPCR drug targets. *Cell.* 2018;172:41–54.e19.

<table>
<tr><td>**2.6**</td><td>**Genetic Association Studies and Neurotransmitter Pathways**</td><td>Jeremy Hall and Jack F. G. Underwood</td></tr>
</table>

OVERVIEW

Over the past 50 years, genomic methodologies have paved the way to a greater understanding of the underlying pathology of mental health disorders. In that time the techniques have developed from candidate gene studies in relatively small samples of patients, to large-scale collaborative studies using array and DNA sequencing approaches. These methodological approaches are outlined in detail in Chapter 7. In particular, genome-wide association studies (GWAS), which examine the association between single-nucleotide polymorphisms (SNPs) and disease, have made great inroads into our understanding of genetic risk for mental health disorders. While SNPs can be used to investigate any part of the genome, here we focus on what they have taught us about the role of neurotransmitter systems in psychiatry.

Genome-wide association study (GWAS) methodologies require internationally collaborative cohorts with many thousands of participants, potentially identifying hundreds of promising relevant associations. Results from these studies support a polygenic model in which many DNA changes across multiple loci contribute to disorder risk. These studies have also implied that genetic risk for mental disorders is attributable to particular molecular pathways. The largest GWAS in psychiatry thus far have been conducted for depression [1, 2], schizophrenia [3, 4] and bipolar disorder [5]. The results of these studies have shown some evidence of genetic association with neurotransmitter systems previously considered central to the origin of these conditions, although there are some notable exceptions [6, 7]. Intriguingly, the GWAS findings have also highlighted novel and hitherto unexpected associations with disease, suggesting new routes for investigation in the development of new therapies and diagnostics (see Table 2.6.1).

2.6.1 Schizophrenia

A long-standing theory for the origin of psychotic symptoms in schizophrenia and related disorders is that they result from disordered dopamine signalling (see

Table 2.6.1 Neurotransmitter-related genes implicated through GWAS by disorder [1–5, 8, 9]

Disorder	Genes implicated by risk variants	Pathway
Schizophrenia	DRD2	Dopamine
	GRM3, GRIN2A	Glutamate and NMDA
	CACNA1C, CACNA1I, CACNB2	Voltage-gated calcium channels
Bipolar	GRIN2A	NMDA
	CACNA1C, CACNB2	Voltage-gated calcium channels
	SCN2A	Voltage-gated sodium channels
	SHANK2	Glutamate and NMDA
Depression	DRD2	Dopamine
	GRM5	Glutamate
	CACNA1E	Voltage-gated calcium channels

Section 9.9.4). This is consistent with the association of the clinical efficacy of drugs having antipsychotic action with their ability to block subcortical dopamine D2 receptors [10–12]. GWAS evidence supports this clinical finding by identifying a significant genetic association for schizophrenia with common variants in the DRD2 gene, which encodes the D2 receptor. These findings also provide genomic support for the primary target of medications with antipsychotic action.

In recent years, abnormalities in glutamatergic neurotransmitter pathways have also been implicated in schizophrenia, potentially interacting with dopamine signalling [10–12]. This theory is supported by the psychotic symptoms that can result from the use of NMDA receptor antagonistic psychotropics, such as ketamine and phencyclidine. GWAS findings have corroborated this view by identifying associations between a number of genes encoding components of the glutamate signalling system and schizophrenia [3, 4]. Specifically, common variants (mainly single-nucleotide polymorphisms (SNPs); see Chapter 7) in a number of key glutamate pathway genes have been found to be associated with schizophrenia. This includes SNPs in the metabotropic glutamate receptor 3 (*GRM3*) gene, and the gene encoding the NMDA receptor subunit GluN2A (*GRIN2A*). Overall, genetic studies provide significant support for the role of the glutamatergic system in schizophrenia, although as yet no commonly available treatments for schizophrenia intentionally target this system.

GWAS approaches have also highlighted new pathways associated with schizophrenia. One major finding has been the association of a number of genes encoding subunits of voltage-gated calcium channels, most notably *CACNA1C*, which encodes the pore-containing subunit of a species of L-type voltage-gated calcium channel, involved in synaptic plasticity [7]. This link suggests a broader involvement of genes implicated in neuronal plasticity in schizophrenia. Other novel associations identified through GWAS include a correlation with immune loci, most significantly the complement C4 component of the innate immune system, which has been shown to play an important role in plasticity during neurodevelopment [3,13]. These recent results provide new potential targets for therapy development.

2.6.2 Bipolar Disorder

GWAS analyses have demonstrated considerable genetic overlap between bipolar disorder and schizophrenia at the level of common variants, reflecting clinical observations that these diagnoses are not always phenomenologically distinct, sharing many symptoms. This genetic overlap results from a wide number of common genetic variants, some of which implicate genes involved in neurotransmission. Convergence is seen on the glutamatergic neurotransmitter system, through the NMDA receptor

gene *GRIN2A*; and on neuronal ion channels, through the voltage-gated calcium-channel gene, *CACNA1C* [5, 7, 8]. Other genes associated with bipolar disorder include: sodium voltage-gated channel alpha subunit 2 (*SCN2A*), which mediates ion transport across cell membranes [5]; SH3 and multiple ankyrin repeat domains 2 (*SHANK2*), which interconnects metabotropic glutamate receptors and NMDA receptors; and the cytoskeleton gene ankyrin 3 (*ANK3*). Together, these genes point towards molecular pathways involved in regulating neuronal excitability [5]. These pathways have been shown to be affected by the mood-stabilising drug lithium, as well as anticonvulsant therapies such as valproate and lamotrigine, potentially linking previous pharmacotherapies to emerging genetic pathway data [5].

2.6.3 Depression

The neurotransmitter system traditionally linked with depression is serotonin, as this is the target of most common medications used to treat depression [14]. Established medications are theorised to predominantly exert their effects by increasing synaptic serotonin levels [15]. However, perhaps surprisingly, the serotonin system has not been implicated by the findings of large GWAS investigations of depression. This suggests a degree of separation between the underlying pathophysiology and genetics of depression, and the main neurotransmitter targeted therapeutically [2].

GWAS in depression have instead shown an association with the *DRD2* gene, implicating altered dopamine function [1, 2]. These studies also suggest an important role for glutamate in the aetiology of depression, highlighting significantly associated polymorphisms in the metabotropic glutamate receptor 5 (*GRM5*) gene [1, 2]. *GRM5* encodes the metabotropic glutamate receptor 5 (*mGluR5*), a G-protein-coupled receptor shown to activate phospholipase C and which may be involved in neural network regulation and synaptic plasticity. Voltage-gated calcium channels have also been implicated in depression through GWAS, specifically the calcium voltage-gated channel subunit alpha-1e (encoded by *CACNA1E*), which affects neuronal excitability, rhythmic activity and synaptic transmission [1].

Together, the findings from GWAS of depression support a greater involvement of synaptic genes in depression than had been previously anticipated from available pharmacological data. This suggests synaptic genes are of great importance across psychiatric disorders.

2.6.4 Other Disorders

Like schizophrenia, ADHD has long been hypothesised to be a clinical manifestation of a disorder of dopamine signalling. Early 'candidate gene' studies examined the dopaminergic and noradrenergic pathways, targets of effective drug therapies in ADHD [16]. These studies implicated five neurotransmitter-related genes: the serotonin transporter gene, *5-HTT*, the serotonin 1B receptor gene, *HTR1B*, the dopamine transporter gene, *DAT1*, and two dopamine receptor genes, *DRD4* and *DRD5* [16]. Studies looking for copy number variants found that a significant number of ADHD patients carried duplications of the alpha-7 nicotinic acetylcholine receptor gene (*CHRNA7*) [17]. Nicotinic neurons modulate dopaminergic neurons, suggesting that disordered nicotinic regulation in ADHD may contribute to symptomatic presentation. GWAS further support the role of dopamine in the pathology of ADHD, implicating the dual specificity protein phosphate 6 (*DUSP6*) gene, which regulates dopamine levels at synapses [18].

In autism, GWAS analyses have highlighted multiple genetic variants involved in neuronal growth, stability and plasticity [19]. Of note are: the neuronal growth regulator 1 (*NEGR1*) gene, which modulates neurite growth and synapse formation in the hippocampus; the calcium-dependent activator protein for secretion (*CADPS*) gene, which encodes a protein involved in exocytosis of neurotransmitters; and the potassium calcium-activated channel subfamily N member 2 (*KCNN2*) gene, which modulates excitability in the central nervous system. GWAS conducted in these disorders are currently smaller than those of schizophrenia, depression and bipolar disorder. It is likely that clearer patterns of genetic association will emerge as larger studies are completed. GWAS studies are focused on common genetic variation. Notably, sequencing studies, which can identify rare deleterious variants (see Chapter 7), have also associated autism and ADHD with such variants affecting genes involved in synaptic processes.

Conclusions and Outstanding Questions

Genetic association studies are revealing molecular pathways involved in mental health disorder pathology. There is considerable overlap between disorders in their genetic and neurotransmitter systems identified by genetic studies, especially in synaptic genes such as *DRD2*, *CACNA1C* and *GRIN2A*. Support for risk variants in glutamatergic and dopaminergic systems validates some pre-existing theories based upon pharmacological studies. Beyond neurotransmitters, GWAS have implicated many other biological pathways for potential development of mental health disorders. These include: neuronal growth, maturation and pruning; neuroinflammation and inflammatory response; and neuronal architecture. A number of common SNPs have been demonstrated to increase risk for all adult-onset mental health disorders. Novel findings, such as widespread associations with voltage-gated calcium channel genes, offer new opportunities for the development of therapies for psychiatric disorders.

Outstanding Questions

- How do the mechanistic pathways beyond the brain implicated by GWAS, such as inflammation, interact with those involving synaptic structure and function?

- What is the therapeutic potential of novel mechanisms such as those involving voltage-gated calcium channels?

- Should we continue to research specific psychiatric disorders when GWAS suggest such a high degree of overlap in terms of genetic and neurotransmitter-based mechanisms?

- To what extent are GWAS investigating persistence of mental disorder rather than its origin?

REFERENCES

1. Howard DM, Adams MJ, Clarke T-K et al. Genome-wide meta-analysis of depression identifies 102 independent variants and highlights the importance of the prefrontal brain regions. *Nat Neurosci*. 2019;22:343–352.

2. Wray NR, Ripke S, Mattheisen M et al. Genome-wide association analyses identify 44 risk variants and refine the genetic architecture of major depression. *Nat Genet*. 2018; 50:668–681.

3. Ripke S, Neale BM, Corvin A et al. Biological insights from 108 schizophrenia-associated genetic loci. *Nature*. 2014;511:421–427.

4. Trubetskoy V, Pardiñas AF, Qi T et al. Mapping genomic loci implicates genes and synaptic biology in schizophrenia. *Nature*. 2022;604(7906):502–508.

5. Mullins N, Forstner AJ, O'Connell KS, Coombes B, Coleman JRI, Qiao Z et al. Genome-wide association study of more than 40,000 bipolar disorder cases provides new insights into the underlying biology. *Nat Genet*. 2021;53(6):817–829.

6. Consortium TN and PAS of the PG, O'Dushlaine C, Rossin L et al. Psychiatric genome-wide association study analyses implicate neuronal, immune and histone pathways. *Nat Neurosci*. 2015;18:199–209.

7. Cross-Disorder Group of the Psychiatric Genomics Consortium. Identification of risk loci with shared effects on five major psychiatric disorders: a genome-wide analysis. *Lancet*. 2013;381:1371–1379.

8. Craddock N, Sklar P. Genetics of bipolar disorder. *Lancet*. 2013;381:1654–1662.

9. Power RA, Tansey KE, Buttenschøn HN et al. Genome-wide association for major depression through age at onset stratification: Major Depressive Disorder Working Group of the Psychiatric Genomics Consortium. *Biol Psychiatry*. 2017;81:325–335.

10. Howes O, McCutcheon R, Stone J. Glutamate and dopamine in schizophrenia: an update for the 21st century. *J Psychopharmacol*. 2015;29:97–115.

11. Laruelle M, Kegels M, Kegeles LS, Abi-Dargham A. Glutamate, dopamine, and schizophrenia. *Ann N Y Acad Sci*. 2003;1003:138–158.

12. Kesby J, Eyles D, McGrath J, Scott J. Dopamine, psychosis and schizophrenia: the widening gap between basic and clinical neuroscience. *Transl Psychiatry*. 2018;8:30.

13. Sekar A, Bialas AR, de Rivera H et al. Schizophrenia risk from complex variation of complement component 4. *Nature*. 2016;530:177–183.

14. Owens MJ, Nemeroff CB. Role of serotonin in the pathophysiology of depression: focus on the serotonin transporter. *Clin Chem*. 1994;40:288–295.

15. Stahl SM. Mechanism of action of serotonin selective reuptake inhibitors: serotonin receptors and pathways mediate therapeutic effects and side effects. *J Affect Disord*. 1998;51:215–235.

16. Faraone SV, Larsson H. Genetics of attention deficit hyperactivity disorder. *Mol Psychiatry*. 2019;24:562–575.

17. Thapar A, Martin J, Mick E et al. Psychiatric gene discoveries shape evidence on ADHD's biology. *Mol Psychiatry*. 2016;21:1202–1207.

18. Demontis D, Walters RK, Martin J et al. Discovery of the first genome-wide significant risk loci for attention deficit/hyperactivity disorder. *Nat Genet*. 2019;51:63–75.

19. Autism Spectrum Disorders Working Group of the Psychiatric Genomics Consortium, Consortium TASDWG of TPG. Meta-analysis of GWAS of over 16,000 individuals with autism spectrum disorder highlights a novel locus at 10q24.32 and a significant overlap with schizophrenia. *Mol Autism*. 2017;8:21.

Ewan St John Smith and
Anne Lingford-Hughes

2.7 Opioids and Common Recreational Drugs

OVERVIEW

Broadly speaking, common recreational drugs, including 'novel psychoactive substances' can be split into stimulants (a drug that generally increases activity in the central nervous system, e.g. cocaine and amphetamines) and depressants (a drug that generally decreases activity in the central nervous system, e.g. ethanol and opioids) (see Table 2.7.1). They may mimic endogenous substances – molecules produced by the body (e.g. opioids), enhance the effect of an endogenous substance at its receptor (e.g. benzodiazepines), or modulate neurotransmitter levels in the synaptic cleft (e.g. inducing neurotransmitter release or preventing neurotransmitter reuptake). It should be remembered that 'polydrug' use is the norm and drug interactions should be considered in relation to impact on mental health. Our knowledge about the impact of drugs of abuse on brain function has substantially increased in the last few decades. Nevertheless, when interpreting the apparent effects of exposure to a drug on brain structure and function, or when comparing the effects of different drugs, it is important to consider the following issues:

- the dose and duration of exposure
- whether an individual is 'substance dependent' (i.e. addiction)
- the impact of age
- whether the changes seen reflect vulnerability to use (e.g. impulsivity) rather than the impact of drug exposure or the effects of 'recovery' with abstinence.

2.7.1 Depressants

2.7.1.1 Opioids

Opioids can be categorised as endogenous (produced by the body, see Section 2.5.1) or exogenous (administered). Many exogenous opioids (e.g. morphine, heroin, fentanyl and methadone) act as full agonists on four main receptors: delta, kappa, mu and the nociception opioid receptor, which are G-protein-coupled receptors (GPCRs); delta, kappa and mu all have receptor subtypes. Some drugs show mixed pharmacology, for instance buprenorphine is a partial agonist at mu receptors, but a delta and kappa antagonist. The mu receptor mediates key functions including pleasure (positive reinforcement), analgesia and respiratory depression while stimulation of kappa receptor results in dysphoria. Therapeutically, opioid analgesia is mediated by several mechanisms including (Figure 2.7.1):

- counteracting the sensitising effects of prostaglandins on peripheral sensory neurons
- inhibiting presynaptic voltage-gated Ca^{2+} channels at the first synapse in the pain pathway in the spinal cord to decrease neurotransmitter release
- hyperpolarising postsynaptic neurons in the spinal cord, making them less excitable.

Table 2.7.1 Effects of substances of abuse

Drug	Acute effects	Chronic effects	Withdrawal	Key brain regions and functions involved
Depressants				
Opioids	Initial euphoria followed by apathy, dysphoria, sedation, disinhibition, psychomotor retardation, impaired attention and judgement, slurred speech, pupillary restriction, drowsiness; in severe cases, reduced consciousness with respiratory depression, to coma	Tolerance develops to all effects, to varying degrees, e.g. still vulnerable to respiratory depression, pupils remain reactive despite substantially blunted euphoria	Dysphoric mood, rhinorrhoea, lacrimation, muscle aches or cramps, abdominal pains, nausea/vomiting, diarrhoea, pupillary dilatation, piloerection (goose-bumps), yawning, insomnia, diarrhoea, fever	Neural mechanisms of impact of opiates on brain function or underpinning opiate addiction are less well studied in humans; neuroadaptations in locus coeruleus underpin many withdrawal symptoms (noradrenergic hyperactivity)
Benzodiazepine	Euphoria, anxiolytic, apathy, aggression, labile mood, impaired attention, anterograde amnesia, impaired psychomotor performance, unsteady gait, slurred speech, sedation to coma	Dysphoria, dysthymia and memory impairment described; dependence develops with tolerance – more to sedative effects than anxiolytic	Tremor of outstretched hands, nausea/vomiting, tachycardia, postural hypotension, psychomotor agitation, headache, insomnia; in severe cases, transient visual, tactile or auditory hallucinations, paranoia, seizures	Benzodiazepines impact on a wide range of brain functions given the ubiquity of GABA-A receptors; effect dependent on which subtype present
Alcohol	Anxiolytic, sedative, disinhibition, aggression, labile mood, impaired attention and judgement, unsteady gait, nystagmus, poor motor control, slurred speech; in severe cases, reduced consciousness to coma	Tolerance develops to all effects, withdrawal becomes evident unless blood alcohol levels maintained; anxiety may increase or emerge *de novo* (e.g. panic disorder), comorbid depression will persist or worsen	Tremor, shaking, sweating, nausea, psychomotor agitation, insomnia, anxiety; in severe cases, seizures and delirium tremens	All brain processes are affected by alcohol though prefrontal cortical and hippocampal function are particularly sensitive to adverse consequences of chronic alcohol exposure In those with alcohol dependence, reduced function in mesolimbic (reward–motivation) pathway to monetary rewards (blunted dopaminergic function likely linked with low mood), but heightened responses to salient (e.g. alcohol related) cues; also dysregulated responses seen in prefrontal cortex in reward processing, to alcohol-related cues
Cannabis	Euphoria, disinhibition, increased appetite, tachycardia, anxiety, agitation, paranoia, altered sense of time, impaired attention and judgement, auditory, visual and tactile hallucinations, depersonalisation, derealisation, conjunctival injection, dry mouth	Chronic intoxication can result in prolonged periods of apathy or amotivational syndrome, which mimics depression; recent evidence suggests increased risk of psychosis, schizophrenia, possibly cognitive impairment	Anxiety, irritability, tremor of outstretched hands, sweating, muscle aches	Cannabis use has been shown to be associated with some structural (e.g. smaller hippocampus; area rich in CB1 receptors) and functional changes (e.g. prefrontal cortex) – however not consistently
Gamma-hydroxybutyrate (GHB) and its precursor gamma-butyrolactone	Euphoria, relaxation, increased sociability and loss of inhibition; muscle relaxant, enhanced libido, increased sexual arousal, can lead to dizziness, blurred vision, hot/cold flushes, excess sweating, confusion, drowsiness, dizziness, myoclonic jerking, vomiting, loss of consciousness, tremors, blackouts and memory lapses, seizures, agitation, death	Changes associated with dependence are unclear	Insomnia, anxiety, tremor, confusion, delirium, hallucinations, tachycardia, hypertension, nausea, vomiting, sweating; can develop severe withdrawal very quickly, requiring urgent hospitalisation	Limited evidence though impaired memory, dorsolateral prefrontal cortex and hippocampal function, activity in salience and default-mode networks have been described in those with multiple GHB comas; also increased activity in limbic areas associated with emotion regulation consistent with its euphoric effects

Table 2.7.1 (cont.)

Drug	Acute effects	Chronic effects	Withdrawal	Key brain regions and functions involved
		Stimulants		
Cocaine, amphetamines	Euphoria, increased energy, hypervigilance, grandiose beliefs, aggression, labile mood, repetitive stereotyped behaviours, auditory, visual or tactile illusions, paranoia, tachycardia, cardiac arrhythmias, perspiration or chills, hypertension or lowered blood pressure, muscular weakness, chest pain, respiratory depression, confusion, dyskinesias or dystonias, sweating, chest pain, pupillary dilatation, psychomotor agitation, weight loss; physical effects include cardiomyopathy, cerebrovascular effects (stroke, haemorrhage) and seizures	Physical effects include cardiomyopathy, cerebrovascular effects (stroke) and weight loss; depressive disorder	Dysphoric mood, anhedonia, lethargy/ fatigue, psychotomor retardation or agitation, craving, increased appetite, insomnia or hypersomnia, bizarre or unpleasant dreams	Many neuroimaging studies showing dysregulation in dopamine system – is main target of stimulants – e.g. lower dopamine receptor D2 availability, blunted amphetamine-induced dopamine release; blunted mesolimbic dopaminergic activity to 'rewarding' tasks, altered prefrontal cortal–striatal function; likely underpins depressive symptoms and increased impulsivity
Ketamine	Is dissociative (severe state known as k-hole) i.e. alters perception; hallucinations, psychedelic-like experiences (mystical insight, spiritual trips, revelations or alternative realities), can lead to a trance-like cataleptic state, unconsciousness, amnesia and deep analgesia, but with intact ocular, laryngeal and pharyngeal reflexes (beneficial when used as an anaesthetic); is also a stimulant – euphoria; nausea and muscle spasms may occur, seizures, respiratory depression and cardiac arrest also described	Chronic use associated with short-term and long-term memory impairment; adverse physical consequences: on urinary system – irreversible damage to bladder that may require surgery; abdominal pain or k-cramps	Specific withdrawal syndrome has not been described, though non-specific symptoms seen: anxiety, tremor, sweating, palpitations, craving	Adverse impact on memory likely due to glutamate antagonism; in animal models ketamine has been shown to release dopamine which may be linked to its impact on mood; ketamine alters prefrontal cortical (particularly dorsolateral prefrontal cortical) function, which likely underpins its psychomimetic and therapeutic effects (including as an antidepressant)
Ecstasy (3,4-methylenedioxy-N-methylamphetamine; MDMA)	Desired: energy, euphoria, empathy, as well as anorexia, tachycardia, bruxism and sweating; hyperthermia; rhabdomyolysis and acute renal failure or hyponatremia complicated by brain oedema, cardiac arrhythmias and cerebral haemorrhage reported; associated with fatal water intoxication; serotonergic syndrome	Concerns that long-term use may result in depression and cognitive impairment are contentious with lack of consistent evidence showing substantial enduring harm from less than heavy use	Dysphoric 'crash' in first few days, anhedonia, reduced energy (like other stimulants)	Functional and structural imaging studies have reported some changes (e.g. reduced serotonin reuptake sites) but only in heavy users and not in moderate users; results are heterogeneous and likely due to different doses taken, other drug use etc.; acutely, ecstasy has been shown to reduce cerebral blood flow and connectivity in brain regions, consistent with its potential therapeutic effects, e.g. in insula, hippocampus, amygdala, somatosensory cortex

Table 2.7.1 (cont.)

Drug	Acute effects	Chronic effects	Withdrawal	Key brain regions and functions involved
Psychedelics: e.g. lysergic acid diethylamide (LSD), *N,N*-dimethyltryptamine, psilocybin, mescaline, 'magic mushrooms'	Visual and auditory pseudohallucinations distortion of sense of time, adverse emotional reactions including fear, anxiety, depression and paranoia, altered short-term memory, impaired concentration, feelings of depersonalisation, potential dangerous behaviours, tachycardia, palpitations, impulsive acts, impaired attention, pupillary dilatation, tremor, dizziness and lack of coordination, blurred vision, sweating, nausea	Flashbacks; anxiety and depression	None recognised	Psychedelics are proposed to acutely alter connectivity in cortical networks (cortex has high levels of 5-HT2A receptors – target for psychedelics) such that connectivity may be greater between a broader range of brain regions, e.g. with visual cortex (associated with hallucinatory activity) or reduced between parahippocampus and retrosplenial cortex (ego-dissolution); these effects are proposed to underpin how psychedelics can alter 'aberrant beliefs' and their therapeutic potential

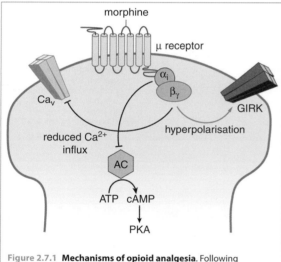

Figure 2.7.1 Mechanisms of opioid analgesia. Following activation of the G-protein-coupled mu (μ) opioid receptor in neurons, some key mechanisms by which analgesia is induced are: (1) G$_{\alpha i}$-mediated inhibition of adenylyl cyclase (AC) activity leading to reduced cAMP synthesis and protein kinase A (PKA) activation, effects that counteract the neuron sensitising effects of prostaglandins; (2) G$_{\beta\gamma}$ subunits inhibit voltage-gated calcium channels (Ca$_v$) in presynaptic neurons leading to reduced Ca^{2+} influx and thus neurotransmission; and (3) G$_{\beta\gamma}$-subunits open G-protein-coupled inwardly rectifying potassium channels (GIRKs) in postsynaptic neurons leading to neuronal hyperpolarisation.

The effects of opioids are not limited to the pain pathway and opioid receptor activation generally inhibits neurotransmission. Effects experienced therefore depend upon opioid receptor expression. Some key effects are:

- activation of mu receptors in the brainstem, resulting in respiratory depression
- activation of opioid receptors expressed by inhibitory GABAergic neurons that synapse onto excitatory glutamatergic nerves, resulting in a switching off of the inhibitory input and hence greater activity of the excitatory nerve
- activation of opioid receptors on GABAergic neurons, providing background or tonic inhibition of mesolimbic dopaminergic neurons, which results in their phasic firing (positive reinforcement).

Many aspects of opioid withdrawal are due to a 'noradrenergic storm', where cessation of long-term mu-opioid receptor-mediated inhibition leads to noradrenergic hyperactivity, as a consequence of neuroadaptations in the locus coeruleus. This is the rationale for using alpha-2-adrenoceptor agonists to treat opioid withdrawal.

2.7.1.2 Benzodiazepines

Benzodiazepines (e.g. diazepam, lorazepam), are positive allosteric modulators of gamma-aminobutyric acid (GABA)-A receptor function, that is, they amplify the effect of the endogenous ligand GABA at GABA-A receptors. GABA-A receptors are pentameric ligand-gated ion channels and benzodiazepines bind at the alpha/gamma subunit interface to enhance the effects of GABA, which means they enhance inhibitory neurotransmission in the brain (Figure 2.7.2). Therapeutically, benzodiazepines

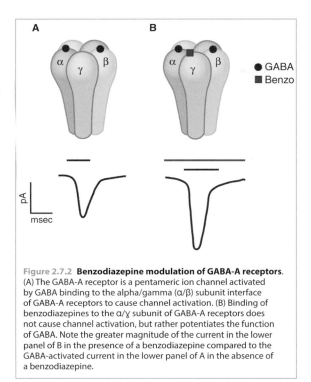

Figure 2.7.2 Benzodiazepine modulation of GABA-A receptors.
(A) The GABA-A receptor is a pentameric ion channel activated by GABA binding to the alpha/gamma (α/β) subunit interface of GABA-A receptors to cause channel activation. (B) Binding of benzodiazepines to the α/γ subunit of GABA-A receptors does not cause channel activation, but rather potentiates the function of GABA. Note the greater magnitude of the current in the lower panel of B in the presence of a benzodiazepine compared to the GABA-activated current in the lower panel of A in the absence of a benzodiazepine.

have a range of uses including as anxiolytics, sedatives and anticonvulsants, but they can be addictive (see Section 9.3).

2.7.1.3 Ethanol (Alcohol)

There is no specific receptor for ethanol, but rather it modulates the function of various neurotransmitter systems. Two key factors are the following:

- the enhancement of the inhibitory neurotransmitters GABA and glycine activity at certain GABA-A and glycine receptors (both are pentameric ion channels and the delta-GABA-A and alpha-1-glycine receptor subunits appear necessary for ethanol's activity)
- inhibition of the N-methyl-D-aspartate (NMDA) receptor for the excitatory neurotransmitter glutamate.

Overall, ethanol has a depressant effect on brain function, which leads to its anxiolytic and sedative effects. The pleasurable effects of alcohol are related to release of endogenous opioids (endorphins), which then increase firing of dopaminergic neurons in the mesolimbic system (see above). Adaptations in the dopaminergic and opioidergic systems likely underpin mood dysregulation

commonly seen in alcohol misuse. Alcohol also has potent neuroinflammatory effects, which likely contribute to neuronal dysfunction and atrophy.

2.7.1.4 Cannabis

The main active ingredient of cannabis is delta-9-tetrahydrocannabinol (THC), which, like endocannabinoids, exerts its effects on cannabinoid receptors, CB1 and CB2 being the most well understood and CB1 being perhaps the most important for psychiatry, considering its comparatively high expression in the brain. Cannabis also contains cannabidiol (CBD), which has antioxidant, anticonvulsant, anti-inflammatory and neuroprotective properties and therefore may have therapeutic utility. CBD has been shown to oppose many of the desired effects of THC, such as the 'high', thus plants are cultivated to have higher THC:CBD content. These strains (e.g. 'skunk') are therefore also associated with greater harm. The CB1 receptor is the main neuronal receptor, CB2 being largely expressed by immune cells. Mechanistically, like opioid receptors, CB1 receptors are GPCRs and, when activated, lead to inhibition of neurotransmission through mechanisms described for opioids. Differential expression of cannabinoid versus opioid receptors largely underpins the differences in effects experienced when taking an opioid- or THC-containing substance. Synthetic cannabinoid receptor agonists (e.g. 'Spice') have been developed as highly potent CB1 receptor agonists with very high affinity.

2.7.1.5 Gamma-Hydroxybutyrate and Its Precursor Gamma-Butyrolactone

The effects of GHB, which is also an endogenous neurotransmitter, are mediated via GABA-B and GHB receptors. Its effects are similar to alcohol and can be stimulatory as well as sedative.

2.7.2 Stimulants

2.7.2.1 Cocaine

Cocaine competitively inhibits the dopamine, noradrenaline and serotonin transporters so that neurotransmitter accumulates at the synapse and neurotransmission is enhanced (Figure 2.7.3A). Cocaine also inhibits voltage-gated Na^+ channels and thus has local anaesthetic activity. The effects observed with cocaine thus result from an increase in dopaminergic, noradrenergic and

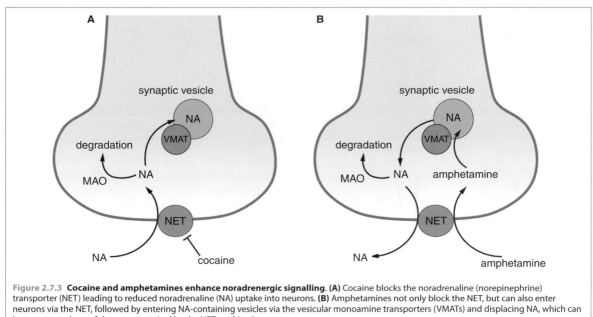

Figure 2.7.3 Cocaine and amphetamines enhance noradrenergic signalling. (A) Cocaine blocks the noradrenaline (norepinephrine) transporter (NET) leading to reduced noradrenaline (NA) uptake into neurons. **(B)** Amphetamines not only block the NET, but can also enter neurons via the NET, followed by entering NA-containing vesicles via the vesicular monoamine transporters (VMATs) and displacing NA, which can be transported out of the nerve terminal by the NET working in reverse.

serotonergic signalling and include euphoria, increased motor activity and enhancement of pleasure, at least initially, followed by neuroadaptations associated with tolerance, which include both up- and downregulation of receptors.

2.7.2.2 Amphetamines

Amphetamines (e.g. dextroamphetamine and methamphetamine) are competitive inhibitors of DAT and NET (not SERT) and thus produce some similar effects to cocaine. However, amphetamines can also infiltrate nerve terminals via DAT/NET and enter into synaptic vesicles via the VMATs, displacing dopamine and noradrenaline, which can then leave the nerve via DAT/NET working in reverse, thus further enhancing dopaminergic and noradrenergic neurotransmission (Figure 2.7.3B). Therapeutically, amphetamine derivatives can be used in the treatment of ADHD.

2.7.2.3 Ketamine

Ketamine is a non-competitive NMDA receptor antagonist (i.e. it does not compete with the binding of the NMDA receptor agonist glutamate, but binds elsewhere to the receptor; in this case, ketamine simply blocks the pore of the NMDA receptor). By blocking NMDA

receptors on inhibitory neurons, ketamine may actually increase glutamatergic activity and increase excitatory neurotransmission. It is a derivative of phencyclidine. Ketamine is used therapeutically as an anaesthetic or analgesic. There is increasing evidence for its efficacy as an antidepressant and the S(+) enantiomer of ketamine, esketamine, has been recently licensed by the US Food and Drug Administration for the treatment of depression, showing greater potency and more rapid elimination than racemic ketamine (a mix of both enantiomers). Ketamine can produce a wide spectrum of positive, negative and cognitive symptoms that have been used as a model to study schizophrenia.

2.7.2.4 Ecstasy

Ecstasy has stimulant and hallucinatory effects, which are largely mediated by increasing serotonin release and preventing its reuptake. There is growing interest in and evidence for using ecstasy to treat post-traumatic stress disorder and other psychiatric disorders.

2.7.2.5 Psychedelics

Psychedelics, such as LSD, psilocybin and mescaline, interact with many different receptors, but modulation of serotonergic signalling is key and all act as agonists of the

5-HT2A receptor. 5-HT2A activation results in neuronal excitation and thus, depending upon where the 5-HT2A receptor is expressed, different effects are observed. For example, 5-HT2A expression by inhibitory neurons in the nigrostriatal pathway results in 5-HT2A activation causing more GABA to be released onto dopaminergic neurons, which may explain the tremor observed in some individuals following LSD consumption.

Conclusions and Outstanding Questions

Whilst we understand a lot about how drugs interact with the brain, we need to understand more about long-term neuroadaptations and relation to drug-related behaviour and mental health during current use as well as once abstinent.

Outstanding Questions

- As polydrug use is the norm in humans, how do different drugs of abuse interact with each other?
- Does prior exposure to one drug of abuse alter how the brain responds to a different class of drug of abuse and how does this influence drug-related behaviour?
- What neurobiological processes underpin withdrawal from drugs of abuse?

FURTHER READING

Abdulrahim D, Bowden-Jones O, on behalf of the NEPTUNE Expert Group. *Guidance on the Management of Acute and Chronic Harms of Club Drugs and Novel Psychoactive Substances*. Novel Psychoactive Treatment UK Network (NEPTUNE), 2015.

Koob GF, Volkow ND. Neurobiology of addiction: a neurocircuitry analysis. *Lancet Psychiatry* 2016; 3(8): 760–773.

National Neuroscience Curriculum Initiative online resources

From "Azalla" to Anandamide: Distilling the Therapeutic Potential of Cannabinoids

Rajiv Radhakrishnan and David A. Ross

3

Basic Techniques in Neuroscience

Rudolf N. Cardinal

3.1 Recording from the Brain

3.1

Recording from the Brain

Rudolf N. Cardinal

OVERVIEW

This chapter reviews briefly some of the fundamental techniques used to study the nervous system in humans and other animals. We begin by considering common methods for measuring brain structure and function, from single-neuron recordings and tissue analysis to whole-brain neuroimaging, touching on some points of clinical relevance. Next, we examine methods for altering brain function experimentally, and consider animal models of psychiatric disease in overview. We examine core ideas in data analysis (including statistics, causality and computational modelling), and conclude with a brief look at key concepts in functional neuroimaging.

The are many ways to record brain function. They differ in what they measure – for example, electrical signals, magnetic signals or chemical concentrations – but they also vary considerably in terms of their resolution and extent. Some techniques have high **spatial resolution**, measuring from small things such as single neurons or even single molecules. In general, these techniques have low **spatial extent**: it's hard to measure trillions of individual neurons simultaneously. Techniques that measure the whole brain at once (i.e. have high spatial extent) typically have lower spatial resolution and cannot distinguish individual neurons. Techniques also vary considerably in their **temporal resolution**, from electrical techniques that can record signals much faster than those generated by neurons, to those that are temporally 'blurry' for technical or physiological reasons, and some that analyse brain tissue from a single moment in time. Measurement techniques vary in **invasiveness**, too.

3.1.1 Single-Unit Electrophysiology and Related Small-Scale Techniques

Neurons receive chemical information from many incoming synapses, convert that information into an electrical signal and propagate that signal as action potentials to their own outgoing synapses. How can those signals be recorded? In the original method of single-unit electrophysiology, a fine hollow glass needle (micropipette) is inserted into a neuron (the 'unit') and connected to an electrical circuit. The electrical potential from this **intracellular electrode** is compared to an electrical 'ground' (reference point) outside the neuron and some distance away. This technique has excellent spatial resolution – a single neuron – and extremely high temporal resolution (Figure 3.1.1A). It can be performed on isolated neurons or brain slices in culture dishes (in vitro) or, with some adaptations, on living brains (in vivo).

A slightly different approach is to measure **local field potentials** (LFPs; Figure 3.1.1B). Here, an electrode is inserted into nervous tissue so that it sits close to several neurons, and measures their summed electrical activity (relative to a distant ground point). These extracellular electrodes can be made of sharpened metal and are more robust than glass micropipettes. Each neuron produces very consistent action potentials, so with the right electrodes and careful signal processing it is possible to distinguish the firing of different cells within the LFP and isolate individual cell responses. This gives **single-cell recording from extracellular electrodes**, the first method to allow neuronal recording in vivo (Figure 3.1.1C).

Single-neuron techniques have been used extensively to determine the stimuli to which different neurons respond (on the sensory side of the nervous system), what actions they command (on the motor side) or what cognitive functions they carry information about (in the middle).

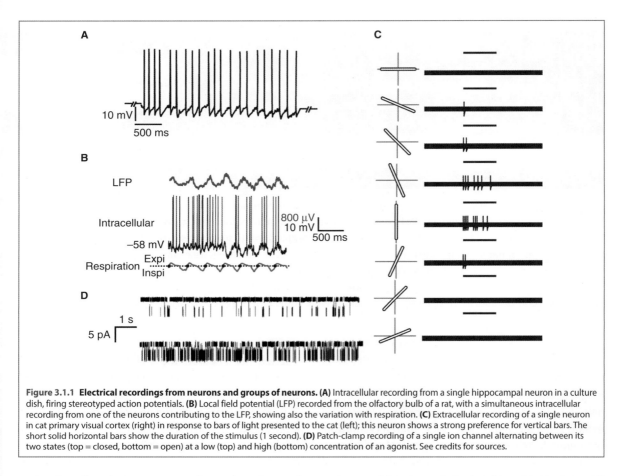

Figure 3.1.1 Electrical recordings from neurons and groups of neurons. (A) Intracellular recording from a single hippocampal neuron in a culture dish, firing stereotyped action potentials. **(B)** Local field potential (LFP) recorded from the olfactory bulb of a rat, with a simultaneous intracellular recording from one of the neurons contributing to the LFP, showing also the variation with respiration. **(C)** Extracellular recording of a single neuron in cat primary visual cortex (right) in response to bars of light presented to the cat (left); this neuron shows a strong preference for vertical bars. The short solid horizontal bars show the duration of the stimulus (1 second). **(D)** Patch-clamp recording of a single ion channel alternating between its two states (top = closed, bottom = open) at a low (top) and high (bottom) concentration of an agonist. See credits for sources.

Single-cell techniques are not limited to electrical recording. For example, neurons can be bathed in dyes that fluoresce in response to calcium entering the cell, or genetically modified to express such calcium indicators. **Optical single-cell imaging** (measuring light emission) can then be used to study calcium signalling.

It is possible to zoom in further: by sucking a very small part of the surface of a neuron onto the tip of a hollow pipette, one can record electrically from single ion channels. This is the 'patch clamp' technique (Figure 3.1.1D).

Nobel prizes were awarded to the following scientists, all relevant to this field:

Sherrington and Adrian (1932): the functions of neurons, including recording from single sensory and motor nerve fibres, all-or-nothing propagation, the concept of communication via synapses, work on reflexes, and mapping of the motor cortex.

Erlanger and Gasser (1944): impulse conduction by different types of nerve fibres.

Eccles, Hodgkin and Huxley (1963): the ionic mechanisms of the action potential and of synaptic transmission.

Hubel and Wiesel (1981): single-cell extracellular recording of visual neurons, and the development of the visual cortex.

Neher and Sakmann (1991): patch clamp and ion-channel operation.

O'Keefe, Moser and Moser (2014): 'place cells' in the hippocampus.

3.1.2 Local Chemical Measurement

A **microdialysis probe** is a small tube that can be inserted into a brain region of interest. Fluid such as artificial cerebrospinal fluid (CSF) is pumped gently in through one port, flows past a semipermeable membrane where it can collect chemicals from the brain, and flows out again. The resulting fluid – the dialysate – is analysed chemically. This is a direct way of measuring neurotransmitters and other molecules in specific brain regions. It can be combined with stimuli to trigger neurotransmitter release (such as a high-potassium dialysis fluid) or used to deliver drugs. Microdialysis is sometimes used in neurological intensive care units to assess brain metabolism.

A related technique is **cyclic voltammetry**: the voltage of an electrode in the brain is varied and the resulting current is measured. The current is influenced by oxidation or reduction of chemicals (such as dopamine) at the electrode's tip, allowing the concentration of those chemicals to be measured. It has much greater temporal resolution than microdialysis, but less chemical specificity.

3.1.3 Post-Mortem Tissue Analysis

There are many techniques for studying individual neurons after death. For example, one might study an animal's behaviour and then measure the activity of an important protein (such as the phosphorylation of a transcription factor) in specific cells using a histological technique such as **immunocytochemistry**, detecting proteins via antibodies. Chemicals of interest can be labelled with radioactive tracers, injected systemically or into the brain and then mapped via **autoradiography**, placing brain slices on radiation-sensitive film.

3.1.4 Brain Recording from the Surface

3.1.4.1 Electroencephalography

Electroencephalography (EEG) measures the collective activity of large swathes of the brain, with very good temporal resolution but poor spatial resolution. The dominant contribution to the **scalp EEG** signal is thought to be from pyramidal neurons of surface cortex. The axons of pyramidal neurons are perpendicular to the cortical surface. For gyri at the surface of the cortex (rather than sulci folded beneath), those axons are also perpendicular to the scalp. Therefore, as currents flow along many

aligned axons, a voltage change is generated at the scalp. The signal from neurons is weakened by its passage through brain, CSF, skull and scalp, and is small compared to many other electrical signals. Practical problems therefore include interference from muscle activity (including the heart) and external signals like mains electricity.

In clinical EEG using the internationally recognised '10–20' system, electrodes are placed on the scalp, separated by either 10% or 20% of the total front–back or left–right distance of the skull (Figure 3.1.2A). The electrical activity at each electrode is compared to another electrode (bipolar recording), or to a reference point or the average of all electrodes (unipolar recording). Each electrical trace that results is called a **channel.** A clinical array uses at least 21 electrodes and 16 channels, but many more may be used to improve resolution. The channels are displayed in a standardised format called a **montage** (Figure 3.1.2B). By convention, 'up' means 'more negative at the first electrode' (or more positive at the second or reference electrode).

EEG is not restricted to the scalp; surgically implanted electrodes (**intracranial EEG**) may be used to discover or map deep epileptogenic foci.

Both **spontaneous** and **evoked** (**event-related**) EEG may be examined. In a spontaneous EEG, the subject sits quietly. Additional provoking techniques are often used clinically to elicit abnormalities, such as hyperventilation, photic (light flash) stimulation, sleep deprivation the night before, and sleep during the recording. In event-related EEG, a stimulus is played to the subject, usually several times, and the average response is measured.

Any time-varying signal, such as an EEG trace, can be analysed in terms of the frequencies it contains. For example, a sine wave (pure tone) contains a single frequency, a piano chord contains more and white noise contains all possible frequencies. EEG signals are often subjected to frequency analysis (Figure 3.1.2C), and the frequency bands are named as in Table 3.1.1.

Electroencephalography is useful for demonstrating **generalised cerebral pathology** such as generalised slowing in encephalopathies and drug-induced sedation, the distinctive but non-specific triphasic waves seen in hepatic and other encephalopathies, or generalised seizure activity. **Focal cerebral pathology** may include epileptiform discharges between overt seizures (though a normal interictal EEG does not exclude epilepsy)

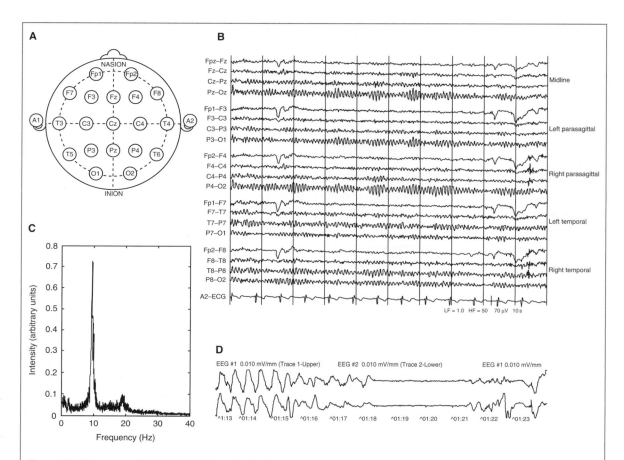

Figure 3.1.2 Electroencephalography. (A) The standard 21 electrodes of the international '10–20' system (see text; nasion front, inion back; Fp frontopolar, F frontal, C central, T temporal, P parietal, O occipital; odd numbers for the left hemisphere and even numbers for the right; greater numbers more laterally; z for zero at the midline). This system has later been extended. **(B)** Normal waking electroencephalography: montage of 10 seconds. The time between vertical lines is 1 second by convention. The 20 channels are grouped into five chains of four channels each, with channels ordered from front (top) to back (bottom) within a chain. From top to bottom the chains are: midline, left parasagittal, right parasagittal, left temporal, right temporal. At the very bottom is the electrocardiogram (ECG). The EEG shows posterior alpha rhythm at about 10 Hz, plus two eye-blink artefacts visible frontally in the 2nd and 9th seconds. Some electrodes are used that are not shown in (A). (LF, low-frequency cutoff in Hz; HF, high-frequency cutoff.) **(C)** Frequency analysis, via fast Fourier transform (FFT), of a waking eyes-closed EEG. Alpha frequencies predominate. **(D)** Two-channel EEG showing the tail end of a seizure induced by electroconvulsive therapy (ECT) (left); the seizure ends abruptly and is followed by postical suppression (centre) as expected, followed by artefacts (right). Not to scale. See credits for sources.

Table 3.1.1 EEG frequency bands

Name	Frequency range in Hz (note: definitions vary quite a bit!)	Comments
Delta (δ)	0.5–4	Delta dominates in (and defines) slow-wave sleep.
Theta (θ)	4–8	Cortical theta appears in drowsy states and light sleep.
Alpha (α)	8–12	Alpha dominates in resting subjects with eyes closed, occipitally; and in rapid eye movement (REM) sleep, frontally.
Beta (β)	12–30	Beta waves dominate in normal eyes-open waking states.
Gamma (γ)	30–100	Gamma waves are a high-frequency signal that is quite hard to measure via a scalp EEG, but is thought to reflect thalamocortical oscillations that may be important in attention.

Table 3.1.2 Some features seen in EEG reports

Feature	Description	Relevance
K complex	A high-amplitude biphasic waveform (a single long delta wave lasting ~1 s) during non-REM (NREM) sleep. Negative (up) then positive (down).	The largest events in a healthy EEG. They are diffuse and reflect cortical 'silence' and oscillatory synchrony. Often followed by sleep spindles. May trigger epileptiform activity in some seizure disorders (e.g. autosomal dominant nocturnal frontal lobe epilepsy). Increased in restless leg syndrome.
Sleep spindle	A burst at 11–16 Hz lasting ~1 s during NREM sleep.	Normal. Predominantly a local thalamocortical phenomenon. Linked to memory consolidation.
Generalised slowing	Global reduction in frequency.	Seen in diffuse encephalopathies (e.g. diffuse encephalitis, metabolic encephalopathy) and drug-induced sedation.
Focal slowing	Slow waves in one area only.	If present continuously, suggests a structural lesion of white matter. Transient focal polymorphic slow-wave activity suggests migraine or a postictal state after a focal seizure. Intermittent rhythmic slow activity frontally (in adults) or occipitally (in children) is non-specific (e.g. seen in metabolic disturbances, diencephalic lesions, hydrocephalus).
Generalised attenuation	Reduction of EEG amplitude everywhere.	Seen in severe encephalopathy and some degenerative disorders (e.g. Huntington's disease). A quiet background with bursts of mixed-frequency activity ('burst-suppression pattern') can be seen in any severe encephalopathy (e.g. after anoxia) or with high-dose sedatives. Complete EEG silence is seen in sedative overdose, hypothermia and neocortical brain death.
Focal attenuation	Reduction of EEG amplitude in one area.	Suggests local cortical destruction.
Spike discharges and sharp waves	Spike discharge (spike): a potential with a sharp contour lasting < 80 ms. Sharp wave: similarly, but lasting 80–200 ms.	Spikes probably reflect excitable cortex. Spike–wave bursts probably involve thalamocortical projections too. Isolated spikes and sharp waves can be normal (and there are many forms of normal spike) but they are more common in patients with epilepsy, interictally. Epileptiform discharges are abnormal paroxysmal events containing spike discharges or sharp waves, sometimes also with slow waves. Epileptiform activity may be focal or generalised (e.g. 'generalised spike–wave activity'), or start focally and generalise. Repetitive sharp and/or slow-wave activity is also seen in other conditions, including brain infections such as herpes simplex encephalitis.
Triphasic waves	Originally called 'blunted spike and wave' – e.g. 'small sharp negative (up), big sharp positive (down), slow negative (up)'.	Distinctive but non-specific: seen in a variety of encephalopathies (such as hepatic encephalopathy, renal failure).

or focal attenuation (reduction in signal amplitude) after local damage. Requesting clinicians often see a narrative summary by an EEG technician and a clinical interpretation by a neurophysiologist, rather than raw EEG data; some EEG 'features' are shown in Table 3.1.2. See Section 9.18 for more on EEG findings in epilepsy. Electroencephalography is also a core component of **polysomnography** to diagnose sleep disorders. Sensory evoked potentials may be used to evaluate the function of sensory pathways. **Seizure monitoring**, usually via simple two-channel EEG, is part of electroconvulsive therapy (ECT) (Figure 3.1.2D).

3.1.4.2 Magnetoencephalography

Magnetoencephalography (MEG) is conceptually similar to EEG, but the equipment is much more complicated (Figure 3.1.3A). All electrical currents produce magnetic fields. Therefore, as neuronal currents flow (giving rise to voltage changes that can be measured via EEG), magnetic fields are produced by the brain. The practical difficulty is in detecting very small magnetic field changes (e.g. about 10^{-14} to 10^{-12} tesla (T)) on the background of the much larger magnetic field of the Earth (about 10^{-5} T). MEG scanners need to be shielded from interference. Historically, superconducting magnetic field detectors were necessary, and superconductors generally need to be very cold (e.g. cooled by liquid helium at −270 °C). This poses the safety challenge of getting liquid helium quite close to someone's head! Newer advances in room-temperature magnetometers are making MEG systems smaller and more portable.

The magnetic fields are at right angles to the electrical currents, so while EEG is most sensitive to groups of cells that 'face the outside' (whose axons are perpendicular

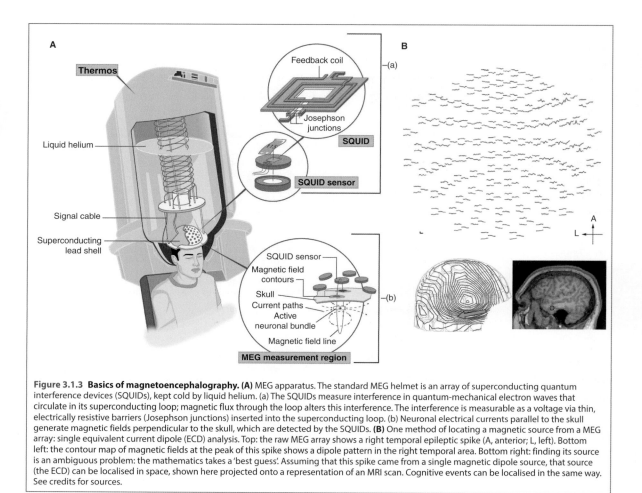

Figure 3.1.3 Basics of magnetoencephalography. (A) MEG apparatus. The standard MEG helmet is an array of superconducting quantum interference devices (SQUIDs), kept cold by liquid helium. (a) The SQUIDs measure interference in quantum-mechanical electron waves that circulate in its superconducting loop; magnetic flux through the loop alters this interference. The interference is measurable as a voltage via thin, electrically resistive barriers (Josephson junctions) inserted into the superconducting loop. (b) Neuronal electrical currents parallel to the skull generate magnetic fields perpendicular to the skull, which are detected by the SQUIDs. **(B)** One method of locating a magnetic source from a MEG array: single equivalent current dipole (ECD) analysis. Top: the raw MEG array shows a right temporal epileptic spike (A, anterior; L, left). Bottom left: the contour map of magnetic fields at the peak of this spike shows a dipole pattern in the right temporal area. Bottom right: finding its source is an ambiguous problem: the mathematics takes a 'best guess'. Assuming that this spike came from a single magnetic dipole source, that source (the ECD) can be localised in space, shown here projected onto a representation of an MRI scan. Cognitive events can be localised in the same way. See credits for sources.

to surface cortex, like 'vertical' neurons in gyri), MEG is most sensitive to groups of cells with axons parallel to the skin (e.g. running transversely in gyri, or perpendicular to the cortex in sulci). Unlike EEG, MEG requires no reference point.

The spatial resolution of MEG is intrinsically better than EEG. Clinical uses therefore include mapping cortex prior to neurosurgery (e.g. for epilepsy; Figure 3.1.3B), but much of its use is in the research domain to measure event-related cortical activity with high spatial and temporal resolution.

 The Nobel Prize in Physics was awarded to Brian Josephson in 1973 for predictions that led to the superconducting quantum interference device (SQUID), used in MEG.

3.1.5 Three-Dimensional Neuroimaging Techniques

3.1.5.1 Computerised Tomography

Computerised tomography (CT) transformed clinical neuroscience by detecting structural abnormalities affecting the brain. It is less sensitive to tissue changes than MRI, except for detecting fresh blood and calcification or bony changes, but it is readily available and quick.

The principle of CT is to measure the penetration of X-rays from a source to an array of detectors. The source and detectors are then rotated around the subject, taking images in many directions. The series of one-dimensional images is then combined mathematically to produce a two-dimensional image, typically an axial 'slice'. The patient is then moved slightly in the superior–inferior direction and another 'slice' is captured, generating a three-dimensional scan. Shades of grey are used to represent tissue density (ordered: air → fat → water → bone → metal), measured in Hounsfield units (defined as –1,000 for air, 0 for water). There are many variations on this basic method, with iodine-based intravenous contrast being a key method for detecting tumours.

CT has always been viewed as a structural imaging technique, but has been extended to a kind of functional imaging in the form of perfusion CT: intravenous contrast is given and its flow through the brain measured to map cerebral blood flow (CBF). This is primarily of use for detecting salvageable tissue in early stroke.

 The Nobel Prize in Physiology or Medicine was awarded to Godfrey N. Hounsfield and Allan M. Cormack in 1979 for their work on computer-assisted tomography.

3.1.5.2 Positron Emission Tomography

In positron emission tomography (PET), subjects are injected with a radioactive isotope, usually ^{18}F (fluorine-18), that decays and emits positrons (anti-electrons).

When a positron is emitted, it travels a short distance (median range ~1 mm for ^{18}F) before hitting an electron in the subject's tissue. When the particle and antiparticle collide, they annihilate each other and a pair of gamma photons is emitted, travelling in opposite directions (Figure 3.1.4A). Detectors around the subject notice the simultaneous arrival of gamma pairs. This locates the annihilation event, and thus the approximate place where the positron was first emitted. The scanner builds a map of positron emissions across the brain.

What this actually measures depends on the tracer that the radioisotope was part of. A common tracer is ^{18}F-fluorodeoxyglucose (^{18}FDG), which is taken up by tissues in the same way as glucose. ^{18}FDG-PET therefore produces a map of glucose utilisation in the brain. Similarly, ^{18}F-fallypride, a dopamine D2/D3 receptor antagonist, can be used to image dopamine D2/D3 receptor occupancy; and so on. Because isotopes like ^{18}F have a fairly short half-life, they need to be made near the patient. Radiotracer production is a significant cost in PET scanning.

At present, the principal clinical use of PET is in CT-PET imaging for cancer: ^{18}FDG-PET measures tissue

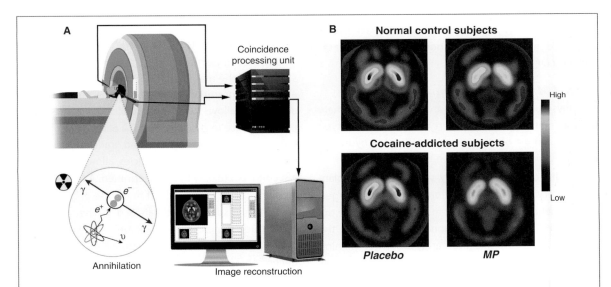

Figure 3.1.4 Positron emission tomography (PET). (A) Principle: the detection of simultaneous gamma (γ) rays arriving at opposite detectors, as a result of a positron (e^+)/electron (e^-) annihilation event (see text). A neutrino (v) is also emitted as ^{18}F decays to ^{18}O. **(B)** Illustration of abnormalities of the dopamine (DA) system in addiction, shown by PET imaging of the DA D2 receptor with the D2 antagonist ^{11}C-raclopride. Images are group averages. More signal indicates more raclopride binding, which indicates more 'free' (unoccupied) D2 receptors, and less synaptic DA. Compared to placebo (left), intravenous methylphenidate (MP, right), which normally causes substantial DA release, reduced D2 receptor availability in controls (top) but not in people with cocaine addiction (bottom), suggesting a reduced capacity for DA release in the cocaine users. See credits for sources.

metabolism and is co-registered with CT (that is, the patient is scanned with two scanners and the two images are aligned in three-dimensional space, giving what looks like a 'coloured-in' CT scan). PET has been widely used for functional neuroimaging in research (Figure 3.1.4B). MRI has largely superseded PET for measuring general 'activity' (better resolution, no ionising radiation) but PET can image chemically specific targets, like receptor occupancy, in a way that MRI cannot.

 The Nobel Prize in Physics was awarded to Carl Anderson in 1936 for the discovery of the positron.

3.1.5.3 Single-Photon Emission Computed Tomography

Single-photon emission computed tomography (SPECT) is similar to PET, but uses tracers that emit gamma rays directly. Gamma cameras capture a 'gamma image' from one or two directions, then rotate (like CT) to capture from many directions, building a three-dimensional image. The resolution is worse than PET, but SPECT is much cheaper. A well-known application of SPECT is ^{123}I-ioflupane imaging of the dopamine transporter (DAT) ('DaTSCAN') for the diagnosis of Parkinson's disease, dementia with Lewy bodies or other diseases affecting DAT density.

3.1.5.4 Magnetic Resonance Imaging

The physics of MRI is complex and we will approximate it. Atomic nuclei have a property called **spin**. The type of nucleus most often scanned in MRI is the hydrogen nucleus, which is a single proton.

Imagine protons in the body, spinning like little planets in every possible orientation. A spinning charged particle behaves like a tiny bar magnet. Once inside the strong static field of an MRI scanner (typically 1–7 T), the protons' axes line up, like a vast array of vertical spinning gyroscopes. If we imagine the patient's head as the 'up' direction and describe three perpendicular axes, x (right), y (forwards) and z (up), then the static field, pointing up, makes the protons spin with an axis in the z direction. More accurately, they align both 'up' and 'down' but with more 'up' than 'down' and, even more accurately, they are in a quantum mixture of the two states – but the basic

description suffices! If a magnetic pulse of the right type from a radiofrequency transmitter is applied to all of the proton gyroscopes, they will suddenly deflect. MRI scanners typically deflect them to 90° (let's say: to the right, in the x direction). When the pulse is switched off, they start to relax or decay back to their starting orientation – but gradually, and in a rotary way, 'precessing' like a gyroscope settling back to its vertical (Figure 3.1.5A). As they do so, their net magnetic field sweeps past the receiver coil and generates current, which the scanner detects.

The most interesting plrt is that the way the protons relax depends on their local chemical environment (e.g. water versus fat). The time T_1 ('spin–lattice relaxation time') measures how long the spins take to settle back to the starting (z) direction – how long the gyroscopes take to return to vertical (Figure 3.1.5A). In contrast, T_2 ('spin–spin relaxation time') measures how long the gyroscopes take to desynchronise (point in different directions) in the x and y plane (Figure 3.1.5A). Different tissues, such as water and fat, have different values of T_1 and T_2. By altering the pulse 'sequence', such as how often the main pulse is delivered (repetition time) and when the scanner adds an extra 180° pulse after the main 90° pulse to create 'echoes' (echo time), MRI scanners can be tuned to be more sensitive to T_1 differences (T1-weighted imaging: bright fat, dark CSF) or T_2 differences (T2-weighted imaging: bright CSF, less-bright fat).

Another important aspect is that by varying the strength of the main magnetic field from head to toe, applying a gradient, the resonance frequencies are altered. This allows the scanner to pick out signals from a particular 'slice' (e.g. one xy slice at a particular location in the z direction). Applying a second gradient, and analysing the resulting signal frequencies, allows positions on a second axis (e.g. x) to be determined. A final dynamic gradient can be used to affect the phase of the protons, giving a third spatial coordinate (e.g. y). The spatial units of the three-dimensional image are called voxels (small cubes that are analogous to square pixels in a two-dimensional image).

Structural MRI is common in clinical practice for detecting disorders of grey and white matter, and can be tuned in many different ways (Figure 3.1.5B). As well as T1- and T2-weighted imaging, sequences can be tuned to emphasise pathology. For example, **fluid-attenuated inversion recovery (FLAIR)** is a pulse sequence designed

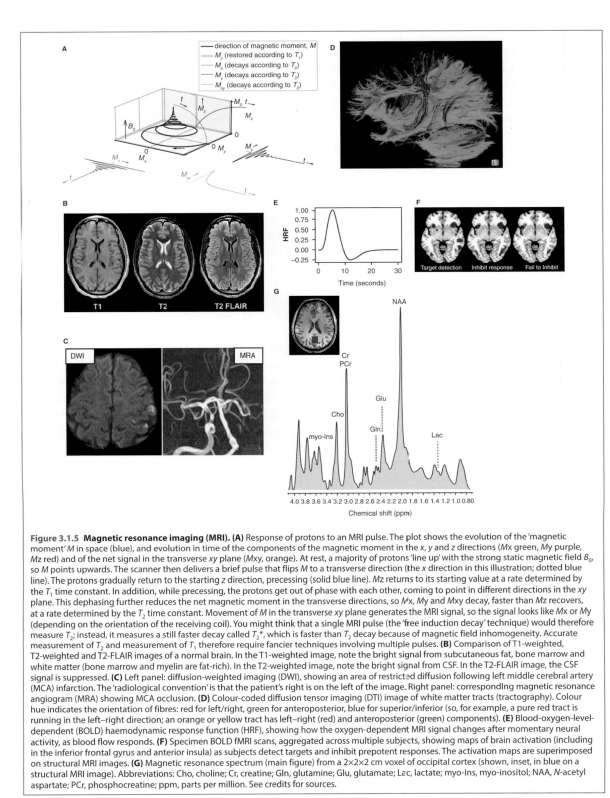

Figure 3.1.5 Magnetic resonance imaging (MRI). (A) Response of protons to an MRI pulse. The plot shows the evolution of the 'magnetic moment' M in space (blue), and evolution in time of the components of the magnetic moment in the x, y and z directions (Mx green, My purple, Mz red) and of the net signal in the transverse xy plane (Mxy, orange). At rest, a majority of protons 'line up' with the strong static magnetic field B_0, so M points upwards. The scanner then delivers a brief pulse that flips M to a transverse direction (the x direction in this illustration; dotted blue line). The protons gradually return to the starting z direction, precessing (solid blue line). Mz returns to its starting value at a rate determined by the T_1 time constant. In addition, while precessing, the protons get out of phase with each other, coming to point in different directions in the xy plane. This dephasing further reduces the net magnetic moment in the transverse directions, so Mx, My and Mxy decay, faster than Mz recovers, at a rate determined by the T_2 time constant. Movement of M in the transverse xy plane generates the MRI signal, so the signal looks like Mx or My (depending on the orientation of the receiving coil). You might think that a single MRI pulse (the 'free induction decay' technique) would therefore measure T_2; instead, it measures a still faster decay called T_2^*, which is faster than T_2 decay because of magnetic field inhomogeneity. Accurate measurement of T_2 and measurement of T_1 therefore require fancier techniques involving multiple pulses. **(B)** Comparison of T1-weighted, T2-weighted and T2-FLAIR images of a normal brain. In the T1-weighted image, note the bright signal from subcutaneous fat, bone marrow and white matter (bone marrow and myelin are fat-rich). In the T2-weighted image, note the bright signal from CSF. In the T2-FLAIR image, the CSF signal is suppressed. **(C)** Left panel: diffusion-weighted imaging (DWI), showing an area of restricted diffusion following left middle cerebral artery (MCA) infarction. The 'radiological convention' is that the patient's right is on the left of the image. Right panel: corresponding magnetic resonance angiogram (MRA) showing MCA occlusion. **(D)** Colour-coded diffusion tensor imaging (DTI) image of white matter tracts (tractography). Colour hue indicates the orientation of fibres: red for left/right, green for anteroposterior, blue for superior/inferior (so, for example, a pure red tract is running in the left–right direction; an orange or yellow tract has left–right (red) and anteroposterior (green) components). **(E)** Blood-oxygen-level-dependent (BOLD) haemodynamic response function (HRF), showing how the oxygen-dependent MRI signal changes after momentary neural activity, as blood flow responds. **(F)** Specimen BOLD fMRI scans, aggregated across multiple subjects, showing maps of brain activation (including in the inferior frontal gyrus and anterior insula) as subjects detect targets and inhibit prepotent responses. The activation maps are superimposed on structural MRI images. **(G)** Magnetic resonance spectrum (main figure) from a 2×2×2 cm voxel of occipital cortex (shown, inset, in blue on a structural MRI image). Abbreviations: Cho, choline; Cr, creatine; Gln, glutamine; Glu, glutamate; Lac, lactate; myo-Ins, myo-inositol; NAA, N-acetyl aspartate; PCr, phosphocreatine; ppm, parts per million. See credits for sources.

to suppress the signal from fluids, and is typically used to suppress the CSF signal. T2-FLAIR images look like T2 but with dark CSF, and are often good for identifying pathology by emphasising more subtle differences in T2 and allowing periventricular changes to be seen more clearly. **Diffusion weighted imaging** (**DWI**) measures the ability of protons to diffuse in water; one clinical application is in detecting early cerebral ischaemia (Figure 3.1.5C). **Diffusion tensor imaging** (**DTI**) extends DWI to measure both a rate of diffusion (per voxel) and a preferred direction of diffusion (per voxel) by combining multiple diffusion-weighted scans. This can be used to map white matter tracts (Figure 3.1.5D), because water diffuses more readily along such tracts than across them. **Magnetic resonance angiography** (**MRA**) delineates blood vessels (Figure 3.1.5C), typically by distinguishing moving from stationary tissue or by using intravascular contrast agents (see below). There are a variety of MRA techniques; some allow fast-flowing (e.g. arterial) blood and slow-flowing (e.g. venous) blood to be isolated selectively, or the direction of blood flow to be shown. Intravenous **gadolinium contrast** may be used to enhance some forms of MRI. Gadolinium influences the MRI signal of nearby protons, appearing bright on T1-weighted images. If gadolinium is given and MRI performed after a short delay, any gadolinium accumulation highlights areas of blood–brain barrier breakdown. By highlighting blood, gadolinium can also be used to enhance MRA and to perform **perfusion** scans, measuring cerebral blood flow. Perfusion scanning is also possible without contrast injections: **arterial spin labelling** involves 'tagging' incoming blood magnetically with an MRI pulse (instead of with gadolinium) and comparing images with and without this tag to show cerebral blood flow. Perfusion MRI can be used to detect stroke and perhaps neurodegenerative disorders.

The main contraindication to MRI is ferromagnetic metal implants, which can be accelerated lethally by the static field in the scanning room.

MRI can also show brain function: **functional MRI** (**fMRI**). The particular innovation most used for fMRI is **blood-oxygen-level-dependent** (**BOLD**) MRI, now very widely used in research (Figure 3.1.5F). This relies on the fact that oxygenated and deoxygenated haemoglobin alter the local magnetic field differently. Neuronal activity indirectly causes an increase in local blood flow and thus an increase in the local oxyhaemoglobin-to-deoxyhaemoglobin ratio, which the scanner detects. This neurovascular process takes several seconds, limiting temporal resolution (Figure 3.1.5E).

MRI was originally developed from nuclear magnetic resonance (NMR) techniques in chemistry, and magnetic resonance has chemical applications in the brain too. **Magnetic resonance spectroscopy** (**MRS**) is a technique for analysing the chemical composition of tissues. Like MRI, MRS typically records signals from protons, though other nuclei can also be used. However, whereas MRI uses frequencies to encode spatial location, MRS uses frequency information to identify differences in the chemical environment of the protons. The chemical environment in which a proton sits – such as the specific molecule or molecular group of which it's a part – influences the local magnetic field, and thus alters the resonance frequencies (termed 'chemical shift', expressed as parts per million, ppm). Different molecular groups have different chemical shift positions. Thus, by analysing the degree to which tissue resonates at different frequencies (the spectrum), a chemical analysis can be performed (Figure 3.1.5G). Since water is very abundant in the brain, techniques are also required to suppress the strong signal from water in order to examine other metabolites. MRS can quantify levels of glutamate, glutamine, gamma-aminobutyric acid (GABA), creatine, lactate and other substances. Its spatial resolution is generally lower than MRI. MRS is used clinically, such as for the analysis of brain tumours, and in a range of research applications.

Pharmacological MRI (**phMRI**) is a different 'chemical' technique: this means examining the effects of drugs on MRI signals, or on fMRI measures during behavioural/cognitive tasks.

Nobel prizes were awarded to the following scientists, all relevant to this area of medicine:

Stern (1943): magnetic moment of the proton.

Rabi (1944): nuclear magnetic resonance (NMR).

Bloch and Purcell (1952): development of NMR for liquids and solids.

Lauterbur and Mansfield (2003): magnetic resonance imaging.

3.2 Perturbing Brain Function

Rudolf N. Cardinal

When scientific studies are observational, based purely on measurement – however sophisticated – the possibility will remain that correlations between two things of interest do not reflect a direct causal connection. For example: suppose you find that a subject's self-report of auditory hallucinations is associated with increased BOLD signal in brain region X. This doesn't prove that there's an abnormality of X (the abnormality might be in region Y, which influences X) or even that activity in X reflects the hallucination itself (perhaps it relates to an emotional response to the hallucination, or to the motor activity required to report it). A true experiment involves manipulating one or more independent variables, with appropriate control conditions, and examining the effects.

In **lesion studies**, regions of the brain are destroyed. This might be through relatively crude neurosurgical techniques such as cutting or heating, which destroy both neuronal cell bodies (grey matter) and 'fibres of passage' (white matter: axons travelling through the region but connecting entirely different regions). Alternatively, excitotoxins might be injected to kill cell bodies selectively, sparing fibres of passage. Suitable control conditions are required, such as identical neurosurgery injecting the saline vehicle without the toxin. Brain regions can also be **inactivated** by infusing inhibitory drugs like GABA agonists locally, or **stimulated** electrically or pharmacologically. Electrical deep brain stimulation (DBS) is used for Parkinson's disease, where it has replaced irreversible lesion procedures, and may have use in other conditions including obsessive–compulsive disorder.

More precise control of neurons has been achieved via **optogenetics**. For example, breeding of experimental animals (to introduce genes into specific cell types) and/or virus injection (to introduce genetic material into specific locations in the brain) can deliver light-sensitive or light-emitting proteins into precise subsets of neurons. These proteins might 'report' neuronal activity optically, or allow neurons to be turned on and off very quickly through laser light shone in through optical fibres. In **chemogenetics**, an artificial 'switch' is localised genetically to specific neurons, then controlled by systemic administration of a drug. These techniques allow the causal role of small groups of neurons to be examined. For example, glutamatergic neurons of the paraventricular thalamus have been shown to control wakefulness: they are more active during wakefulness than sleep (measured via light-emitting calcium sensors), while activating them induces wakefulness (via light-controlled stimulation) and inhibiting them reduces wakefulness (via chemically controlled inhibitory receptors). These neurons are in turn controlled by orexin (hypocretin) neurons in the hypothalamus. Similarly, dopamine neurons have been controlled optogenetically to test theories of the role of dopamine in reward/reinforcement. As always, appropriate control conditions are required (e.g. for non-selective effects of light, or of the chemical that is supposedly inactive except in the presence of the target gene).

Relatively large-scale manipulation of human brain function can be achieved via electromagnetic stimulation. The use of electroconvulsive therapy (**ECT**) is the best known (see Section 9.19). Repetitive transcranial magnetic stimulation (**rTMS**) involves the delivery of brief magnetic pulses to the scalp and thus part of the brain. It has approval from the US Food and Drug Administration (FDA) for refractory depression and is generally supported by the UK National Institute for Health and Care Excellence. Transcranial direct current stimulation (**tDCS**) involves the application of weak direct current to the scalp; it is being investigated for depression. See Section 9.20 for more on brain stimulation. Other electrical interventions affect brain function less directly. These include vagus nerve stimulation, in which an implanted pacemaker-like device stimulates the vagus nerve, usually unilaterally. Vagus nerve stimulation is effective for refractory epilepsy and has been investigated for some time as a therapy for depression (with FDA approval but limited evidence).

Obviously, all **psychotropic drugs** affect brain function, as do **behavioural** and **cognitive** interventions!

 An ignoble Nobel Prize was awarded to Egas Moniz in 1949 for prefrontal leucotomy (lobotomy) for severe mental illness.

Rudolf N. Cardinal

3.3 Animal Models of Psychiatric Disease

Psychiatric diseases have been amongst the hardest to model well in animals. Nonetheless, important advances in human treatments have followed from animal models. Animal models are used to understand more about human disease where human testing would be impossible or unethical. The species used depends on the question. For example, *Drosophila* (fruit flies) have a very short generation time, so are suited to genetic studies involving very simple behaviour. *Xenopus* tadpoles have been widely used to study neurodevelopment. Zebrafish are vertebrates amenable to genetic investigation and have many similarities to mammals. Much psychology research has historically used rats and birds to study more complex behaviour – along with many other species, famously including Pavlov's dogs. Rats are used widely for neurosurgical measurement and manipulation, with mice often favoured for mammalian genetics. Non-human primates have a prefrontal cortex that is most similar to that of humans, so are used when other species cannot be – with all animal experimentation following the 'three Rs' of replacement, reduction and refinement to minimise their use.

Traditionally, an animal model is considered a good one if it is valid in several ways. A model has **face validity** if it 'looks like' what it's purporting to measure – if its signs or symptoms resemble those of the human. For example, in

rodents, the **elevated plus maze** task (see Table 3.3.1) is a model of anxiety. It involves a +-shaped platform, elevated above the floor. Two arms of the cross are enclosed at the sides, and two are open. Healthy animals prefer the closed arms and spend more time there (equivalently: they avoid the open arms). Anxiety-related behaviour (e.g. freezing, defaecation) is commoner in the open arms, and plasma corticosteroid levels are higher in rats confined to the open arms than to the closed arms. Anxiolytic drugs such as benzodiazepines shift behaviour towards the open arms, and anxiogenic drugs like caffeine shift behaviour towards the closed arms. In any experiment, there should be appropriate control conditions: for example, in a pharmacological experiment involving injection of a drug, where that drug is dissolved in a saline 'vehicle', the control condition might be an injection of saline. **Construct validity** means that the model measures what it claims to be measuring – for example, that it has similar underlying biology. This is rarer, but an example is the Huntington's disease transgenic mouse, which produces aberrant huntingtin protein and exhibits aspects of the Huntington's disease phenotype. **Predictive validity** means that the model predicts which treatments will work in humans. Many models have significant caveats.

Examples are shown in Table 3.3.1.

Table 3.3.1 A few examples of animal models of neuropsychiatric diseases

Disease	Specimen models	Description/comments
Depression	Forced swim test Chronic mild stress	In the forced swim test (FST), a rat is forced to swim for 15 minutes, and then tested the next day; the acute stress produces immobility and the rat just floats rather than trying to escape. Chronic stress produces long-lasting behavioural changes resembling depression in some ways (compare the concept of learned helplessness). These models predict the effects of several types of clinically effective drugs with antidepressant action – but have substantial limitations. For example, immobility in the FST is often anthropomorphised as 'despair' but may be no such thing (indeed, it may be adaptive), and acute tests such as this do not model depression itself.
Anxiety	Elevated plus maze Novelty-suppressed feeding	The elevated plus maze is described in the main text. Novelty-suppressed feeding measures a rodent's unwillingness to eat in an unfamiliar environment (via latency to eat). It detects the effect of benzodiazepines and a variety of drugs with antidepressant action.
Schizophrenia	Amphetamine-induced sensitisation Methylazoxymethanol acetate on rodent embryonic day 17 (MAM-E17)	Amphetamine is psychotogenic in humans, and humans with schizophrenia show altered dopamine release after amphetamine. Repeated amphetamine administration in rodents leads to sensitisation: an increase in stereotyped behaviours and impairment of prepulse inhibition (PPI). (PPI is where a weak stimulus, such as a quiet sound, inhibits the startle response to a subsequent strong stimulus, such as a loud sound. PPI may be related to the ability to filter out sensory stimuli and is also impaired in schizophrenia.) Amphetamine sensitisation may model some positive symptoms of schizophrenia, but does not capture the negative and cognitive symptoms well. The MAM-E17 model is a developmental model: a DNA-alkylating agent given during embryonic development causes schizophrenia-like changes manifesting in adolescence (e.g. social withdrawal, hypersensitivity to amphetamine and alterations in hippocampal glutamatergic neurotransmission).
Huntington's disease	R6/2 transgenic mouse	These mice express part of the human Huntington's disease gene with a high level of C–A–G (cytosine, adenine, guanine) triplet repeats. They develop progressive motor and cognitive impairments with neurodegeneration including neuronal atrophy.
Parkinson's disease	6-hydroxydopamine (6-OHDA) lesion	The toxin 6-OHDA kills dopaminergic neurons. When injected into the nigrostriatal dopamine pathway unilaterally, rodents develop 'hemiparkinsonian' motor deficits (with turning behaviour in response to dopaminergic drugs that can be quantified).

The Nobel Prize in Physiology or Medicine was awarded to Arvid Carlsson in 2000 for his work on dopamine as a neurotransmitter and its role in movement – with Greengard (postsynaptic response) and Kandel (synaptic mechanisms of memory). Carlsson also developed the first selective serotonin reuptake inhibitor.

3.4 Data Analysis and Computational Modelling

Rudolf N. Cardinal

All data analysis – all statistics – involves a mathematical 'model'. This **statistical modelling** can be very simple. If we hypothesise that male and female gerbils differ in weight, we might use a model like *weight_for_this_gerbil = mean_weight + sex_effect_for_this_gerbil + error_for_ this_gerbil*, or more generally (across all the gerbils we measure): *weight = mean_weight + sex_effect + error*. By 'error', or 'residual', we mean 'what's left after we're done explaining'. We could compare this to a simpler model, *weight = mean_weight + error*, in which sex plays no explanatory role. If our model is any good – if sexes differ in weight – then the model with *sex_effect* will predict better than the model without.

Many statistical tests are more complex, involving many predictors. They all involve describing the data with a mathematical model. In our gerbil example, we might add a predictor like *strain*, or *age*, and we might allow for the possibility that the two sexes gain weight at different rates by including an interaction term, *sex × age* ('the effect of age on weight depends on sex', or 'the effect of sex on weight depends on age'). Statistical modelling like this is usually an example of **generalised linear modelling**, which encompasses techniques like *t* tests, linear regression, analysis of variance (ANOVA) and covariance (ANCOVA), logistic regression and so forth.

In traditional 'frequentist' statistics, a **null hypothesis** is tested (giving a *p* value: 'How likely is this pattern of data, if only chance processes are operating?'). Models may also be built, used and compared in a **Bayesian** way (e.g. 'How likely is our hypothesis, given the data and our model, including estimates of our previous knowledge?').

Large data sets can bring statistical '**power**' (being less likely to 'miss' real changes, or lower '**type II error**') and the ability to detect smaller changes. However, large and complex data sets can also bring the temptation to ask more questions. For example, if one subdivides the brain into thousands of voxels in an fMRI experiment, it's simple to ask thousands of questions ('Does my task affect voxel 1? Voxel 2? Voxel 2,817?'). Asking lots of statistical questions increases the likelihood that at least one true null hypothesis is rejected (that is, being more likely to declare something significant spuriously, or higher '**type I error**'). One must correct for **multiple comparisons** in such situations (adjusting the *p* value or the threshold at which it is considered 'significant', *a*). Alternatively, Bayesian statistical approaches do not suffer from this problem in the same way.

Correlation does not imply **causation**: showing that *X* predicts *Y* doesn't tell you that changes in *X* caused the changes in *Y*. Knowledge about causation must come from the real world that your model represents. For example, if you had randomised subjects to different values of *X* and measured *Y* in a true experiment, you could be much more confident of causation.

Statistical models can explicitly include the researcher's hypotheses about causal relationships, as in **structural equation modelling** (**SEM**), in which proposed causal links between several variables are built, and the strengths of these links estimated from the data. While this allows competing models to be compared and tested (some models may fit better than others), and may strengthen the evidence for causal relationships, no analytical technique can magically prove causation and SEM is no exception.

Sometimes, special clues can be used to test for causation without a direct experiment. One is **Mendelian randomisation**, which is conceptually complex but sometimes powerful. Suppose you wish to test whether smoking (the **exposure** of interest) causes heart disease (the **outcome**). Perhaps, however, smokers also show other unhealthy behaviours that might affect heart disease (potential **confounding factors**). Since environmental factors can't affect your genetic sequence, we may be able to make use of genetic variation as a natural 'experiment'. The concept is to 'vary' genotype as if in an experiment, thus affecting exposure, and see if the outcome is altered. This requires three assumptions. (1) You need a genetic polymorphism that is associated with the exposure (e.g. if gene *M* makes you smoke more than gene *L*). This association might be sought through genome-wide association studies. (2) The genotype must not be associated with the confounding factors (e.g. the gene does not affect how likely you are to drink more alcohol or to be sedentary or have high cholesterol, and the confounding factors do not affect the gene across generations via choice of mate). (3) The gene must have no effect on the outcome except via the exposure. (Sometimes this is testable: e.g. among non-smokers, the gene should not be associated with heart disease.) If all three assumptions are met, and you find that gene *M* is associated with higher rates of heart disease than gene *L*, it is likely that it is the smoking that causes the difference. This technique has been used in psychiatry, for example to examine the effects of sleep pattern (exposure) on psychiatric disorders (outcomes), of smoking on the risk of bipolar disorder, of cannabis use on schizophrenia, and so on. However, sometimes the underlying assumptions are hard to test.

Predictive models may also be trained by *machine learning (ML)*, in which a computer algorithm is used to build the model. The algorithm attempts to find good predictors or combinations of predictors. There are many ML methods and this area is growing in popularity, but ML is not infallible. As well as difficulties with learning and performance, including the problem of knowing which algorithm to pick, ML-trained models can be hard to interpret and may generalise poorly to new data.

Computational modelling of behaviour is a slightly different kind of modelling. Here, we tell a computer program how we think the brain is operating: the computer simulates brain function in a very simplified way. We might tell the model: 'When you receive reward, strengthen the tendency to repeat your last behaviour' (habit learning). We might allow the model a **parameter** that controls how much it should strengthen that habit. Our model might also involve more complex phenomena, like a calculation of the expected consequences of potential actions. Once we've described the model, we fit it to real-life behaviour by allowing the computer to 'tune' its parameters to get the best fit to the choices made by a real subject. We might also compare several models to see which is best (remembering that adding more flexibility will generally improve the fit, so we should include a penalty for being too complex – Occam's razor). Why is this technique useful? It can improve our explanations, allowing descriptions of behaviour to be compared directly, and interpreting (for example) drug effects in terms of parameters of the model. It can also give us the values of hidden quantities 'inside' the model, which we can then relate to neuroimaging. For example, if reward prediction error (RPE) is hypothesised to be aberrant in psychosis, we can predict moment-by-moment RPE using a computational model, then take those RPE values and relate them to fMRI BOLD signals from specific brain regions. See Section 5.7 on how computational models of learning have been used to understand psychiatric disorders.

3.5 Functional Neuroimaging and Connectivity

Rudolf N. Cardinal

In correlative neuroimaging research, traditional designs relate brain activity (measured, for example, with EEG, MEG, PET or BOLD fMRI) to performance of some behavioural or cognitive task, suitably adapted for the physical requirements of the scanning process. In **block designs**, periods of time when a subject is performing some task are compared with periods during which they're not (an important question being: 'What are they doing instead?'). For example, one would expect that 'time spent watching a chequerboard pattern' would involve more activation of visual cortex than 'time spent watching a grey screen', and indeed it does; one can map visual cortex in this way. In **event-related designs**, a stimulus is presented (e.g. 'You won £5!') many times; the brain signal is measured before, during and after the event; and these signals are averaged over trials to detect the response evoked by the stimulus. With **computational models of behaviour**, as above, we might relate brain activity to continuously changing variables in the model.

All whole-brain neuroimaging techniques generate vast quantities of data, and care must be taken to balance type I statistical errors (false 'discoveries' simply as a consequence of many comparisons) against type II errors (missing genuine effects) – see Section 3.4 above.

In **resting state fMRI**, the subject is scanned while doing 'nothing', usually with the aim of measuring interrelationships between activity in different brain areas. The BOLD signal varies over time throughout the brain. The correlation between the time-varying BOLD signals from area X and from area Y can be taken as a measure of **functional connectivity** between those two regions – on the basis that if they talk to each other their activity will be (positively or negatively) correlated. In this way, a functional connectivity network map of the brain can be derived, and compared between health and disease. Those brain regions which are most active when subjects are awake, but not performing an explicit task, are called the **default-mode network**; its interpretation is debated. Functional connectivity can also be assessed during performance of specific tasks (see Section 5.18).

FURTHER READING

Single-Cell Recording and Much More

Kandel ER (ed.) (2013). *Principles of Neural Science*, 5th ed. McGraw-Hill.

EEG and MEG

Goetz CG (ed.) (2007). *Textbook of Clinical Neurology*, 3rd ed. Saunders Elsevier.

Pizzella V et al. (2014). Magnetoencephalography in the study of brain dynamics. *Funct Neurol* **29**: 241–253.

Three-Dimensional Neuroimaging with a Clinical Emphasis

Yousem DM, Grossman RI (2010). *Neuroradiology: The Requisites*, 3rd ed. Mosby/Elsevier.

Perturbing Brain Function

Cusin C, Dougherty DD. (2012). Somatic therapies for treatment-resistant depression: ECT, TMS, VNS, DBS. *Biol Mood Anxiety Disord* **2**: 14.

Feldman RS et al. (1997). *Principles of Neuropsychopharmacology*. Sinauer Associates.

Harrington M. (2011). *The Design of Experiments in Neuroscience*, 2nd ed. SAGE.

Park HG, Carmel JB. (2016). Selective manipulation of neural circuits. *Neurotherapeutics* **13**: 311–324.

Animal Models of Psychiatric Disorders

Feldman RS et al. (1997). *Principles of Neuropsychopharmacology*. Sinauer Associates.

McGonigle P. (2014). Animal models of CNS disorders. *Biochem Pharmacol* **87**: 140–149.

Data Analysis and Statistics

Harrington M. (2011). *The Design of Experiments in Neuroscience*, 2nd ed. SAGE.

Howell DC. (2010). *Statistical Methods for Psychology*, 7th ed. Thomson Wadsworth.

Computational Modelling of Mental Illness

Adams RA et al. (2016). Computational psychiatry: towards a mathematically informed understanding of mental illness. *J Neurol Neurosurg Psychiatry* **87**: 53–63.

Functional Connectivity

Fornito A et al. (2016). *Fundamentals of Brain Network Analysis*. Elsevier/Academic Press.

Mendelian Randomisation

Davies NM et al. (2018). Reading Mendelian randomisation studies: a guide, glossary, and checklist for clinicians. *BMJ* 362: k601.

Credits and Licensing

National Neuroscience Curriculum Initiative online resources

"Not Dead Yet!" – Confronting the Legacy of Dualism in Modern Psychiatry

Christopher W. T. Miller, David A. Ross and Andrew M. Novick

Scanning for Justice With Functional Magnetic Resonance Imaging

Stephanie Yarnell, Alexander Westphal and David A. Ross

Computational Psychiatry: Embracing Uncertainty and Focusing on Individuals, Not Averages

Adam M. Chekroud, Chadrick E. Lane and David A. Ross

Out of the Cave, Into the Light? Modeling Mental Illness With Organoids

Erik A. Levinsohn and David A. Ross

Nanovesicles: A Novel Window Into Neuronal Functioning

Tara M. Thompson-Felix and David A. Ross

This "stuff" is really cool: Brandon Kitay, *"Dude, There's A Fly In My Beer!"* on animal models in psychiatry

This "stuff" is really cool: Brandon Kitay, *"The Connectome"* on brain wiring and courtship behaviour in flies

This "stuff" is really cool: Alfred Kaye, *"Neural Surveillance"* on calcium channel imaging

4

Neuroanatomy

4.1 Fundamentals

Laith Alexander

OVERVIEW

Neuroanatomy is the study of the structure of the nervous system. Starting with an overview of important terminology and the embryological origins of the nervous system, this section describes its basic anatomy at different levels of organisation: macroscopic, microscopic and circuit-level. The fluid compartments within the nervous system are also reviewed.

4.1.1 Terminology and Organisation of the Nervous System

At the macroscopic level, the nervous system can be divided into the **central nervous system** (**CNS**), consisting of the brain and spinal cord, and **peripheral nervous system** (**PNS**), consisting of spinal nerves and cranial nerves (with their branches).

At the histological level, **grey matter** contains primarily cell bodies, and **white matter** contains primarily myelinated nerve fibres, whose fatty sheaths ensure the integrity and speed of action potential conduction.

At the circuit level, small-scale **local circuits** and large-scale inter-regional **networks** exist. Networks can be defined structurally using tract tracing and structural imaging techniques, or functionally with electrophysiological and functional imaging techniques.

Structures in the brain are defined in three planes relative to the long axis of the **body** (a straight line from head to toe) corresponding to *x*, *y* and *z* directions (Figure 4.1.1A).

- The **sagittal** (*x*) plane moves from left to right. Structures towards the midline are **medial** and structures away from the midline are **lateral**.
- The **coronal** (*y*) plane moves from front to back, or **anterior** to **posterior**.
- Finally, the **axial** or **transverse** (*z*) plane is horizontal. Structures towards the top are **superior** and structures towards the bottom are **inferior**.

The terminology can become confusing because some anatomical terms – **ventral**, **dorsal**, **rostral** (also termed **cranial**) and **caudal** – are defined relative to the long axis of the **CNS** rather than the body. The CNS long axis is not a straight line: it has a bend in it at the junction between the brain and the brainstem, called the **cephalic flexure** (Figure 4.1.1B). Owing to the bend, ventral is towards the floor in the brain but towards the front of the body in the brainstem and spinal cord, and dorsal is towards the roof in the brain but towards the back of the body in the brainstem and spinal cord. Rostral is towards the nose in the brain but towards the head in the brainstem and spinal cord, and caudal is towards the occiput in the brain but towards the coccyx in the brainstem and spinal cord.

Other important terminology includes:

- **afferent** projections (axonal connections from one area to another), which travel towards a region of interest
- **efferent** projections, which travel away from a region of interest
- **ipsilateral**, which refers to the same side as a region of interest
- **contralateral**, which refers to the opposite side to a region of interest.

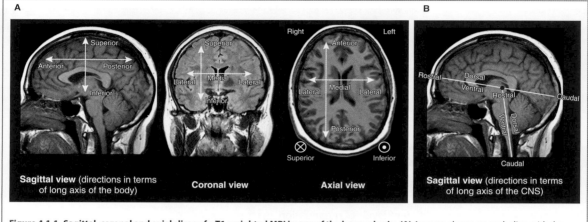

Figure 4.1.1 Sagittal, coronal and axial slices of a T1-weighted MRI image of the human brain. (A) Axes are shown on each slice, with the directions labelled relative to the long axis of the body. The axial section is viewed from the feet, looking superiorly. **(B)** Here, directions are labelled relative to the long axis of the CNS, which bends at the cephalic flexure (red dot). The rostral direction is sometimes referred to as 'cranial'.

4.1.2 Embryology of the Nervous System

The best way to understand the anatomy of the nervous system is to understand the basics of its embryological development (see also Section 8.1). **Neurulation** is the initial stage in this process and occurs between days 21 and 28 of development. During neurulation, part of the **ectoderm** – the outermost layer of cells in the embryo – folds into a hollow **neural tube**, which will form the brain and spinal cord (Figure 4.1.2A).

The folding during neurulation is initiated and maintained by signalling from the mesodermal **notochord** (despite its importance in development, the notochord forms only the nucleus pulposus of the intervertebral discs in adult life). As folding progresses, the neural tube closes off and separates from the overlying ectoderm with some cells being 'pinched off' in the process, termed **neural crest cells**. These ectodermal cells migrate and form the **peripheral nervous system**, in addition to other structures.

After neurulation, the neural tube then undergoes extensive **patterning** along all three axes, ultimately resulting in a fully developed CNS. Patterning refers to the process by which initially equivalent cells in an embryonic tissue develop complex and heterogeneous forms and functions, through genetic programs, gradients of signalling molecules and local cell–cell signalling.

Patterning in the rostral–caudal direction involves rostral parts of the tube swelling and folding to form the **brain**, consisting of three vesicles (Figure 4.1.2B): the **forebrain** (prosencephalon); the **midbrain** (mesencephalon); and the **hindbrain** (rhombencephalon). Eventually, the three vesicles become five: the forebrain forms two separate swellings, called the telencephalon (cortex and basal ganglia) and the diencephalon (thalamus and hypothalamus); the rhombencephalon forms the metencephalon (pons and cerebellum) and myelencephalon (medulla). The hollow portion of the tube becomes the ventricles – the lateral ventricles are associated with the telencephalon; the third ventricle is associated with the diencephalon; the cerebral aqueduct with the mesencephalon; and the fourth ventricle is associated with the rhombencephalon. The caudal neural tube forms the **spinal cord**, and the hollow portion here shrinks to become the **spinal canal**.

Patterning in the dorsal–ventral direction is poorly understood in the brain. In the spinal cord there is differentiation of grey matter into the **dorsal horn** and **ventral horn**, mediated by complex signalling from the base of the neural tube called the floorplate.

In the medial–lateral direction (also known as 'radial'), neurons begin their development in the **ventricular zone** (next to the hollow portion of the neural tube) where **neural stem cells** are found. As the neurons develop, they migrate outwards through subventricular and intermediate zones (populated by glial cells), to the

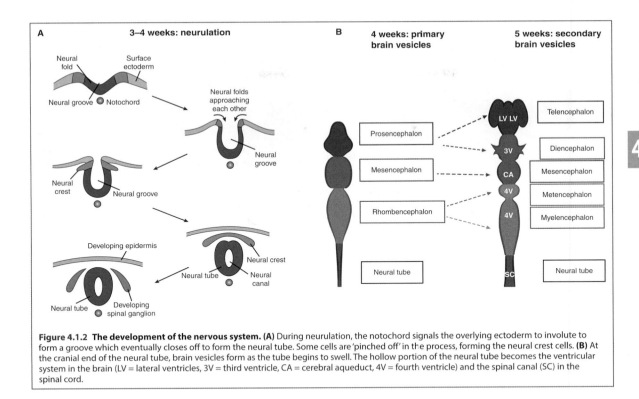

Figure 4.1.2 The development of the nervous system. (A) During neurulation, the notochord signals the overlying ectoderm to involute to form a groove which eventually closes off to form the neural tube. Some cells are 'pinched off' in the process, forming the neural crest cells. **(B)** At the cranial end of the neural tube, brain vesicles form as the tube begins to swell. The hollow portion of the neural tube becomes the ventricular system in the brain (LV = lateral ventricles, 3V = third ventricle, CA = cerebral aqueduct, 4V = fourth ventricle) and the spinal canal (SC) in the spinal cord.

cortical plate. Radial glial cells, with cell bodies next to the ventricles and very long fibres, act as scaffolds upon which developing neurons migrate.

4.1.3 The Macroscopic Organisation of the Nervous System

Macroscopically, the nervous system is divided into central and peripheral nervous systems. The **CNS** consists of the brain and spinal cord. The **PNS** consists of the voluntary nervous system (with sensory and motor functions) and the involuntary or autonomic nervous system (with visceral sensory and visceral motor functions, incorporating the **parasympathetic** and **sympathetic** nervous system).

4.1.3.1 The Central Nervous System

THE BRAIN

The brain is divided into the **forebrain**, the **midbrain** and the **hindbrain**. The 'brainstem' refers to the midbrain and hindbrain, excluding the cerebellum.

THE FOREBRAIN

The forebrain consists of the telencephalon and the diencephalon. The **telencephalon** (cerebrum) consists of the **cerebral cortex**, underlying white matter and **subcortical structures** such as the basal ganglia (see Section 4.2). The **diencephalon** includes the **thalamus** and **hypothalamus**.

The **cerebral cortex** consists of two **hemispheres**, left and right, separated by the longitudinal fissure. The **dominant hemisphere** controls language comprehension and production, typically being the left hemisphere in both right- and left-handed people (although there is a greater frequency of right-hemisphere dominance in left-handed people) [1]. Each hemisphere contains four **lobes: frontal**, **parietal**, **occipital** and **temporal** (Figures 4.1.3A and 4.1.3B). All human cortex is folded into sulci (grooves) and gyri (ridges).

Cerebral cortex can be divided functionally into the **primary sensory cortices** (vision, hearing, smell, touch, taste), **primary motor cortex** and **association cortex**.

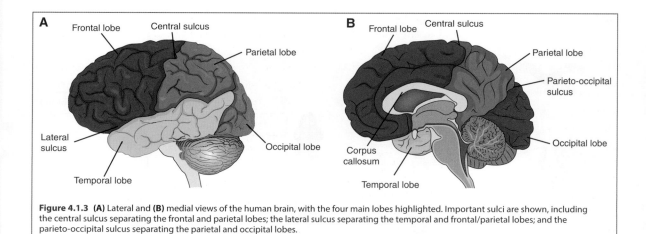

Figure 4.1.3 (A) Lateral and **(B)** medial views of the human brain, with the four main lobes highlighted. Important sulci are shown, including the central sulcus separating the frontal and parietal lobes; the lateral sulcus separating the temporal and frontal/parietal lobes; and the parieto-occipital sulcus separating the parietal and occipital lobes.

The primary sensory cortices deal with one sensory modality and the primary motor cortex with motor information. The association cortex, the most common type, deals with multimodal sensory integration and sensorimotor integration. Areas of cortex involved in the comprehension and production of **language** are typically highlighted separately owing to their unique function (see Section 5.17). The functions of cortex within each lobe are shown in Table 4.1.

The **thalamus** is a diencephalic structure and comprises symmetrical cores of grey matter sitting either side of the midline, deep in each hemisphere. It has bidirectional connections to the cerebral cortex and brainstem, with roles in sensorimotor and limbic processing together with arousal. The **hypothalamus** sits inferior to the thalamus, with several nuclei. Its four functions are fighting, fleeing, feeding and fornicating (four Fs). Additionally, one of its nuclei – the suprachiasmatic nucleus – is important in

Table 4.1.1 The functions of the cerebral cortex in the four lobes of the human brain

Lobe	Type of cortex	Specific examples	Function
Frontal	Primary motor Primary sensory Association Language	Primary motor cortex (precentral gyrus) Gustatory cortex Lateral and medial prefrontal cortex Premotor and supplementary motor areas Frontal eye fields Anterior cingulate cortex Broca's area (inferior frontal gyrus of dominant hemisphere)	Motor output Taste Executive function Motor planning Saccadic eye movements Emotion, decision making, autonomic regulation Language production
Temporal	Primary sensory Association Language	Primary auditory cortex (superior temporal gyrus) Olfactory cortex (piriform cortex) Auditory association cortex Inferotemporal cortex and fusiform gyrus Temporal pole Perirhinal, entorhinal and parahippocampal cortices Insula (border with frontal lobe) Wernicke's area (superior temporal gyrus of dominant hemisphere)	Hearing Smell Memory, sound processing Object recognition and face recognition Semantic memory Object recognition and spatial memory Interoception Language comprehension
Parietal	Primary sensory Association	Primary somatosensory cortex (postcentral gyrus) Somatosensory association cortex Lateral and anterior intraparietal areas, parietal reach region	Somatosensation Integration of somatosensory information Motor planning, eye movements
Occipital	Primary sensory Association	Visual cortex, V1 Visual association areas V2–V4	Processing of static and moving objects Further processing of visual form (ventral) and integrating vision with motor and sensory information (dorsal)

circadian rhythms (see Section 5.2.2). The hypothalamus is connected to the pituitary gland via the infundibular stalk, conducting the body's 'hormonal orchestra' (see Section 6.1 for more on hypothalamic and pituitary anatomy and function).

THE MIDBRAIN

The midbrain forms the most rostral part of the brainstem. Rostrally, it is continuous with the thalamus and hypothalamus. Caudally, it is continuous with the pons. The **tegmentum** refers to the part of the midbrain ventral to the **cerebral aqueduct**. The **tectum** is dorsal to the cerebral aqueduct, containing the **superior** and **inferior colliculi** involved in eye movements and auditory processing, respectively. The nuclei of the oculomotor (III) and trochlear (IV) cranial nerves are found in the midbrain, together with **dopaminergic neurons** of the **substantia nigra** and the **ventral tegmental area**.

The midbrain is effectively part of the brain that connects the forebrain with the rest of the brainstem. You will hear the term **cerebral peduncles** used to refer to the 'stalks' connecting the forebrain and brainstem and, generally speaking, the cerebral peduncles refer to all of the midbrain except for the colliculi.

THE HINDBRAIN

The hindbrain includes the pons superiorly and medulla inferiorly, together with the cerebellum posteriorly. The pons and medulla contain several important cranial nerve nuclei, as well as bundles of ascending and descending fibres. Extending throughout the pons, medulla and midbrain is a 'core' of streaked grey matter referred to as the **reticular formation**, responsible for arousal, containing monoaminergic, cholinergic and histaminergic nuclei (Section 4.6).

THE SPINAL CORD

The spinal cord (Figure 4.1.4A) is enclosed within the bony **spinal column**, which is divided into **cervical** (C1–C7), **thoracic** (T1–T12), **lumbar** (L1–L5), **sacral** (S1–S5) and **coccygeal** (Co1–Co4) vertebrae. Paired **spinal nerves** emerge at each level and exit the spinal column through **intervertebral foramina**. Nerves C1 to C7 exit *above* the corresponding vertebrae, spinal nerve C8 exits below vertebra C7, and all other nerves (T1–S5) exit *below* the corresponding vertebrae. The spinal cord ends at the level of L1/L2 of the spinal column in a tapering called

the **conus medullaris**, with the remaining nerves forming the **cauda equina** and exiting out of their respective foramina.

The grey matter of the spinal cord (Figure 4.1.4B) is divided into the **dorsal horn** where afferent sensory information arrives, and the **ventral horn** where efferent motor information leaves. In the thoracic spinal cord, there is a **lateral horn**, which contains sympathetic cell bodies.

The white matter is arranged into ascending and descending tracts (Figure 4.1.4B). Ascending information includes **pain, temperature** and **crude touch** information via the **anterolateral spinothalamic** tract, and **vibration, proprioception** and **fine touch** information via the **dorsal column–medial lemniscal** tract. See Section 5.5 for more on pain perception.

Descending tracts are grouped into **pyramidal tracts** (which originate in the cortex) and **extrapyramidal tracts** (which originate in the brainstem; note the confusing similar terminology that 'extrapyramidal symptoms' relate to dysfunction in the basal ganglia).

The **corticospinal tract** is the main pyramidal tract. The cell bodies are located in the primary motor cortex, called **upper motor neurons**. The axons descend and, in the medulla, form the **medullary pyramids**. Most of the fibres (85–90%) then cross over the midline at the **motor decussation** in the inferior part of the medulla and descend in the contralateral spinal cord; the remainder remain uncrossed until the spinal level of their termination where they cross.

Extrapyramidal tracts include the **vestibulospinal, reticulospinal, rubrospinal** and **tectospinal** tracts. These pathways are important in postural control and controlling proximal muscles, originating from different nuclei within the brainstem. The vestibulospinal and reticulospinal tracts mostly travel ipsilaterally, whereas the rubrospinal tract crosses the midline and travels contralaterally. The tectospinal tract controls contralateral movements of the head in relation to visual stimuli.

4.1.3.2 The Peripheral Nervous System

The peripheral nervous system is grouped into the **voluntary nervous system** and the **autonomic** (or involuntary) **nervous system**. Processing in the former enters conscious awareness, whereas processing in the latter is largely unconscious although it has a profound effect on behaviour.

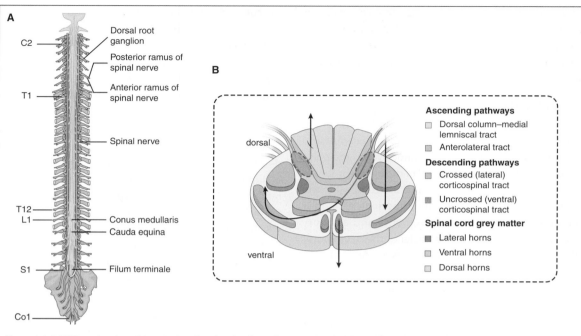

A

C2
Dorsal root ganglion
Posterior ramus of spinal nerve
Anterior ramus of spinal nerve

T1

Spinal nerve

T12
L1
Conus medullaris
Cauda equina

S1
Filum terminale

Co1

B

dorsal

ventral

Ascending pathways
☐ Dorsal column–medial lemniscal tract
☐ Anterolateral tract

Descending pathways
☐ Crossed (lateral) corticospinal tract
☐ Uncrossed (ventral) corticospinal tract

Spinal cord grey matter
☐ Lateral horns
☐ Ventral horns
☐ Dorsal horns

Figure 4.1.4 (A) Posterior view of the spinal cord enclosed within its bony canal, with the meningeal layers peeled away. The conus medullaris is the inferior tapering of the spinal cord where it ends at L1, with the cauda equina consisting of the remaining spinal nerves that have not yet left the bony spinal canal. The filum terminale is an extension of the dura mater, connecting the meningeal sac to the coccyx. **(B)** A cross-section of the spinal cord is shown, taken at the mid-thoracic level. The grey matter is divided into dorsal, lateral and ventral horns. The major ascending (sensory) and descending (motor) pathways are indicated.

Peripheral nerves often contain fibres from both branches. Thirty-one pairs of **spinal nerves** arise from the spinal cord, and 12 pairs of **cranial nerves** arise from the midbrain, pons and medulla. Spinal and cranial nerves form many individual branches, and some spinal nerves intermingle in complex structures called **nerve plexuses**.

SPINAL NERVES

Spinal nerves form from the union of the **dorsal** (sensory) and **ventral** (motor) **roots** of the spinal cord, and divide into **dorsal** (mixed) and **ventral** (mixed) **rami**, which contain several types of nerve fibres. **Somatic sensory and somatic motor** fibres are part of the voluntary nervous system, whereas **visceral sensory and visceral motor** fibres are part of the autonomic nervous system.

Somatic sensory fibres carry pain, temperature, proprioception, touch and vibration information to the spinal cord. Their cell bodies reside in the **dorsal root ganglia** of the spinal cord.

Somatic motor fibres carry information to **skeletal** (voluntary) **muscles** of the body. Their cell bodies reside in the ventral horn of the spinal cord, and their axons

terminate at the **neuromuscular junction** where they synapse with skeletal muscle fibres.

The visceral motor neurons of the autonomic nervous system can be divided into **parasympathetic** ('rest and digest') and **sympathetic** ('fight-or-flight') components. Their cell bodies reside in the brain and spinal cord. Parasympathetic outputs originate from **cranio-sacral** regions of the CNS ('cranio' referring to the cranial nerves, see below), whereas sympathetic outputs are **thoraco-lumbar**, forming the **sympathetic chains** either side of the spinal column.

The visceral sensory nervous system senses stimuli from the internal organs, such as stretch, pain and chemical irritation of the viscera. Their cell bodies reside in the dorsal root ganglia. They are responsible for sensations such as hunger and nausea.

CRANIAL NERVES

Cranial nerves also contain multiple fibre types, similar to peripheral nerves. Additional distinctions are made between (1) 'general' somatic sensory fibres versus 'special' sensory fibres of vision, hearing and smell; and

(2) motor fibres innervating structures derived from embryological somites (somatic motor) versus those derived from the branchial, or facial, arches (branchial motor). Visceral motor fibres carried by cranial nerves are parasympathetic (carried in cranial nerves III, VII, IX and X); any sympathetic innervation of the head ascends from the sympathetic chain. Table 4.1.2 outlines the functions of cranial nerves by fibre type.

The vagus nerve (X) has received particular interest in psychiatry, as a bidirectional neural 'highway' between the brain and body. By this means, activity within the heart and gut can impact upon the brain, and vice versa. The vagus nerve is the principal means by which the CNS and the **enteric nervous system** communicate, forming the neural component of the gut–brain axis. The importance of the gut–brain axis is beginning to be understood, and may even underlie some of the antidepressant effects of selective serotonin reuptake inhibitors [2]. In **vagal nerve stimulation therapy**, a subcutaneous pulse generator is used to stimulate the vagus nerve in the neck, as a 'bottom-up' approach to try and modulate the brain's neural circuitry.

Table 4.1.2 The cranial nerves and their functions

Cranial nerve	Major nuclei	Type of fibre	Specific function	Clinical relevance
I – Olfactory	Olfactory bulb	Special sensory	Smell	Anosmia is a non-motor symptom of Parkinson's disease
II – Optic	Lateral geniculate nucleus (thalamus)	Special sensory	Vision	Visual field defects
III – Oculomotor	Oculomotor nucleus (midbrain)	Somatic motor	Eye movements – all muscles except superior oblique and lateral rectus Eyelid elevation – levator palpebrae superioris	Damage results in 'down and out' appearance of the eye
	Edinger–Westphal nucleus (midbrain)	Visceral motor (parasympathetic)	Pupillary constriction via ciliary ganglion	Pupillary dilation if damaged
IV – Trochlear	Trochlear nucleus (midbrain)	Somatic motor	Eye movements – superior oblique muscle	Damage results in vertical and torsional diplopia (e.g. going down stairs, tilting head)
V – Trigeminal *Ophthalmic division (V1)* *Maxillary division (V2)* *Mandibular division (V3)*	Motor trigeminal nucleus (pons)	Branchial motor	Muscles of mastication	Trigeminal neuralgia
	Spinal trigeminal nucleus (spans brainstem)	General somatic sensory	Touch, pain, temperature sensation of the face, tongue, cornea	
VI – Abducens	Abducens nucleus (pons)	Somatic motor	Eye movements – lateral rectus muscle	Damage results in horizontal diplopia
VII – Facial	Facial nucleus (pons)	Branchial motor	Muscles of facial expression, platysma, stapedius	Facial nerve palsy
	Salivatory nucleus (pons/medulla)	Visceral motor	Submandibular, sublingual and lacrimal glands	
	Nucleus of the solitary tract (medulla)	Visceral sensory (chorda tympani)	Taste to anterior 2/3 of the tongue	
	Spinal trigeminal nucleus	General somatic sensory	A small area of the external ear around the external auditory meatus	
VIII – Vestibulocochlear	Cochlear nuclei and vestibular nuclei (pons/medulla)	Special sensory	Hearing and balance	Conductive and sensorineural hearing loss, vertigo
IX – Glossopharyngeal	Ambiguus nucleus (medulla)	Branchial motor	Stylopharyngeus	
	Salivatory nucleus (pons/medulla)	Visceral motor	Parotid gland	
	Nucleus of the solitary tract (medulla)	Visceral sensory	Taste and sensation from posterior 1/3 of the tongue; carotid bodies and carotid sinus	

Table 4.1.2 (cont.)

Cranial nerve	Major nuclei	Type of fibre	Specific function	Clinical relevance
X – Vagus	Ambiguus nucleus (medulla)	Branchial motor	Soft palate, pharynx	Mediates the 'mind–body' connection, including heart–brain and gut–brain interactions
	Dorsal motor nucleus (medulla)	Visceral motor	Control of thoracic and abdominal viscera	
		General somatic sensory	External auditory meatus	Vagal nerve stimulation therapy for depression
	Nucleus of the solitary tract (medulla)	Visceral sensory	Sensation of thoracic and abdominal viscera	
XI – Accessory	Ventral horns of C2–C5	Branchial motor	Sternocleidomastoid and trapezius	Torticollis and dystonia
XII – Hypoglossal	Hypoglossal nucleus	Somatic motor	Muscles of the tongue	

4.1.3.3 The Meningeal Layers Covering the Central Nervous System

Within the CNS, neural tissue is covered by three membranes called the meninges; from outermost to innermost, these are the **dura mater**, **arachnoid mater** and **pia mater** (in the brain, the dura mater forms two layers: the 'periosteal' and 'meningeal' layers). The meninges contain immune cells and are one route by which the immune system and nervous system can communicate to influence behaviour or immune responses (see Section 6.4).

The meningeal layers are continuous with the coverings of peripheral nerves, as spinal/cranial nerves carry coverings with them as they leave the CNS. In the spinal cord, the meningeal sac ends at S1, with an extension of dura mater called the **filum terminale** (seen in Figure 4.1.4A) connecting the meninges to the coccyx.

Spaces between meningeal layers are either **actual** spaces or **potential** spaces (i.e. where the layers are normally pressed together but can be pushed apart by pathological events such as a bleed). The **subarachnoid space** is an important actual space where cerebrospinal fluid circulates.

4.1.4 The Microscopic Organisation of the Central Nervous System

As mentioned, the CNS is arranged into grey and white matter. Grey matter contains neurons, glial cells and dendrites/synapses. White matter contains neuronal axons and glial cells. Understanding the microscopic architecture of the nervous system has been particularly important when trying to parcellate (i.e. separate into distinct areas) the grey matter of the human cerebral cortex.

4.1.4.1 Cytoarchitectonics Parcellates the Grey Matter of the Brain

Cytoarchitectonics is a term used to describe the **cellular** architecture of the nervous system, particularly when studying the grey matter of the brain. It focuses on differences in the **layered appearance** of the grey matter in the cerebral cortex.

There are three **phylogenetic types** of cortex based on the appearance of the layers:

- **Allocortex** is evolutionarily ancient, containing three to five layers.
- **Mesocortex** is a 'transitional cortex' between allocortex and neocortex, containing three to six layers.
- **Neocortex** is the most prevalent and evolutionarily recent cortex, generally containing six layers. Layers I–IV receive afferent inputs and layers V and VI are efferent. Layer IV contains **granule cells**. So-called **granular cortex** has a well-developed layer IV; other areas have a thinner layer IV and are termed **agranular** (minimal to no layer IV) or **dysgranular** (thin layer IV).

A more detailed cytoarchitectonic appraisal of the brain's microscopic appearance is Korbinian Brodmann's classification of the cerebral cortex into 52 numbered **Brodmann areas** [3] (Figure 4.1.5). Similarities and differences in microscopic appearance of the cortex are presumed to have functional relevance. This is crucial when translating experimental results across species (such as rodents, non-human primates and humans), where similarities in the cytoarchitectonic appearance of brain regions are often presumed to reflect analogous function. Additionally, the highly regularised cytoarchitectural appearance of some brain regions such as the cerebellum – which resemble repeated electronic circuits on a chip – has inspired the development of **computational models** of their function [4].

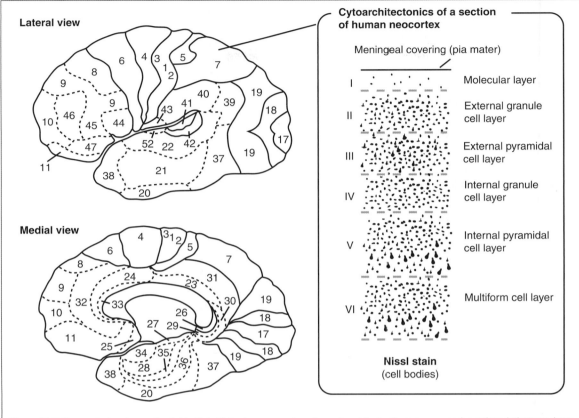

Figure 4.1.5 The cerebral cortex can be divided into 52 Brodmann areas based on cytoarchitectural appearance, each numbered. The inset shows an example of Nissl (cell body) staining of human neocortex, showing its six-layered appearance.

4.1.4.2 Myeloarchitectonics Parcellates Grey Matter by Studying Fibre Arrangements

Myeloarchitectonics is a complementary approach to cytoarchitectonics, and delineates cortical regions based on the organisation of the **myelinated fibre bundles** (looking at the 'white matter' within the grey matter). It was pioneered by Oskar Vogt and Cecile Vogt-Mugnier in the early twentieth century [5], working in the same laboratory as Brodmann. They noted that the myelinated fibres were arranged in two principal directions – radial and tangential – and classified over 180 myeloarchitectonic subdivisions of the human cerebral cortex based on the relative proportions and organisation of the fibres.

4.1.5 Circuit-Level Organisation within the Nervous System

A neural circuit is a group of neurons which communicate using synapses and neurotransmitters to subserve a specific function. Neural circuits are often studied at the **local level** but can be studied at the whole-brain, or **network/connectomic** level.

Local neural circuits are often studied in the context of **information processing models**, which try to explain how neurons process incoming information. Local neural circuits mediate functions such as **feedforward/feedback** control, **lateral inhibition**, **pattern completion** and **associative learning**.

Over larger scales, we can explore both structural and functional connections across different regions within the brain, forming **neural networks** or **neural systems**, and ultimately a '**connectome**', detailing all the brain's intimate connections. Structural approaches include **tractography**, using **structural neuroimaging** techniques to identify major white matter tracts in the brain (Section 4.5). Functional approaches assess **functional connectivity**, utilising **functional neuroimaging** to identify brain regions with correlated or anti-correlated activity.

An example of a neural system particularly relevant to psychiatry is the **limbic system**. This is a network of medial structures sitting close to the midline ('limbus' meaning border in Latin), thought to mediate emotion and memory. The concept of the limbic system was articulated in 1949 by Paul MacLean [6], expanding on **Papez's loop** [7] (Figure 4.1.6). Papez's loop is a circuit between the cingulate cortex, the parahippocampal cortex, the hippocampus, the mamillary bodies and the thalamus that was thought to be responsible for emotion and memory. MacLean expanded this circuitry to emphasise the distributed nature of emotional processing by including the **amygdala**, **ventral striatum** and **prefrontal cortex**.

Later in this book, you will come across several other neural circuits – defined both structurally and functionally – which are thought to perform specific functions (Chapter 5).

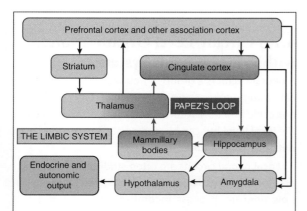

Figure 4.1.6 An example of a neural circuit – the limbic system. Papez's loop (shown in blue) was the initial instantiation of a neural circuit proposed to mediate emotion and memory. In 1949, Paul MacLean expanded this circuit to form a distributed system called the limbic system.

4.1.6 Fluid Compartments in the Central Nervous System

The fluid compartments in the nervous system include **arterial blood**, **venous blood**, **cerebrospinal fluid** (CSF) and interstitial fluid.

4.1.6.1 Arterial Supply

The brain's arterial supply is dual: the **anterior circulation** is derived from the **internal carotid arteries**, and the **posterior circulation** is derived from the **vertebrobasilar arteries**. The anterior and posterior circulations anastomose (join) at the base of the brain, forming the **Circle of Willis** (Figure 4.1.7A). The anterior circulation includes the **anterior cerebral arteries** and **middle cerebral arteries**. The posterior circulation includes the **posterior cerebral arteries** together with arteries supplying the brainstem and the cerebellum.

The cerebral arterial cortical territories are shown in Figure 4.1.7B. As these arteries branch into arterioles and capillaries, they supply the brain with oxygen and nutrients. The **blood–brain barrier** is a highly selective boundary between the peripheral blood and the brain's parenchyma, limiting the substances that can cross it (Figure 4.1.7C). Its components include:

- capillary endothelial cells, with **tight gap junctions** in between cells (unlike most capillaries elsewhere in the body)
- the basal lamina separating endothelial cells from the brain parenchyma
- **pericytes**, a type of glial cell which can locally regulate blood flow
- **astrocytes** and **astrocytic foot processes**, which maintain the integrity of the blood–brain barrier.

There are some areas of the brain not shielded by the blood–brain barrier, in particular the **circumventricular organs** such as the **area postrema** (involved in vomiting, so it is important that this area can freely sense blood-borne toxins) and the **organum vasculosum of the lamina terminalis** (involved in thirst and regulating serum osmolality).

The spinal cord is supplied by one anterior and two posterior spinal arteries, derived from the vertebral arteries.

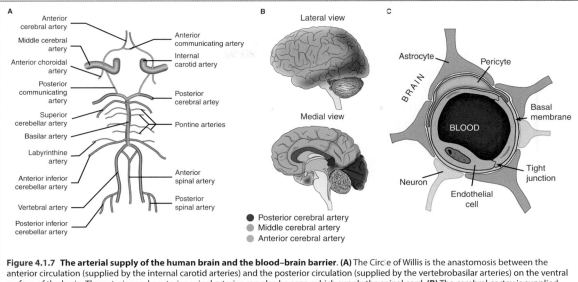

Figure 4.1.7 The arterial supply of the human brain and the blood–brain barrier. (A) The Circle of Willis is the anastomosis between the anterior circulation (supplied by the internal carotid arteries) and the posterior circulation (supplied by the vertebrobasilar arteries) on the ventral surface of the brain. The anterior and posterior spinal arteries can also be seen, which supply the spinal cord. **(B)** The cerebral cortex is supplied by the posterior (red), middle (green) and anterior (blue) cerebral arteries, whose territories are depicted on the medial and lateral views of the human brain. **(C)** The blood–brain barrier is a barrier between circulating blood and the brain's parenchyma. Its main components include the capillary endothelial cells with tight junctions, the capillary basement membrane, astrocytic foot processes and pericytes. (Illustration by Kollath Graphic Design, reproduced with permission.)

4.1.6.2 Venous Drainage

As is the case in the peripheral circulation, capillaries in the brain aggregate into venules, which form veins. In the brain, however, veins drain into **venous sinuses** (Figure 4.1.8A), which form in the space between the periosteal and meningeal dural layers. The venous sinuses ultimately drain into the internal jugular veins.

The spinal cord is drained by anterior and posterior spinal veins.

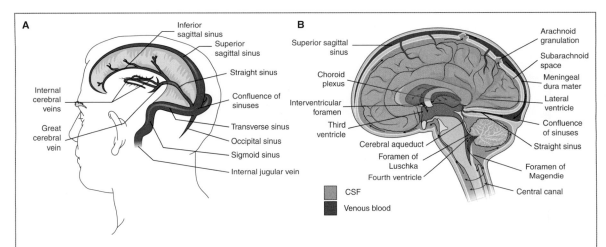

Figure 4.1.8 Dural venous sinuses and CSF circulation. (A) The venous blood of the brain drains via cerebral veins into the dural venous sinuses, which are hollow spaces formed at points of separation between two layers of dura mater (periosteal and meningeal). The venous sinuses meet at the confluence of sinuses and drain via the transverse and sigmoid sinuses into the internal jugular vein. **(B)** The CSF circulation of the brain and spinal cord. CSF is produced in the choroid plexuses lining each ventricle and circulates through the ventricular system: from the lateral ventricles, through the interventricular foramina (also called the foramina of Monro) to the third ventricle, and then through the cerebral aqueduct to the fourth ventricle. CSF can then continue into the spinal canal or pass through the lateral foramina of Luschka and medial foramen of Magendie to enter the subarachnoid space. CSF is reabsorbed into the venous sinuses via the arachnoid granulations and the glymphatic system.

4.1.6.3 Cerebrospinal Fluid

CSF bathes the brain and the spinal cord, with a total volume of between 100 and 200 ml. CSF originates from filtered plasma in the **choroid plexus**, found in the brain's ventricles. The CSF in the ventricular system is continuous with the spinal canal (Figure 4.1.8B).

The CSF also leaves the ventricular system via the **foramen of Magendie** (one medial) and **foramina of Luschka** (two lateral) in the fourth ventricle, and enters the **subarachnoid space**, where it bathes the brain and spinal cord. The CSF then re-enters the vasculature via two main routes:

- **arachnoid granulations**, which are protrusions of the arachnoid mater into the venous sinuses
- the **glymphatic system** [8], where CSF flows along periarterial spaces, mixes with the brain's interstitial fluid and then drains along perivenous spaces

REFERENCES

1. Knecht, S. et al. (2000). Handedness and hemispheric language dominance in healthy humans. *Brain* 123, 2512–2518.

2. McVey Neufeld, K.-A. et al. (2019). Oral selective serotonin reuptake inhibitors activate vagus nerve dependent gut–brain signalling. *Sci Rep* 9, 14290.

3. Brodmann, K. (1909). *Vergleichende Lokalisationslehre der Grosshirnrinde* [*Localisation in the Cerebral Cortex*]. Verlag von Johann Ambrosius Barth (3rd edition of *Localisation in the Cerebral Cortex* published by Springer, 2006, translated by Laurence J. Garey).

4. Marr, D. (1969). A theory of cerebellar cortex. *J Physiol* 202, 437–470.

5. Vogt, C. Vogt, O. (1919). Allgemeinere Ergebnisse unserer Hirnforschung [General results of our brain research]. *J Psychol Neurol* 25, 292–398.

6. Maclean, P. D. (1949). Psychosomatic disease and the 'visceral brain'; recent developments bearing on the Papez theory of emotion. *Psychosom Med* 11, 338–353.

7. Papez, J. (1937). A proposed mechanism of emotion. *J Neuropsychiatry*, doi:10.1176/jnp.7.1.103.

8. Xie, L. et al. (2013). Sleep drives metabolite clearance from the adult brain. *Science* 342, 10.1126/science.1241224.

4

<table>
<tr><td>**4.2**</td><td>**The Basal Ganglia**</td><td>Guilherme Carvalhal Ribas,
Andre Felix Gentil and Eduardo
Carvalhal Ribas</td></tr>
</table>

OVERVIEW

Neuroimaging techniques have demonstrated a neuroanatomical basis for various psychiatric disorders. In particular, alterations in the structure and function of the prefrontal cortex and limbic system have been implicated in depression, anxiety, and addiction. Insights about the neural etiology of psychiatric disorders can foster the design of appropriate treatment plans targeting specific neural substrates. This section discusses specifically the anatomy and function of the basal ganglia, a group of brain structures involved in modulating motor and executive functions, including the organization of cortical connections and pathways involved in goal-directed behaviors. The following sections provide information on the anatomy of the temporal and frontal lobes, including their surfaces, gyri and white matter connections within the cerebral hemispheres. Finally, ascending neurotransmitter systems are described in detail.

4.2.1 Anatomy of the Basal Ganglia

Anatomically, the basal ganglia refer to the dorsal striatum, ventral striatum, globus pallidus, substantia nigra and subthalamic nucleus. The putamen and globus pallidus form the lentiform or lenticular nucleus, with the globus pallidus situated medially and basally in relation to the putamen (Figure 4.2.1) (Mello, 1997; Ribas, 2018). The primary role of the basal ganglia is to modulate motor function (Section 5.6) and executive functions (Section 5.15). The basal ganglia are also critical to reward (Section 5.9) and in the development of habits (Section 5.8).

Through evolution, in order to enlarge without a proportional increase of the size of the skull, the brain itself, many of its deep structures and the lateral ventricles have bent around both thalami, forming a 'C' shape. In parallel, both ancient corpora striata (comprising the caudate, putamen, globus pallidus and nucleus accumbens) were dorsally divided by the fan-shaped developing internal capsule fibres without the division of their ventral portions.

The dorsal striatum corresponds medially to the caudate nucleus and laterally to the putamen, with the internal capsule fibres in between. The anterior and basal portions of the dorsal striatum are continuous with the ventral striatum (Figure 4.2.1B). The caudate nucleus forms an arch around the thalamus and bulges in the lateral wall of the lateral ventricle. Its large anterior head constitutes the lateral wall of the anterior horn of the ventricle, its narrower body corresponds to the lateral wall of the ventricular body and its tail encircles the thalamus posteriorly and laterally. The tail then runs along the roof of the inferior horn of the ventricle.

The ventral-striato-pallidal region, previously also known as the innominata substance (Heimer, 1995), is instrumental in reward and arousal. It includes the nucleus accumbens, the ventral part of the globus pallidus, the magnocellular nucleus of the basal forebrain (nucleus basalis of Meynert) and fibers travelling from the amygdala toward the septal region, the hypothalamus, the thalamus and to the bed nucleus of the stria terminalis, located under the head of the caudate nucleus. The ventral-striato-pallidal region is delimited superiorly by the anterior limb of the internal capsule and posteriorly by the anterior commissure, which passes along a groove of the globus pallidus ventral aspect.

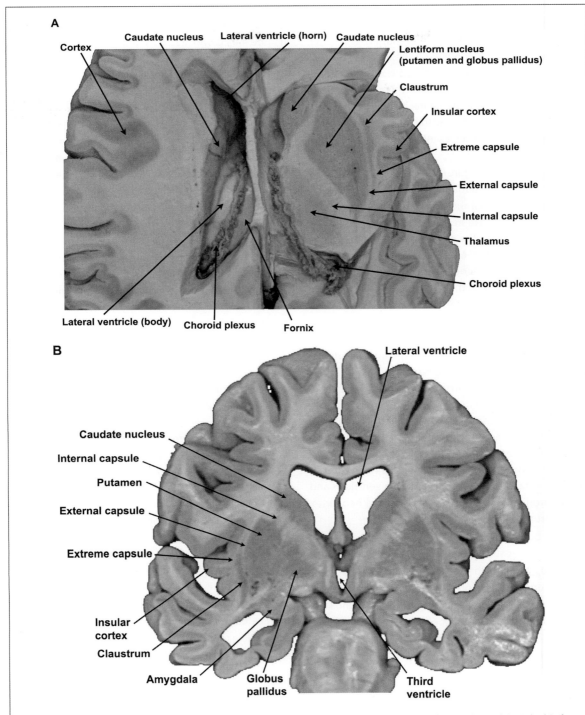

A

Cortex

Caudate nucleus

Lateral ventricle (horn)

Caudate nucleus

Lentiform nucleus
(putamen and globus pallidus)

Claustrum

Insular cortex

Extreme capsule

External capsule

Internal capsule

Thalamus

Choroid plexus

Lateral ventricle (body)

Choroid plexus

Fornix

B

Lateral ventricle

Caudate nucleus

Internal capsule

Putamen

External capsule

Extreme capsule

Insular
cortex

Claustrum

Amygdala

Globus
pallidus

Third
ventricle

Figure 4.2.1 (A) Axial dissection of the brain. At the left hemisphere, an axial (horizontal) cut was made inferior to the trunk (main body) of the corpus callosum, opening the lateral ventricle and offering a superior view of the structures related to this cavity. At the right hemisphere, an axial cut was made more inferiorly through the central core of the brain, revealing its structures (insular cortex, basal ganglia, thalamus and white matter capsules). **(B) Coronal dissection of the brain.** A coronal cut was made at the level of the amygdala, revealing the anatomy of the basal ganglia and adjacent structures.

The ventral striatum system (Figures 4.2.2E, 4.2.2F), unlike the rest of the cerebral cortex, is responsible for connecting the allocortex (three- or four-layered cortex including the hippocampus) and the mesocortex (the transitional areas between the allocortex, including the amygdala, and the neocortex) directly to the hypothalamus. Although related with neural activity processed in anterior cortical areas, the ventral striatum also participates in perceptual processes integrated in more posterior cerebral regions.

The insular cortex (Figure 4.2.2A), basal ganglia (claustrum, lentiform and caudate nuclei), their surrounding fibres (internal, external and extreme capsules) and thalamus define together a morphological block in each hemisphere, referred to as the central core of the brain. This block is primarily supplied by perforating arteries, with the lenticulostriate arteries passing anteriorly through the ventral striatum and the thalamoperforating arteries located more posteriorly (Ribas, 2018).

When seen from above, this block has a biconvex configuration, with its lateral aspect given by the insular cortex and its medial aspect by the intraventricular surfaces of the caudate nucleus and thalamus. The anterior portion of the insula is related to the head of the caudate nucleus while its posterior portion is related to the thalamus. There is an anatomical continuity between each thalamus and the mesencephalon (midbrain), and therefore each central core is morphologically equivalent to a true head of each half of the brainstem, surrounded by the ventricles and supratentorial cisterns and encircled by the neocortex and centrum semiovale.

The subcortical white matter of the insula represents the extreme capsule (Figure 4.2.2B) and is constituted by short association fibres, also known as U fibres. These U fibres connect the insular gyri among themselves and pass underneath the anterior and superior limiting sulci to reach the frontoparietal operculum and underneath the inferior limiting sulcus of the insula to reach the temporal operculum (Ribas, 2015).

Underneath the extreme capsule there is the fine lamina of grey matter that constitutes the claustrum (Figure 4.2.2C and 4.2.2D). While the ventral portion of the claustrum is sparse and composed by small islands of grey matter, its dorsal portion is thicker and better defined (Fernández-Miranda, 2008).

Proceeding inward, the external capsule lies medial to the claustrum, and is constituted dorsally by fibres originated from the claustrum (claustro-cortical fibres) and ventrally by the uncinate fasciculus and the inferior fronto-occipital fasciculus (Figure 4.2.2C). The lentiform nucleus, formed by the putamen and globus pallidus (Figures 4.2.2E, 4.2.2F), is covered laterally by the external capsule and medially by internal capsule fibres.

The frontal cortex projects through the basal ganglia, then to the thalamus, thence back to the cortex. These interconnections are topographically organised in a series of parallel pathways or loops (Alexander, 1986; Haber, 2003). Together, these circuits control all aspects of goal-directed behaviours, from their motivation, the cognition that organises them, to their execution:

- the orbital and medial prefrontal cortices are involved in emotion and motivation and project to the most ventral aspect of the basal ganglia
- the dorsolateral prefrontal cortex is involved in higher cognitive processes or 'executive functions' and projects to an intermediate region of the basal ganglia
- premotor and motor areas, involved in motor planning and the execution of those plans, project to the most dorsal aspect of the basal ganglia (Haber, 2003; Ribas, 2010).

Various neurological and psychiatric conditions can arise due to dysfunctions within neural circuits that relay in basal ganglia neurons, including movement disorders, addiction and Tourette syndrome, among others (Koestler, 1967; LaPlane, 1989; McGuire, 1994; Middleton, 2000; Teixeira, 2006). The basal ganglia are particularly implicated in apathy/anhedonia (Section 5.13) and in obsessive–compulsive disorder, where they are a target for therapeutic stimulation (see Section 9.6).

4

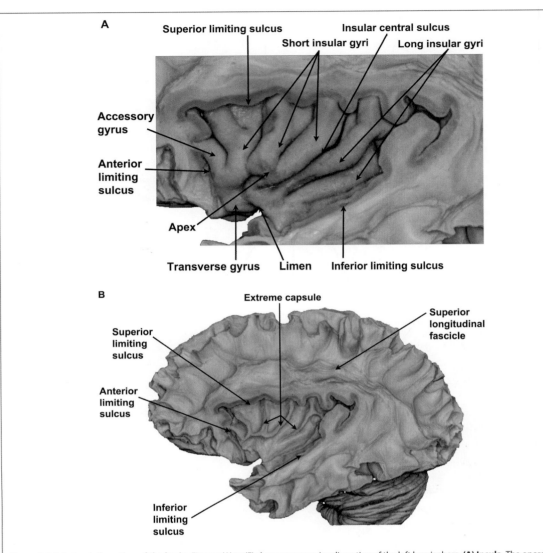

Figure 4.2.2 Lateral dissection of the brain. Figures (A) to (F) show a progressive dissection of the left hemisphere. **(A) Insula.** The opercula (Latin for 'cover,' i.e. the cortex covering the insula) were removed, and the insular cortex is shown. The anterior limiting sulcus bounds the insula anteriorly; the short insular gyrus is also known as the anterior insula; the long insular gyrus as the posterior insula. **(B) Extreme capsule.** The insular cortex was removed (decorticated) and the extreme capsule is shown, composed of short association fibres. These fibres connect the insular gyri together and also to the opercula, by passing underneath the anterior, superior and inferior limiting sulci. Further deep-fibre dissection at the frontal, parietal and temporal lobes reveals the superior longitudinal fascicle. **(C) Claustrum.** The removal of the extreme capsule deep to the insula exposes the claustrum and three main white matter fibre bundles at this region, organised in an antero-posterior sequential disposition: uncinate fascicle (which connects the hippocampus and amygdala to frontal cortex), inferior fronto-occipital fascicle and claustro-cortical fibres. Some claustro-cortical fibres have been removed, creating small 'windows' where the putamen can be seen directly underneath these fibres. **(D) Putamen.** The claustrum and claustro-cortical fibres were removed, revealing the putamen, and some fibres of the inferior fronto-occipital fascicle were resected, exposing underneath fibres that belong to the lateral extension of the anterior commissl. **(E) Globus pallidus and ventral striatum.** The globus pallidus is seen after the putamen was removed. The grey matter indicated by the asterix (*) extends from the (removed) putamen, and medially will merge with the grey matter that extends from the caudate nucleus (constituting the ventral striatum). **(F) Internal capsule.** The projection fibres located inside a circle defined by the outer margin of the lentiform nucleus (putamen and globus pallidus) are named internal capsule. Outside this region and toward the cerebral lobes, the projection fibres are named the corona radiata. The double asterix (**) indicates the location of the ventral striatum (removed), composed of the grey matter that extends from the putamen (laterally) and the caudate nucleus (medially) to merge ventrally. The optic radiation, which includes Meyer's loop, is the part of the radiation which sweeps back into the temporal lobe.

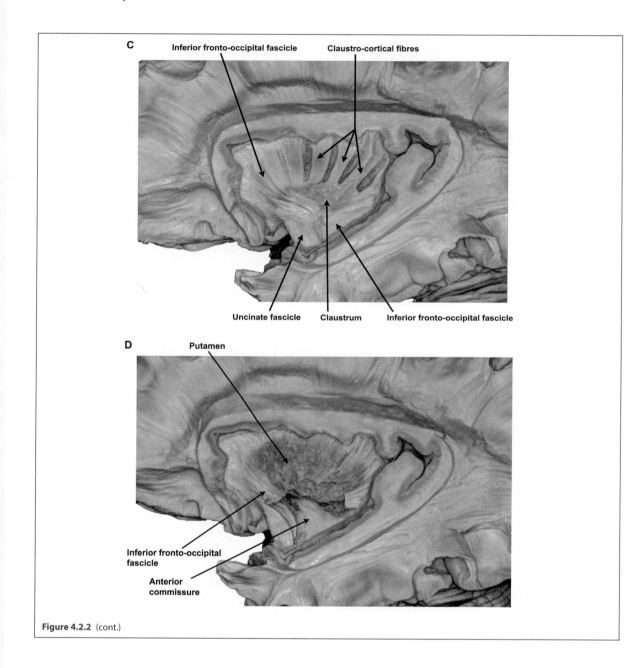

Figure 4.2.2 (cont.)

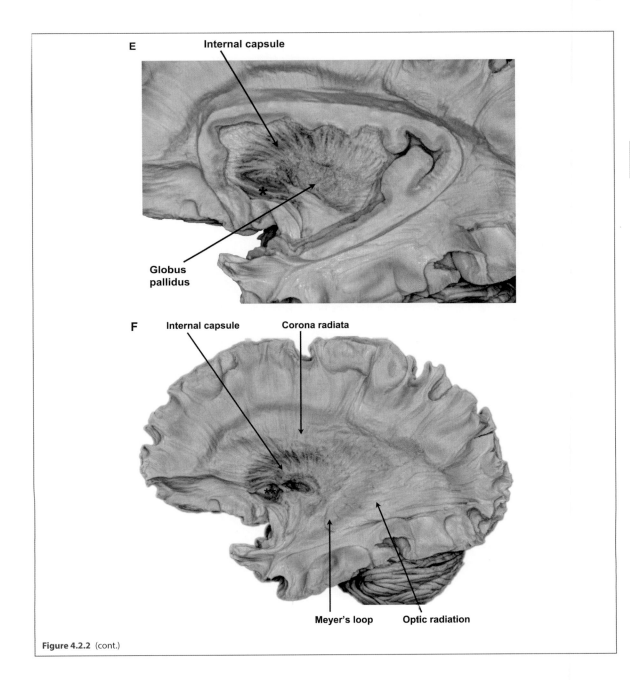

E

Internal capsule

Globus
pallidus

F

Internal capsule   Corona radiata

Meyer's loop   Optic radiation

Figure 4.2.2 (cont.)

REFERENCES

Alexander GE (1986). Parallel organization of functionally segregated circuits linking basal ganglia and cortex. *Ann Rev Neurosci* 9: 357–381.

Fernández-Miranda JC, Rhoton AL Jr, Kakizawa Y, Choi C, Alvarez-Linera J (2008). The claustrum and its projection system in the human brain: a microsurgical and tractographic anatomical study. *J Neurosurg* 108(4): 764–774.

Haber SN (2003). The primate basal ganglia: parallel and integrative networks. *J Chem Neuroanat* 26: 317–330.

Heimer L (1995). *The Human Brain and Spinal Cord: Functional Neuroanatomy and Dissection Guide*, 2nd ed. Springer Verlag.

Koestler A (1967). *The Ghost in the Machine*. MacMillan.

Laplane D, Levasseur M, Pillon B et al. (1989). Obsessive–compulsive and other behavioural changes with bilateral basal ganglia lesions: a neuropsychological, magnetic resonance imaging and positron tomography study. *Brain* 112(Pt 3): 699–725.

McGuire PK, Bench CJ, Frith CD et al. (1994). Functional anatomy of obsessive–compulsive phenomena. *Br J Psych* 164(4): 459–468.

Mello E, Villares J (1997). Neuroanatomy of the basal ganglia. *Psychiatr Clin North Am* 20(4): 691–704.

Middleton FA, Strick PL (2000). Basal ganglia and cerebellar loops: motor and cognitive circuits. *Brain Res Rev* 31(2–3): 236–250.

Ribas EC, Yagmurlu K, Wen HT, Rhoton AL Jr (2015). Microsurgical anatomy of the inferior limiting insular sulcus and the temporal stem. *J Neurosurg* 122(6): 1263–1273.

Ribas EC, Yağmurlu K, de Oliveira E, Ribas GC, Rhoton A (2018). Microsurgical anatomy of the central core of the brain. *J Neurosurg* 129(3): 752–769.

Ribas GC (2010). The cerebral sulci and gyri. *Neurosurg Focus* 28(2): E2.

Teixeira AL, Malheiros JA, de Oliveira JT, Nicolato R, Correa H (2006). Limbic encephalitis manifesting as a psychotic disorder. *Rev Bras Psiquiatr* 28(2): 163–164.

4.3 The Temporal Lobes

Guilherme Carvalhal Ribas,
Andre Felix Gentil and Eduardo
Carvalhal Ribas

The temporal lobes are situated inferiorly to the lateral (Sylvian) fissure and are limited posteriorly by an imaginary line running from the superomedial portions of the parieto-occipital sulcus to the preoccipital notch, which is located approximately 5 cm from the occipital pole (Figure 4.3.1A). Each temporal lobe has three surfaces: lateral (composed by the superior, middle and inferior temporal gyri), opercular (inside the Sylvian fissure) and basal (lying on the floor of the cranial middle fossa). (Ribas, 2010, 2015, 2018). The medial temporal lobe includes the hippocampus and amygdala, implicated in memory (Section 5.14) and emotion (Section 5.10), while the lateral temporal lobe is particularly important in language (Section 5.17).

The superior temporal gyrus always continues posteriorly to the supramarginal gyrus encircling the terminal portion of the lateral (Sylvian) fissure (Figure 4.3.1A). The middle temporal gyrus is often partially connected to the angular gyrus. The inferior temporal gyrus extends along the inferolateral margin of the cerebral hemisphere and continues to the inferior occipital gyrus, over the preoccipital notch (Figure 4.3.1A, Ribas, 2010).

Within the temporal opercular surface there is a voluminous transverse gyrus that originates around the midpoint of the superior temporal gyrus. It is oriented diagonally toward the posterior vertex of the floor of the Sylvian fissure, with its longest axis oriented toward the ventricular atrium. This is the transverse gyrus of Heschl (Figure 4.3.1A), and together with the most posterior aspect of the superior temporal gyrus, constitutes the primary auditory cortical area (Williams and Warwick, 1980). In the dominant hemisphere, the posterior part of the superior temporal gyrus corresponds to the so-called Wernicke area, particularly related to language comprehension.

The basal surface of the temporal lobe is constituted laterally by the inferior surface of the inferior temporal gyrus, and medially by the fusiform gyrus (involved in recognition, including face recognition), with the temporo-occipital sulcus separating them. Medially, the fusiform gyrus is delimited by the collateral sulcus, separating it from the parahippocampal gyrus, already part of the limbic lobe (Figure 4.3.1B).

Anteriorly, the parahippocampal gyrus bends over itself and forms a triangular shape called an uncus ('hook') (Figure 4.3.1C). It is separated from the temporal pole by the rhinal sulcus.

The cortex of the medial temporal lobe includes important subdivisions of the limbic system, including the hippocampus and entorhinal cortex (the major input to the hippocampus). Areas of neocortex adjacent to these limbic regions are grouped together as the medial temporal association cortex.

The amygdala (or amygdaloid body) lies within the anterior half of the uncus, immediately anterior to the head of the hippocampus, which lies inside the posterior half of the uncus, and constitutes the anterior wall of the temporal horn of the lateral ventricle (Figure 4.3.1D and 4.3.1E). It continues superiorly with the base of the globus pallidus, creating a figure of eight or hourglass when seen in the coronal plane (Wen et al., 1999; Ture et al., 1999, 2000) (Figures 4.3.1D and 4.3.1E). Nuclei of the amygdala project to, and receive fibres from neocortical areas, predominantly of the temporal lobe, and possibly also from the inferior parietal cortex.

Three distinct parts compose the amygdala. The basolateral part receives afferents from the cerebral cortex and thalamic nuclei and, similarly to the rest of the cortex, projects fibers to the ventral striatum and thalamus (Heimer and Van Hoesen, 2006). The smaller olfactory part receives afferent fibers from the adjacent temporal olfactory cortex, and projects mainly to the centromedial part of the amygdala and to the hypothalamus. The centromedial part, in turn, receives afferents

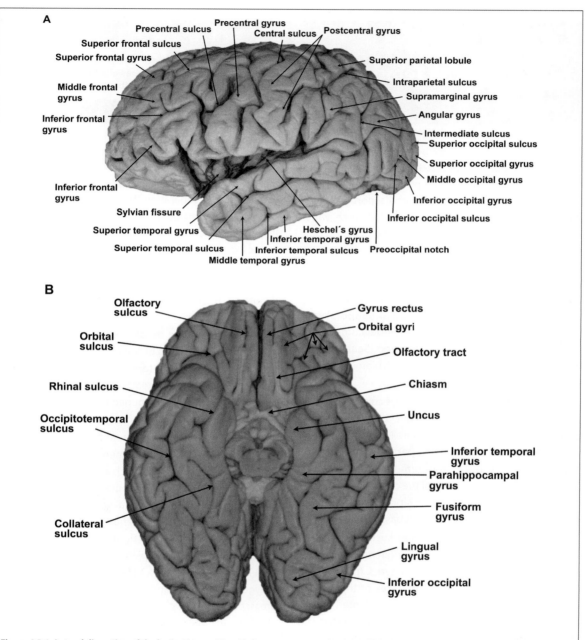

A

Precentral gyrus
Precentral sulcus
Central sulcus
Postcentral gyrus
Superior frontal sulcus
Superior frontal gyrus
Superior parietal lobule
Middle frontal gyrus
Intraparietal sulcus
Supramarginal gyrus
Inferior frontal gyrus
Angular gyrus
Intermediate sulcus
Superior occipital sulcus
Superior occipital gyrus
Middle occipital gyrus
Inferior frontal gyrus
Inferior occipital gyrus
Sylvian fissure
Inferior occipital sulcus
Superior temporal gyrus
Heschel´s gyrus
Preoccipital notch
Superior temporal sulcus
Inferior temporal gyrus
Inferior temporal sulcus
Middle temporal gyrus

B

Olfactory sulcus
Gyrus rectus
Orbital sulcus
Orbital gyri
Olfactory tract
Rhinal sulcus
Chiasm
Occipitotemporal sulcus
Uncus
Inferior temporal gyrus
Parahippocampal gyrus
Fusiform gyrus
Collateral sulcus
Lingual gyrus
Inferior occipital gyrus

Figure 4.3.1 Lateral dissection of the brain. Figures (A) to (E) show a progressive dissection of the left hemisphere. **(A) Cortical sulci and gyri.** The lateral surface of the brain is exposed and its main sulci and gyri can be identified. **(B) Basal dissection of the brain.** The basal surface of the brain is shown and its main sulci and gyri can be identified. **(C) Medial view of limbic structures.** Some limbic structures are shown, demonstrating that together they form the shape of a ring around the central core of the brain, particularly the thalamus (removed here). **(D) Lateral view of limbic structures.** Lateral view of the structures in (B), showing the amygdala and the hippocampus inside the parahippocampal gyrus, and the fornix constituted by fibres from the hippocampus. Fibre dissection was performed at the cingulate gyrus, and the cingulum can be identified inside this region (fibres projecting from the cingulate to the entorhinal cortex). Also seen are the lateral ventricular choroid plexus and subiculum (part of the hippocampal flation). **(E)** Lateral and enlarged view of limbic structures, showing the fibres from the hippocampus surface join posteriorly and form the fornix. The amygdala can be displaced anteriorly, revealing its separation from the hippocampus.

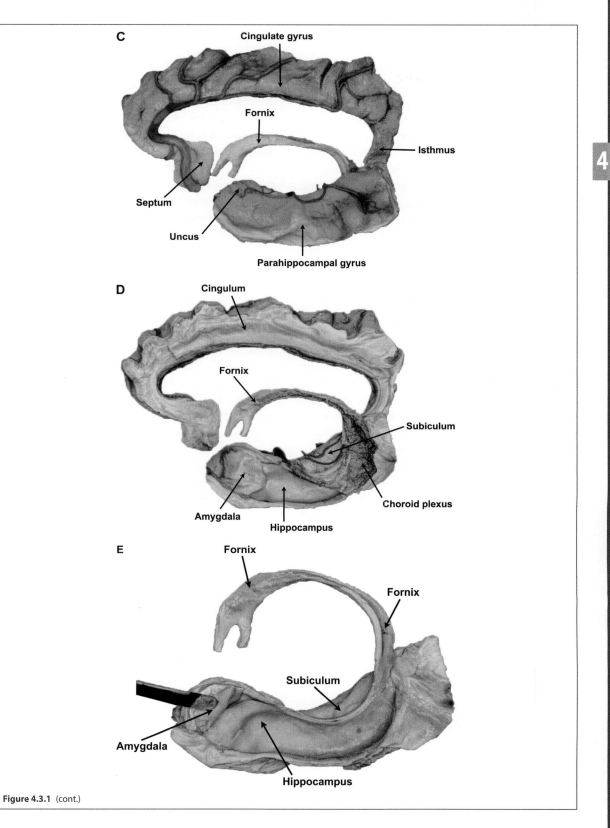

Figure 4.3.1 (cont.)

from the hippocampal formation, insula, orbitofrontal cortex and midline thalamic nuclei (particularly related to interoceptive information), and projects to the septal region, hypothalamus, thalamus and brainstem (Heimer and Van Hoesen, 2006).

The centromedial portion of the amygdala extends both posteriorly and ventrally to reach the bed nucleus of the stria terminalis in the posterior striatum, immediately inferior to the head of the caudate nucleus. The semicircular arrangement of these structures around the caudate nucleus and thalamus creates a ring around the internal capsule and thalamus, referred to as the extended amygdala (de Olmos and Heimer, 1999; Heimer and Van Hoesen, 2006). The disposition of the extended amygdala is particularly relevant to its role in regulating emotions and behaviour. It receives inputs mainly from the limbic lobe and, through its projections to the hypothalamus and brainstem, the entire extended amygdala exerts influence on the neural areas that generate the autonomic, endocrine and somatomotive components of emotional experiences, modulating thirst, eating and sexual activity, among other behaviours. A direct pathway between the amygdala and the thalamus is responsible for non-specific, fast and intense autonomic responses to external stimuli, explaining, for example, abrupt reactions of fear to certain situations (Le Doux, 1994, 2003).

During evolution, the hippocampus suffered a postero-inferior displacement around the thalamus, giving rise to the fornix of white matter connecting to the ipsilateral mammillary body of the hypothalamus (through posterior–anterior commissure fibres of the fornix) and the septal region (through pre-commissural forniceal fibres) (Figure 4.3.1C and 4.3.1D). The cleft between the fornix and the thalamus constitutes the choroidal fissure (Williams and Warwick, 1980; Nagata et al., 1988). The hippocampus, fornices and adjacent cortical areas are responsible for information storage, and therefore participate in memory and learning processing (Kandel et al., 1991; Duvernoy, 1998; Squire et al., 2003). The intimate topographic and functional relationship between the amygdala and the hippocampus also allows for processes of memory storage to include their respective emotional charge.

It is interesting to note that the hippocampal cortex maintains a primitive arrangement with the white substance situated external to the grey matter, equivalent to the white matter arrangement in the medulla and brainstem: it is covered by the so-called alveus, the white matter fibres which aggregate to form the fimbria of the fornix. Further evolutionary development of the neocortex and corpus callosum, covering the telencephalic ventricles, resulted in the hippocampus being the only intraventricular cortical surface, situated in the medial wall of each temporal ventricular horn.

In relation to the thalamus, the mammillothalamic tract is found at its anterior aspect, the field of Forel is at its basal limit, and the internal capsule at its lateral border. The subthalamic and red nuclei are found inferior to the thalamus.

REFERENCES

de Olmos JS, Heimer L (1999). The concept of ventral striatopallidal system and extended amygdala. *Ann N Y Acad Sci* 877: 1–32.

Duvernoy MH (1998). *The Human Hippocampus: Functional Anatomy, Vascularization, and Serial Section with MRI*, 2nd ed. Springer.

Heimer L, Van Hoesen GW (2006). The limbic lobe and its output channels: implications for emotional functions and adaptive behavior. *Neurosci Biobehav Rev* 30(2): 126–147.

Kandel ER, Schwartz JH, Jessell TM, eds (1991). *Principles of Neural Science*, 3rd ed. Elsevier.

LeDoux J (1994). Emotion, memory and the brain: the neural routes underlying the formation of memories about primitive emotional experiences, such as fear, have been traced. *Sci Am* 270(6): 50–57.

LeDoux J (2003). The self: clues from the brain. *Ann N Y Acad Sci* 1001: 295–304.

Nagata S, Rhoton AL, Barry M (1988). Microsurgical anatomy of the choroidal fissure. *Surg Neurol* 30: 3–59,

Ribas GC (2010). The cerebral sulci and gyri. *Neurosurg Focus* 28(2): E2.

Ribas GC (2015). The cerebral hemispheres. In *Gray's Anatomy*, 41st ed. Elsevier.

Ribas GC (ed.) (2018). *Applied Cranial-Cerebral Anatomy*. Cambridge University Press.

Squire LR, Bloom FE, McConnell SK et al. (2003). *Fundamental Neuroscience*, 2nd ed. Elsevier Academic Press.

Ture U, Yasargil DC, Al-Mefty O, Yasargil MG (1999). Topographic anatomy of the insular region. *J Neurosurg* 90(4): 730–733.

Ture U, Yasargil MG, Friedman AH, Al-Mefty O (2000). Fiber dissection technique: lateral aspect of the brain. *Neurosurgery* 47(2): 417–426.

Wen HT, Rhoton AL Jr, de Oliveira E et al. (1999). Microsurgical anatomy of the temporal lobe: Part I: mesial temporal lobe anatomy and its vascular relationships and applied to amygdalohippocampectomy. *Neurosurgery* 45(3): 549–591.

Williams PL, Warwick R, eds. (1980). *Gray's Anatomy*, 36th ed. Saunders.

4

<table>
<tr></tr>
</table>

4.4 The Frontal Lobes

Guilherme Carvalhal Ribas,
Andre Felix Gentil and Eduardo
Carvalhal Ribas

The frontal lobes are the largest and most anterior parts of each cerebral hemisphere. They are limited posteriorly by the central sulcus, anteriorly by the cerebral supraciliary margin, medially by the interhemispheric fissure, and laterally and inferiorly by the lateral (Sylvian) fissure (see Figure 4.3.1 in the previous section; Ribas, 2015). The dorsal surface of the frontal lobes is constituted posteriorly by the precentral gyrus, and anteriorly by the longitudinal superior, middle and inferior frontal gyri, converging in front to constitute the frontal pole. The ventral surface is constituted by the orbital and rectus gyri. The medial frontal surface faces the falx cerebri, the crescent-shaped fold of dura mater which separates the hemispheres.

The frontal lobe is responsible for planning and executing motor and executive functions (see Section 5.6 and Section 5.15 respectively). The precentral gyrus corresponds to Brodmann's area 4 and contains the primary motor cortex. This gyrus is topographically organised with the contralateral head (face) represented most inferiorly and laterally, the arm and hand represented on its upper lateral aspect, and the leg and foot represented on the medial surface, therefore corresponding to the classical motor homunculus described by Penfield and Rasmussen (1950).

The premotor and the supplementary motor areas are placed anteriorly to the MI and are active in the planning and organisation of movements (Brodal, 2010). The premotor cortex corresponds to the superolateral surface (Brodmann's area 6) anterior to the precentral sulcus and can be subdivided into a dorsal area (mostly related to the middle frontal gyrus) and a ventral area (mostly within the inferior frontal gyrus).

The ventral premotor cortex within the opercular part of the inferior frontal gyrus has been related to vocalisation bilaterally (Duffau, 2011), and also classically to speech production in the dominant hemisphere. The supplementary motor area lies in the posterior and medial aspect of the superior frontal gyrus, just anterior to the paracentral lobule. The frontal eye field (Brodmann's areas 6, 8 and 9), a cortical region associated with eye movements, is also found anteriorly to the primary motor cortex, at the posterior aspect of the middle and superior frontal gyri.

The prefrontal cortex modulates sensory information projected by the thalamus to neocortical areas, acting as a main center of organisation and planning of complex cognitive behaviour, including orchestration of emotional reactions, executive function and social expression. The prefrontal cortex exerts intense regulatory activity on the extended amygdala (Heimer and Van Hoesen, 1995; Marino, 1996; MacLean, 1997; Duvernoy, 1998; LeDoux, 2003).

On the orbital (i.e. above the eyes) surface of each frontal lobe, the deep olfactory sulcus harbors the olfactory bulb and olfactory tract (Figure 4.3.1B). Medial to the olfactory sulcus is the long and narrow gyrus rectus, considered the most anatomically constant of the cerebral gyri, which is continuous with the superior frontal gyrus along the medial aspect of the frontal pole. Lateral to the olfactory sulcus are the orbital gyri, which account for the greatest proportion of the fronto-basal surface. The H-shaped orbital sulcus delineates the anterior, posterior medial and lateral orbital gyri. The most anterior and basal aspects of both frontal lobes are related with judgement and volitional complex aspects of behaviour.

The olfactory system is composed, at each hemisphere, by the olfactory bulb, the olfactory tubercle, the prepiriform and pirifrom (or periamygdaloid) cortices and the cortical nuclei of the amygdala. The olfactory bulbs phylogenetically and embryologically correspond to rostral (towards the nose) extensions of both telencephalic masses, and display neurons in a cortical laminar fashion, which receive efferent fibres from the olfactory receptors. The olfactory tract extends posteriorly from the bulb: the efferent projections from the olfactory bulb are directed to the anterior olfactory nuclei and the olfactory tubercle, and continue laterally to the olfactory cortex, which is subdivided into prepiriform and piriform (or periamygdaloid) cortices, and certain nuclei of the amygdaloid complex. Fibres from the lateral olfactory area connect to diencephalic centers and to the extended amygdala (MacLean, 1990; Finger, 1994; Heimer and Van Hoesen, 2006).

Immediately in front of the lamina terminalis (the anterior wall of the third ventricle), and under the rostrum of the callosum, lie the subcallosal gyri (both paraterminal gyri) harboring the septal nuclei. The septal nuclei receive afferents mainly from the hippocampus and subiculum of the parahippocampal gyrus through the indusium griseum (grey matter on the upper surface of the callosum) and the fornix (pre-commissural fibres of the fornix). They relay efferents mostly to the hypothalamus, midbrain and habenula (involved in pain and reward processing) via the medullary stria of the thalamus (Mesulam, 1987).

Functionally, the septal nuclei connect limbic structures to the hypothalamus, midbrain and extend to the ventral striatum. Clinically, lesions to the septal area result in a syndrome characterised by exaggerated reactions to environmental stimuli and consequent behavioural changes.

Due to its large anatomical extension and functional heterogeneity, neurological symptoms and signs caused by frontal affectations can vary significantly according to their site, comprising a clinical spectrum that varies from absolutely no signs or symptoms to complete hemiplegias and severe cognitive dysfunction, more frequently related to bilateral frontal lesions.

4

REFERENCES

Brodal P (2010). *The Central Nervous System, Structure and Function*, 4th ed. Oxford University Press.

Duffau H (2011). *Brain Mapping: from Neural Basis of Cognition to Surgical Applications*. Springer-Verlag.

Duvernoy MH (1998). *The Human Hippocampus: Functional Anatomy, Vascularization, and Serial Section with MRI*, 2nd ed. Springer.

Finger S (1994). *Origins of Neuroscience*. Oxford University Press.

Heimer L (1995). *The Human Brain and Spinal Cord: Functional Neuroanatomy and Dissection Guide*, 2nd ed. Springer Verlag.

Heimer L, Van Hoesen GW (2006). The limbic lobe and its output channels: implications for emotional functions and adaptive behavior. *Neurosci Biobehav Rev* 30(2): 126–147.

LeDoux J (2003). The self: clues from the brain. *Ann N Y Acad Sci* 1001: 295–304.

MacLean PD (1990). *The Triune Brain in Evolution*. Plenum.

Marino R Jr. (1975). *Fisiologia das emoções*. Sarvier. 18.

Martin JH (1996). *Neuroanatomy, Text and Atlas*, 2nd ed. Appleton and Lange Co.

Mesulam MM (1987). Patterns in behavioral neuroanatomy: association areas, the limbic system, and hemisphere specialization. In *Principles of Behavioral Neurology*. FA Davis, pp. 1–70.

Penfield W, Rasmussen T (1950). *The Cerebral Cortex of Man*. Macmillan,

Ribas GC (2015). The cerebral hemispheres. In *Gray's Anatomy*, 41st ed. Elsevier.

4.5

White Matter Pathways

Guilherme Carvalhal Ribas, Andre Felix Gentil and Eduardo Carvalhal Ribas

The white matter within the cerebral hemispheres is composed of myelinated fibre bundles (tracts or fasciculi), named according to their course and connections. Association fibres link different cortical areas within the same hemisphere, commissural fibres connect cortical areas between hemispheres and projection fibres connect the cerebral cortex with the corpus striatum, diencephalon, brainstem and spinal cord.

4.5.1 Association Fibres

There are two types of association fibres: short (arcuate or 'U') linking adjacent gyri (Figure 4.5.1; see also Figure 4.2.2), and long, connecting more distant gyri within the same hemisphere. The latter are grouped in bundles and the most significant are discussed below.

The superior longitudinal fasciculus (see Figure 4.2.2B) is a complex association system of different subsets of fibres, being macroscopically composed by the frontoparietal or horizontal segment, temporoparietal

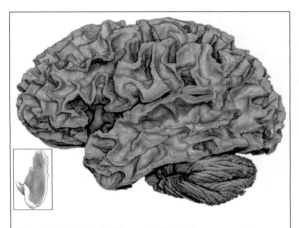

Figure 4.5.1 Cortical white matter. The brain was prepared for white matter fibre dissection by Klinger's technique (freezing method) and the cortical grey matter was removed (decortication). The short association fibres (or U fibres) visible here are the most superficial fibres and are located directly underneath all cerebral cortex. A U-fibre is shown at the figure inset.

or vertical segment, and temporo-frontal segment or arcuate fasciculus. The superior longitudinal fasciculus has been related to language function in the dominant hemisphere, connecting the Broca and Wernicke areas by an indirect and more superficial pathway relayed at the inferior parietal lobule as well as a direct and deeper pathway corresponding to the arcuate fasciculus (Duffau, 2008).

The frontoparietal segment runs deeply underneath the frontal gyri towards the parietal lobe posteriorly. According to diffusion tensor imaging (DTI) findings (see Section 3.1.5), this segment is subdivided into three components: superior longitudinal fasciculus I, connecting the superior parietal lobule and the precuneus with the premotor and prefrontal cortices; superior longitudinal fasciculus II, connecting the angular gyrus with the dorsal premotor and prefrontal areas; and superior longitudinal fasciculus III, connecting the supramarginal gyrus with the ventral premotor and prefrontal cortex (Broca's area) (Makris et al., 2005; Catani, 2011; Thiebaut de Schotten et al., 2011). The temporoparietal or vertical segment of the superior longitudinal fasciculus connects the posterior portions of the superior and middle temporal gyri (Wernicke area) with the inferior parietal lobule. The temporo-frontal segment (arcuate fasciculus) connects more diffuse areas of the posterior aspect of the temporal lobe with the posterior aspect of the frontal lobe.

The inferior fronto-occipital fascicle (Figure 4.2.2C) is an associative bundle that connects frontal regions to the temporal and occipital lobes, having a ventral trajectory which runs underneath the insula (Ribas, 2018). Findings from intraoperative brain electrical stimulation during awake neurosurgeries suggest that the superior longitudinal fasciculus is more particularly related with phonological aspects of language, while the inferior fronto-occipital fascicle is more related with its semantic aspects (Duffau, 2008). The uncinate fasciculus is a hook like-shaped associative bundle which connects the anteromedial temporal lobe with the orbitofrontal region (Figure 4.2.2C). Both the uncinate and the inferior fronto-occipital fascicle converge like a funnel beneath the apex of the insula, with the uncinate positioned anterior to the inferior fronto-occipital fascicle. They also intertwine with the extreme and external capsules, incorporating the most ventral fibres.

The inferior longitudinal fasciculus (Figure 4.5.2) runs mostly along the depth of the fusiform gyrus and connects the basal aspects of the temporal and occipital lobes. The inferior longitudinal fasciculus is particularly implicated in face recognition and its emotional significance (Tavor, 2014).

The cingulum (Figures 4.3.1D and 4.5.3) lies within the depth of the cingulate and parahippocampal gyri, projecting the cingulate gyrus into the entorhinal cortex and connecting different components of the limbic system.

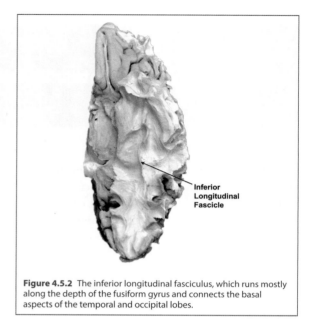

Figure 4.5.2 The inferior longitudinal fasciculus, which runs mostly along the depth of the fusiform gyrus and connects the basal aspects of the temporal and occipital lobes.

4.5.2 Commissural Fibres

The corpus callosum is the largest brain fibre pathway, containing up to 200 million fibres. At midline, it is a well-defined arch connecting the cortex of both hemispheres and extending for approximately 10 centimetres, divided into a rostrum, genu, trunk and splenium (Figure 4.5.3), and its commissural fibres connect the frontal, parietal and occipital lobes, as well as some parts of the temporal lobes.

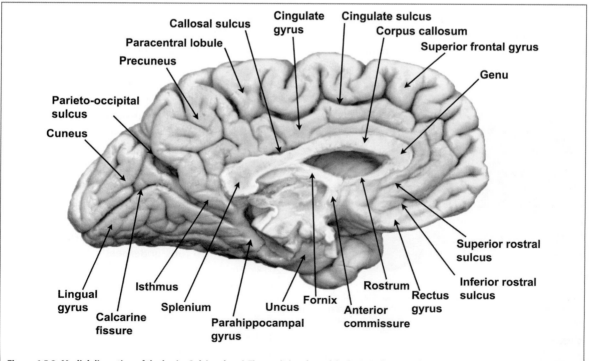

Figure 4.5.3 Medial dissection of the brain. Sulci and gyri. The medial surface of the brain is shown and its main sulci and gyri can be identified.

Interhemispheric callosal connections are not a simple linking of loci between both hemispheres, and only the areas related to midline representation are linked to the contralateral hemisphere through callosal fibres. This is clearly the case for the visual areas, where only the cortex containing the representation of each midline retinal zone is linked to its contralateral counterpart, and in somatic areas, where only the trunk representation is callosally linked, while the peripheral limb areas (hand and foot) are not (Williams and Warwick, 1980).

These connections that link the same or similar areas of both hemispheres are termed homotopic connections, and the corpus callosum also interconnects bilateral heterogeneous cortical areas through heterotopic connections. These may serve to connect functionally similar but anatomically different loci, and/or to connect functional areas of one hemisphere with contralateral regions that are specialised in a confined unilateral function.

The inner surface of the corpus callosum is concave along its longest axis, is attached to both membranes that constitute the septum pellucidum along its trunk, genu and rostrum, and along the splenium is fused to both crura of the fornices and to the hippocampal commissure that runs between them.

The superior surface of the callosal trunk is covered by a thin layer of grey matter, the indusium griseum, extending anteriorly around the genu and then into the paraterminal gyrus below the rostrum.

The anterior commissure (Figures 4.2.2D and 4.5.3) is a compact bundle of myelinated fibres, which runs within the basal forebrain and projects anteriorly to interconnect olfactory structures, and laterally fans out to interconnect both temporal lobes, linking structures that are not interconnected by the corpus callosum. The anterior commissure was the main commissure for ancient reptiles, and regressed together with the olfactory pathways throughout phylogeny. In humans, its function is not completely understood.

The hippocampal commissure or commissure of the fornix functionally connects both hippocampi. It is situated underneath and intimately attached to the splenium, overhanging the pineal region. The pineal is an unpaired, midline neuroendocrine gland located immediately posterior to the third ventricle and produces the sleep-promoting hormone melatonin.

The habenular commissure lies between both habenula, which are small protuberances of the medial surface of both thalami, within the posterior aspect of the lateral wall of the third ventricle. Since the pineal gland is superiorly attached to the habenular commissure, and inferiorly attached to the posterior commissure, the pineal recess of the third ventricle is located between the two commissures.

The habenular nuclei receive limbic inputs through the stria medullaris thalami (which is formed mainly by fibres of the fornix, stria terminalis and medial forebrain bundle) and send efferent outputs to the interpeduncular nucleus (through the fasciculus retroflexus of Meynert) and to the rostral salivatory nuclei in the floor of the fourth ventricle, which activate reflex salivation (Brodal, 1981).

There are clinical and experimental data which relate these small diencephalic structures with specific functions. For example, a correlation of the habenula with reward expectation and depression has been described (Matsumoto and Hikosaka, 2007). However, it is still not well established whether these structures and connections are really functional in humans or if they only correspond to vestigial structures (i.e. evolutionary remnants).

4.5.3 Projection Fibres

Projection fibres connect the cerebral cortex with lower levels in the brain and spinal cord (Figure 4.2.2F). They include large numbers of both corticofugal (going away from the cortex) and corticopetal (going towards the cortex) fibres, which converge from all directions to form the dense subcortical white matter mass named the corona radiata, intersecting the commissural fibres of the corpus callosum and other association tracts along their trajectories within the centrum semiovale.

The corona radiata is continuous with the internal capsule of the lentiform nucleus, and inferiorly to the lentiform nucleus it continues as the cerebral peduncle (Figure 4.2.2F). The fibres of the internal capsule are disposed in a radial pattern, converging medial to the lenticular nucleus, and are classically subdivided in relation to this nucleus: it includes an anterior limb (between the head of the caudate and the putamen), a genu (that corresponds to its most medial fibres, adjacent to the interventricular foramen and which includes the corticobulbar tract), a posterior limb (between both the body of the caudate and thalamus medially and the putamen laterally, and which includes the corticospinal tract and the superior thalamic radiation), the retrolentiform part (which includes the auditory thalamic radiations), and the sublentiform part (which includes most of the optic radiations) (Figure 4.5.1).

4.5.4 Papez's Circuit and the Limbic Lobe

Paul Broca, in 1877, described the 'great limbic lobe' as comprising the cingulate and parahippocampal gyri (Figure 4.5.3), and the 'limbic fissure' as comprising the cingulate and collateral sulci, having adopted the term limbic (from the Latin *limbus*: border, ring around) since these structures are located around the top of the brainstem in all mammals (Broca, 1877).

In 1937, James Papez suggested a key circuit in the brain that he thought to be essential for our emotions, which was later shown to be a circuit more particularly related with memory. This pathway involves several connected parts of the brain: it starts at the hippocampal formation, goes through the fornix, passes the mamillary body and proceeds via the mammillothalamic tract to the anterior nuclei of the thalamus, reaches the cingulum via anterior thalamic projections in the internal capsule, and finally loops back to the hippocampal formation via the parahippocampal gyrus and the entorhinal cortex. This view was adopted and enlarged by Paul MacLean in 1949, who proposed the concept of a visceral brain, consisting of the olfactory areas, cingulate gyrus, parahippocampal gyrus and hippocampus, as responsible for the basic functions of eating, drinking and sexual behaviour (Papez, 1937; MacLean, 1949; Papez, 1958). In subsequent publications, MacLean adopted the term proposed by Broca and defended the concept of a 'limbic system' (MacLean, 1978). Further studies showed that the original Papez's circuit is more particularly related to short-term memory than to emotion (Brodal, 1981).

The most recent international anatomical terminology grouped the cingulate and the parahippocampal gyri as composing the limbic lobe (Federative Committee on Anatomical Terminology, 1998). However, it is currently accepted that the structures that compose the limbic system itself can be characterised as a series of 'C'-shaped curves, centered on the thalamus and hypothalamus in each hemisphere. Anatomically, five 'C' curves can be described from medial to lateral (Williams and Warwick, 1980):

(1) cingulate gyrus and parahippocampal gyrus (Figure 4.5.3)

(2) medullary stria of the thalamus, habenular nuclei tract and interpeduncular tract

(3) centromedial amygdala, its dorsal component that characterises the stria terminalis and its sublentiform ventral component (all together corresponding to the extended amygdala)

(4) fimbria, crura, body and pillar of the fornix, which connect the hippocampus to the mamillary body

(5) hippocampus and longitudinal striae (induseum griseum), which connect the hippocampus with the paraterminal gyrus.

REFERENCES

Broca P (1877). Sur la circonvolution limbique et la scissure limbique. *Bull Soc d'Anth* 12: 646–657.

Brodal A (1981). *Neurological Anatomy in Relation to Clinical Medicine*, 3rd ed. Oxford University Press.

Catani M, Jones DK, ffytche DH (2005). Perisylvian language networks of the human brain. *Ann Neurol* 57(1): 8–16.

Duffau H (2008). The anatomo-functional connectivity of language revisited. New insights provided by electrostimulation and tractography. *Neuropsychologia* 46: 927–934.

Federative Committee on Anatomical Terminology (1998). *Terminologia Anatomica: International Anatomical Terminology*. Thieme.

MacLean PD (1949). Psychosomatic disease and the visceral brain: recent developments bearing on the Papez theory of emotion. *Psychosom Med* 11(6): 338–353.

MacLean PD (1978). Challenges of the Papez heritage. In Livingston KE, Hornykiewicz O, eds. *Limbic Mechanisms: The Continuing Evolution of the Limbic System Concept*. Plenum Press, pp. 1–15.

Makris N, Kennedy DN, McInerney S et al. (2005). Segmentation of subcomponents within the superior longitudinal fascicle in humans: a quantitative, in vivo, DT-MRI study. *Cereb Cortex* 15(6): 854–869.

Matsumoto M, Hikosaka O (2007). Lateral habenula as a source of negative reward signals in dopamine neurons. *Nature* 447: 1111–1115.

Papez J (1937). A proposed mechanism of emotion. *Arch Neurol Psychiatry* 38: 725–743.

Papez JW (1958). Visceral brain, its component parts and their connections. *J Nerv Ment Dis* 126(1): 40–55.

Ribas GC, ed. (2018). *Applied Cranial-Cerebral Anatomy*. Cambridge University Press.

Tavor I, Yablonski M, Mezer A, Rom S, Assaf Y, Yovel G. (2014) Separate parts of occipito-temporal white matter fibers are associated with recognition of faces and places. *Neuroimage* 86:123–30.

Thiebaut de Schotten M, Dell'Acqua F, Forkel SJ et al. (2011). A lateralized brain network for visuospatial attention. *Nat Neurosci* 14:1245–1246.

Williams PL, Warwick R, eds. (1980). *Gray's Anatomy*, 36th ed. Saunders.

4

4.6   **Ascending Neurotransmitter Systems**

Jeffrey W. Dalley and
Rebecca P. Lawson

OVERVIEW

In this section, we describe key functions of neurons in the brain that synthesise and release noradrenaline (NA), serotonin (5-hydroxytryptamine; 5-HT), dopamine (DA), and acetylcholine (ACh). As classic 'neuromodulators', these widely researched neurotransmitter systems ascend from posterior and ventral regions of the brain and work by optimising the performance of brain networks without inhibiting or exciting neurons directly. Traditionally considered in the context of 'non-specific' arousal states (i.e. sleep and wakefulness) and the 'reticular activating system' (Moruzzi and Magoun, 1949), the ascending neurotransmitter systems contribute to a surprisingly diverse array of behavioural and cognitive functions via specific pathways in the brain. These pathways arise from discrete clusters of neurons in the midbrain and forebrain (Figure 4.6.1). As the loci for clinically effective drugs to treat neuropsychiatric conditions such as depression, schizophrenia and attention deficit hyperactivity disorder, the ascending neurotransmitter systems are a major success story for the 'receptor revolution' in neuropsychiatry. For more on the synaptic physiology of these neurotransmitters, see Section 2.4.

4.6.1 Noradrenaline

Noradrenergic neurons arise from the blue-pigmented locus coeruleus in the brainstem and innervate wide expanses of the forebrain, including the entire cerebral cortex, amygdala, hippocampus and hypothalamus (Poe et al., 2020). Locus coeruleus neurons receive multiple inputs (e.g. medulla, amygdala, lateral hypothalamus, prefrontal cortex), and form a highly branched fibre system that innervates several regions of the brain simultaneously. Key to understanding their function, locus coeruleus neurons have different modes of activity, either transient **phasic activation** or longer-lasting **tonic activity** (see the glossary). These distinct states of activation fall on a continuum, from sleep and quiet wakefulness, to immediate stress-related

responses, to more intense behavioural reactions involving co-activation of the amygdala and other limbic regions (Atzori et al., 2016). Single neurons in the locus coeruleus respond best to stimulus intensity, as well as novelty and other highly salient stimuli. Locus coeruleus neurons facilitate the reliability of spike timing to sensory stimuli (Sara, 2009) and operate in a conditional manner to boost signal-to-noise processing in cortical regions; that is, how locus coeruleus activity affects other neurons is dependent not only on the sensory stimulus but also on its context. To illustrate this point, locus coeruleus stimulation enhanced the normal inhibitory response of hippocampus neurons to an arbitrary auditory tone in the rat. However, when the tone was paired with food, thus becoming a conditioned stimulus, the same auditory tone activated hippocampal neurons. This response was potentiated by concurrent locus coeruleus stimulation (Segal and Bloom, 1976).

GLOSSARY

Phasic neuronal activity reflects a rapid but relatively transient burst of action potentials from a neuron, often aligned to the onset of a salient stimulus, which increases the release of a neurotransmitter in terminal brain regions by many orders of magnitude.

Tonic neuronal activity reflects a spontaneous and continuous train of action potentials from a neuron, often driven by an underlying pacemaker-like current across the neuronal membrane, resulting in a steady background release of neurotransmitter in terminal brain regions.

Reward prediction error is the difference between a reward that is received and the reward that is predicted to be received, based on prior learning. When rewards are fully predicted, there is no reward prediction error, and dopaminergic neurons do not respond.

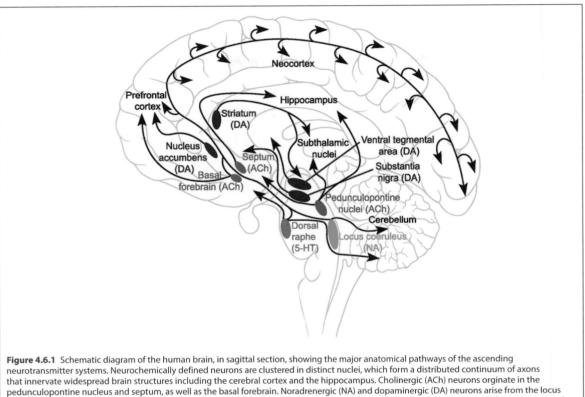

Figure 4.6.1 Schematic diagram of the human brain, in sagittal section, showing the major anatomical pathways of the ascending neurotransmitter systems. Neurochemically defined neurons are clustered in distinct nuclei, which form a distributed continuum of axons that innervate widespread brain structures including the cerebral cortex and the hippocampus. Cholinergic (ACh) neurons orginate in the pedunculopontine nucleus and septum, as well as the basal forebrain. Noradrenergic (NA) and dopaminergic (DA) neurons arise from the locus coeruleus and substantia nigra/ventral tegmental area, respectively. The latter then project to the striatum and nucleus accumbens. Serotonergic (5-HT) neurons arise in the raphe nucleus. Adapted from Mei et al. (2022).

The locus coeruleus–NA system, behind the blood–brain barrier, is analogous to the sympathetic nervous system in the periphery in that it uses similar catecholamine chemicals and responds quickly to real or perceived stressors in the environment which have behavioural relevance. However, on successful negotiation of the stressor, the locus coeruleus–NA system rapidly habituates, unlike the sympathetic nervous system. It is thought that this dynamic mode of activation signals sudden changes in the environment, which necessitate increased alertness and rapid learning, consistent with the hypothesised role of NA in encoding 'unexpected uncertainty' (Yu and Dayan, 2005). Accordingly, stressor-evoked changes in locus coeruleus–NA activity enable adaptive adjustments in alertness, increased attentional focus to contextually salient stimuli (Aston-Jones et al., 1999) and the consolidation of salient emotional memories (Cahill et al., 1994) – see Section 5.14 for more on memory consolidation. However, the adaptive role of NA in stress is self-limiting; in animals, chronic forms of uncontrollable stress

cause a sharp depletion of NA in the brain and produce behaviours resembling depression (Weiss et al., 1970). In humans, the misestimation of 'unexpected uncertainty' is also implicated in the pathophysiology of affective disorders (Browning et al., 2015). See Section 6.2 for more on the neurobiology of stress and Section 5.7 for more on the role of unexpected uncertainty in psychiatric disorders.

4.6.2 Serotonin

The brain serotonin (5-HT) systems arise from the raphe nuclei located along the midline of the brainstem. The dorsal and median raphe nuclei supply the majority of 5-HT fibres to the forebrain, including the amygdala, hippocampus, basal ganglia and hypothalamus, where transmission is mediated by a complex array of 5-HT receptors (Sharp and Barnes, 2020). 5-HT is uniform in its distribution in the cortex, but curiously is concentrated in occipital (visual) areas, where it is thought to play a role in enhancing thalamocortical transmission. Raphe nuclei neurons activate during movement and by intense visual stimuli but more classically during the transition from wakefulness to non-rapid-eye-movement (NREM) sleep. During rapid-eye-movement (REM) sleep, 5-HT neurons fall silent, so 5-HT is thought to play an inhibitory role in the switch from NREM to REM sleep. Other regulatory roles of 5-HT neurons include appetite control and energy balance via interactions with the hypothalamus and mood states, guided by 5-HT signalling in the limbic forebrain. Drugs that reduce 5-HT transmission cause hypophagia while drugs that boost synaptic levels of 5-HT (e.g. selective serotonin reuptake inhibitors) remediate depression but can also lead to weight gain. See Section 5.1 for more on appetite.

5-HT neurons play a key role in how individuals cope with stress. In situations that compromise stress controllability (i.e. when stressors are intense, unpredictable and unavoidable), the activity of raphe nuclei neurons greatly increases. These neurons are much less active if the stress is of equal intensity, but controllable. Effective stress coping depends on a specific pathway emanating from the medial prefrontal cortex that terminates in the raphe nuclei. Experiments in rats using intracerebral injections of muscimol to pharmacologically suppress the medial prefrontal cortex show that when stress is controllable, stress-induced activation of the raphe nuclei is inhibited by the prefrontal cortex, in turn blocking the behavioural effects of stress (Amat et al., 2005). This is consistent with the hypothesis that the prefrontal cortex signals and conveys to the 5-HT system how controllable a stressor is. In humans, the acute cortisol response to both physical and psychological stressors is associated with 5-HT receptor binding in many brain regions, including the medial prefrontal cortex (Steinberg et al., 2019), and reducing levels of 5-HT via tryptophan depletion lowers mood following an uncontrollable stress test. One intriguing possibility is that, if stress continues, 5-HT neurons eventually become 'exhausted' and release less neurotransmitter, which could in turn lead to maladaptive outcomes such as depression. Low levels of 5-HT are also linked to increased impulsivity, especially impulsive aggression, and cause individuals to become behaviourally disinhibited (Soubrie, 1986). In addition, selective depletion of 5-HT in the orbitofrontal cortex results in behavioural inflexibility, or an inability to adaptively switch when stimulus–reward associations are altered.

The myriad roles supported by 5-HT extend to learning and memory. Recognised by Kandel as a key neurotransmitter underlying learning in the sea mollusc *Aplysia*, selective 5-HT receptor ligands (e.g. 5-HT4, 5-HT6 and 5-HT7) have been widely researched as potential cognitive enhancers in schizophrenia and Alzheimer's disease (Svob Strac et al., 2016).

4.6.3 Dopamine

Dopamine is perhaps the most widely studied neurotransmitter in the brain. Formally identified as a neurotransmitter by Carlsson in the late 1950s, DA neurons form dense projections from the midbrain to the caudate, putamen (in rodents the dorsal striatum), nucleus accumbens (in rodents the ventral striatum) and the prefrontal cortex. Within the midbrain, DA cell bodies cluster to form two principal nuclei – the substantia nigra and ventral tegmental area – from which discrete pathways emerge. The nigrostriatal pathway, comprising substantia nigra DA axons, innervates the caudate and putamen and controls motor function and motor-skill learning. The nigrostriatal pathway selectively degenerates in Parkinson's disease. The ventral tegmental area projects to the frontal cortex, including the prefrontal cortex and cingulate gyrus, via the mesocortical pathway, but only sparsely innervates caudal regions of the cerebral cortex. Ventral tegmental area neurons also project to various structures involved in reward learning and motivation, namely the nucleus accumbens, amygdala, hippocampus and olfactory cortex via the mesolimbic pathway. DA neurons in the arcuate and periventricular nucleus of the hypothalamus merge within the tuberoinfundibular pathway to regulate the release of prolactin and other hormones from the pituitary gland.

Myriad functions have been ascribed to the DA systems and superficially these appear to reflect what their terminal regions do. For example, DA inputs to the anterior (frontal) parts of the cerebral cortex contribute to working memory, whereas DA inputs to the caudate and putamen support movement initiation and control, as well as habit-based learning. In more ventral regions of the striatum, mesolimbic DA neurons mediate the reinforcing and incentive motivational effects of natural and synthetic rewards (e.g. food, sex, drugs), including subjective feelings of 'wanting' as opposed to 'liking' (Morales and

Berridge, 2020). This division between wanting and liking reactions separates purely incentive-motivational processes (i.e. anticipation, excitement and even craving) from the hedonic (pleasurable) or desirable effects of rewards. However, it would be misleading to suggest that such functions are strictly localised to particular cortical and striatal regions, given the existence of topographically organised 'loops' connecting the cortex with the underlying striatum. Moreover, the caudate and putamen are not solely concerned with motor functions, and neurons responsive during working memory tasks also exist in the nucleus accumbens, a region that is not the exclusive repository of reward-sensitive neurons within the broader striatum. Such discrepancies question the logic of ascribing functions to DA based on the specific regions to which DA neurons project.

A broader consensus has been reached for DA functioning as a teaching signal. In a series of groundbreaking studies, Schultz showed that DA neurons respond with a burst of action potentials (a phasic-like response) when rewards are presented during the early stages of classical conditioning. However, with repeated pairings of a stimulus with reinforcement, DA neurons cease to respond, implying that DA neurons code a **reward prediction error** (Schultz, 2007) (see the glossary). This process is referred to as 'temporal difference learning' and may underlie the activation or invigoration of motor actions in the presence of reward-conditioned stimuli. This is distinct from the responses of the locus coeruleus–NA system, which is thought to signal when a previously learned association changes unexpectedly or becomes volatile. See Sections 5.7 and 5.9 for more on the role of DA in learning and reward. DA neurons also code reward uncertainty and respond to aversive stimuli, often with a decrease in activity. Thus, midbrain DA neurons are well placed to enable adaptive reinforcement learning to reward and punishment. The balance of these processes may underlie reward-related disorders such as drug addiction (see Section 9.3) and the motivational aspects of mood disorders (Section 5.13.4). See also Section 9.9.4 for the role of DA in psychosis.

4.6.4 Acetylcholine

Acetylcholinergic neurons are clustered in the brainstem within the pedunculopontine nucleus and laterodorsal tegmental nucleus and innervate regions including the thalamus, which mediate sleep, wakefulness, motor function, learning and reward. A second grouping of cholinergic neurons lie more anteriorly in the basal forebrain and include the nucleus basalis of Meynert (or magnocellularis in rats), diagonal band of Broca and the medial septum (Mesulam et al., 1983). The nucleus basalis of Meynert is implicated especially in attentional functions, mediated by the prefrontal and parietal cortices, and learning, dependent on the amygdala. Diagonal band neurons project to the neocortex and modulate recognition memory, dependent on the perirhinal cortex in the medial temporal lobe, whereas cholinergic neurons in the medial septum modulate cognitive functions, dependent on the hippocampus.

Interest in the brain cholinergic systems intensified in the mid-1970s following the discovery that ACh was depleted in the temporal neocortex of patients with Alzheimer's disease. The cholinergic hypothesis of Alzheimer's disease formalised a link between the degeneration of cholinergic fibres and some of the cognitive deficits of this disorder, including memory loss (Perry, 1986), and justified the use of cholinesterase inhibitors as therapeutic interventions to boost cholinergic function. However, early clinical trials appeared to show better effects for tests of attention than recognition memory, suggesting that the effects of cholinergic drugs depend on the precise extent of degenerative cell loss in different cortical regions, and therefore the time course of the disease. Nevertheless, cognitive deficits associated with dementia of the Lewy-body type and Parkinson's disease, where profound cortical cholinergic loss is evident, can be mitigated by anticholinesterase drugs. See Chapter 10 for more on ACh in neurodegenerative disorders.

The finding that the antimuscarinic agent scopolamine exerts rapid and sustained antidepressant and anti-anxiety effects led to renewed interest in the cholinergic system as a key player in the neurochemistry of major depression (Furey and Drevets, 2006); however, there is debate over whether these effects on mood actually result from indirect modulation of N-methyl-D-aspartate (NMDA) receptor function rather than effects on cholinergic signalling. Cholinergic drugs have also been proposed as a potential treatment for the general cognitive impairments seen in other psychiatric disorders such as schizophrenia, presumably via modulation of the brain's frontoparietal attention system. Several studies have shown that ACh acts on the sensory cortex to enhance the signal-to-noise ratio, consistent with heightened attention. Theoretical models of ACh function suggest that it also plays a crucial role in learning by reporting on 'expected uncertainty' – the reliability of specific cues within the environment (Yu and Dayan, 2005). Here, ACh is thought to work in concert with NA, which would signal when cues had become unreliable so as to suggest a change of context had occurred (cf. unexpected uncertainty; Figure 4.6.2).

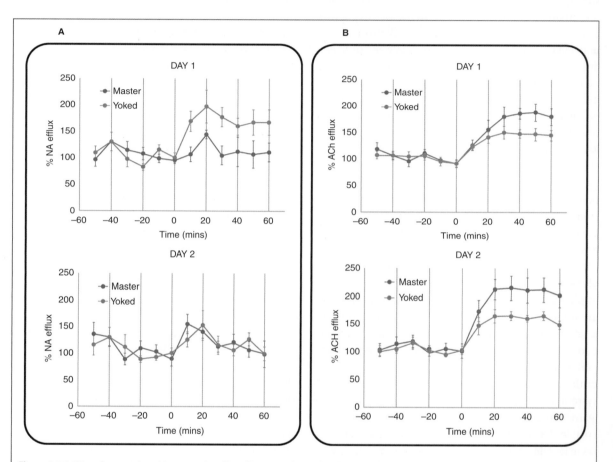

Figure 4.6.2 NA and uncertainty. Measuring the efflux of **(A)** NA and **(B)** ACh in the rat prefrontal cortex with the technique of in-vivo microdialysis. The Master animals (blue) are performing a sustained visual attention task, and receive rewards or punishment (no reward) if they make correct or incorrect responses, respectively. In contrast, the Yoked animals (orange) – having previously been trained to perform the task themselves – now unexpectedly only receive rewards or punishment in a manner controlled by the Master animals (i.e. there is a sudden change in context). In all cases the task starts at time 0, after a 60-minute baseline period. The Master animals must sustain attention across both day 1 and day 2 to perform the task, and show an increase in ACh efflux in both testing sessions but no change in NA. The Yoked animals show an increase in NA in Day 1 when they are adjusting to the new context, and this normalises by the second testing session on day 2. These data suggest that ACh is critically involved in the maintenance of attention and taskset in the Master animals (cf. expected uncertainty) whereas NA is signalling the sudden change in the task rules for the Yoked animals (cf. unexpected uncertainty). Adapted from Dalley et al. (2001).

Table 4.6.1 Main psychological and cognitive functions of the ascending neurotransmitters

Neurotransmitter	Key cognitive functions
Serotonin (5-HT)	Involved in emotion processing and mood. Strongly implicated in the pathogenesis of depression (some drugs used for depression raise serotonin levels) and how individuals cope with stress (especially uncontrollable stress). Also critically involved in the regulation of sleep and appetite. Low 5-HT has also been associated with impulsivity, behavioural inflexibility and risk-taking behaviour.
Dopamine (DA)	Strongly associated with reward mechanisms in the brain, especially the computation of surprise – or prediction errors – involved in reward and punishment learning. Elevated DA has been associated with schizophrenia; some drugs used for psychosis block the action of DA. Also linked to general salience processing, uncertainty and the invigoration of behaviour towards motivationally relevant stimuli.
Noradrenaline (NA)	Plays a key role in stress and the adaptive responses to stressors in the environment. Drugs targeting the reuptake of both 5-HT and NA are widely used to treat a range of psychiatric disorders including depression. Supports the adaptive processing of salient stimuli that command attention and increase arousal. Theoretically linked to encoding 'unexpected uncertainty' – sudden changes in context that indicate the need for new learning.
Acetylcholine (ACh)	Responsible for some memory functions and linked to the cognitive impairments associated with Alzheimer's disease. Has consistently been implicated in the maintenance of attention and boosting the signal-to-noise-ratio of sensory processing (similar to NA). Critically involved in 'expected uncertainty' of learning. Drugs acting on the ACh system are used to treat the cognitive impairments associated with some neuropsychiatric disorders.

Conclusions

The overlapping and broadly distributed nature of pathways established by the ascending neurotransmitter systems (Table 4.6.1) belie their remarkable functional specificity in the central nervous system. Their nuclei of origin integrate diverse inputs from sensory, limbic and cortical regions of the brain, and optimise perceptual, cognitive and behavioural aspects of brain function by broadcasting neurochemical signals throughout the forebrain. Rather than conveying hard-wired 'information', the ascending neurotransmitters can more intuitively be conceptualised as 'switches' or teaching signals, which alter the state of brain networks (Azizi, 2020). A clearer understanding of how each of the ascending neurotransmitter systems optimises the computations carried out by their terminal fields may yield deeper insights into a range of neuropsychiatric disorders in which impaired chemical neuromodulation is implicated.

REFERENCES

Amat J, Baratta MV, Paul E et al. (2005). Medial prefrontal cortex determines how stressor controllability affects behavior and dorsal raphe nucleus. *Nat Neurosci* 8(3): 365–371. doi:10.1038/nn1399

Aston-Jones G, Rajkowski J, Cohen J (1999). Role of locus coeruleus in attention and behavioral flexibility. *Biol Psychiatry* 46(9): 1309–1320. doi:10.1016/s0006-3223(99)00140-7

Atzori M, Cuevas-Olguin R, Esquivel-Rendon E et al. (2016). Locus ceruleus norepinephrine release: a central regulator of CNS spatio-temporal activation? *Front Synaptic Neurosci* 8: 25. doi:10.1177/1073858420974336

Azizi SA (2020). Monoamines: dopamine, norepinephrine, and serotonin, beyond modulation, "switches" that alter the state of target networks. *Neuroscientist* 28(2) doi:10.1177/1073858420974336

Browning M, Behrens TE, Jocham G, O'Reilly JX, Bishop SJ (2015). Anxious individuals have difficulty learning the causal statistics of aversive environments. *Nat Neurosci* 18(4): 590–596. doi:10.1038/nn.3961

Cahill L, Prins B, Weber M, McGaugh JL (1994). Beta-adrenergic activation and memory for emotional events. *Nature* 371(6499): 702–704. doi:10.1038/371702a0

Dalley JW, McGaughy J, O'Connell MT et al. (2001). Distinct changes in cortical acetylcholine and noradrenaline efflux during contingent and noncontingent performance of a visual attentional task. *J Neurosci* 21(13): 4908–4914. www.ncbi.nlm.nih.gov/pubmed/11425918

Furey ML, Drevets WC (2006). Antidepressant efficacy of the antimuscarinic drug scopolamine: a randomized, placebo-controlled clinical trial. *Arch Gen Psychiatry* 63(10): 1121–1129. doi:10.1001/archpsyc.63.10.1121

Mei J, Muller E, Ramaswamy S (2022). Informing deep neural networks by multiscale principles of neuromodulatory systems. *Trends Neurosci* 45(3): 237–250. doi: 10.1016/j.tins.2021.12.008

Mesulam MM, Mufson EJ, Wainer BH, Levey AI (1983). Central cholinergic pathways in the rat: an overview based on an alternative nomenclature (Ch1-Ch6). *Neuroscience* 10(4): 1185–1201. doi:10.1016/0306-4522(83)90108-2

Morales I, Berridge KC (2020). 'Liking' and 'wanting' in eating and food reward: brain mechanisms and clinical implications. *Physiol Behav* 227: 113152. doi:10.1016/j.physbeh.2020.113152

Moruzzi G, Magou HW (1949). Brain stem reticular formation and activation of the EEG. *Electroencephalogr Clin Neurophysiol* 1(4): 455–473. www.ncbi.nlm.nih.gov/pubmed/18421835

Perry EK (1986). The cholinergic hypothesis ten years on. *Br Med Bull* 42(1): 63–69. doi:10.1093/oxfordjournals.bmb.a072100

Poe GR, Foote S, Eschenk O et al. (2020). Locus coeruleus: a new look at the blue spot. *Nat Rev Neurosci* 21(11): 644–659. doi:10.1038/s41583-020-0360-9

Sara SJ (2009). The locus coeruleus and noradrenergic modulation of cognition. *Nat Rev Neurosci* 10(3): 211–223. doi:10.1038/nrn2573

Schultz W (2007). Behavioral dopamine signals. *Trends Neurosci* 30(5): 203–210. doi:10.1016/j.tins.2007.03.007

Segal M, Bloom FE (1976). The action of norepinephrine in the rat hippocampus. IV. The effects of locus coeruleus stimulation on evoked hippocampal unit activity. *Brain Res* 107(3): 513–525. doi:10.1016/0006-8993(76)90141-4

Sharp T, Barnes NM (2020). Central 5-HT receptors and their function: present and future. *Neuropharmacology* 177: 108155. doi:10.1016/j.neuropharm.2020.108155

Soubrie P (1986). [Serotonergic neurons and behavior]. *J Pharmacol* 17(2): 107–112. www.ncbi.nlm.nih.gov/pubmed/2875217

Steinberg LJ, Rubin-Falcone H, Galfalvy HC et al. (2019). Cortisol stress response and in vivo PET imaging of human brain serotonin 1A receptor binding. *Int J Neuropsychopharmacol* 22(5): 329–338. doi:10.1093/ijnp/pyz009

Svob Strac D, Pivac N, Muck-Seler D (2016). The serotonergic system and cognitive function. *Transl Neurosci* 7(1): 35–49. doi:10.1515/tnsci-2016-0007

Weiss JM, Stone EA, Harrell N (1970). Coping behavior and brain norepinephrine level in rats. *J Comp Physiol Psychol* 72(1) 153–160. doi:10.1037/h0029311

Yu AJ, Dayan P (2005). Uncertainty, neuromodulation, and attention. *Neuron* 46(4): 681–692. doi:10.1016/j.neuron.2005.04.026

4

5

Neural Circuits

| 5.1 | **Appetite** | I. Sadaf Farooqi |

OVERVIEW

Clinically, it is well recognised that neuropsychiatric disorders – and the drugs we use to treat them – frequently affect appetite. While our precise understanding of how specific disorders affect appetite and weight regulation is still at an early stage, we now have a framework that can in part explain the findings from genetic, experimental and clinical studies. The ultimate goal of eating is to obtain and then store enough energy to survive and reproduce as a species – as such, the neural circuits that defend against starvation are hard-wired in our brains. Adipose tissue-derived hormones, which provide information about nutritional state and hormonal and neural signals generated by meal consumption, act in combination on neuronal circuits in the hypothalamus and brainstem which express specific receptors and ion channels on their cell surface (Figure 5.1.1). The function of these neurons can also be regulated by a range of neurotransmitters (e.g. serotonin, dopamine, histamine, noradrenaline), which are released by neurons that project widely throughout the brain. In this way the neural circuits which regulate appetite are intricately connected to the circuits that regulate mood, anxiety and behaviour.

5.1.1 The Neuroanatomy of Appetite

The primary function of the hypothalamus is to maintain homeostasis by integrating internal and external sensory inputs and then modulating pituitary hormone secretion, autonomic nervous system activation and behaviour to restore physiological set-points. Hypothalamic appetite circuits receive inputs from, and project to, multiple parts of the brain, allowing them to respond to innate biological signals and environmental cues (such as sight, smell and taste) to modulate hunger (drive to eat) and satiety (fullness after a meal), to maintain body weight over time (Waterson and Horvath, 2015). In addition to this homeostatic regulation of eating behaviour driven by energy demands, hedonic food intake (i.e. consumption of food beyond the need for energy), in response to the rewarding properties of food, is an important contributor to appetite (Kenny, 2011). Imaging studies in humans and and experimental studies in animals have indicated that food reward is encoded by opioidergic pathways mediating liking (pleasure/palatability), whereas the wanting

of food (incentive motivation) appears to be mediated by dopaminergic circuits (Berridge, 1996; Pecina et al., 2003). Activation of midbrain dopaminergic neurons has been implicated in the motivating, rewarding, reinforcing and incentive salience properties of natural stimuli such as food and water, as well as drugs of abuse. See Section 4.6.3 for more on dopaminergic pathways and Section 5.9 for their role in reward.

5.1.2 Leptin: The Master Regulator of Appetite

The molecular mechanisms by which appetite and weight are regulated were first revealed in 1994, with the discovery of the hormone leptin. Leptin is made in adipose tissue in proportion to the amount of fat stored, and it circulates in the blood to reach the brain. Mice that are unable to make leptin due to a genetic defect (*ob/ob* mice) exhibit an intense drive to eat and develop severe obesity, which can be reversed by central injections of leptin (i.e. injections into the brain). Similarly, children with homozygous

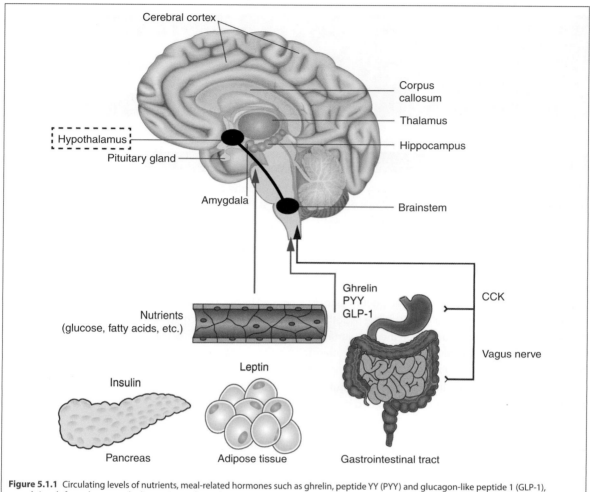

Figure 5.1.1 Circulating levels of nutrients, meal-related hormones such as ghrelin, peptide YY (PYY) and glucagon-like peptide 1 (GLP-1), neural signals from the gut and adipose tissue-derived hormones such as leptin act on neurons in the hypothalamus to regulate appetite. These hypothalamic circuits project to other brain regions as shown.

mutations that disrupt the production of leptin have intense hyperphagia leading to severe childhood-onset obesity, which can be reversed by synthetic leptin therapy (van der Klaauw and Farooqi, 2015). Leptin's physiological role is to signal nutritional depletion, such that fasting or weight loss results in a fall in leptin levels, which then triggers an increase in energy intake and reduced energy expenditure to restore energy homeostasis. Leptin levels fall in people who diet and in those who lose weight. This fall in leptin triggers hyperphagia and rebound weight gain (commonly referred to as yo-yo dieting). However, the rebound hyperphagia triggered by a fall in leptin levels appears to be suppressed in disorders such as anorexia nervosa or severe depression, where a loss of

appetite and low body weight can be maintained for long periods of time. These observations suggest that brain regions outside of the hypothalamus can, in certain disorders or physiological states, suppress the normal adaptive response to nutrient deprivation. The mechanisms by which they do so are unknown to date. Leptin is a permissive factor for the development of puberty and for the maintence of fertility. As such, low leptin levels in women with anorexia nervosa explain amennorhoea, which can be reversed with weight regain and/or leptin supplementation in clinical trials (Welt et al., 2004).

As the key signal of nutritional state, leptin also plays a role in food reward. In the absence of leptin, functional MRI studies have shown that images of any food elicit high liking scores and marked activation of the antero-medial ventral striatum (nucleus accumbens and caudate nucleus) and posterolateral ventral striatum (putamen and globus pallidus) (Farooqi et al., 2007), brain regions known to be involved in reward-related behaviours. Treatment with leptin in this setting increases the ability to discriminate between the rewarding properties of food and, at the neuronal level, reduces activation in the ventral striatum. These findings are consistent with experiments in animals which show that leptin plays a role in mediating the rewarding properties of food by changing the electrical activity of dopaminergic neurons (DiLeone et al., 2012). Thus, in people who are dieting or deprived of nutrients (or have no leptin), food is intensely rewarding (often described as cravings). This behavioural response facilitates the drive to seek food to restore energy homeostasis. Leptin levels are high in most obese people and in this group treatment with additional leptin does not lead to weight loss, in keeping with leptin's primary role being to defend against starvation.

5.1.3 Leptin-Responsive Neural Circuits

The physiological effects of leptin are mediated through neural circuits in the hypothalamus and other brain regions,

where the leptin receptor is highly expressed. Hunger is modulated by the effects of leptin on primary neurons in the hypothalamus, which express pro-opiomelanocortin (POMC), which is processed to yield melanocortin peptides (alpha-, beta- and gamma-melanocyte stimulating hormone). These bind to melanocortin 4 receptors (MC4R), expressed on second-order neurons (Figure 5.1.2); their activation decreases food intake (see Section 2.5 for more on neuropeptides). Inherited mutations that disrupt POMC, MC4R (the commonest genetic cause of obesity) and other genes in this pathway can cause severe childhood-onset obesity characterised by increased hunger and impaired satiety (van der Klaauw and Farooqi, 2015). Interestingly, this pathway is also involved in food preference. In clinical studies, MC4R deficiency is associated with an increased preference for dietary fat and a reduced preference for sucrose (van der Klaauw et al., 2016). The neural mechanisms that mediate these behaviours are not known although studies in rodents have implicated regions such as the amygdala, nucleus accumbens and parabrachial nucleus (Figure 5.1.3). There is evidence from imaging studies that these and other pathways are disrupted in neurodegenerative disorders such as frontotemporal dementia, which is characterised by a marked preference for sweet foods (Ahmed et al., 2014).

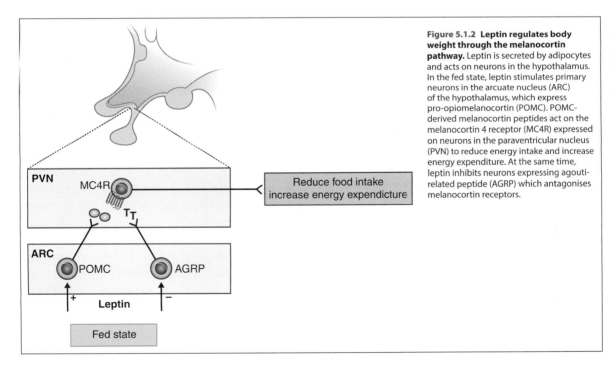

Figure 5.1.2 Leptin regulates body weight through the melanocortin pathway. Leptin is secreted by adipocytes and acts on neurons in the hypothalamus. In the fed state, leptin stimulates primary neurons in the arcuate nucleus (ARC) of the hypothalamus, which express pro-opiomelanocortin (POMC). POMC-derived melanocortin peptides act on the melanocortin 4 receptor (MC4R) expressed on neurons in the paraventricular nucleus (PVN) to reduce energy intake and increase energy expenditure. At the same time, leptin inhibits neurons expressing agouti-related peptide (AGRP) which antagonises melanocortin receptors.

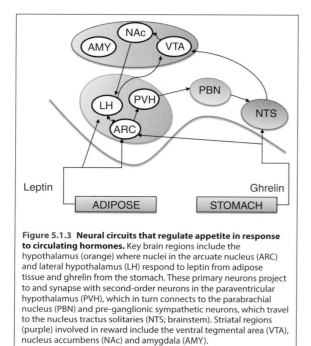

Figure 5.1.3 Neural circuits that regulate appetite in response to circulating hormones. Key brain regions include the hypothalamus (orange) where nuclei in the arcuate nucleus (ARC) and lateral hypothalamus (LH) respond to leptin from adipose tissue and ghrelin from the stomach. These primary neurons project to and synapse with second-order neurons in the paraventricular hypothalamus (PVH), which in turn connects to the parabrachial nucleus (PBN) and pre-ganglionic sympathetic neurons, which travel to the nucleus tractus solitaries (NTS; brainstem). Striatal regions (purple) involved in reward include the ventral tegmental area (VTA), nucleus accumbens (NAc) and amygdala (AMY).

Neurons in the hypothalamic melanocortin pathway project throughout the brain and are themselves modulated by neurons which arise in other brain regions. An increasing understanding of these neural connections is providing new insights into the multiple links that exist between brain pathways which regulate appetite and those which regulate mood, anxiety and behaviour. Disruption of these neural pathways in some genetic disorders can result in disordered appetite (usually hyperphagia) and disordered behaviour. For example, Prader–Willi syndrome is caused by chromosomal deletions that result in the loss of neurons expressing brain-derived neurotrophic factor and oxytocin, two molecules which regulate appetite, weight, social interaction and aggressive behaviour. Patients have hyerphagia from childhood and a spectrum of behavioural conditions.

5.1.4 Peripheral Peptides That Affect Appetite

Peripheral peptides such as cholecystokinin from the stomach, glucagon-like peptide 1 (GLP-1) and gastric inhibitory polypeptide from entero-endocrine cells of the small intestine, insulin from the pancreas and peptide YY and oxytomodulin from the large intestine

are secreted in response to eating a meal and/or the presence of nutrients in the intestinal lumen. Their release contributes to satiety and meal termination, together with neural signals from the vagus nerve (which innervates the digestive system) and the enteric nervous system (a mesh-like system of neurons in the gastrointestinal tract, which can act relatively independently of the brain) (Clemmensen et al., 2017) (Figure 5.1.1). Ghrelin is a hormone produced by entero-endocrine cells, mainly in the stomach, and increases food intake – it is often known as the 'hunger hormone'. Infusion studies in healthy volunteers have shown that ghrelin and other gut-derived regulators of energy homeostasis also act on brain reward circuits, most notably on the mesoaccumbens dopamine system, to increase or decrease the incentive value of food depending on energy requirements (Malik et al., 2008).

5.1.5 Drugs That Affect Appetite and Mood

Many centrally acting drugs used in the treatment of neurological and psychiatric disorders target neurotransmitters and neuropeptides that are involved in the regulation of appetite – opioid receptors, dopamine, serotonin and/or noradrenaline – with the broad principle being to increase concentrations at the synaptic cleft. Commonly prescribed drugs with antidepressant and anxiolytic action, such as selective serotonin reuptake inhibitors (SSRIs), often affect appetite. This is not surprising as, in addition to their involvement in anxiety, fear and emotion (Marcinkiewcz et al., 2016), serotoninergic neurons play a critical role in the suppression of eating, acting through the serotonin 2C (5-HT2C) receptor, which is expressed on melanocortin circuits (Marston et al., 2011). As such, some SSRIs, e.g. fluoxetine, increase the amount of serotonin that is available to act at the 5-HT2C receptor, thereby causing decreased appetite. Indeed, agonists of this receptor have been used as weight-loss treatments in obesity. Serotonin and noradrenaline reuptake inhibitors (e.g. venlafaxine) can affect appetite and may also increase lipolysis (fat utilisation) to decrease weight by enhancing release of noradrenaline in sympathetically innervated tissues such as adipose tissue. In clinical practice, it can be challenging to predict the effect of a particular drug with antidepressant/anxiolytic action on appetite and weight as many of these drugs lack specificity and therefore target multiple receptors, which can have opposing effects, leading to weight gain in some patients and weight loss in others. Drugs that inhibit monoamine oxidase (MAO inhibitors), the enzyme that breaks down serotonin, noradrenaline and dopamine, similarly can affect appetite and weight. Drugs used for depression such as mirtazapine have a different mechanism of action, which is likely to explain why patients often have increased appetite and gain weight. Mirtazapine blocks presynaptic alpha-2-adrenergic autoreceptors, increasing the release of noradrenaline, and blocks 5-HT2 and 5-HT3 receptors. Bupropion inhibits the reuptake of both noradrenaline and dopamine and can be used for weight-loss therapy. Notably, the combination of bupropion and naltrexone, an opioid receptor antagonist with high affinity for the mu-opioid receptor, increases the activity of POMC neurons to the extent that it has been used as a treatment for obesity.

Second-generation drugs with antipsychotic action are well known to cause increased hunger and weight gain (in up to 60% of patients). While the majority of drugs in this class act by inhibiting dopaminergic transmission, many (including clozapine and olanzapine, which have the most weight-promoting effects) have additional antagonistic effects on serotonin, histamine and muscarinic cholinergic receptors. The discovery that people with mutations in the 5-HT2C receptor develop hyperphagia and obesity and social anxiety demonstrates that this particular receptor plays a critical role in mediating anxiety. These studies may pave the way for the design of more specific drugs which target some receptor subtypes but not others, allowing for greater clinical precision. These findings have additional relevance as the degree of 5-HT2C receptor antagonism associated with drugs used for psychosis in cells correlates with the degree of weight gain seen when those drugs are used in clinical studies (Matsui-Sakata et al., 2005) and in clinical practice. 5-HT2C receptors also play a role in the handling of glucose by the liver, which may explain the increased risk of type 2 diabetes in people chronically treated with these drugs.

Many drugs of abuse also target the same neural pathways. The well-known appetite-stimulating effects of plant-derived cannabinoids are mediated by the cannabinoid receptor type 1 (CB1R) in the hypothalamus and brainstem, which modulates eating behaviour in response to both leptin and ghrelin (Koch, 2017). Based on this known mechanism of action, the CB1R antagonist rimonabant was proposed as a treatment for obesity. In clinical trials, it was shown to be effective, but in clinical practice the drug caused low mood and increased suicidal ideation, which ultimately led to its withdrawal from use (King, 2010). Several drugs used in the treatment of epilepsy, such as sodium valproate, can cause weight gain by increasing levels of the inhibitory neurotransmitter gamma-aminobutyric acid. Sodium valproate also blocks voltage-gated ion channels, thereby altering the function of multiple neuronal populations at the same time. Cumulatively, it is clear that there is a substantial unmet need for drugs which more precisely target the receptors and neuronal populations whose function is affected in a particular condition to deliver safe and effective treatments for patients.

5.1.6 Appetite and Thirst

The hypothalamus plays a critical role in the regulation of thirst and fluid balance. Our classical framework for understanding thirst has focused on homeostatic mechanisms, which drive increased intake of water in response to a fall in blood osmolality and increased intake of both water and salts to recover blood volume (detected by changes in serum sodium levels). Dehydration or volume loss lead to the release of antidiuretic hormone (ADH or vasopressin) by the pituitary gland which causes water reabsorption by the kidney, concentrating the urine until fluids are consumed. However, recent studies using sophisticated genetic tools applied to study neurons within the lamina terminalis in mice have shown that there is a network of neurons in the subfornical organ, the organum vasculosum lamina terminalis and the median preoptic nucleus which can regulate drinking behaviour in animals that are not dehydrated. Some of these neural circuits express receptors which are known to regulate hunger and fullness, such as the GLP-1 receptor, providing the first insights into circuits which link eating and drinking. It is now clear that there are circuits which mediate the action of drinking/gulping water and additional circuits which regulate fluid intake to correct dehydration (Zimmerman et al., 2017). This emerging area of research has the potential to provide insights into clinical disorders, such as psychogenic polydipsia, which are poorly understood at present.

Conclusions and Outstanding Questions

In summary, as we build a detailed understanding of the neural circuits that regulate appetite, there remains a clear need to understand how those circuits can be targeted in a specific way to develop safe and effective medicines for neuropsychiatric disease whilst minimising effects on appetite and weight that will invariably occur when shared pathways are targeted. Similarly, drugs that target these pathways for obesity often have effects on mood and behaviour. Neurotransmitters like dopamine, serotonin and noradrenaline act on a myriad of receptors that are expressed on neurons in many brain regions. These ciruits are involved in arousal, movement and appetite – behaviours that are fundamental for survival. They are hard-wired in the brain but their activation and inhibition can also be modulated by environmental and physiological stimuli. Understanding how these pathways work, how their function is disturbed in health (e.g. stress, nutrient deprivation) and in disease will be vital to finding new ways to both prevent and treat disorders of brain development, neuropsychiatric and neurodegenerative disease as well as severe obesity.

Outstanding Questions

- How do concentrations of neurotransmitters and their function change at the onset and during the course of neuropsychiatric disease?

- Which receptors mediate these effects and how can they be targeted to design safer, more effective drugs?

- Can combination therapy offset the weight gain seen in patients treated with drugs with antipsychotic action and will this improve adherence with treatment?

- Why and how does disruption of these circuits cause such a heterogeneous clinical presentation?

Addressing these questions may pave the way for a better understanding of the fundamental mechanisms that underpin common neuropsychiatric disorders and the mechanism of action of treatments.

REFERENCES

Ahmed RM, Irish M, Kam J et al. (2014). Quantifying the eating abnormalities in frontotemporal dementia. *JAMA Neurol* 71: 1540–1546.

Berridge KC (1996). Food reward: brain substrates of wanting and liking. *Neurosci Biobehav Rev* 20: 1–25.

Clemmensen C, Muller TD, Woods SC et al. (2017). Gut–brain cross-talk in metabolic control. *Cell* 168: 758–774.

Dileone RJ, Taylor JR, Picciotto MR (2012). The drive to eat: comparisons and distinctions between mechanisms of food reward and drug addiction. *Nat Neurosci* 15: 1330–1335.

Farooqi IS, Bullmore E, Keogh J et al. (2007). Leptin regulates striatal regions and human eating behavior. *Science* 317: 1355.

Kenny PJ (2011). Reward mechanisms in obesity: new insights and future directions. *Neuron* 69: 664–679.

King A (2010). Neuropsychiatric adverse effects signal the end of the line for rimonabant. *Nature Rev Cardiol* 7: 602.

Koch M (2017). Cannabinoid receptor signaling in central regulation of feeding behavior: a mini-review. *Front Neurosci* 11: 293.

Malik S, Mcglone F, Bedrossian D, Dagher A (2008). Ghrelin modulates brain activity in areas that control appetitive behavior. *Cell Metab* 7: 400–409.

Marcinkiewcz CA, Mazzone CM, D'Agostino G et al. (2016). Serotonin engages an anxiety and fear-promoting circuit in the extended amygdala. *Nature* 537: 97–101.

Marston OJ, Garfield AS, Heisler LK (2011). Role of central serotonin and melanocortin systems in the control of energy balance. *Eur J Pharmacol* 660: 70–79.

Matsui-Sakata A, Ohtani H, Sawada Y (2005). Receptor occupancy-based analysis of the contributions of various receptors to antipsychotics-induced weight gain and diabetes mellitus. *Drug Metab Pharmacokinet* 20: 368–378.

Pecina S, Cagniard B, Berridge KC, Aldridge JW, Zhuang X (2003). Hyperdopaminergic mutant mice have higher "wanting" but not "liking" for sweet rewards. *J Neurosci* 23: 9395–9402.

van der Klaauw AA, Farooqi IS (2015). The hunger genes: pathways to obesity. *Cell* 161: 119–132.

van der Klaauw AA, Keogh JM, Henning E et al. (2016). Divergent effects of central melanocortin signalling on fat and sucrose preference in humans. *Nat Commun* 7: 13055.

Waterson MJ, Horvath TL (2015). Neuronal regulation of energy homeostasis: beyond the hypothalamus and feeding. *Cell Metab* 22: 962–970.

Welt CK, Chan JL, Bullen J et al. (2004). Recombinant human leptin in women with hypothalamic amenorrhea. *N Engl J Med* 351: 987–997.

Zimmerman CA, Leib DE, Knight ZA (2017). Neural circuits underlying thirst and fluid homeostasis. *Nat Rev Neurosci* 18(8): 459–469.

National Neuroscience Curriculum Initiative online resources

Eat to Live or Live to Eat? The Neurobiology of Appetite Regulation

Kathryn R. Kinasz, David A. Ross and Joseph J. Cooper

Clinical neuroscience conversations: *The Neuroscience Behind Appetite*

Kathryn Kinasz, MD and Joseph Cooper

Ute Stead and Stephen M. Stahl

5.2 Sleep

OVERVIEW

Sleep is a naturally recurring state of reduced activity and altered consciousness, which is relatively easily reversible [1–3]. While asleep, our awareness and ability to respond to stimuli are decreased. For centuries, sleep was considered a passive state with an unknown function [4]. However, in contrast to outer appearances, sleep is an active brain state with distinct changes in brain wave activity and physiological function, accompanying the different stages of sleep [1–5]. It is only in recent decades that we have started to uncover some of the complex neural systems underlying the regulation of sleep, although many aspects still remain a mystery [4, 6, 7]. In this section we look at the characteristics of sleep and its different stages. This is followed by an outline of the neural circuits involved in regulation of sleep, wakefulness and arousal, and the mechanisms underlying the circadian rhythm. Finally, the effects of sleep deprivation are discussed. Sleep disorders, the role of sleep in psychiatric conditions and the effects of medication on sleep will be discussed in a later chapter, in Section 9.16.

5.2.1 Stages of Sleep and Assessment of Sleep

The first neurophysiological evidence of differing brain activity between wakefulness and sleep was recorded with electroencephalography (EEG) in 1928 by Hans Berger [4]. In 1953, Kleitman and Aserinsky described two different aspects of the sleep state by monitoring eye movements and EEG patterns: rapid eye movement (REM) sleep, with characteristic saccadic eye movements, and non-rapid-eye-movement (NREM) sleep [4].

Today, it is possible to examine sleep stages and sleep disorders in far greater detail through the use of polysomnography. This involves an overnight sleep study, during which brain activity is monitored by EEG, eye movements are recorded by electro-oculogram and muscle activity by electromyogram. Breathing (effort sensor), oxygen saturation (pulse oximeter), heart rate and rhythm (ECG) are also monitored (Figure 5.2.1) [8, 9].

Humans undergo several sleep cycles throughout the night. A sleep cycle usually starts with NREM sleep, which progresses through stages N1–3, representing increased depths of sleep [1–3]. The cycle then reverses and moves from deep to lighter sleep, which is then followed by a period of REM sleep. NREM and REM sleep alternate in cycles taking about 90 minutes. REM sleep increases in length and frequency towards the morning, while deep sleep reduces [1, 2, 8]. Brief awakenings are a normal aspect of sleep and usually occur during the lighter sleep stages or following REM sleep. Sleep patterns and requirements change over the lifespan, with total sleep time and the proportions of both REM and deep sleep all decreasing with advancing age [1].

The pattern of sleep stages is referred to as 'sleep architecture' and can be depicted in a hypnogram, showing stages of NREM sleep (N1-3) alternating with REM sleep (Figure 5.2.2) [1–3, 8].

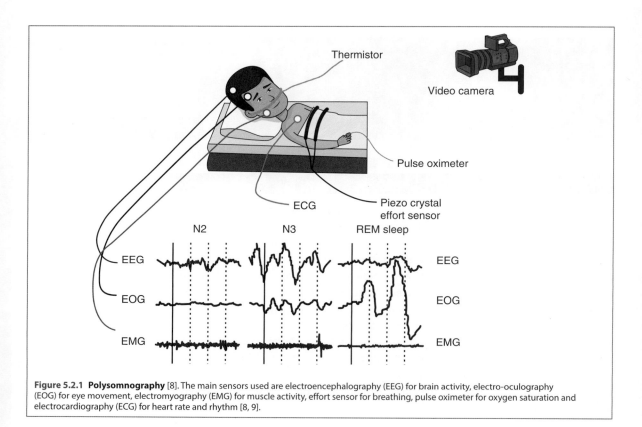

Figure 5.2.1 Polysomnography [8]. The main sensors used are electroencephalography (EEG) for brain activity, electro-oculography (EOG) for eye movement, electromyography (EMG) for muscle activity, effort sensor for breathing, pulse oximeter for oxygen saturation and electrocardiography (ECG) for heart rate and rhythm [8, 9].

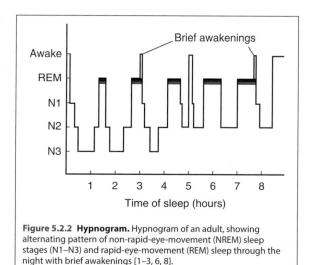

Figure 5.2.2 Hypnogram. Hypnogram of an adult, showing alternating pattern of non-rapid-eye-movement (NREM) sleep stages (N1–N3) and rapid-eye-movement (REM) sleep through the night with brief awakenings [1–3, 6, 8].

A summary of characteristics and key features of the sleep stages can be found in Table 5.2.1.

5.2.2 Two-Process Model of Sleep Regulation

The two-process model suggests two separate processes which interact in a synergistic way [11, 12] (Figure 5.2.3):

- The **homeostatic sleep drive (process S)** builds up during wakefulness throughout the day and dissipates while asleep at night [1, 13]. Slow-wave (or delta-) sleep increases with time spent awake and is a marker for the homeostatic sleep drive [11]. Rising adenosine levels seem to be involved in increasing sleep drive (see Section 5.2.3.2).

- The **circadian process (process C)** promotes wakefulness during the day and sleep at night [11]. The suprachiasmatic nucleus plays an important role in coordinating the circadian rhythm (see Subsection 5.2.4). Melatonin and core body temperature are its main markers. Melatonin secretion starts at onset of darkness, peaks in the early hours of the morning and subsides at dawn. It is inhibited by light [1, 13]. Core body temperature reduces overnight [11].

Table 5.2.1 A summary of different sleep stages [1–3, 6, 9, 10]

Stage	Typical relationship to total sleep time	EEG		Associated features
Wakefulness	Variable	Relaxed wakefulness Eyes closed: predominantly occipital alpha rhythm (8–13 Hz) [2, 9, 10] Eyes open: low voltage, mixed frequency [9]		- Voluntary movements - Rapid eye movements, blinking (eyes open) [2, 9, 10] - No or slow eye movements (eyes closed) [2, 9] - Normal or increased muscle tone [2, 9, 10]
N1	5% [2]	Low voltage, mixed frequency [3, 8, 10] Disappearance of alpha waves and emergence of theta waves (4–7 Hz) [2, 9, 10]		- Easily roused [4] - Slow eye movements [2, 9, 10] - Decrease in muscle tone [2, 9, 10] - Hypnic myoclonus at sleep onset [2, 4] - Stage increased in disturbed sleep [2] - Not considered restorative [2]
N2	50% [2]	Low voltage, mixed frequency [8] Sleep spindles and K-complexes [2, 4, 9, 10]		- Intermediate sleep stage [4] - Low muscle tone [2, 9, 10] - Movements common [4] - Reduced sympathetic tone [6] - Reduced heart rate [3, 4] - Lowered body temperature [3, 4] - Relative autonomic stability [3]
N3	12.5–20% [2] Mostly present in first half of the night [2]	High voltage, slow frequency: Delta waves (0.5–2 Hz) [4, 10]		- Deepest sleep stage [2, 3] - Requires higher stimulus for arousal than other stages [2, 3, 6] - Also referred to as 'slow wave sleep (SWS)', or delta sleep [3, 4] - Duration is linked to prior time awake ('homeostatic sleep pressure') and reduces over course of the night, reflecting dissipating sleep need [6] - Movements uncommon [4] - Low muscle tone [9, 10] - No eye movements [9, 10] - Parasomnias more common [4] - Considered most restorative sleep stage [2]
R (REM sleep)	20–25% [4] More prominent in last third of the night, with increasing duration and frequency [2, 6]	Low voltage, mixed frequency activity [9] Desynchronised pattern [9] Possible alpha waves (similar to waking, but 1–2 Hz slower) [2, 9, 10] Possible 'sawtooth' waves [9, 10]		- Follows N2 sleep stage [6] - Most dreaming occurs in this stage ('dream sleep') [3, 4, 6] - Variation in sympathetic activity, with irregular heart rate and breathing [2, 4, 6] REM sleep has 'tonic' features, which are present throughout the REM period, and intermittently occurring 'phasic' components Tonic features: - Loss of muscle tone (atonia), except diaphragm (to maintain respiration), muscles controlling eye movements and muscles of the middle ear [2, 6] - Muscle atonia thought to prevent acting out dreams [2, 6] - Reduced thermoregulation [2] - Penile tumescence (males), vaginal engorgement (females) [2, 3] - Constriction of pupils [2] Phasic features: - Rapid eye movements (REM) [2, 6, 9, 10] - Fluctuations in breathing and heart rate [6] - Brief bursts of muscle activity on EMG [9, 10]

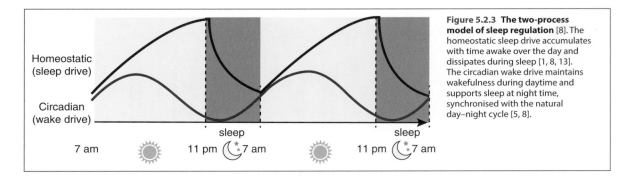

Figure 5.2.3 **The two-process model of sleep regulation** [8]. The homeostatic sleep drive accumulates with time awake over the day and dissipates during sleep [1, 8, 13]. The circadian wake drive maintains wakefulness during daytime and supports sleep at night time, synchronised with the natural day–night cycle [5, 8].

Alignment of these processes ensures regular sleep and wakeful periods in keeping with the natural day–night cyclce, while it also optimises the function of many other circadian physiological processes [1, 8, 11–16].

5.2.3 Neural Circuits Regulating Sleep and Wakefulness

In recent years, significant progress has been made in identifying more of the neural circuits underlying the regulation of wakefulness and sleep, and this remains an area of intense research [5, 6, 14, 15, 17, 18]. Figures 5.2.4 and 5.2.5 show the main brain regions and associated neuromodulators involved.

5.2.3.1 *Arousal and Wake-Promoting Systems*

Several systems have been identified as promoting and regulating wakefulness and arousal. The main pathways project from the brainstem to the cortical and other

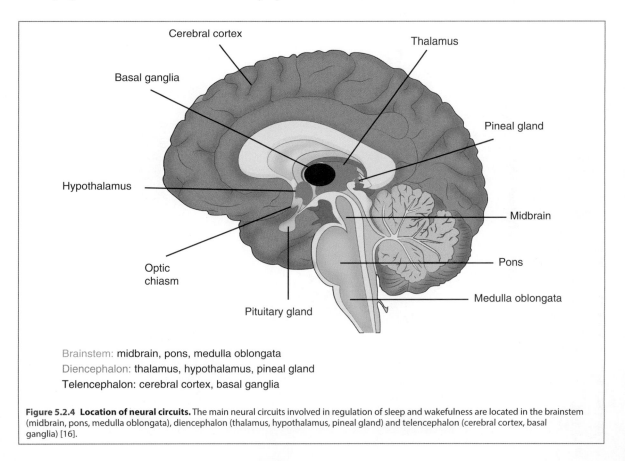

Brainstem: midbrain, pons, medulla oblongata
Diencephalon: thalamus, hypothalamus, pineal gland
Telencephalon: cerebral cortex, basal ganglia

Figure 5.2.4 **Location of neural circuits.** The main neural circuits involved in regulation of sleep and wakefulness are located in the brainstem (midbrain, pons, medulla oblongata), diencephalon (thalamus, hypothalamus, pineal gland) and telencephalon (cerebral cortex, basal ganglia) [16].

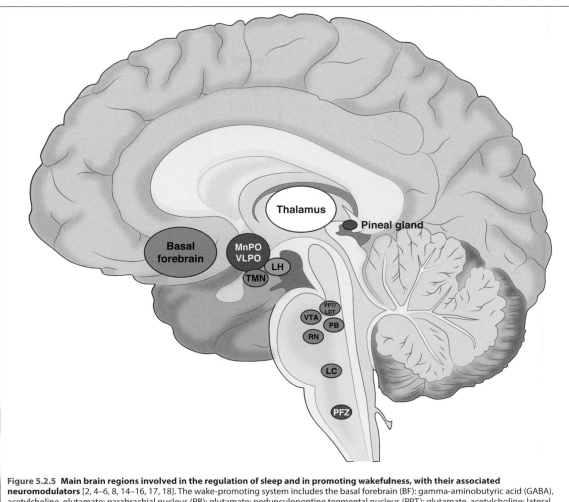

Figure 5.2.5 Main brain regions involved in the regulation of sleep and in promoting wakefulness, with their associated neuromodulators [2, 4–6, 8, 14–16, 17, 18]. The wake-promoting system includes the basal forebrain (BF): gamma-aminobutyric acid (GABA), acetylcholine, glutamate; parabrachial nucleus (PB): glutamate; pedunculopontine tegmental nucleus (PPT): glutamate, acetylcholine; lateral dorsal tegmental nucleus (LDT): acetylcholine; tuberomammillary nucleus (TMN): histamine; raphe nucleus (RN): serotonin; locus coeruleus (LC): noradrenaline; ventral tegmental area (VTA): dopamine, GABA, glutamate; lateral hypothalamus (LH): hypocretin/orexin. The main regions of the sleep-promoting system are the ventrolateral preoptic area (VLPO): GABA, galanin; median preoptic nucleus (MnPO): GABA; parafacial zone (PFZ): GABA; pineal gland: melatonin.

brain regions via a large ventral pathway, which innervates the hypothalamus, basal forebrain and cortex, and also via a dorsal pathway, which projects to the thalamus and cortex [5, 6, 14, 16]. Historically, the ascending monaminergic and cholinergic arousal systems were considered the main wake-promoting systems [5]. It was thought that the inhibitory neurotransmitter gamma-aminobutyric acid (GABA) was mainly involved in sleep promotion [5]. However, more recent advances suggest that specific GABAergic neurons and glutamate play a crucial role in promoting wakefulness, while monaminergic and cholinergic systems have a modulatory function

[5, 6, 17]. It is important to note that all these systems interact with each other in complex ways and despite significant progress made in research, many aspects of these regulatory systems remain unexplained.

GABAERGIC AND GLUTAMATERGIC AROUSAL SYSTEM

Several wake-promoting glutaminergic and GABAergic neural pathways have been proposed. One such pathway originates from glutamatergic neurons in the pedunculopontine and parabrachial nuclei in the brain-stem, and it projects to the basal forebrain

[5, 6, 17]. The basal forebrain is a region strongly implicated in arousal. It contains cholinergic, glutamatergic and GABAergic neurons, with direct projections to the cortex [5, 6, 17] (Figure 5.2.6). These three types of neurons all increase arousal and cortical activation, but a specific subgroup of GABAergic neurons (parvalbumin positive neurons) has been suggested as the main driver of wakefulness in the basal forebrain [5, 6, 17]. This is reflected in an increased pattern of activity in this group of neurons during wakefulness. In general GABAergic neurons show functional heterogeneity, with other populations of GABA neurons appearing to reduce arousal and presenting with increased activity in NREM sleep [5, 6, 17].

ASCENDING CHOLINERGIC AND MONAMINERGIC SYSTEMS

The cholinergic and monaminergic neurotransmitter systems are believed to have a modulating function on the arousal system, mediating the arousal level and

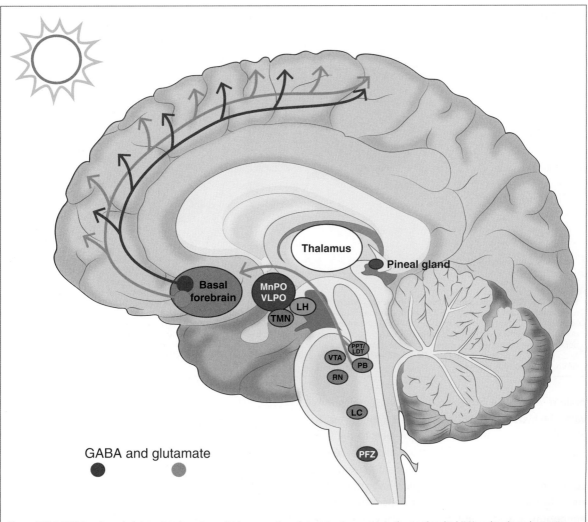

Figure 5.2.6 GABAergic and glutamatergic systems. Wake-promoting glutamatergic neurons in the parabrachial (PB) and pedunculopontine tegmental nucleus (PPT) innervate the basal forebrain [5, 6, 17]. GABAergic and glutamatergic neurons located in the basal forebrain project to the cortex, increasing arousal and cortical activation [5, 6, 17]. Specific (parvalbumin positive) GABAergic neurons have been suggested as one of the main drivers for promoting wakefulness in the basal forebrain [5, 6, 17]. Other abbreviations: GABA, gamma-aminobutyric acid; LC, locus coeruleus; LDT, lateral dorsal tegmental nucleus; LH, lateral hypothalamus; MnPO, median preoptic nucleus; PFZ, parafacial zone; PPT, pedunculopontine tegmental nucleus; RN, raphe nucleus; TMN, tuberomammillary nucleus; VLPO, ventrolateral preoptic area; VTA, ventral tegmental area.

wake-related behaviours such as attention, motivation, learning, reward and mood [5, 6, 8, 16, 17].

The cholinergic system consists of **acetylcholine**-containing neurons, which are located in the pedunculo-pontine tegmental and the laterodorsal tegmental nuclei, and in the basal forebrain [16] (Figure 5.2.7A). Cholinergic neurons are most active in wakefulness and REM sleep [18].

The monaminergic system has widespread projections across the central nervous system and includes histamine, noradrenaline, serotonin and dopamine neurons. With the exception of dopamine, monamines are most active during wakefulness, showing reduced activity in NREM sleep and almost none in REM sleep [6].

The tuberomammillary nucleus is the only source of **histamine** in the brain [5] (Figure 5.2.7B). Histamine is thought to play a role in promoting general arousal and maintaining wakefulness [5, 6, 16]. Centrally acting histamine H1 antagonists have a sedating effect and have long been used as sleep aids [5].

Noradrenaline neurons are widely distributed in the brainstem, but the locus coeruleus is the main source of ascending noradrenaline projections [6, 16] (Figure 5.2.7C). Noradrenaline increases arousal in general, and especially in response to stressors, as well as novel and salient stimuli [5, 6].

Serotonin neurons are located in the dorsal and median raphe nucleus and project widely to brain regions involved in sleep–wakefulness regulation and other regions [6, 16] (Figure 5.2.7D). Serotonin is thought to increase arousal and suppress REM sleep, but its effects are variable in view of the high number of receptor subtypes [16, 18].

The effects of **dopamine** seem location and pathway specific. Dopaminergic neurons located in the ventral tegmental area appear to play a role in promoting wakefulness [6] (Figure 5.2.7E). Dopamine neurons show increased activation in response to salient stimuli, such as rewards, and under conditions of high motivation [5, 6]. Unlike other monoamines, they are most active during wakefulness and REM sleep [6, 16]. Stimulants, such as amphetamines and modafinil, enhance dopamine signalling and are known to increase arousal [5, 6].

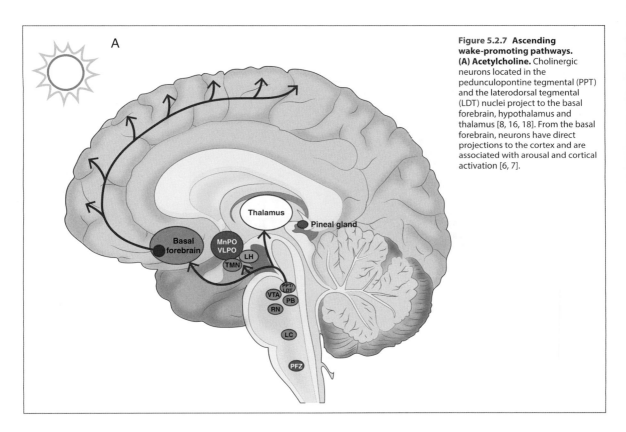

Figure 5.2.7 Ascending wake-promoting pathways. (A) Acetylcholine. Cholinergic neurons located in the pedunculopontine tegmental (PPT) and the laterodorsal tegmental (LDT) nuclei project to the basal forebrain, hypothalamus and thalamus [8, 16, 18]. From the basal forebrain, neurons have direct projections to the cortex and are associated with arousal and cortical activation [6, 7].

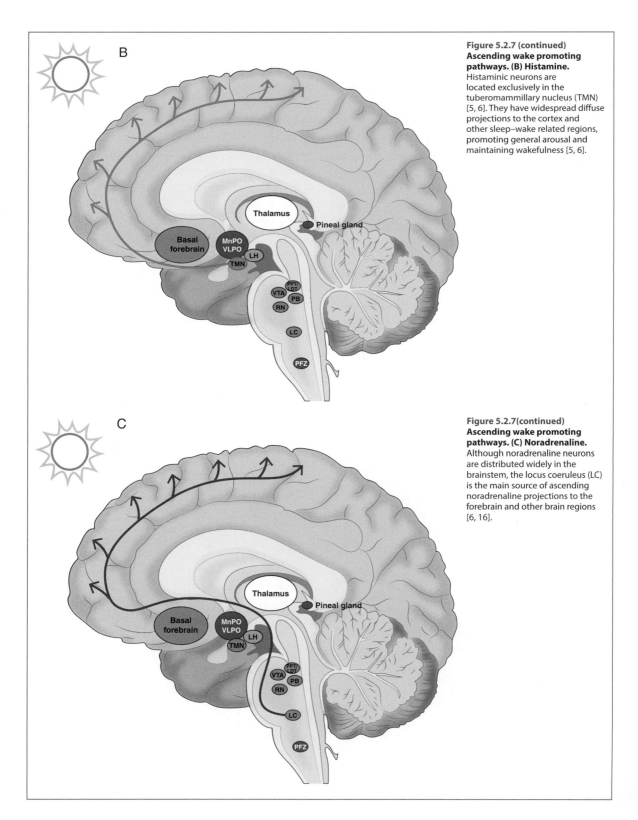

Figure 5.2.7 (continued)
Ascending wake promoting pathways. (B) Histamine.
Histaminic neurons are located exclusively in the tuberomammillary nucleus (TMN) [5, 6]. They have widespread diffuse projections to the cortex and other sleep–wake related regions, promoting general arousal and maintaining wakefulness [5, 6].

Figure 5.2.7(continued)
Ascending wake promoting pathways. (C) Noradrenaline.
Although noradrenaline neurons are distributed widely in the brainstem, the locus coeruleus (LC) is the main source of ascending noradrenaline projections to the forebrain and other brain regions [6, 16].

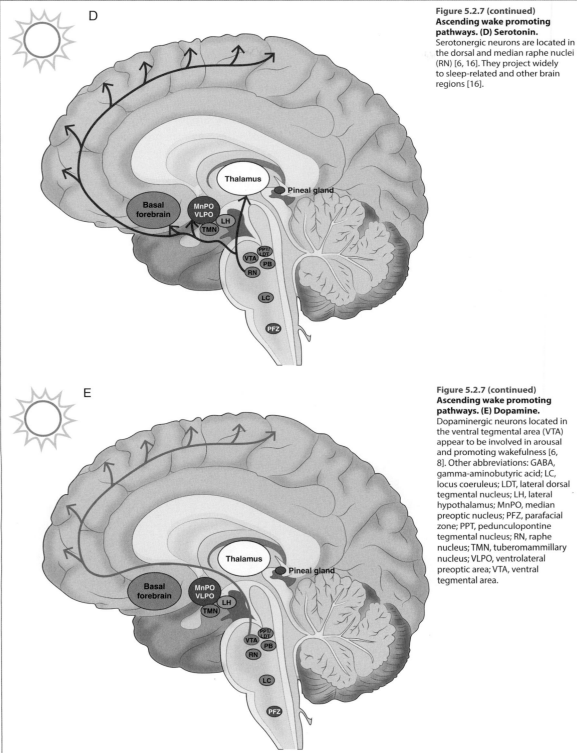

**Figure 5.2.7 (continued)
Ascending wake promoting
pathways. (D) Serotonin.**
Serotonergic neurons are located in
the dorsal and median raphe nuclei
(RN) [6, 16]. They project widely
to sleep-related and other brain
regions [16].

**Figure 5.2.7 (continued)
Ascending wake promoting
pathways. (E) Dopamine.**
Dopaminergic neurons located in
the ventral tegmental area (VTA)
appear to be involved in arousal
and promoting wakefulness [6,
8]. Other abbreviations: GABA,
gamma-aminobutyric acid; LC,
locus coeruleus; LDT, lateral dorsal
tegmental nucleus; LH, lateral
hypothalamus; MnPO, median
preoptic nucleus; PFZ, parafacial
zone; PPT, pedunculopontine
tegmental nucleus; RN, raphe
nucleus; TMN, tuberomammillary
nucleus; VLPO, ventrolateral
preoptic area; VTA, ventral
tegmental area.

HYPOCRETIN (OREXIN) SYSTEM

Hypocretin and orexin are different names for the same neurotransmitter. Hypocretin/orexin neurons are located in the lateral hypothalamus and project widely throughout the brain to the wake-promoting areas (Figure 5.2.8) [6, 14, 16, 19]. The hypocretin/orexin system is essential for regulating and stabilising the sleep and wakefulness system, including REM sleep, and for maintaining arousal [5, 6, 19]. However, hypocretin/orexin neurons are not necessarily required for the generation of sleep or wakefulness [5]. This system integrates a wide range of information about general arousal, metabolic state, circadian factors, homeostatic sleep pressure and inputs from the limbic system [7, 19]. Depending on which state is favoured, hypocretin/orexin neurons either activate wake-promoting networks, leading to sustained arousal and suppression of REM sleep, or remain silent and thereby support the maintenance of sleep [19]. Hypocretin/orexin neurons are most active during wakefulness, especially in explorative and goal-directed

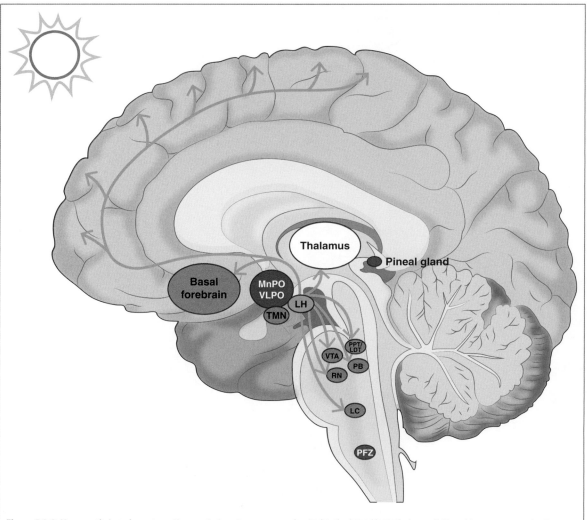

Figure 5.2.8 Hypocretin/orexin system. Hypocretin/orexin neurons are located in the lateral hypothalamus (LH) and have strong projections to wake- and arousal-promoting regions across the brain [5, 8]. The system plays a crucial role in stabilising the sleep–wake cycle, sustaining regular wakefulness and maintaining increased levels of arousal if required [5, 6, 8]. Structures involved include: parabrachial nucleus (PB), pedunculopontine tegmental nucleus (PPT), lateral dorsal tegmental nucleus (LDT), tuberomammillary nucleus (TMN), raphe nucleus (RN), locus coeruleus (LC), ventral tegmental area (VTA) and lateral hypothalamus (LH).

behaviour, and are mostly silent during sleep [5, 6, 19]. Stimulation of hypocretin/orexin neurons suppresses REM sleep [6, 19].

Narcolepsy is a neurological disorder with markedly reduced hypocretin/orexin cells in the hypothalamus [8]. This results in an instability of sleep and wakefulness states. Features of narcolepsy include excessive daytime sleepiness, difficulties in maintaining wakefulness and abnormal REM sleep (see Section 9.16.1) [6, 8].

5.2.3.2 Regulation of NREM Sleep

The ventrolateral preoptic area and the median preoptic nucleus in the anterior hypothalamus play an important role in the onset and maintenance of sleep. They contain GABAergic neurons, and galanin producing neurons in the ventrolateral preoptic area, which innervate and inhibit the major wake- and arousal-promoting areas (Figure 5.2.9) [6, 16]. Conversely, the arousal-promoting regions project to the ventrolateral preoptic area and

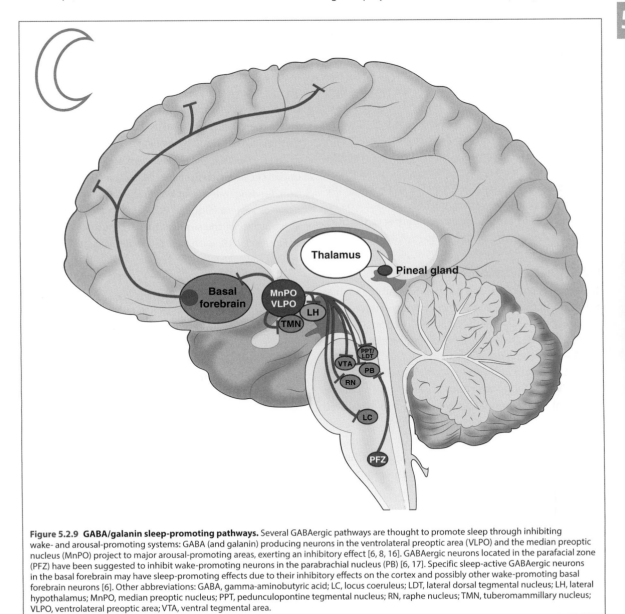

Figure 5.2.9 GABA/galanin sleep-promoting pathways. Several GABAergic pathways are thought to promote sleep through inhibiting wake- and arousal-promoting systems: GABA (and galanin) producing neurons in the ventrolateral preoptic area (VLPO) and the median preoptic nucleus (MnPO) project to major arousal-promoting areas, exerting an inhibitory effect [6, 8, 16]. GABAergic neurons located in the parafacial zone (PFZ) have been suggested to inhibit wake-promoting neurons in the parabrachial nucleus (PB) [6, 17]. Specific sleep-active GABAergic neurons in the basal forebrain may have sleep-promoting effects due to their inhibitory effects on the cortex and possibly other wake-promoting basal forebrain neurons [6]. Other abbreviations: GABA, gamma-aminobutyric acid; LC, locus coeruleus; LDT, lateral dorsal tegmental nucleus; LH, lateral hypothalamus; MnPO, median preoptic nucleus; PPT, pedunculopontine tegmental nucleus; RN, raphe nucleus; TMN, tuberomammillary nucleus; VLPO, ventrolateral preoptic area; VTA, ventral tegmental area.

inhibit the sleep-active neurons [6, 14, 16]. Hence, arousal-promoting and sleep-promoting systems have inhibitory effects on each other, allowing relatively rapid change in sleep and wakeful states. This is referred to as the 'flip-flop switch' [6, 8, 14–16]. In addition, sleep-active GABAergic neurons originating in the parafacial zone and the basal forebrain are thought to have sleep-promoting effects (Figure 5.2.9) [6, 17].

Extended periods of wakefulness lead to increased homeostatic sleep pressure. Several neurochemical agents are believed to play a role in homeostatic sleep regulation, but the exact mechanisms are not fully understood. One of these agents is adenosine. Adenosine levels in the basal forebrain have been found to increase during sustained wakefulness and to decrease as sleep progresses [6, 7, 14, 16, 18]. In the basal forebrain, the effects are thought to be mediated by adenosine A1 receptors, inhibiting wake-promoting neurons. Adenosine A2A receptors in the ventrolateral preoptic area and other brain regions also appear to contribute to increased sleepiness [7, 14, 16]. The observation that caffeine, a non-specific antagonist of adenosine receptors, has strong arousal-promoting effects supports adenosine's role in promoting sleep [6, 7, 16, 18].

5.2.3.3 Regulation of REM Sleep

REM sleep is characterised by specific features such as dreaming, activated EEG pattern, rapid eye movements and muscle atonia (see Table 5.2.1). The function and regulation of REM sleep is an evolving area of research and the underlying mechanisms are still not fully understood. Glutamate neurons located in the subcoeruleus region (ventral to locus coeruleus) appear to play an important role in regulating REM sleep and associated features, such as muscle atonia [6, 17, 20]. This seems to be in concert with specific GABAergic neurons and other neuromodulators, including glycine, acetylcholine, melanin-concentrating hormone and the monamines [6, 17, 20].

5.2.4 Circadian Rhythm

Like many organisms, humans are naturally able to maintain a rhythm of sleep and wakefulness independent of external cues [8, 21]. Without these cues, the natural circadian sleep–wake rhythm in humans is about 24.2 hours [21]. Hence, adjusting to the 24-hour day–night cycle requires daily 'entrainment'. This also allows the circadian rhythm to adjust to seasonal daylight change and other phase shifts, for example jet lag and shift work [21, 22]. The most powerful signal for the daily adjustment of the 'circadian clock' (see Subsection 5.2.4.1) is light, although other cues, such as food, exercise and social interaction contribute to synchronisation [8, 21, 22].

5.2.4.1 Suprachiasmatic Nucleus

In humans, the main circadian pacemaker is the suprachiasmatic nucleus, located just above the optic chiasm in the anterior hypothalamus [23]. Although many tissues and cells can generate circadian rhythms independently, the suprachiasmatic nucleus is considered the 'circadian master clock', responsible for maintaining a consistent rhythm in central and peripheral tissues [6, 8, 13, 22, 23].

In addition to sleep, various other processes are also under circadian control, including temperature regulation, feeding, release of hormones and the autonomic nervous system (Figure 5.2.10) [6, 22–24]. The main in- and outputs of the suprachiasmatic nucleus are shown in Figure 5.2.10, with hypothalamic structures shaded in blue.

5.2.4.2 Molecular Regulation of the Circadian Clock

At the individual cell level, cells in the suprachiasmatic nucleus, as well as those in many peripheral tissues, are able to generate their own circadian rhythm. The molecular mechanism of these intracellular clocks consists of a series of genetic transcription–translation feedback loops [6, 8, 13, 22, 24].

A number of genes (expressed in italics) have been identified, coding for proteins (expressed in capital letters) that are either part of the feedback loops or modulate them. These include: *Per1*, *Per2* and *Per3* (period), *Cry1* and *Cry2* (plant cryptochrome gene homologues), *Clock* (circadian locomotor output cycles kaput), *Bmal1* (brain and muscle Arnt-like 1) and *Ck1ε* (casein kinase epsilon), amongst many others [13, 22, 24].

Transcription factors play a role in regulating the expression of genes by binding to a promoter region of

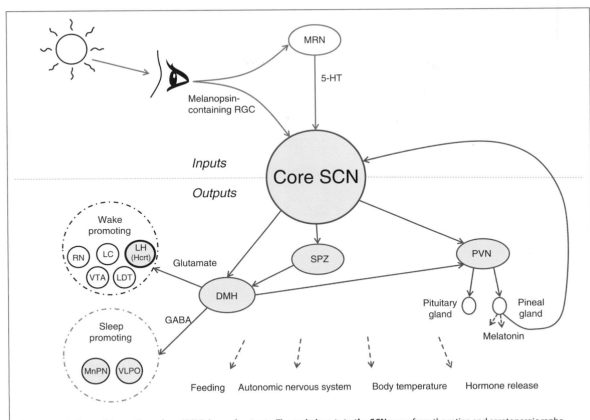

Figure 5.2.10 Suprachiasmatic nucleus (SCN): in- and outputs. The **main inputs to the SCN** come from the retina and serotonergic raphe nucleus (RN). When light hits melanopsin-containing retinal ganglion cells (RGC), the light information is transmitted to the SCN core via the retinohypothalamic tract [6, 22, 23]. From the median raphe nucleus (MRN), serotonergic non-photic signals are transmitted to the SCN [6, 22, 23]. The **main outputs of the SCN** are to the subparaventricular zone (SPZ), with a secondary projection to the dorsomedial hypothalamic nucleus (DMH) [13, 23]. Glutamatergic neurons in the DMH activate the wake-promoting circuits, in particular the hypocretin/orexin neurons, while GABAergic neurons project to sleep-promoting areas [6, 13, 23]. The DMH and the SCN project to the paraventricular hypothalamic nucleus (PVN), which stimulates the nocturnal release of melatonin from the pineal gland via multisynaptic pathways [6, 23]. The cyclical release of melatonin supports the circadian alignment of peripheral and central tissues expressing melatonin receptors. This includes a feedback loop back to the SCN [6, 22, 23]. Several hormones are under similar circadian control, for example the peak of cortisol release is in the morning [13, 22, 23]. Other abbreviations: DMH, dorsomedial hypothalamic nucleus; GABA, gamma-aminobutyric acid; Hcrt, hypocretin/orexin; LC, locus coeruleus; LDT, lateral dorsal tegmental nucleus; LH, lateral hypothalamus; MnPO, median preoptic nucleus; PFZ, parafacial zone; PPT, pedunculopontine tegmental nucleus; PVN, paraventricular nucleus; VLPO, ventrolateral preoptic area; VTA, ventral tegmental area.

DNA and turning the expression of a gene either on or off [8]. One of the main transcription factors in the molecular clock is the protein complex CLOCK/BMAL1, which promotes the transcription of many clock-controlled genes [8, 13]. As part of the negative feedback loop, the protein products of these genes accumulate across the day and form complexes, which eventually inhibit CLOCK/BMAL1 and their own production [13, 24]. Once these complexes have degraded, transcription can start again. In this way, an oscillating circadian rhythm over 24 hours

is established [13]. A range of other feedback loops, genes and proteins are involved in modulating and stabilising the molecular clock [6, 8, 13, 22, 24]. Figure 5.2.11 shows the molecular regulation of the circadian clock.

Disturbances of the molecular clock have been suggested as a factor in mental and physical illness [8, 22].

In 2017, the Nobel Prize in Physiology or Medicine was awarded jointly to Hall, Rosbash and Young for discovering these molecular mechanisms many years earlier [25].

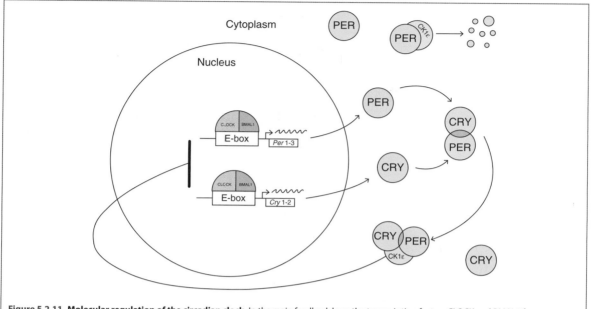

Figure 5.2.11 Molecular regulation of the circadian clock. In the main feedback loop the transcription factors CLOCK and BMAL1 form a heterodimer and bind to the E-box promoter of clock-controlled genes, including those expressing *Per* and *Cry* genes [8, 13, 24]. The protein products PER and CRY accumulate during the day and form complexes (e.g. CRY–PER), which after entering the nucleus, eventually inhibit the activity of CLOCK/BMAL1, and therefore reduce their own transcription in a negative feedback loop [8, 13, 22, 24]. Additional feedback loops and key proteins regulate the period length and precision of the molecular circadian clock, allowing the system to respond to internal and external influences [13, 24]. One such protein is casein kinase 1 epsilon (CK1ε). This affects the nuclear translocation of the CRY–PER complex, and also binds to PER, leading (through phosphorylation) to its degradation [13, 24]. In this way it modifies the period length of the molecular clock [13, 22, 24].

5.2.5 Effects of Sleep Deprivation

The optimal duration of sleep remains a topic of debate. It varies with age and there are significant interindividual differences. In adults, sleep duration of less than 7 hours or more than 9 hours has been associated with adverse health outcomes, with increasing effects at the extremes [8].

Sleep deprivation occurs either acutely, with an extended wake period, or more chronically, with an accumulative restriction of sleep [26, 27]. Cognitive impairment effects are similar, whether subsequent to acute or chronic sleep deprivation [26–28]. These include slowing of cognitive and psychomotor processes, and the impairment of attention, executive function, decision-making capacity and working memory [13, 26–28]. Individuals tend to underestimate their level of sleepiness and functional impairment [26, 27].

Historic studies of healthy volunteers undergoing prolonged periods of acute sleep deprivation (e.g.

several days without sleep) have shown elevated stress reactions, mood changes and eventually progression to psychotic-like experiences [26, 28–30].

The effects of sleep deprivation increase with duration of sleep loss, and extended sleep opportunities are required for performance to recover and sleepiness to abate [26].

Chronic lack and disturbance of sleep are associated with significant mental and physical health problems. These include mood and anxiety disorders, cardiovascular disease and metabolic disorders such as obesity and diabetes [8, 13, 26]. The underlying mechanisms appear complex and multifactorial. Autonomic nervous system abnormalities, hormonal changes leading to metabolic dysfunction, altered immune response and genetic factors are all thought to contribute to the health effects of sleep disruption [8, 13, 26, 31].

Conclusions and Outstanding Questions

In this section we have gained some insight into the complex neural processes regulating wakefulness and sleep, including the remarkable ability to switch from one state to the other. A range of intricate mechanisms allow the system to adapt to changes in environment and internal states, and the circadian rhythm system ensures synchronisation with the natural day–night cycle. However, despite significant scientific advances, many aspects of these systems are still waiting to be uncovered. There is increasing awareness that sleep is important for virtually all aspects of human life, and studies show that chronic lack or disturbance of sleep has a significant impact on health and well-being.

Outstanding Questions

- Many neurochemical agents and mechanisms involved in the regulation of sleep and wakefulness are also implicated in psychiatric disorders. What is the relationship between mental health and sleep with regard to underlying processes? Will a better understanding open up new treatment approaches?

- With extended periods of sleep deprivation, increasing cognitive impairment and psychiatric features have been observed. What are the underlying mechanisms mediating these effects?

5

REFERENCES

1. Muza R. Normal sleep. In Selsick H (ed.). *Sleep Disorders in Psychiatric Patients*. Springer-Verlag, 2018, pp. 3–25.

2. Harvard Medical School, Division of Sleep Medicine. Healthy Sleep. http://healthysleep.med.harvard.edu/healthy/ (accessed 19 November 2019).

3. Royal College of Psychiatrists. TrOn trainees online: The physiology of arousal and sleep. www.rcpsych.ac.uk/training/your-training/training-resources/trainees-online (accessed 19 November 2019).

4. Pelayo R, Dement WC. History of sleep physiology and medicine. In Kryger M, Roth T, Dement WC. *Principles and Practice of Sleep Medicine*, 6th ed. Elsevier, 2017, pp. 3–14.

5. Eban-Rothschild A, Appelbaum L, de Lecea L. Neuronal mechanisms for sleep/wake regulation and modulatory drive. *Neuropsychopharmacology* 2018; 43: 937–952.

6. Scammell TE, Arrigoni E, Lipton JO. Neural circuitry of wakefulness and sleep. *Neuron Rev* 2017; 93: 747–765.

7. Brown RE, Basheer R, McKenna JT, Strecker RE, McCarley RW. Control of sleep and wakefulness. *Physiol Rev* 2012; 92(3): 1087–1187.

8. Stahl SM, Morrissette DA. *Stahl's Illustrated Sleep and Wake Disorders*. Cambridge University Press, 2016.

9. Caskardon MA, Rechtschaffen A. Monitoring and staging human sleep. In Kryger M, Roth T, Dement WC (eds.). *Principles and Practice of Sleep Medicine*, 4th ed. Elsevier, 2005, pp. 1359–1377.

10. Berry RB, Quan SF, Abreu AR et al. *The AASM Manual for the Scoring of Sleep and Associated Events: Rules, Terminology and Technical Specifications. Version 2.6*. American Academy of Sleep Medicine, 2020.

11. Borbely AA. A two-process model of sleep regulation. *Human Neurobiol* 1982; 1: 195–204.

12. Borbely A, Daan S, Wirz-Justice A, Deboer T. The two-process model of sleep regulation: a reappraisal. *J Sleep Res* 2016; 25: 131–143.

13. Foster RG. Sleep, circadian rhythms and health. *Interface Focus* 2020; 10: 20190098. http://dx.doi.org/10.1098/rsfs.2019.0098.

14. Saper CB, Scammel TE, Lu J. Hypothalamic regulation of sleep and circadian rhythms. *Nature* 2005; 437: 1257–1263.

15. Saper BC, Fuller PM, Pedersen NP, Lu J, Scammel TE. Sleep state switching. *Neuron* 2010; 68(6): 1023–1042.

16. McGinty D, Szymusiak R. Neural control of sleep in mammals. In Kryger M, Roth T, Dement WC (eds.). *Principles and Practice of Sleep Medicine*, 6th ed. Elsevier, 2017, pp. 62–77.

17. Saper C, Fuller P. Wake–sleep circuitry: an overview. *Curr Opin Neurobiol* 2017; 44: 186–192.

18. Holst C, Landolt H-P. Sleep–wake neurochemistry. *Sleep Med Clin* 2018; 13: 137–146.

19. de Lecea L, Huerta R. Hypocretin (orexin) regulation of sleep-to-wake transitions. *Front Pharmacol* 2014; 5(16): 1–7.

20. Freigne JJ, Torontali ZA, Snow MB, Peever JH. REM sleep at its core: circuits, neurotransmitters, and pathophysiology. *Front Neurol* 2015; 6: 123.

21. Abbott SM, Reid KJ, Zee PC. Circadian disorders of the sleep–wake cycle. In: Kryger M, Roth T, Dement WC (eds.). *Principles and Practice of Sleep Medicine*, 6th ed. Elsevier, 2017, pp. 414–423.

22. Hickie IB, Naismith SL, Robillard R et al. Manipulating the sleep–wake cycle and circadian rhythms to improve clinical management of major depression. *BMC Medicine* 2013; 11(79): 1–27.

23. Gooley JJ, Saper CB. Anatomy of the mammalian circadian system. In Kryger M, Roth T, Dement WC (eds.). *Principles and Practice of Sleep Medicine*, 6th ed. Elsevier, 2017, pp. 343–350.

24. Rosenwasser AM, Turek FW. Physiology of the mammalian circadian system. In Kryger M, Roth T, Dement WC (eds.). *Principles and Practice of Sleep Medicine*, 6th ed. Elsevier, 2017, pp. 351–361.

25. The Nobel Prize. The Nobel Prize in Physiology or Medicine 2017. www.nobelprize.org/prizes/medicine/2017/press-release/

26. Banks S, Dorrian J, Basner M, Dingers DF. Sleep deprivation. In Kryger M, Roth T, Dement WC (eds.). *Principles and Practice of Sleep Medicine*, 6th ed. Elsevier, 2017, pp. 49–55.

27. Van Dongen HPA, Maislin G, Mullington JM, Dinges DF. The cumulative cost of additional wakefulness: dose–response effects on neurobehavioural functions and sleep physiology from chronic sleep restriction and total sleep deprivation. *Sleep* 2003; 26(2): 117–126.

28. Goel N, Rao H, Durmer J, Dinges DF. Neurocognitive consequences of sleep deprivation. *Semin Neurol* 2009; 29(4): 320–339.

29. Reeve S, Sheaves B, Freeman D. The role of sleep dysfunction in the occurrence of delusions and hallucinations: a systematic review. *ClinPsychol Rev* 2015; 42: 96–115.

30. Waters F, Chiu V, Atkinson A, Blom JD. Severe sleep deprivation causes hallucinations and a gradual progression toward psychosis with increasing time awake. *Front Psychiatry* 2018; 9: 303.

31. Van Cauter E, Spiegel K, Tasali E, Leproult R. Metabolic consequences of sleep and sleep loss. *Sleep Med* 2008; 9(01): 23–28.

5

5.3	**Sex and Sex Hormones**	Glenda Gillies

OVERVIEW

Sex and gender are of increasing interest and importance in clinical medicine, and psychiatry in particular. A large body of scientific evidence from animal and human studies demonstrates widespread sex differences in neurochemistry, connectivity and structure in virtually all brain regions with consequences for emotional and behavioural regulation [1–3]. We also understand that mental illness is associated with changes in the structure, neurochemistry and function of the brain, which will be superimposed on the innate brain sex differences. These biological differences are thought to contribute to differences between men and women in the prevalence, age at onset, symptomatology, progression, pathology and therapeutic responsiveness manifest in neuropsychiatric, neurological and neurodegenerative disorders [1, 2, 4] (Table 5.3.1). A better understanding of brain sex differences will be critical to advancing our understanding of mental disorders in both sexes, enabling the development of different and improved preventive, diagnostic and treatment approaches that benefit both men and women.

5.3.1 Origins of Brain Sex Differences

5.3.1.1 Hormones and Genes

The hypothalamus is the central regulator of reproduction: in females its circuitry supports ovulation, whereas in males it does not, and it controls stereotypical reproductive behaviours that are unique to males or females. The mechanisms that programme these hard-wired sex differences – that are critical for survival of the species – inevitably lead to sex differences in other brain regions not directly linked to reproduction. Specifically, in males, testosterone stimulates development of male internal and external genitalia early in gestation: at a later stage of development, testosterone masculinises/defeminises the brain at a time when neurodevelopmental processes (neurogenesis, gliogenesis, migration, programmed cell death) are critically sensitive (Figure 5.3.1A). In females, production of ovarian hormones is relatively quiescent until the lead-up to puberty, which is thought to be the main period for hormonal feminisation of the brain. However, these programmed sex differences are not completely manifest until after puberty when testosterone in males and oestrogens and progesterone in females exert differential activational effects on brain circuitry. Sex chromosomal genes will also differentially influence the activity of XX (female) and XY (male) cells (Figure 5.3.1B) [5]. The protein-coding genes exclusive to the Y chromosome (estimated to be around 60 in number) will only be expressed in male cells. In females, epigenetic mechanisms silence the protein-coding genes on one of the X chromosomes (estimated to be around 800 genes), but around 25% of these genes escape inactivation, leading to higher expression in females. Additionally, environmental factors trigger sex- and brain region-specific epigenetic changes in the brain. Collectively these hormonal, genetic and epigenetic influences lead to sex differences in neuronal projection pathways, innervation density, connectivity and neurotransmitter control in regions such as the hypothalamus, hippocampus, amygdala, prefrontal cortex and midbrain dopaminergic systems. Such neurobiological changes impact on the regulation of many behaviours, including those

Table 5.3.1 Sex differences in brain disorders

Condition	Prevalence male:female ratio	Nature
Male sex bias		
Autism; related disorders	4 to 5 : 1	Social impairment dominates in males; affective symptoms dominate in females.
Attention deficit hyperactivity disorder	2 to 3 : 1	Greater hyperactivity, externalising, impulsivity in males; greater internalising, inattention and cognitive impairment in females.
Schizophrenia	1.5 : 1	Earlier age at onset, more severe pathological symptoms, poorer prognosis in males; more affective symptoms in females.
Drug abuse, addiction	Perceived male bias is changing as sociocultural factors change	Differences evident in all phases with women escalating more rapidly to addiction and more likely to relapse following abstinence. Severity of withdrawal symptoms may depend on nature of addiction (e.g. females > males for drug abuse and smoking; males > females for alcohol).
Parkinsosn's disease	1.5 to 2 : 1	Males have earlier onset, greater parkinsonian motor features, sleep disturbances and associative cognitive impairments. Females present with a milder phenotype, slower decline in motor impairments; more prominent tremor, postural impairment and depressive symptoms. Sex-specific changes in gene expression in surviving dopaminergic neurons.
Stroke	Male bias declines in old age	Earlier onset in males.
Female sex bias		
Major depression	1 : 2	Differences emerge after puberty.
Anxiety	1 : 2	Greater linkage with major depression in females.
Panic disorder	1 : 2.5	Higher frequency and severity of panic attacks in women.
Obsessive–compulsive disorder	1 : 1.5	Sex differences in the characteristics and symptoms.
Post-traumatic stress disorder	1 : 2	Females have more severe symptoms and are more susceptible to childhood trauma.
Eating disorders (anorexia nervosa, bulimia)	1 : 3 to 4	Puberty is a critical risk period for girls; limited findings in boys suggest a lesser role for puberty.
Alzheimer's disease	1 : 1.5 to 2 emerges in old age	Earlier onset in females. Sex differences in neuropathological and behavioural disturbances.

For original references, see reviews [1-3].

involved in reproduction, cognition, mood, stress and fear responses. Accordingly, certain tests of specific brain functions do reveal sex differences in performance that accord with known structural and neurochemical differences. Equally, however, men and women may perform similarly on cognitive tests, despite differences in the connectivity of underlying circuitry. The latter may arise as a result of compensatory mechanisms, which preserve equal functions in the face of sex differences in physiological conditions (sex hormones and chromosomes) [6].

5.3.1.2 Sex and Gender

Biological sex is defined and traditionally assigned at birth on the basis of phenotype (male vs female genitalia) and genotype (sex chromosome complement – XX or XY in females and males, respectively), giving rise to biological sex differences. In contrast to the binary nature of sex, which is common across species, gender is a continuum and uniquely human. Gender is shaped by sociocultural norms and experience (environment) and defines an individual's innermost self as identifying with stereotypic maleness/masculinity or femaleness/femininity. Sex and gender, therefore, powerfully overlap, such that gender equity and gender roles impact on the epidemiology of mental disorders and the sex differences manifest therein. This creates likely insurmountable difficulties in identifying a purely biological component in sex differences in the human brain in health and disease. The very nature of gender precludes its investigation in preclinical (animal) studies, although the power of animal studies to identify how sex influences brain structure, function and dysfunction cannot be denied.

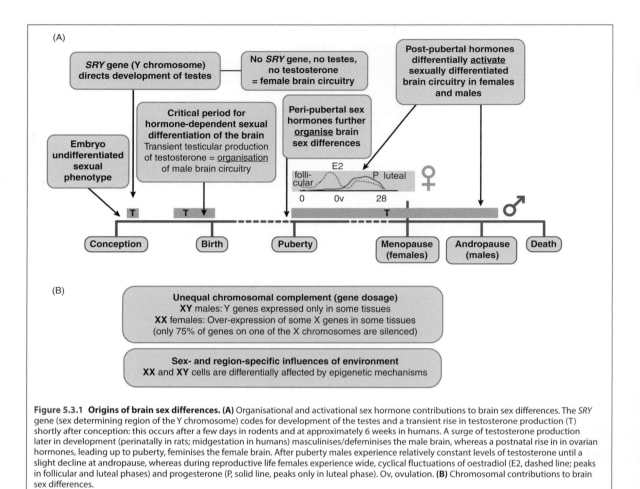

Figure 5.3.1 Origins of brain sex differences. (A) Organisational and activational sex hormone contributions to brain sex differences. The *SRY* gene (sex determining region of the Y chromosome) codes for development of the testes and a transient rise in testosterone production (T) shortly after conception: this occurs after a few days in rodents and at approximately 6 weeks in humans. A surge of testosterone production later in development (perinatally in rats; midgestation in humans) masculinises/defeminises the male brain, whereas a postnatal rise in in ovarian hormones, leading up to puberty, feminises the female brain. After puberty males experience relatively constant levels of testosterone until a slight decline at andropause, whereas during reproductive life females experience wide, cyclical fluctuations of oestradiol (E2, dashed line; peaks in follicular and luteal phases) and progesterone (P, solid line, peaks only in luteal phase). Ov, ovulation. **(B)** Chromosomal contributions to brain sex differences.

5.3.2 Sex Differences and Hormonal Influences in the Healthy Brain: Examples from Midbrain Dopaminergic Systems

The midbrain dopaminergic pathways (Figure 5.3.2) provide clear illustrations of sex differences in central systems at neurochemical, structural and behavioural levels. Table 5.3.2 summarises some brain sex differences and how they are influenced by sex hormones, focusing on midbrain dopaminergic systems. These systems (as shown in Figure 5.3.2) are pivotal regulators of normal adaptive behaviours and cognition, malfunction of which contributes significantly to brain disorders that, themselves, show sex bias [7].

In addition to examining the effects of the ovarian hormones, oestrogen and progesterone, in women, and testicular androgens in men, it is also relevant to investigate the effects of androgens in females and oestrogens and progestogens in males, because in both sexes oestrogen, androgen and progestogen receptors (ERs, ARs and PRs, respectively) are widely expressed in the brain. Moreover, the brain itself can synthesise its own oestrogens, androgens and other steroids (neurosteroids) *de novo* from cholesterol or from circulating gonadal or adrenal presursors, such as conversion of testosterone or dehydroepiandrosterone (DHEA) to oestradiol by central aromatase (Figure 5.3.3) [10].

Broadly speaking, findings in the normal female midbrain dopaminergic systems demonstrate that

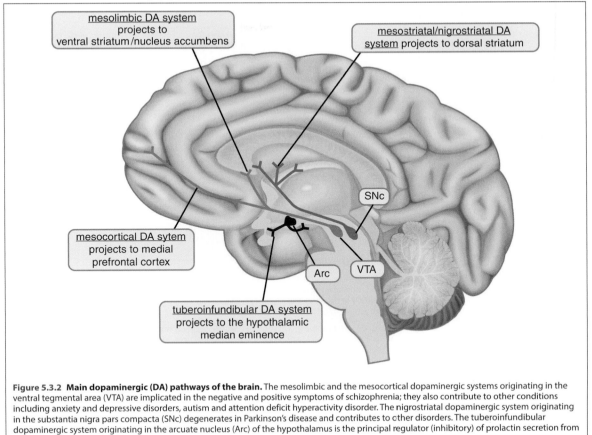

Figure 5.3.2 Main dopaminergic (DA) pathways of the brain. The mesolimbic and the mesocortical dopaminergic systems originating in the ventral tegmental area (VTA) are implicated in the negative and positive symptoms of schizophrenia; they also contribute to other conditions including anxiety and depressive disorders, autism and attention deficit hyperactivity disorder. The nigrostriatal dopaminergic system originating in the substantia nigra pars compacta (SNc) degenerates in Parkinson's disease and contributes to other disorders. The tuberoinfundibular dopaminergic system originating in the arcuate nucleus (Arc) of the hypothalamus is the principal regulator (inhibitory) of prolactin secretion from the anterior pituitary gland.

physiological levels of oestradiol are positive activators of these systems. In females and males, the effects of testosterone may be positive, negative or absent and influenced by whether testosterone is acting via ARs or, after aromatisation, via ERs. Similarly varied findings emerge from studies of other systems and brain regions, such as the hippocampus, amygdala and cortex. Clearly, the situation is complex: hormonal influences depend not only on the neural circuitry under study, but also on the sex of the individual. These results forcefully demonstrate that evidence gained in one sex may not be applicable to the other.

5.3.3 Impact of Sex Hormones on Psychiatric Disorders and Their Sex Bias

5.3.3.1 Role in Pathophysiology in Adolescence and Adulthood

While genetic factors contribute to susceptibility and differences in central nervous system disorders between men and women, both the external and internal environments, especially the sex hormone milieu, play a significant role. Puberty is a time of notable remodelling

Table 5.3.2 Neurochemical, structural and behavioural sex differences in the normal, adult midbrain dopaminergic systems and the activational (reversible) influences of sex steroid hormones

Key system	Test feature	Differences (typical male/female advantage)	Impact of sex hormones (where reported)
Humans			
Mesolimbic dopaminergic system	NAc dopaminergic activity, rewarding effect of psychoactive drugs (amphetamine, cocaine)	f > m	Varies across menstrual cycle; maximum as E2 levels rise in mid-follicular phase
Mesocortical dopaminergic system /prefrontal processes	Verbal memory: visuospatial memory	f > m	+ve effect of E2, −ve effect of T in f; +ve effect of T in m after aromatisation to E2
	Manual dexterity	f > m	+ve effect of E2, −ve effect of T in f
	Mental re-orientation spatial memory	m > f	+ve effect of DHT (non-aromatisable androgen), no effect of E2 in m; no effect of androgens in f
	Target-directed motor skills	m > f	
	DA synthetic capacity, DAT density, D2 receptor affinity	f > m	
Nigrostriatal dopaminergic system	In vivo imaging of caudate and putamen dopaminergic activity in cognitive and motor functioning	f > m	
	SNc gene expression (laser capture microdissection in post-mortem brain)	Sex differences in expression of genes for signal transduction, neuronal maturation (f > m) and genes implicated in Parkinson's disease pathogenesis (alpha-synuclein, PINK-1)	
Rodents (rats or mice)			
Mesocortical dopaminergic system/prefrontal processes	VTA volume, number of VTA DA neurons projecting to medial prefrontal cortex, DA axon density, extracellular resting DA levels	f > m	−ve effect of T, no effect of E2 in m
	DA-dependent operant spatial working memory, T-maze acquisition, novel object recognition		+ve effect of T, no effect of E2 in m
	DA-dependent tests of motivation		−ve effect of Cx reversed by E2, not T in m
Mesolimbic dopaminergic system	DA uptake and release, synthesis and turnover, DA fibre density and responses to psychoactive drugs (amphetamine, cocaine)	f > m	+ve effect of E2 in f; no effect of Cx, T, DHT or E2 in m
	Haloperidol-induced catalepsy	f > m	
Nigrostriatal dopaminergic system	Number of SNc dopaminergic neurons	m > f	
	Synthesis, metabolism and release of DA		+ve effect of E2 in f; −ve effect of E2 (synthesised from T) on TH gene expression in m
	Striatal DA loss in 6-OHDA lesion model of PD	m > f	Protective effect of E2 in f. −ve effect of E2 in m after aromatisation of circulating E2

Abbreviations: Cx, corticosteroids; D2, dopamine 2; DA, dopamine; DAT, dopamine transporter; E2, oestradiol, the main circulating oestrogen in non-pregnant females (others include oestriol and oestrone); f, females; m, males; mPFC, medial prefrontal cortex; NAc, nucleus accumbens; 6-OHDA, 6-hydroxydopamine; SNc, substantia nigra pars compacta; T, testosterone; TH, tyrosine hydroxylase (dopamine synthetase); VTA, ventral tegmental area; +ve, positive; −ve, negative. For original references see reviews [3, 7–9].

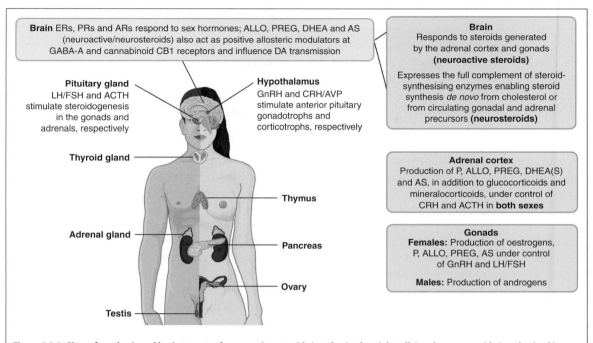

Brain ERs, PRs and ARs respond to sex hormones; ALLO, PREG, DHEA and AS (neuroactive/neurosteroids) also act as positive allosteric modulators at GABA-A and cannabinoid CB1 receptors and influence DA transmission

Brain
Responds to steroids generated by the adrenal cortex and gonads **(neuroactive steroids)**

Expresses the full complement of steroid-synthesising enzymes enabling steroid synthesis *de novo* from cholesterol or from circulating gonadal and adrenal precursors **(neurosteroids)**

Pituitary gland
LH/FSH and ACTH stimulate steroidogenesis in the gonads and adrenals, respectively

Hypothalamus
GnRH and CRH/AVP stimulate anterior pituitary gonadotrophs and corticotrophs, respectively

Adrenal cortex
Production of P, ALLO, PREG, DHEA(S) and AS, in addition to glucocorticoids and mineralocorticoids, under control of CRH and ACTH in **both sexes**

Thyroid gland

Thymus

Gonads
Females: Production of oestrogens, P, ALLO, PREG, AS under control of GnRH and LH/FSH

Males: Production of androgens

Adrenal gland

Pancreas

Ovary

Testis

Figure 5.3.3 Sites of synthesis and brain targets of neuroactive steroids (synthesised peripherally) and neurosteroids (synthesised in the brain). Gonads: The ovaries synthesise and release oestrogens (oestradiol, the main circulating oestrogen in non-pregnant, cycling women, and the less potent oestriol and oestrone) and progesterone (P). They also produce allopregnenolone (ALLO, synthesised from progesterone) and pregnenolone (PREG, an intermediate in the biosynthesis of most steroid hormones, including the sex hormones) as well as androstenedione (AS, an androgen). The testes produce androgens, principally testosterone (T), and the weaker AS. The production of all these gonadal steroids is under the control of the hypothalamic gonadotropin releasing hormone (GnRH) acting on the anterior pituitary gland to release the gonadotropins (luteinising hormone, LH, and follicle-stimulating hormone, FSH). **Adrenals:** At adrenarche (occurring just before puberty) the adrenal cortex begins, and continues throughout life, to synthesise and secrete P, ALLO, PREG, dehydroepiandrosterone and its sulphate (DHEA(S), weak androgenic and oestrogenic activities). **Brain:** The brain expresses the full complement of steroid-synthesising enzymes, enabling local biosynthesis of steroids *de novo* from cholesterol or circulating gonadal or adrenal precursors, including metabolism of testosterone or DHEA to oestradiol by aromatase. In the healthy brain, aromatase is expressed in neurons, not glia; in response to injury, aromatase is upregulated in astrocytes, leading to local increases in synaptic oestradiol levels and neuroprotection. **Brain targets:** The classical, intracellular, nuclear receptors for oestrogens, androgens and progestogens (ERs, ARs, PRs) as well as non-classical, membrane-bound, rapidly acting G-protein-coupled receptors, are widely distributed throughout male and female brains. Neuroactive/neurosteroids also act as positive modulators at GABA-A and cannabinoid CB1 receptors and modulate dopaminergic transmission. Other abbreviations: ACTH, adrenocorticotrophic hormone; AVP, arginine vasopressin; CRH, corticotrophin-releasing hormone; GABA-A, gamma-aminobutyric acid.

in the brain and many sex differences in brain structure emerge during adolescence. This is associated not only with the dramatic rise in circulating sex hormones, but also with an increase in the incidence of and sex bias in mental illnesses, implying a hormonal contribution to differences in the rates and characteristics of psychiatric disorders in men and women [11]. Clinically, the hormonal contribution has been investigated primarily in women, focusing on how changes (puberty, menopause, pregnancy, postpartum, therapy) and cyclical (menstrual) fluctuations in circulating levels impact on psychiatric symptoms. In men, the relatively stable circulating levels of testosterone throughout adulthood provide little

clue to sex-hormone influences. Premenstrual dysphoric disorder (PMDD), a very severe form of premenstrual syndrome affecting as many as 1 in 20 women, has been proposed as a candidate hormone-specific (and sex-specific) disorder, with evidence of impaired sensitivity of emotional and cognitive brain networks mediated by ovarian hormones [12, 13]. Postpartum obsessive–compulsive disorder and manic episodes are other sex-specific disorders where dramatic hormonal reductions appear to contribute. Symptoms mostly subside as stable, pre-pregnancy conditions return. These examples indicate that sex hormones are causally related to primary neuropsychiatric disorders.

In conditions affecting both men and women but where there is a female advantage (lower morbidity), oestradiol emerges as having significant protective effects, thereby contributing to sex bias. For example, in women with schizophrenia who were free of antipsychotic medication at the time of testing, psychotic symptoms lessened in mid-cycle when oestradiol levels are high. The higher level of oestradiol in younger cycling women delays the onset and improves the course of schizophrenia, benefits that are lost at menopause [14]. In contrast, oestrogen withdrawal (prior to menses; after menopause; discontinuation of oral contraception or hormone replacement therapy) can precipitate psychosis, even in healthy women. Similar evidence for a protective effect of oestrogens is found in women suffering from Parkinson's disease [8]. Although there is not a female advantage in Alzheimer's disease, endogenous oestradiol is thought to be protective [15]. There are conflicting reports as to whether circulating levels of oestradiol are lower in females with Alzheimer's disease compared with controls. However, recent work using PET imaging with radiolabelled aromatase inhibitors has revealed the widespread distribution of the aromatase enzyme (oestrogen synthetase) in the human brain, expression of which was found to be reduced in women with Alzheimer's disease [15]. We now know that brain levels of neurosteroids may vary independently of circulating levels due to local production of neurosteroids in the brain (Figure 5.3.3) [10, 16]. Therefore, it has been proposed that an age-related decline in brain levels of oestradiol in women may be more significant for Alzheimer's disease pathology than circulating levels [15]. Interestingly, single-nucleotide polymorphisms in the aromatase gene (*CYP19*) are among genetic factors associated with the risk for developing Alzheimer's disease. In men, however, an age-related decline in both circulating and central levels of testosterone (not oestradiol) has been linked to Alzheimer's disease.

In conditions where women fare worse than men, such as anxiety, major depression, panic disorders and post-traumatic stress disorder (PTSD), the focus for sex bias has been on reactivity to stress. A heightened stress response, involving central effects of corticotrophin-releasing hormone (CRH), as well as dysregulation of the hypothalamic–pituitary–adrenal (HPA) axis, has been identified in these conditions [17, 18]. The popular description of the stress response as fright, flight or fight (males) or tend and befriend (females) highlights the sex-specific nature of the response. Human and experimental evidence suggests a greater sensitivity to stressors in females, as well as sex differences in endocrine and behavioural responses (quantitative or qualitative). These arise from different patterns of activation in stress-responding circuitry in males and females (including hypothalamus, hippocampus, amygdala, medial prefrontal cortex and mesocorticolimbic dopaminergic systems). These differences impact on attention, arousal, fear and learning [19, 20]. Moreover, these parameters change with fluctuations in ovarian hormones. The female bias in anxiety and stress-related disorders appears at puberty and lasts until menopause, and women are more likely to experience symptoms during periods of marked hormonal changes (premenstrual, postpartum, perimenopausal) [21]. Thus, fluctuations in ovarian hormones are implicated in the aetiology of anxiety disorders in women. Interestingly, hypogonadal men with low testosterone are at greater risk of developing anxiety- and stress-related disorders, and testosterone replacement can reduce anxiety and depression, indicating opposite influences of gonadal hormones in men and women [21].

In contrast to oestradiol, relatively little attention has been given to a role for progesterone in brain health and dysfunction. There are suggestions in the literature that high levels of progesterone enhance memory and ameliorate effects of stress [21]. However, progesterone also has countering effects on oestrogenic activity, most notably on endometrial proliferation, accounting for its inclusion with an oestrogen in oral contraception. Its effects on stress responses can also be positive or negative over the ovarian cycle as the relative concentrations of the two hormones change. For example, stress was reported to increase amygdala activity when both oestradiol and progesterone were high, but decrease amygdala activity when only oestradiol was high [22]. Such observations highlight the difficulties in ascribing exact roles to each hormone in isolation.

Of growing interest, progesterone can also be metabolised in the brain to the neurosteroid allopregnanolone (ALLO), a positive modulator of gamma-aminobutyric acid (GABA)-A receptors, with anxiolytic properties (in rats) and an ability to reduce HPA axis reactivity and amygdala responsivity to aversive stimuli (in humans)

[21, 22]. Furthermore, an involvement of progesterone and/or ALLO has been suggested for emotional memory formation, mood disorders [23] and PTSD [21]. It may be that the greater exposure of women to fluctuations in oestradiol, progesterone and ALLO leads to instability in emotion regulation, making women more vulnerable than men to anxiety disorders [22].

5.3.3.2 Sex-Specific Effects of Early Adverse Developmental Environments

Exposure to stressors and stress hormones in early life is a recognised factor affecting resilience versus vulnerability to developing neuropsychiatric disorders in later life (Table 5.3.3) [9]. The timing and nature of the stressor, as well as sex, is critical in determining which parameters are

Table 5.3.3 Early-life factors and disease susceptibility

Epidemiological and clinical evidence		
Examples of early-life stressors	Increased disease risk in later life (males vs females)	Prominent disruptions/potential contributory factors
Occuring to a greater extent in males compared with females		
Obstetric complications	Schizophrenia (20–30% attributable to adverse in utero environment), attention deficit hyperactivity disorder, autism	Notable changes in prefrontal cortex and subcortical dopamine activity indicate sensitivity of midbrain dopamine systems to adverse environment Circulating E2 levels in women appear to ameliorate psychotic symptoms in schizophrenia, likely contributing to reduced susceptibility Exposure to raised levels of steroids, especially androgens, in amniotic fluid are associated with autism and linked to greater male susceptibility
Exposure of mothers during pregnancy to: • natural disasters (e.g. famine and malnutrition) • bereavement • conflicts in relationships • low socioeconomic status • infections • repeated exposure to elevated levels of glucocorticoids given to mature fetal lungs in cases of threatened premature delivery		
Occuring to a greater extent in females compared with males		
Factors *in utero* leading to low birthweight (markers of intrauterine metabolic distress) Childhood abuse, neglect; family strife Trauma at various stages of life	Anxiety, depression Bulimia Anorexia Post-traumatic stress disorder	Hyper-reactivity of HPA stress axis, associated with glucocorticoid resistance in brain regions regulating negative feedback (especially hippocampus); increased central CRH activity; reduced central activity of oxytocin (pro-social peptide); decreased hippocampal and mPFC volumes; increased amygdala volumes and reactivity to emotional cues Fluctuating hormone levels after puberty further enhance stress reactivity in women, likely contributing to enhanced susceptibility Impulsivity, difficulty in emotional control Malnutrition and suppression of HPG axis impact brain function Hyperactivity in fear and threat networks
Preclinical evidence (animal models)		
Broad range of stressors in experimental animals to model clinical situations, e.g. perinatal oxygen deprivation, maternal stressors during pregnancy (physical restraint, infection/LPS), antenatal/postnatal glucocorticoid exposure, newborn maternal separation	Sex-specific changes in vigilance, emotional regulation, fear conditioning, memory, learning and cognition Gonadectomy and HRT differentially affect responses in males and females	Sex-specific changes in brain networks influencing neuroendocrine and autonomic control, physiological and behavioural responses to stress in later life

Abbreviations: CRH, corticotrophin-releasing hormone; E2, oestradiol; HPA, hypothalamic–pituitary–adrenal; HRT, hormone replacement therapy; LPS, lipopolysaccharide; mPFC, medial prefrontal cortex.

affected. For example, it appears that the male brain may be more susceptible to *in utero* events, in part because they coincide with a period of particular synaptic plasticity due to the organisational (masculinising) effects of testosterone. The developing female brain appears more sensitive to stressors and trauma at a later developmental time-point, which may coincide with hormonal organisation of feminising processes (see Section 5.3.1 and Section 8.4). Brain regions particularly responsive to developmental disruption appear to be those regulating endocrine, behavioural and emotional responses to stress. Sex-specific changes in HPA reactivity appear to be one consequence [24–26], and differences will be further amplified by fluctuations in ovarian hormones in later life. In humans, antenatal exposure to inappropriately elevated levels of glucocorticoid stress homones is linked to hyperactivity and distractibility in children, which is associated with alterations in dopaminergic signalling. The mesocorticolimbic dopaminergic systems are key to stress coping strategies, enabling the storage and recall of appropriate behaviours on future encounters with the perceived threat or stressor. Rodent studies have identified sexually dimorphic changes within the adult mesocorticolimbic dopaminergic systems following antenatal glucocorticoid exposure, which affect some behaviours in females, not males (motivational arousal) and others in males, not females (pre-attentional processing/pre-pulse inhibition). These have potential behavioural correlates in depression (female bias) and schizophrenia (male bias) [9]. Notably, these sex-specific behavioural effects are accompanied by sex-specific changes in neurochemical markers of dopaminergic transmission. Differential capacities in males and females to adapt to early-life challenges may thus lead to differential vulnerabilities and resilience to psychopathologies in later life [9].

5.3.4 Sex Hormones as Treatments for Psychiatric Disorders

There are many claims for the efficacy of hormonal therapy. Prominent among them are the use of oestrogens in depression (primarily in the perimenopausal context and PMDD) [27], Alzheimer's disease [15], Parkinson's disease [3] and schizophrenia (as adjuncts to improve antipsychotic treatment) [14]. Of the neurosteroids (see Figure 5.3.3), DHEA(S) and pregnenolone show some potential in schizophrenia [28], but ALLO has received most attention as a potential target for treatment of multiple neurological disorders, including Alzheimer's disease, Parkinson's disease, traumatic brain injury and multiple sclerosis as well as anxiety-related disorders [29]. Consequently, brexanolone, a synthetic version of ALLO, received US Food and Drug Administration approval in 2019 as the first treatment for postpartum depression, which carries potentially severe, life-threatening consequences for mother and child. However, there remain significant pharmacokinetic and pharmacodynamic challenges, because ALLO has to be administered by intravenous injection and requires careful monitoring by healthcare professionals due to significant side effects (sedation, loss of consciousness).

In the main, however, the clinical utility of hormone therapy for brain disorders remains to be proven and for most claims there is a counter-claim. There are many reasons which could account for this, especially the diversity in experimental and trial design. It is often the case that clinical investigations into the efficacy and validity of homone therapy are inadequately powered and controlled, representing no more than pilot studies providing no clear answers. Some preclinical and clinical studies fail to analyse male and female data separately, or do not clearly state the sex, despite incontrovertible evidence that male and female responses may differ (Table 5.3.2), such that efficacy in one sex may not be transferrable to the other [3, 30]. Dosage and timing are further critical considerations: steroids have infamous bell-shaped dose–response curves, with low and high concentrations having different effects to median concentrations [8, 27, 31], and there may only be a small window for efficacy [29, 32].

Perhaps one of the greatest challenges to realising the clinical effectiveness of hormone-based therapies is how to achieve selectivity. When aiming for effects in the brain, sex steroid hormones have a wide range of unwanted effects throughout the body, including masculinisation/feminisation of secondary sexual characteristics, oncogenic effects (breast, uterus, prostate) and cardiovascular effects. This can be avoided to a large extent by the use of selective oestrogen and androgen receptor modulators (SERMs and SARMs, respectively). For example, the SERM raloxifene (agonist in bone; antagonist in uterus and breast) is used in post-menopausal women at risk of bone fractures. The realisation that the effects and mechanisms of action of sex hormones in the brain are region-, cell type- and receptor subtype-specific (e.g. ER alpha versus ER beta) offered significant hope for developing SERMs and SARMs that are not only brain specific, but region or pathway specific, and hence disease specific. That promise of neuroSERMs/SARMs has not yet materialised, but there is evidence that existing SERMs have important central actions. For example, tamoxifen, used for its antagonist properties in ER-dependent breast cancer (but agonist in uterus and bone), may have value in managing episodes of mania and as an adjunct to dopamine antagonists in bipolar disorder [33]. Whether this is attributable to its ER activity is unclear, because it also blocks protein kinase C, an established mechanism of action of other treatments, such as lithium or valproate, and has antioxidant and free-radical scavenging properties. Potential uses for SARMs include positive effects on mood, cognitive impairment and post-menopausal female sexual dysfunction. Whether SARMs may help in sexual dysfunction associated with psychiatric disorders (see Section 5.3.5) remains to be tested. Interestingly, rodent data indicate that SERMs targeting ER beta may have effective antidepressant action via an ability to reduce CRH and arginine vasopressin release.

Brain steroid biosynthetic enzymes that synthesise or metabolise steroids offer further potential for selective modulation within the brain. The aromatase gene is of considerable interest, because it contains a brain-selective promoter. A better understanding of promoter regulation, therefore, offers the opportunity to selectively alter brain oestrogen levels, which could be further boosted via delivery of biosynthetic precursors, such as DHEA(S), which has minimal peripheral effects [3]. Interestingly, evidence suggests that selective serotonin reuptake inhibitors may act as brain steroidogenic stimulants, increasing levels of ALLO at low doses that are inactive on serotonin reuptake. Development of related compounds lacking effects on serotonin, but maintaining neurosteroidogenic capacity, may, therefore, help treat disorders where neurosteroid capacity is downregulated, such as major depression and PTSD [10, 34], and reduce side effects associated with elevated serotonin levels (see Section 5.3.5, Table 5.3.4).

Collectively, current research findings offer numerous new avenues for developing (neuro)endocrine-targeted novel therapies for treating brain disorders.

5.3.5 Sex Disturbances Related to Psychiatric Disorders

Individuals with mental health problems commonly present with a spectrum of sexual dysfunction, ranging from problems with libido, penile erection, vaginal lubrication and orgasm to infertility, which may be a consequence of the disease itself and/or medications. With regard to primary disease processes, changes in the hypothalamic–pituitary–gonadal (HPG) axis leading to a hypogonadal state (low levels of oestrogens or testosterone), or psychopathological factors affecting arousal and attentional processes, are likely contributors. Thus, in mood disorders, a lack of desire and interest in sex may be part of the more general anhedonia resulting from disruptions to the reward system. Equally, as glucocorticoids, the products of the HPA stress axis, are well known to downregulate the HPG axis, hyper-reactivity of the HPA axis in psychiatric disorders may also contribute to sexual dysfunction. In a group of antipsychoic-naive women with schizophrenia, sexual dysfunction has been attributed to elevated levels of prolactin, an established inhibitor of the HPG axis, leading to a hypo-oestrogenic state [14]. Prolactin release from the anterior pituitary gland is under inhibitory control by the tuberoinfundibular dopaminergic (TIDA) system (Figure 5.3.2) acting via dopamine 2 (D2) receptors on the lactotroph (prolactin-secreting) cells. It is unclear whether this system, along with the mesolimbic and mesocortical dopamine pathways, is disrupted in schizophrenia, but antenatal exposure of rats to raised glucocorticoid levels reprogrammes the TIDA in a sexually dimorphic manner [35], suggesting that disruptions in prolactin regulation may be present in disorders where exposure to stressors *in utero* (Table 5.3.3) contributes to pathology. Healthy sexual functioning requires inhibition of fear and threat networks, which may be difficult for people with anxiety disorders and trauma. For example, these networks are hyperactive in PTSD, where arousal appears to be associated with fear and danger. Some PTSD patients may avoid sexual behaviour to prevent the rise in arousal, which could rekindle fear-related memories. Consequently, cognitive–behavioural therapies rather than medication may help [36]. Sexual dysfunction is also prevalent in eating disorders [37]. The physiological consequences of malnutrition include suppression of the HPG axis and amenorrhoea. Anorexia also features negative attitudes to to the body and sexual intimacy, leading to avoidance

Table 5.3.4 Potential mechanisms whereby psychoactive drugs cause sexual dysfunction

Rates of sexual dysfunction	Examples	Likely mechanism of action
Drugs used to treat psychosis		
High	Classical medications (e.g. haloperidol, amisulpiride, paliperidone)	Principal antagonistic effect at D2 receptors (1) dampens mesolimbic dopamine transmission (reducing sexual desire) and (2) blocks inhibitory effect of tuberoinfundibular dopamine system on prolactin secretion from anterior pituitary lactotrophs; elevated circulating prolactin levels suppresses HPG (reduced circulating oestrogen and testosterone levels), with detrimental effects on all aspects of sexual activity cycle. High prolactin levels may also induce gynaecomastia and galactorrhoea, especially embarrassing in men.
Low	Atypical antipsychotic medications (e.g. clozapine, olanzapine, quetiapine, aripiprazole, ziprasidone)	Antagonistic effects at serotonin (5-HT) receptors (especially 5-HT2A); relatively lower D2 receptor antagonism, with reduced effects on prolactin levels. Consequently, effects on all aspects of sexual activity cycle are ameliorated.
Drugs used to treat depression, anxiety, obsessive–compulsive disorder		
High	SSRIs TCAs SNRIs (e.g. venlafaxine)	Increased extracellular levels of 5-HT inhibit sexual behaviour via either direct effects on central regulatory pathways (especially regulating erection and orgasm) or by suppressing mesolimbic dopamine transmission (reducing sexual desire) and tuberoinfundibular dopamine transmission (increasing anterior pituitary release of prolactin, causing suppression of HPG axis and circulating levels of oestrogen and testosterone), affecting all aspects of the sexual activity cycle.
Low to negligible	Agomelatine (agonist at melatonin receptors; antagonist at 5-HT2C receptors) Bupropion (NDRI) Mirtazapine SARIs (nefazodone, vortioxetine)	Varied pharmacological profiles, with few unwanted effects on sexual function.

Abbreviations: D2, dopamine 2 (receptor); HPG axis, hypothalamic–pituitary–gonadal axis; NDRI, noradrenaline and dopamine reuptake inhibitor; SARI, serotonin antagonist (5-HTA receptor) and reuptake inhibitor; SNRI, serotonin and noradrenaline reuptake inhibitor; SSRI, selective serotonin reuptake inhibitor; TCA, tricyclic antidepressant.

of sexual activity, whereas in bulimia impulsivity and difficulties in controlling emotions can be associated with extreme and sometimes self-harming sexual activity, followed by shame, withdrawal and avoidance. In bipolar disorder, a sparse literature supports the anecdotal clinical observations that hypersexuality may be uniquely associated with both the manic and hypomanic phases of bipolar disorder, although hyposexuality may also be seen in depressive episodes [38].

Whether or not sexual dysfunction is present as a primary component of any given psychiatric disorder, it is a well-known consequence of taking psychoactive medications [36]. While the precise underlying mechanisms remain to be determined, the ability of medications with antipsychotic action to antagonise dopamine D2 receptors and drugs used for depression to enhance setotonergic activity plays a key role [39], and newer drugs with reduced effects on these neurotransmitter systems have lesser consequences for sexual activity (Table 5.3.4). Hence, switching to one of these newer drugs is one option to ameliorate the problem of sexual dysfunction, often to such an extent

that medication is discontinued. Other options include lowering the dose of medication to the point where only the unwanted effect, but not the clinical effectiveness, is reduced. Adding in a dopamine agonist (e.g. bromocriptine, cabergoline) is likely to counter antipsychotic efficiency. Some adjuncts to treatment have, however, had some success in reducing aspects of sexual dysfunction. These include adding in sex-hormone replacement therapy to reverse hypogonadism, or inhibitors of cyclic guanosine monophosphate-specific phosphodiesterase-5 (e.g. sildenafil, tadalafil), which enhance nitric oxide-dependent vasodilation and increase blood flow to the penis (enabling erection) as well as to clitoral and vaginal tissues.

The continuing improvement of psychoactive drugs is critically important, because sexual dysfunction has considerable impact on patients' well-being, self-esteem and quality of life, and may lead to patients discontinuing medication. Its relevance, however, is often neglected, partly because of sociocultural taboos in discussing intimate issues and partly because of the relative inexperience of clinicians in approaching such matters. In recognition of the problem, guidelines for assessing sexual dysfunction are now beginning to appear.

5.3.6 Gender Identity

In most individuals, gender identity aligns with the spectrum of masculinity/femininity of their phenotypic sex assigned at birth (cisgender) but, for transgender people, this is not the case, which can lead to feelings of distress. This is currently termed gender dysphoria, receiving a DSM-5 classification [40]. It may be declassified as a disorder as preconceptions of the binary nature of gender erode. Indeed, preliminary neuroimaging research indicates that brain morphology and activation patterns at rest and during cognitive performance are more congruent with gender identity than birth sex in untreated male-to-female (MTF) and female-to-male (FTM) transgender people, indicating that the trans brain may have innate qualities related to brain development [41]. This is further reinforced by the knowledge that hormonally directed gonadal and brain sex differentiation are independent events, separated by a significant time period in development (Figure 5.3.2A), providing a scientific rationale for a biological basis in the mismatch between the two.

Gender-affirming hormone thrapy (GAHT) plays an important role in allowing transgender people to achieve their desired phenotype, which may lead to psychological improvements [41]. In MTF people this comprises devirilisation with cyproterone acetate (androgen antagonist) followed by feminisation with high-dose oestrogens and long-acting gonadotropin-releasing hormone (GnRH) agonists to suppress the HPG axis and androgen production. FTM people receive high-dose progestogens for HPG suppression and defeminisation, followed by testosterone for virilisation [13]. Long-acting GnRH agonists may also be employed to suppress puberty in certain gender non-conforming minors. This will temporarily halt the development of secondary sexual characteristics that accord with their natal sex assignment and extend the temporal window to affirm their gender identification. Current investigations provide short-term evidence for GAHT-induced changes in structure and neural activation in various brain regions and indicate a slight reduction in the rates of anxiety, depression and suicide risk following GAHT, although rates remain significantly higher than those for the cisgender population. Longer-term follow-up studies are needed to address the safety of such treatments. GAHT generates a hormonal environment that

is incongruous for individuals whose brains have developed under the influence XX or XY genes and the ensuing developmental hormonal milieu. It involves creation of a hypo-oestrogenic, hyperandrogenic environment in FTM XX individuals and a hypoandrogenic, hyper-oestrogenic environment in MTF XY individuals. Such states are known to have deleterious effects on the brain and behaviour, as well cardiovascular and oncogenic effects, in cisgender females and males. These are causes for concern and require comprehensive longitudinal studies.

Conclusions and Outstanding Questions

This chapter briefly summarises the abundant evidence for biological sex differences in brain structure, function and connectivity and how this is shaped and maintained by sex hormones, with implications for sex differences in normal behavioural, cognitive and emotional responses as well as vulnerability and resilience to the risk of developing psychiatric and neurological disorders. As a corollary to a potential role in psychopathology, we have considered the pros and cons of hormone-based therapies in psychoactive disorders as well as their use in gender-affirming therapy in transgender individuals. Ultimately, our growing understanding of sex, sex hormones and psychiatric disorders highlights the absolute necessity to further erode the sex and gender bias currently present in neuroscience and mental health research in order to optimise treatments for every sex and gender [30].

Outstanding Questions

- What is the aetiology of disease and how does it differ between sexes and genders?
- What are the neural mechanisms underlying functional brain changes induced by sex hormones, their mimics and neurosteroids?
- How can we create steroid-hormone-based therapies that are brain, system and neurotransmitter selective, and hence disease specific?
- Can we selectively modulate brain steroid biosynthetic enzymes to harness the therapeutic potential of neurosteroids?
- Are the onset, progress and patterns of psychiatric symptoms influenced by hormonal events and can manipulations of hormone levels maximise clinical responsiveness to current treatments (e.g. cognitive–behavioural therapy)?

REFERENCES

1. L. Cahill. Why sex matters for neuroscience. *Nat Rev Neurosci* 2006; 7:477–484.

2. K. P. Cosgrove, C. M. Mazure, J. K. Staley. *Biol Psychiatry* 2007; 62: 847–855.

3. G. E. Gillies, S. McArthur. Estrogen actions in the brain and the basis for differential action in men and women: a case for sex-specific medicines. *Pharmacol Rev* 2010; 62: 155–198.

4. D. R. Rubinow, P. J. Schmidt. Sex differences and the neurobiology of affective disorders. *Neuropsychopharmacology* 2019; 44: 111–128.

5. M. M. McCarthy, A. P. Arnold. Reframing sexual differentiation of the brain. *Nature Neuroscience* 2011; 14: 677–683.

6. G. J. De Vries. Minireview: sex differences in adult and developing brains: compensation, compensation, compensation. *Endocrinology* 2004; 145: 1063–1068.

7. G. E. Gillies, K. Virdee, S. McArthur et al. Sex-dependent diversity in ventral tegmental dopaminergic neurons and developmental programming: A molecular, cellular and behavioral analysis. *Neuroscience* 2014; 282: 69–85.

8. G. E. Gillies, I. S. Pienaar, S. Vohra et al. Sex differences in Parkinson's disease. *Front Neuroendocrinol* 2014; 35: 370–384.

9. G. E. Gillies, K. Virdee, I. Pienaar et al. Enduring, sexually dimorphic impact of *in utero* exposure to elevated levels of glucocorticoids on midbrain dopaminergic populations. *Brain Sci* 2016; 7(1): 5.

10. R. C. Melcangi, S. Giatti, L. M. Garcia-Segura. Levels and actions of neuroactive steroids in the nervous system under physiological and pathological conditions: sex-specific features. *Neurosci Biobehav Rev* 2016; 67: 25–40.

11. T. Paus, M. Keshavan, J. N. Giedd. Why do many psychiatric disorders emerge during adolescence? *Nat Rev Neurosci* 2008; 9: 947–957.

12. M. Altemus. Hormone-specific psychiatric disorders: do they exist? *Arch Womens Ment Health* 2010; 13: 25–26.

13. S. Toffoletto, R. Lanzenberger, M. Gingnell et al. Emotional and cognitive functional imaging of estrogen and progesterone effects in the female human brain: a systematic review. *Psychoneuroendocrinology* 2014; 50: 28–52.

14. A. Riecher-Rössler. Oestrogens, prolactin, hypothalamic–pituitary–gonadal axis, and schizophrenic psychoses. *Lancet Psychiatry* 2017; 4: 63–72.

15. C. J. Pike. Sex and the development of Alzheimer's disease. *J Neurosci Res* 2017; 95: 671–680.

16. Y. C. Huang, C. F. Hung, P. Y. Lin et al. Gender differences in susceptibility to schizophrenia: potential implication of neurosteroids. *Psychoneuroendocrinology* 2017; 84: 87–93.

17. S. Wichmann, C. Kirschbaum, C. Böhme et al. Cortisol stress response in post-traumatic stress disorder, panic disorder, and major depressive disorder patients. *Psychoneuroendocrinology* 2017; 83: 135–141.

18. A. N. Hoffman, A. N. Taylor. Stress reactivity after traumatic brain injury: implications for comorbid post-traumatic stress disorder. *Behav Pharmaco* 2019; 30: 115–121.

19. B. M. Kudielka, C. Kirschbaum. Sex differences in HPA axis responses to stress: a review. *Biol Psychol* 2005; 69: 113–132.

20. D. A. Bangasser, B. J. Wicks. Sex-specific mechanisms for responding to stress. *Neurosci Res* 2017; 95: 75–82.

21. L. Y. Maeng, M. R. Milad. Sex differences in anxiety disorders: interactions between fear, stress, and gonadal hormones. *Horm Behav* 2015; 76: 106–117.

22. S. H. Li, B. M. Graham. Why are women so vulnerable to anxiety, trauma-related and stress-related disorders? The potential role of sex hormones. *Lancet Psychiatry* 2017; 4: 73–82.

23. T. Bäckström, M. Bixo, M. Johansson et al. Allopregnanolone and mood disorders. *Prog Neurobiol* 2014; 113: 88–94.

24. R. M. Gifford, R. M. Reynolds. Sex differences in early-life programming of the hypothalamic–pituitary–adrenal axis in humans. *Early Hum Dev* 2017; 114: 7–10.

25. C. Heim, E. B. Binder. Current research trends in early life stress and depression: review of human studies on sensitive periods, gene–environment interactions, and epigenetics. *Exp Neurol* 2012; 233: 102–111.

26. J. W. Roh, H. J. Park, U. Kang. Hormones and psychiatric disorders. *Clinic Psychopharmacol Neurosci* 2007; 5: 3–13.

27. M. Chávez-Castillo, V. Núñez, M. Nava et al. Depression as a neuroendocrine disorder: emerging neuropsychopharmacological approaches beyond monoamines. *Adv Pharmacol Sci* 2019; 2: 7943481.

28. M. S. Ritsner. The clinical and therapeutic potentials of dehydroepiandrosterone and pregnenolone in schizophrenia. *Neuroscience.* 2011; 191: 91–100.

29. R. W. Irwin, C. M. Solinsky, R. D. Brinton. Frontiers in therapeutic development of allopregnanolone for Alzheimer's disease and other neurological disorders. *Front Cell Neurosci* 2014; 8: 203.

30. L. M. Howard, A. M. Ehrlich, F. Gamlen F et al. Gender-neutral mental health research is sex and gender biased. *Lancet Psychiatry* 2017; 4: 9–11.

31. M. B. Solomon, J. P. Herman. Sex differences in psychopathology: of gonads, adrenals and mental illness. *Physiol Behav* 2009; 97: 250–258.

32. M. Singh, J. W. Simpkins, H. A. Bimonte-Nelson et al. Window of opportunity for estrogen and progestin intervention in brain aging and Alzheimer's disease. *Brain Res* 2013; 1514: 1–2.

33. J. Palacios, A. Yildiz, A. H. Young et al. Tamoxifen for bipolar disorder: systematic review and meta-analysis. *J Psychopharmacol* 2019; 33: 177–184.

34. G. Pinna, E. Costa, A. Guidotti. SSRIs act as selective brain steroidogenic stimulants (SBSSs) at low doses that are inactive on 5-HT reuptake. *Curr Opin Pharmacol* 2009; 9: 24–30.

35. S. McArthur, Z. L. Siddique, H. C. Christian et al. Perinatal glucocorticoid treatment disrupts the hypothalamo-lactotroph axis in adult female, but not male, rats. *Endocrinology* 2006; 147: 1904–1915.

36. Barata BC. Affective disorders and sexual function: from neuroscience to clinic. *Curr Opin Psychiatry* 2017; 30: 396–401.

37. V. Kravvariti, F. Gonidakis . [Eating disorders and sexual function]. *Psychiatriki* 2016; 27: 136–143.

38. I. Kopeykina, H. J. Kim, T. Khatun et al. Hypersexuality and couple relationships in bipolar disorder: a review. *J Affect Disord* 2016; 195: 1–14.

39. M. K. de Boer, S. Castelein, D. Wiersma et al. The facts about sexual (dys)function in schizophrenia: an overview of clinically relevant findings. *Schizophr Bull* 2015; 41: 674–686.

40. American Psychiatric Association. *Diagnostic and Statistical Manual of Mental Disorders*, 5th ed. (DSM-5). American Psychiatric Association, 2013.

41. H. B. Nguyen, J. Loughead, E. Lipner et al. What has sex got to do with it? The role of hormones in the transgender brain. *Neuropsychopharmacology* 2019; 44: 22–37.

National Neuroscience Curriculum Initiative online resources

Sex Differences and Personalized Psychiatric Care

Kristen L. Eckstrand, Michael John Travis, Erika E. Forbes, and Mary Louise Phillips

Premenstrual Dysphoric Disorder: From Plato to Petri Dishes

Erica B. Baller and David A. Ross

This "stuff" is really cool: Erica Baller, *"Menstrual Mysteries"*

Herbert E. Covington III and
Klaus A. Miczek

5.4 **Violence and Aggression**

OVERVIEW

Many aggressive and violent behavioural phenotypes (described clinically) are seen across much of the class Mammalia. Here we discuss how the early focus on explaining such behaviours with reference to specific brain regions and single monoaminergic neurotransmitters has matured into an understanding based on neurogenetic networks with different molecular constituents underlying different kinds of aggression. Some of the aminergic and peptidergic neurotransmitter targets that are used clinically significantly reduce bursts of aggressive and violent behaviours. However, long-term treatment strategies remain challenging for clinicians when controlling persistent aggressive syndromes. Current therapies for managing violence, at least in clinical settings, will be enhanced by preclinical experimental efforts that pinpoint more exact pharmacodynamics within neural circuits underlying specific aggressive behaviours. A comprehensive appreciation of the neuroscience of excessive aggression is necessary to begin understanding the complex framework in which patterns of community violence appear.

5.4.1 Transition from Adaptive to Maladaptive Aggression: Types of Aggression

Violence is a global burden with substantial consequences for physical, social and mental health of the individual and the immediate and wider social surroundings [1]. The term 'violence' refers to intense, harmful aggressive acts in the clinical and legal literature, whereas ethologists (scientists studying behaviour of all species) most often study 'aggression' as behavioural adaptation in conflict situations. Violence in and of itself has not been categorised as a disorder, but can be a symptom of many psychopathologies including antisocial personality disorder, intermittent explosive disorder, borderline personality disorder, alcohol and substance use disorder, conduct disorder, post-traumatic stress disorder, as well as psychotic disorders – particularly when comorbid with alcohol and substance use disorders. While such diagnoses are most often associated with self-inflicted, family and intimate partner violence, the strongest predictor of

community violence is *not* mental illness, but an earlier incidence of violence [2]. Patterns of aggression by an individual are often unpredictable and varied in terms of their releasers or triggers, rate of occurrence, intensity and duration [3].

The clinical distinction between **reactive** and **proactive** aggression is based on motivational factors that comprise the distal and proximal antecedents of aggressive **actions** and their **outcomes**. One could argue that there is a distinct neurobiology underlying each of these forms of aggression, but each appears to share considerable overlap within a top-down circuitry model (see Figure 5.4.1). Reactive, 'hot' acts of aggression involve intense affect, impulsivity or hostility. These acts occur with a short latency and mobilise the sympathetic nervous system followed by activation of the hypothalamic–pituitary–adrenal (HPA) stress axis. Dysregulation of negative emotions appears to predispose individuals towards reactive forms of violence. This explosive, arousing type of aggression is linked to excessive neural activity in subcortical and limbic areas with corresponding deficits in more **dorsal** components of the prefrontal cortex – where executive functions originate and conscious experiences of emotions are assembled – with little direct, immediate oversight over the amygdala complex [4, 5]. In fact, violent offenders inherently express higher baseline levels of amygdala–**ventral** prefrontal cortical connectivity. Overall, such data point to neural mechanisms that engender susceptibility to violence during social encounters that should ordinarily elicit only modest 'emotional' demands [6]. These neural events are now being investigated at the cellular and molecular level (see below).

In contrast, 'cold', premeditated or predatory aggression serves as an instrumental means to an end. Like reactive aggression, neuroimaging studies demonstrate that amygdala activity is exaggerated in such violent offenders, while cortical connectivity remains more or less intact. Premeditated aggression as compared to reactive aggression leads to significantly smaller surges in blood corticosteroid levels. Individuals scoring high on the **Hare Psychopathy Checklist – Revised** are remarkably prone to carrying out instrumental antisocial behaviours [7]. Most of these individuals meet the criteria for antisocial personality disorder, display deficits in general arousal and dysregulated amygdala activity during emotional challenges, and exhibit impairments in aversive conditioning like that of passive avoidance learning – learning not to do something that is punished [8]. Psychopathy and also sociopathy are characterised by a **trait** for maladaptive aggression that can be both reactive and proactive, which complicates pinpointing an ontological and biological basis for different types of aggression, or for reliably classifying explosive and premeditated patterns of violence.

5.4.2 Translational Models of Maladaptive Aggression

In the Darwinian tradition, studies on the evolutionary origins of aggressive behaviour have focused on its adaptive nature, such as securing resources within a patrolled and defended territory, selecting mates, attaining social rank/status and group identity. Among socially organised mammalian species, aggression is phylogenetically conserved, and rare acts of intense violence can occur, as illustrated by the lethal raids of chimpanzees directed at neighboring troops [9]. Animal models of violence have translational validity (i.e. good correspondence to human

pathology) in that animals can also exhibit behaviours that deviate from species-typical aggression. Ethological analyses have identified excessive, maladaptive aggression in most mammalian species by (1) low provocation thresholds (a shortened latency to initiate attack), (2) injurious attack sequences (high intensity), (3) more frequent and prolonged attack bouts (failure to stop), (4) attacks directed towards an inappropriate target (e.g. juveniles), (5) a disregard for the long-term consequences of an attack and (6) a disregard for an opponent's appeasement signals (e.g. submission [3]).

In parallel to instrumental and reactive types of aggression in humans, experimental preparations that allow for quantitative and qualitative analyses have identified two categories of animal aggression that are critical for empirical analyses: agonistic and predatory acts. **Agonistic acts** occur in territorial conflicts or in the establishment and maintenance of dominance hierarchies and are typically directed against members of the same species. **Predatory acts** extend beyond a familiar context, may be directed against animals of other species and are motivated by challenges to homeostasis like hunger. Agonistic behaviours, involving increased autonomic signs of affect, have been further subdivided into **offensive** and **defensive** fighting in all species ranging from reptiles and fish to primates [10]. Classic early experimental approaches used *in vivo* electrical stimulation through microelectrodes implanted within discrete sites in the medial and lateral hypothalamic nuclei: stimulation at these sites evoked affective defence *or* predatory attack, respectively [11]. Interestingly, hypothalamic neural ensembles that become active during the initiation, performance and termination of fights are further shaped by experience [12]. This hypothalamic plasticity determines the likelihood of future attacks and the probability of expressing other social behaviours. The past century of aggression research has provided a comprehensive map of the neural architecture supporting activities that range from social approach to forceful attacks. Aggression is the result of a consistent pattern of neural activity in a 'survival circuit' – a network that is constantly being updated by experience of success and failure [13].

5.4.3 Neural Networks

Experimental work in animals is gradually revealing a precise role for certain neural circuits that mediate

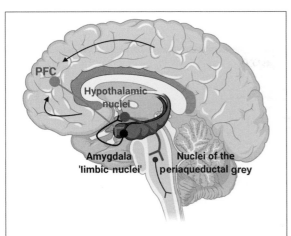

Figure 5.4.1. A 'top-down' model of aggressive behaviour. Orbital frontal, dorsolateral and ventromedial cortical nuclei collectively determine the degree of control over aggression that is assembled to exert inhibitory feedback onto deeper 'limbic' structures. Unless inhibited by circuits initiated in the prefrontal cortex (PFC), the medial amygdala is poised to deliver strong pro-aggressive signals to hypothalamic targets that orchestrate the intensity and duration of specific behavioural actions. Those decisive actions of the hypothalamic nuclei are delivered to corresponding motor neurons organised within the brainstem. Dysregulation of this circuit at any point can generate what is considered maladaptive aggression or pathological violence. For instance, dysregulated PFC–amygdala connectivity has been linked to impulsive, reactive aggressive outbursts, whereas hyper-activation of amygdala–paralimbic structures can be associated with both reactive and 'cold' aggression. Highly conserved mammalian structures like the hypothalamic nuclei once considered to be 'hard-wired' in fact show substantial plasticity – they gradually fine-tune and amplify their neural activity to drive repeated aggressive behavioural routines. Thus, interactions between cell ensembles in the diencephalon and brainstem areas like the periaqueductal grey can be modified by social experiences. Areas like the PFC that are enriched in modulators and receptors for amine neurotransmitters, particularly serotonin, have been useful for curbing self-inflicted or close-interpersonal aggression. The underlying mechanisms for most types of violence including self-inflicted, familial, intimate partner and community directed acts of aggression are in need of precise delineation.

agonistic and predatory aggression. Current evidence suggests that the neural circuits controlling species-typical attacks and threats overlap and interact with those involved in many other prominent adaptive social behaviours like sex, parenting, bonding and play [14]. Yet, there is still much to be learned about the cortical mechanisms that enable executive control over aggressive behaviour for most animal species, despite a wealth of studies demonstrating the critical role of information transmission between the medial, basal, lateral and central amygdala, preoptic area, bed nucleus of the stria terminalis, lateral septum, anterior hypothalamic nucleus, paraventricular nucleus of the hypothalamus, perifornical

region of the lateral hypothalamus, ventral portion of the pre-mammillary nucleus, ventral lateral portion of the ventromedial hypothalamus and supra-mammillary nuclei (see Figure 5.4.2). Activity in the neural circuitry connecting these nuclei contributes to the initiation, performance and termination of aggressive sequences, as described below.

5.4.3.1 Cortical Control

The orbital frontal cortex is crucial for assimilating contextual, historical and sensory details to formulate decisions about the orchestration of offensive and defensive behaviours. A functioning orbital frontal cortex is required for impulse control over aggressive displays that originate from limbic nuclei, particularly the amygdaloid complex. This anterior medial prefrontal cortical nucleus is less active in psychopathy, and in healthy individuals when making impulsive decisions. Anger-induced states of attenuated orbital frontal cortex activity are inversely related to increased amygdala responses, and lesions of the orbital frontal cortex often lead to acquired sociopathy [17]. Such findings support the hypothesis that limbic and diencephalic structures are governed by the prefrontal cortex in a 'top-down' hierarchical system of emotional regulation (see Figure 5.4.1). In species-typical aggression, less is known about cellular and molecular mechanisms in cortical structures than in limbic nuclei, but changes in cellular markers of functional activity within the cortex indicate an important and dynamic role for this area during fighting. For example, adaptations in catecholamine uptake have been demonstrated in the cerebral cortex of mice after only a single aggressive experience [18]. Furthermore, the initiation of an attack, its execution and the cessation of a fighting bout can be significantly modulated by descending cortical projections onto limbic and brainstem structures. Such observations support a role for dysregulation of top-down control of typical adaptive fighting in excessive aggression.

5.4.3.2 Midbrain and Brainstem Control

In mice, the ventral portion of the pre-mammillary nucleus provides excitatory stimulation of the supra-mammillary nuclei and ventral lateral portion of the ventromedial hypothalamus, which respectively modulate attack duration and the total number of attacks during a fight [19]. Steroid receptor-expressing neurons, particularly oestrogen receptor alpha-positive cells in the ventral

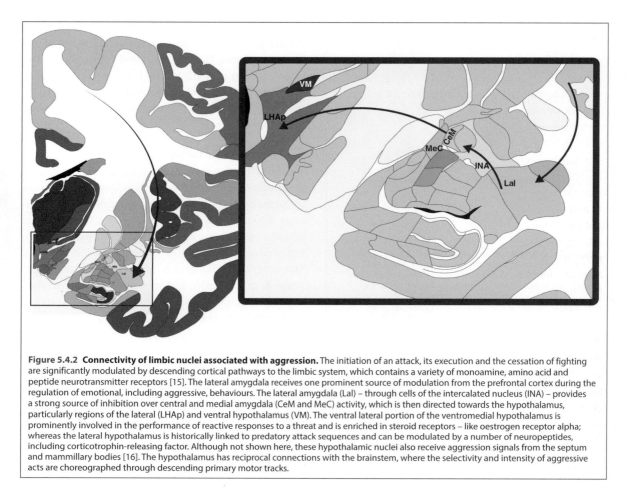

Figure 5.4.2 Connectivity of limbic nuclei associated with aggression. The initiation of an attack, its execution and the cessation of fighting are significantly modulated by descending cortical pathways to the limbic system, which contains a variety of monoamine, amino acid and peptide neurotransmitter receptors [15]. The lateral amygdala receives one prominent source of modulation from the prefrontal cortex during the regulation of emotional, including aggressive, behaviours. The lateral amygdala (LaI) – through cells of the intercalated nucleus (INA) – provides a strong source of inhibition over central and medial amygdala (CeM and MeC) activity, which is then directed towards the hypothalamus, particularly regions of the lateral (LHAp) and ventral hypothalamus (VM). The ventral lateral portion of the ventromedial hypothalamus is prominently involved in the performance of reactive responses to a threat and is enriched in steroid receptors – like oestrogen receptor alpha; whereas the lateral hypothalamus is historically linked to predatory attack sequences and can be modulated by a number of neuropeptides, including corticotrophin-releasing factor. Although not shown here, these hypothalamic nuclei also receive aggression signals from the septum and mammillary bodies [16]. The hypothalamus has reciprocal connections with the brainstem, where the selectivity and intensity of aggressive acts are choreographed through descending primary motor tracks.

lateral portion of the ventromedial hypothalamus appear to shape the strength and quality of these attacks [20]. The excitability of these hypothalamic nuclei adapts with repeated fighting experiences. Daily bouts of aggression fine-tune ensembles of neurons expressing oestrogen receptor alpha, suggesting that specific cell populations active during the execution of a fight become increasingly more specialised following a winning experience [12].

More evidence for a hierarchical neural organisation of species-typical aggression is obtained from studies focused on midbrain structures, including the periaqueductal grey. Recordings from the dorsal periaqueductal grey reveal its functional activation during fights, and electrical stimulation of this region rapidly evokes intense affective defence responses [21]. Neuronal tracing studies have identified descending second-order glutamatergic periaqueductal grey projections (i.e. a pathway

with one intervening synapse) to the pontine nucleus, raphe magnus and locus coeruleus, which modulate arousal, sympathetic tone and motor aspects of the well-characterised feline 'affective defence'. Ascending attack-promoting tracts densely target areas of the ventromedial hypothalamus, which, as mentioned above, also coordinates elements of defensive responses through reciprocal connections to the periaqueductal grey.

5.4.4 Neurotransmitters and Modulators

The integrity and intensity of acts and postures during confrontations depend on the coordinated functional connectivity between medullary, mesencephalic (midbrain) and diencephalic structures (mainly thalamus and hypothalamus). Cortical and striatal contributions during aggressive outbursts encode events as they unfold and contribute to planning future actions. This activity coincides with dopamine and serotonin release in cortical and limbic structures during the initiation of social encounters that range from subordination to offensive aggression [22]. These amine neurotransmitters are key in linking actions to outcomes during fights and contribute to the motivation to engage in or instigate future fights. Within the mesencephalon, the abundant expression of steroids, neuropeptides and their receptors (i.e. testosterone, oestrogen, opioids, corticotrophin-releasing hormone, oxytocin, vasopressin) that converge on and modulate the monoamines are equally important for stabilising patterns of social behaviour, particularly aggression. The immediate functional role of any given neurotransmitter within a circuit is determined by a combination of their distal trait determinants (e.g. inherited genetic and epigenetic regulation of RNA and protein expression) and proximal (i.e. more immediate) physiological states (e.g. sympathetic tone, glucose availability, etc.). Despite these complexities, detailed analysis of the molecular, cellular and circuit mechanisms underlying the expression of aggressive behaviours has been aided by technological advances, particularly the use of transgenic rodent models (animals with targeted gene mutations), which allow us to test the causal contribution of individual genes to aggressive behaviour.

5.4.4.1 Serotonin

The recognition of a 'fight-or-flight' syndrome and its relationship to the hypothalamus [23] was followed by systematic investigations of midbrain and brainstem structures, most prominently the raphe nuclei, locus coeruleus and tegmentum (ventral midbrain) for their role in aggressive behaviour. Of the amine neurotransmitters originating from these structures, serotonin was initially identified as having a role in the inhibitory control of aggressive and violent acts [24]. This early work established the 'serotonin deficiency hypothesis', which simplistically portrayed serotonin as a civilising neurohumour. Violent outbursts were considered a result of generalised deficits in this transmitter function as a result of environmental, genetic or a nuanced combination of both factors. Accordingly, it was thought that restoring levels of serotonin would prove useful for inhibiting violent acts. As evidence, the 1990s provided a series of high-profile papers devoted to a single monoamine gene approach

to the study of aggression, in a 'bottom-up' conceptualisation of this behaviour. Several decades' worth of studies now detail a more intricate and realistic view of serotonin's inactivation, synthesis, release, transport and receptor binding (including a vastly complex expression profile for serotonin receptors throughout the brain) on phases of fighting performance. Serotonin has at least 14 receptor subtypes – linked to metabotropic or ionotropic signalling cascades – which are distributed throughout the mammalian central nervous system. Modulation of aggression by these diverse receptor populations in limbic structures and neocortical areas stems primarily from the firing patterns of serotonergic neurons ascending from the dorsal raphe nucleus. Animal studies from invertebrates to humans have revealed that serotonin is critically involved in the onset and cessation of many types of aggression, including impulsive attacks, hostile and excessive fighting, and even predation.

Impulsive forms of human aggression are attributed to dysregulation of interactions between the prefrontal cortex and amygdala. Anger that is provoked occurs with significant activation within the amygdala. This immediate amygdala activity is soon followed by increased prefrontal cortical activation, at least in healthy subjects. The prefrontal cortex response inhibits activity in the amygdala and, without this inhibitory modulation, exaggerated emotional responses such as aggression can occur. An important stabilising factor for typical prefrontal cortex–amygdala connectivity is serotonin transmission [25]. Thus, alterations in the bioavailability of serotonin can disturb prefrontal cortex–amygdala connectivity and escalate aggressive behaviours. High levels of trait aggression are also reported to occur with disruptions in prefrontal cortex–amygdala functional connectivity. In cases of dementia where high levels of aggression can persist for months or even years, successful pharmacotherapeutic management strategies include selective serotonin reuptake inhibitors citalopram and sertraline, as well as the serotonin 1B receptor partial agonist buspirone [26].

Variants in the gene coding for monoamine oxidase A (MAO-A, which catalyses the breakdown of serotonin) can serve as a predictor of trait aggression. Complete knockdown of this gene in the case of Brunner syndrome results in abnormally high aggression (and severe delinquency), which is paradoxically associated with *excessive* brain serotonin levels (going against the simplistic serotonin deficiency hypothesis of aggression). More subtle variations in serotonin transmission can be driven through numerous polymorphisms in the **MAO-A uVNTR domain** (upstream variable-number tandem repeat domain, that is, person-to-person variation in the number of repeats of a short genetic sequence in the regulatory regions of the gene before the gene transcription start site). A strong gene–environment interaction appears to exist, such that intense childhood trauma in those individuals who have variants associated with low MAO-A gene expression (MAOA-L carriers) can increase vulnerability to heightened aggression. Neurobiological models have attempted to explain how this allelic risk factor, through a blunting of serotonergic tone, could impact amygdalar activity [27].

5.4.4.2 Dopamine

The violence expressed by a subpopulation of institutionalised patients is routinely managed with drugs that have antipsychotic action, particularly compounds with a high selectivity for dopamine D2 receptors [28]. The anti-aggressive pharmacotherapeutic profile of these drugs is compromised by their marked sedative and motor side effects. Thus, these compounds are useful for immediate control of aggressive behaviours but do not provide a promising maintenance strategy for long-term recurring violence. Recent clinical studies on persistent excessive aggression that sometimes (albeit rarely) emerges with psychosis have found promising results with second-generation drugs used for psychosis such as clozapine, olanzapine and risperidone [29]. These compounds significantly reduce aggression during psychotic outbursts. In addition to their actions on dopamine receptors, these compounds may achieve efficacy through their actions at histaminergic, cholinergic and noradrenergic receptor subtypes. But, as with first-generation drugs with antipsychotic action, side effects remain problematic. Disentangling the exact mechanisms responsible for the anti-aggressive effects of typical and atypical medication with antipsychotic action has been hindered by their wide-ranging effects on sensory, motor and motivational functions. Research focusing on the relationship between a patient's specific aggressive tendencies as they are matched with specific drugs used for psychosis may help to elucidate the neural underpinnings of violent psychiatric symptoms.

An intriguing line of research has demonstrated that aggression can serve as a potent reward in most mammalian species, including people [30]. One function of the mesocorticolimbic dopamine system is to encode the probability of reward outcomes and signal when errors occur in these predictions [31] . Phasic dopamine activity in the striatum and prefrontal cortex increases when offensive and defensive aggressive acts are anticipated, initiated and terminated. In mice, blockade of dopamine D1 and D2 receptors in the ventral striatum reduces both motivated 'operant' responses, leading to the opportunity to fight, and the intensity of aggressive bouts [32], highlighting dopamine's non-selective range of effects on motivation and motor output. Psychomotor stimulant administration or selective optogenetic stimulation of dopamine neurons in the ventral tegmental area significantly escalates aggression in rodent studies, underscoring the need to further understand this neurotransmitter's function as it precisely relates to the initiation of aggressive outbursts.

5.4.4.3 Noradrenaline

Another catecholamine, noradrenaline, has a particularly important role in both generalised arousal and specific 'aggressive arousal'. The anticipation of aggression and violence is associated with intense excitement of sympathetic tone as well as behaviour. These anticipatory responses are initiated when a cluster of noradrenergic neurons within the locus coeruleus become activated. This same cluster of neurons is, however, active when attention is directed toward any salient stimulus. For example, significant rises in noradrenaline are also observed when simply witnessing aggressive confrontations [33]. Not surprisingly, beta blockers like propranolol, metropolol or pindolol are quite effective calming agents in the context of potentially intense aggressive outbursts [34]. Noradrenaline receptor antagonism (like dopamine receptor antagonism) has strong sedative effects, but beta-receptor blockade, either alone or in combination with selective dopamine receptor antagonists, is a promising avenue for treating violence associated with psychosis.

Studies on generalised anticipatory arousal have the potential to shed light on the neurobiology of specific *types* of arousal. The anticipation for a fight is likely upheld by neural circuits that differ from neural circuits promoting sexual behaviours and other natural rewards. Similarly, the neural circuitry of fight seeking is different from the neural mechanisms that underlie the *performance* of a fight [30]. Pharmacological tools that can selectively target the motivational aspects of violence should be a primary focus of experimental efforts. As just one example, alcohol, when consumed at intoxicating doses that significantly disrupt coordinated behaviour, continues to escalate attempts at violence. This is reflected in the overwhelming percentage of violent crimes associated with alcohol consumption. Such data highlight a critical need to understand the specific neurobiology of aggressive motivation.

5.4.5 From Neuroscience to Treatment Strategies

Contemporary science on the neural basis of aggression and violence has the potential to advance the currently limited treatment strategies and diagnostic approaches to the various forms of aggression seen in psychiatry. Modulators of monoamine function continue to be one source of significant interest. Polymorphisms in gene products that regulate the bioavailability of monoamines (e.g. MAO-A) and the serotonin-transporter-linked promoter region (5-HTTLPR) have been closely associated with patterns of childhood, adolescent and adult aggression and violence, particularly after experiencing early-life trauma. Other modulators of dopamine, noradrenaline and serotonin synaptic transmission, including neuropeptides and steroids, are also promising pharmacotherapeutic targets. Recently, intranasal brain-penetrant oxytocin administrations have made it possible to study the role of this neuropeptide in clinical experimental settings of human aggression. While a role for these modulators of classical neurotransmitter actions is compelling, there is still much to be learned about large individual differences in the effects of any single hormone, peptide or protein in psychiatric disease, as highlighted by the following observations:

- MAO-A is most active early on during child development before MAO-B assumes a more prominent role in the synaptic regulation of monoamines. A role for MAO-A in aggression has emerged as significant in individuals with a history of early child abuse, highlighting complex gene–environment interactions and the importance of critical periods early in life.

While not all individuals with both risk factors are abnormally aggressive there may be promise for MAO inhibitors or selective serotonin reuptake inhibitors for curbing episodic aggression in the context of child and adolescent mental health services.

- The short allele for the serotonin (5-HT) transporter *5-HTT* gene, which is associated with decreased gene expression (and would be expected to increase synaptic serotonin), is often present in abnormal aggression. Paradoxically, low cerebral spinal fluid concentrations of serotonin – reflecting summed brain serotonergic activity – have also been associated with heightened aggression. Complex epigenetic processes that determine levels of serotonin receptor expression in cortical and subcortical cell clusters may underlie these apparently conflicting results.

- Oxytocin is often viewed as exerting pro-social effects, as its administration increases ratings of trustworthiness in economic games, and this peptide reduces aggression while facilitating intimate social bonds in animal models. Oxytocin can, however, drive these effects through intensifying social competence. Evidence suggests a bidirectional relationship between increasing familiarity with a social stimulus and the putative pro-social effects of oxytocin. In fact, the more unfamiliar, different or distant a social stimulus is, the more likely oxytocin will generate a ethnocentric-like response (i.e. the tendency to view one's own group as superior to other groups) [35].

Conclusions and Outstanding Questions

Much more work is clearly needed to clarify the role of genetic predispositions, traits and states of individuals and their response to candidate mechanisms for the treatment of different kinds of human aggression. Preclinical studies have already begun to outline a plethora of candidate mechanisms targeting receptors for glutamate and GABA in cortical, diencephalic (such as the habenula) and brainstem nuclei as well as other neuropeptides and hormones (e.g. [36, 37]). The functional connectivity between neural populations imbedded within multiple circuits that mediate arousal, motivation and reward processes, otherwise known as survival circuits, have been critically implicated in the dysregulation of behavioural processes, including violence. Selectively modulating the state of any one aspect of these circuit dynamics is the current challenge.

While pharmacological treatments that dampen many components (e.g. drugs with anticonvulsant, anxiolytic and antipsychotic action) of these survival circuits are considerably effective, they each come with a range of off-target and prominent sedative effects.

Outstanding Questions

- The past 100 years have witnessed the world's population increase by about 6 billion. This exceptional growth parallels swiftly evolving complex social interactions. Considering that the development, organisation, and plasticity of neocortex is shaped more by environmental factors and less by genetic endowment, we should ask how closely scientific efforts will track the impact of evolving social demands on individual patterns of aggression. Transpositional elements, retroviruses, allelic polymorphisms in the regulatory (non-coding) regions of genes, histone modifications, and other epigenetic regulatory mechanisms in brain, point toward a potentially deep range of significant interaction effects occurring between molecular events and environmental conditions.

- Childhood measures of cognitive and behavioural performance estimate the probability of later successes. Straightforward enrichment approaches bolster the fulfilment of social and educational milestones. Likewise, environmental factors like poor nutrition, lack of familial support, limited educational resources, lower socioeconomic status, and ineffective forms of punishment negatively bias developmental trajectories. How much effort will be devoted to further elucidating critical periods of brain development relating to the biological basis of aggression? Implementation of enrichment strategies at crucial timepoints may significantly diminish rates of maladaptive aggression.

REFERENCES

1. James SL, Abate D, Abate KH et al. Global, regional, and national incidence, prevalence, and years lived with disability for 354 diseases and injuries for 195 countries and territories, 1990–2017: a systematic analysis for the Global Burden of Disease Study 2017. *Lancet* 2018: 392: 1789–1858.

2. Ahonen L, Loeber R, Brent DA. The association between serious mental health problems and violence: some common assumptions and misconceptions. *Trauma Violence Abuse* 2019: 20(5): 613–625.

3. Miczek KA, de Boer SF, Haller J. Excessive aggression as model of violence: a critical evaluation of current preclinical methods. *Psychopharmacology (Berl)* 2013: 226: 445–458.

4. Davidson RJ, Putnam KM, Larson CL. Dysfunction in the neural circuitry of emotion regulation: a possible prelude to violence. *Science* 2000: 289: 591–594.

5. LeDoux JE, Brown R. A higher-order theory of emotional consciousness. *Proc Natl Acad Sci USA* 2017: 114: E2016–E2025.

6. Siep N, Tonnaer F, van de Ven V et al. Anger provocation increases limbic and decreases medial prefrontal cortex connectivity with the left amygdala in reactive aggressive violent offenders. *Brain Imaging Behav* 2019: 13: 1311–1323.

7. Hare RD, Neumann CS (2008). Psychopathy as a clinical and empirical construct. *Annu Rev Clin Psychol* 4: 217–246.

8. Blair RJ. The roles of orbital frontal cortex in the modulation of antisocial behavior. *Brain Cogn* 2004: 55: 198–208.

9. Wrangham RW, Glowacki L. Intergroup aggression in chimpanzees and war in nomadic hunter–gatherers: evaluating the chimpanzee model. *Hum Nat* 2012: 23: 5–29.

10. Scott JP. *Aggression*. University of Chicago Press. 1958.

11. MacDonnell M, Flynn JP. Sensory control of hypothalamic attack. *Anim Behav* 1966: 14: 399–405.

12. Remedios R, Kennedy A, Zelikowsky M et al. Social behaviour shapes hypothalamic neural ensemble representations of conspecific sex. *Nature* 2017: 550: 388–392.

13. LeDoux J. Rethinking the emotional brain. *Neuron* 2012: 73: 653–676.

14. Ferguson JN, Young LJ, Insel TR. The neuroendocrine basis of social recognition. *Front Neuroendocrinol* 2002: 23: 200–224.

15. Dedic N, Kuhne C, Jakovcevski M et al. Chronic CRH depletion from GABAergic, long-range projection neurons in the extended amygdala reduces dopamine release and increases anxiety. *Nat Neurosci* 2018: 21: 803–807.

16. Leroy F, Park J, Asok A et al. A circuit from hippocampal CA2 to lateral septum disinhibits social aggression. *Nature* 2018: 564: 213–218.

17. Blair RJ. The neurobiology of impulsive aggression. *J Child Adolesc Psychopharmacol* 2016: 26: 4–9.

18. Welch BL, Hendley ED, Turek I. Norepinephrine uptake into cerebral cortical synaptosomes after one fight or electroconvulsive shock. *Science* 1974: 183: 220–221.

19. Stagkourakis S, Spigolon G, Williams P et al. A neural network for intermale aggression to establish social hierarchy. *Nat Neurosci* 2018: 21: 834–842.

20. Falkner AL, Lin D. Recent advances in understanding the role of the hypothalamic circuit during aggression. *Front Syst Neurosci* 2014: 8: 168.

21. Adams DB. Cells related to fighting behavior recorded from midbrain central gray neuropil of cat. *Science* 1968: 159: 894–896.

22. Miczek KA, Fish EW, De Bold JF, De Almeida RM. Social and neural determinants of aggressive behavior: pharmacotherapeutic targets at serotonin, dopamine and gamma-aminobutyric acid systems. *Psychopharmacology (Berl)* 2002: 163: 434–458.

23. Bard P. A diencephalic mechanism for the expression of rage with special reference to the sympathetic nervous system. *Am J Physiol* 1928: 84: 490–515.

24. Brown GL, Goodwin FK, Ballenger JC, Goyer PF, Major LF. Aggression in humans correlates with cerebrospinal fluid amine metabolites. *Psychiatry Res* 1979: 1: 131–139.

25. Klasen M, Zvyagintsev M, Schwenzer M et al. Quetiapine modulates functional connectivity in brain aggression networks. *Neuroimage* 2013: 75: 20–26.

26. Siegel A, Bhatt S, Bhatt R, Zalcman SS. The neurobiological bases for development of pharmacological treatments of aggressive disorders. *Curr Neuropharmacol* 2007: 5: 135–147.

27. Buckholtz JW, Meyer-Lindenberg A. MAOA and the neurogenetic architecture of human aggression. *Trends Neurosci* 2008: 31: 120–129.

28. Itil TM, Wadud A. Treatment of human aggression with major tranquilizers, antidepressants, and newer psychotropic drugs. *J Nerv Ment Dis* 1975: 160: 83–99.

29. Correll CU, Yu X, Xiang Y, Kane JM, Masand P. Biological treatment of acute agitation or aggression with schizophrenia or bipolar disorder in the inpatient setting. *Ann Clin Psychiatry* 2017: 29: 92–107.

30. Covington HE 3rd, Newman EL, Leonard MZ, Miczek KA. Translational models of adaptive and excessive fighting: an emerging role for neural circuits in pathological aggression. *F1000Res* 2019: 8: 963.

31. Schultz W. Dopamine reward prediction–error signalling: a two-component response. *Nat Rev Neurosci* 2016: 17: 183–195.

32. Couppis MH, Kennedy CH. The rewarding effect of aggression is reduced by nucleus accumbens dopamine receptor antagonism in mice. *Psychopharmacology (Berl)* 2008: 197: 449–456.

33. Henley ED, Moisset B, Welch BL. Catecholamine uptake in cerebral cortex: adaptive change induced by fighting. *Science* 1973: 180: 1050–1052.

34. Ratey JJ, Gordon A. The psychopharmacology of aggression: toward a new day. *Psychopharmacol Bull* 1993: 29: 65–73.

35. De Dreu CK, Greer L, Van Kleef GA, Shalvi S, Handgraaf MJ. Oxytocin promotes human ethnocentrism. *Proc Natl Acad Sci USA* 2011: 108: 1262–1266.

36. Newman EL , Smith KS, Takahashi A et al. Alpha2-containing GABA(A) receptors: a requirement for midazolam-escalated aggression and social approach in mice. *Psychopharmacology (Berl)* 2015: 232: 4359–4369.

37. Golden SA , Heshmati M, Flanigan M et al. Basal forebrain projections to the lateral habenula modulate aggression reward. *Nature* 2016: 534: 688–692.

5.5 **Nociception and Pain**

Ewan St John Smith and
Michael C. Lee

OVERVIEW

Chronic pain ranks among the top causes of years lived with disability worldwide [1]. Management is challenging because it is difficult to relieve pain as a sensation. Analgesics play a limited role and can be harmful, for example opioid prescription in chronic pain is now linked to considerable harm and even deaths through overdose. Depression and anxiety disorders are common in patients with chronic pain, hence management may require joint expertise from multiple healthcare disciplines.

The International Association for the Study of Pain defines nociception as 'the neural process of encoding noxious stimuli', and pain as 'an unpleasant sensory and emotional experience associated with, or resembling that associated with, actual or potential tissue damage'. Essentially, nociception is a detect-to-protect physiological function that prevents or limits overt damage to the body [2], whereas pain is a sensation that encompasses sensory and emotional components.

5.5.1 Nociception

Nociception is vital to survival, and when impaired it is associated with tissue damage, a common example being diabetic foot [3]. Nociceptors are specialised sensory neurons, which detect temperatures, mechanical forces and chemicals that threaten tissue integrity. Stimulus detection depends upon a diverse range of receptors found at nerve terminals, and an individual nociceptor's function will depend upon the receptors it expresses because different receptors detect different stimuli. For example, the transient receptor potential vanilloid 1 (TRPV1) ion channel is activated by noxious heat (> 42 °C), protons (an acidic extracellular environment is associated with tissue damage) and capsaicin, the substance giving chili pepper its hot taste (Figure 5.5.1).

Molecular analyses show that different types of sensory neurons can be classified by numerous factors, including their transcriptome (gene expression). This could lead to therapeutics targeting nociceptor subgroups driving specific qualities of pain [4, 5]. For example, certain voltage-gated sodium-channel subtypes that are important for signal conduction along the neuron (Na_V1.7–1.9), are almost exclusively expressed by nociceptors. Extremely rare genetic mutations can cause gain or loss of channel function, resulting in extreme pain (erythromelalgia) or painlessness (congenital insensitivity to pain), respectively [6].

5.5.2 Functional Neuroanatomy of Pain

The neuroanatomical pain pathway begins with the nociceptor, a pseudo-unipolar neuron with peripheral and central terminals; nociceptor cell bodies are located in the dorsal root ganglia (nociceptors that innervate the body) or trigeminal ganglia (nociceptors that innervate the head) and each cell's axon bifurcates into a peripheral and central axonal branch, which terminate in the peripheral organ (e.g. skin, muscle etc.) and spinal cord, respectively. The central terminal synapses with spinal dorsal horn neurons. Only a small proportion of nociceptors synapse with spinal cord projection neurons, that is, those that run directly to the brain. Other nociceptors synapse onto interneurons to modulate the pain signal. Those nociceptors synapsing with projection neurons

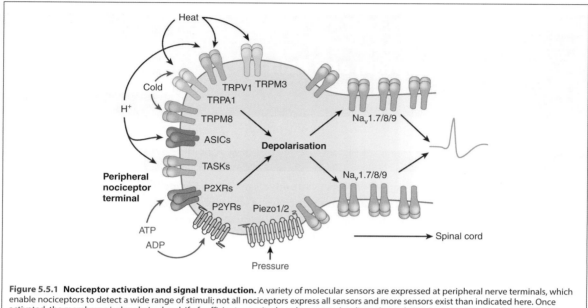

Figure 5.5.1 Nociceptor activation and signal transduction. A variety of molecular sensors are expressed at peripheral nerve terminals, which enable nociceptors to detect a wide range of stimuli; not all nociceptors express all sensors and more sensors exist than indicated here. Once activated, the membrane is depolarised and, if of sufficient magnitude, voltage-gated sodium channels (Na_V) are activated leading to action potential generation and transmission of the signal to the central nervous system. Abbreviations: ADP, adenosine diphosphate; ASIC, acid-sensing ion channel; ATP, adenosine triphosphate; P2XR, purinergic ATP-gated ionotropic receptor; P2YR, purinergic G-protein-coupled receptor; TASK, TWIK (tandem of pore domains in a weak inward rectifying K channel)-related acid-sensitive potassium channel; TRP, transient receptor potential (A1, V1, M3 and M8 are all different subtypes).

connect directly to the brain because the projection neuron decussates in the spinal cord and then connects to the brain via ascending tracts (Figure 5.5.2A):

- the neo-spinothalamic tract projects from the spinal cord to the thalamus, where third-order neurons in the ventroposterior lateral nucleus of the thalamus comprise the final relay to the primary somatosensory cortex;

- spinal neurons also project to limbic or emotional brain regions, for example to the amygdala via the parabrachial nuclei in the brainstem.

Hence, information from nociceptors is processed within the central nervous system to generate sensory-discriminatory and affective-motivational aspects of pain.

Most nociceptors synapse with spinal cord interneurons that communicate with spinal projection neurons, but are also subject to descending control from neurons in the brainstem, e.g. nuclei in the rostral-ventromedial medulla or the periaqueductal grey (Figure 5.5.2B). Descending control explains how mood, expectations and beliefs shape the perception of pain, for example pain relief afforded by placebo [7]. Regarding pain sensations,

there is still debate regarding the existence of a primary 'pain' or 'nociceptive' cortical area [8], analogous to those for other senses of sight, hearing or touch. Pain is perhaps more akin to itch, hunger and thirst, other sensations that are accompanied by a strong behavioural drive. These sensations may thus share a common neurobiology [9].

5.5.3 Pain and Disease

Nociceptive pain is protective and includes increased sensitivity to pain (hyperalgesia) caused by tissue inflammation. This occurs after tissue trauma (e.g. surgery) or results from chronic diseases such as rheumatoid arthritis. Inflammation involves influx of leucocytes (white blood cells), which release inflammatory mediators such as cytokines (e.g. tumour necrosis factor alpha). These cytokines act on peripheral nerve terminals to enhance their responsiveness, that is, peripheral sensitisation. Sustained signalling from nociceptors also leads to sensitisation of neurons in the central nervous system, which cause pain at locations beyond the site of tissue injury (secondary hyperalgesia). Treatment focuses on suppressing inflammation (e.g. non-steroidal anti-inflammatory

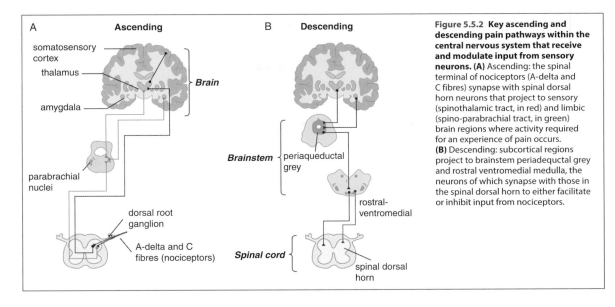

Figure 5.5.2 Key ascending and descending pain pathways within the central nervous system that receive and modulate input from sensory neurons. (A) Ascending: the spinal terminal of nociceptors (A-delta and C fibres) synapse with spinal dorsal horn neurons that project to sensory (spinothalamic tract, in red) and limbic (spino-parabrachial tract, in green) brain regions where activity required for an experience of pain occurs. **(B)** Descending: subcortical regions project to brainstem periadequtal grey and rostral ventromedial medulla, the neurons of which synapse with those in the spinal dorsal horn to either facilitate or inhibit input from nociceptors.

drugs (NSAIDs) or corticosteroids), or treating the primary disease (e.g. disease-modifying antirheumatic drugs, which include monoclonal antibodies, some of which disrupt cytokine signalling). These can prevent tissue destruction (e.g. joints in rheumatoid arthritis), but neuronal hyperactivity may still persist to maintain pain.

Neuropathic pain is that caused by a lesion or disease of the somatosensory pathways, either peripherally or centrally [10]. Clinically, there is loss of sensory function in the affected body region, but patients also report spontaneous pain, described as 'shooting' or 'electric'. Neuropathic pain is challenging to manage and often resistant to conventional analgesics such as NSAIDs or opioids (see Section 2.7 for more details). Pharmacological options are limited, but evidence from randomised controlled trials favours medications with anticonvulsant (e.g. pregabalin) and antidepressant action (e.g. tricyclics or serotonin and noradrenaline reuptake inhibitors), with these agents being clinically recommended [10]. Preclinical research has elucidated mechanisms for neuronal hyperexcitability in neuropathic pain and demonstrated hyperactivity of immune cells (microglia), so therapeutics with novel mechanisms of action are being developed [11].

Many chronic pain disorders are defined solely on symptoms, meaning that they lack overt injury to the nervous system or an active inflammatory process, so-called **nociplastic pain** [12]. Examples include irritable bowel syndrome, fibromyalgia and non-specific back pain. The neurobiological mechanisms for these heterogeneous disorders are poorly understood but failure of descending control is strongly implicated [13] (see Section 9.13 on medically unexplained symptoms). The prognoses for these pain disorders are generally poor, with polypharmacy being common because of associated depressive symptoms or anxiety disorders. An interdisciplinary approach to pain management is required, including input from psychiatry, alongside other healthcare specialities involved in pain management.

5.5.4 Psychiatric Diagnoses and Chronic Pain

Physical disability, mood and anxiety disorders are highly prevalent in patients with chronic pain. The approach in pain clinics is one that optimises emotional and physical function for self-management. Current evidence supports cognitive behavioural therapy, and there is increasing evidence for 'third-wave' methods, such as mindfulness practice (including tai chi, yoga) for chronic pain [14–16]. The focus shifts from primary provision of comfort (pain relief) to other goals of health care, including longevity, physical functioning and quality of life.

Diagnoses of personality disorders, substance misuse and post-traumatic stress disorder can complicate pain management considerably due to potential for reduced self-management. Similarly, pain is difficult to assess in psychiatric disorders that affect cognition or communication, for example schizophrenia or dementia, and options for self-management are limited. Psychiatrists play a key role in multi/inter-disciplinary clinics given the prevalence of psychiatric comorbidities in chronic pain and the challenges of pain management in psychiatric disorders [17].

Conclusions and Outstanding Questions

The molecular mechanisms underpinning the sensation of pain are complex and vary from one form of pain to another, which explains why pain management remains a significant clinical challenge. Psychiatric comorbidities, such as anxiety, are highly prevalent in those experiencing chronic pain, and this needs to be considered when providing holistic patient care. From a clinical care perspective, it also needs to be remembered that an individual presenting with certain psychiatric conditions can complicate pain assessment and management.

Outstanding Questions

- What molecular mechanisms drive different forms of pain? Furthering such understanding could lead to more targeted medications, with fewer side effects than those currently in use.

- What determines the inter-individual disparity in analgesia efficacy? A better understanding of the reasons for differential responses to drug treatment and other forms of pain management could lead to more personalised medicine, for example based upon better understanding of the genetics of certain pain conditions.

REFERENCES

1. GBD 2016 Disease and Injury Incidence and Prevalence Collaborators. Global, regional, and national incidence, prevalence, and years lived with disability for 328 diseases and injuries for 195 countries, 1990–2016: a systematic analysis for the Global Burden of Disease Study 2016. *Lancet* 2017; 390(10100): 1211–1259.

2. St John Smith E. Advances in understanding nociception and neuropathic pain. *J Neurol* 2018; 265(2): 231–238.

3. Mishra SC, Chhatbar KC, Kashikar A, Mehndiratta A. Diabetic foot. *BMJ* 2017; 359: j5064.

4. Zeisel A, Hochgerner H, Lönnerberg P et al. Molecular architecture of the mouse nervous system. *Cell* 2018; 174(4): 999–1014.e22.

5. Hockley JRF, Taylor TS, Callejo G et al. Single-cell RNAseq reveals seven classes of colonic sensory neuron. *Gut* 2019; 68: 633–644.

6. Bennett DLH, Woods CG. Painful and painless channelopathies. *Lancet Neurol* 2014; 13(6): 587–599.

7. Wager TD, Atlas LY. The neuroscience of placebo effects: connecting context, learning and health. *Nat Rev Neurosci* 2015; 16(7): 403–418.

8. Lee MC, Tracey I. Imaging pain: a potent means for investigating pain mechanisms in patients. *Br J Anaesth* 2013; 111(1): 64–72.

9. Critchley HD, Garfinkel SN. Interoception and emotion. *Curr Opin Psychol* 2017; 17: 7–14.

10. Colloca L, Ludman T, Bouhassira D et al. Neuropathic pain. *Nat Rev Dis Primers* 2017; 3: 17002.

11. Inoue K, Tsuda M. Microglia in neuropathic pain: cellular and molecular mechanisms and therapeutic potential. *Nat Rev Neurosci* 2018; 19(3): 138–152.

12. Fitzcharles MA, Cohen SP, Clauw DJ et al. Nociplastic pain: towards an understanding of prevalent pain conditions. *Lancet* 2021; 397(10289): 2098–2110.

13. Schmidt-Wilcke T, Clauw DJ. Fibromyalgia: from pathophysiology to therapy. *Nat Rev Rheumatol* 2011; 7(9): 518–527.

14. Wang C, Schmid CH, Rones R et al. A randomized trial of tai chi for fibromyalgia. *NEJM* 2010; 363(8): 743–754.

15. Turk DC, Swanson KS, Tunks ER. Psychological approaches in the treatment of chronic pain patients: when pills, scalpels, and needles are not enough. *Can J Psychiatry* 2008; 53(4): 213–223.

16. Wang C, Schmid CH, Fielding RA et al. Effect of tai chi versus aerobic exercise for fibromyalgia: comparative effectiveness randomized controlled trial. *BMJ* 2018; 360: k851.

17. Goesling J, Lin LA, Clauw DJ. Psychiatry and pain management: at the intersection of chronic pain and mental health. *Curr Psychiatry Rep* 2018; 20(2): 12.

National Neuroscience Curriculum Initiative online resources

Your System Has Been Hijacked: The Neurobiology of Chronic Pain

Erica B. Baller and David A. Ross

Cannabinoids and Pain: Weeding Out Undesired Effects With a Novel Approach to Analgesia

Joao P. De Aquino and David A. Ross

What to say: *Cannabinoids and Pain: Weeding Out Undesired Effects With a Novel Approach to Analgesia*

This "stuff" is really cool: Erica Baller, *"Sos: Your System's Been Hijacked!"* *on circuit changes in chronic pain*

<table>
<tr><td>**5.6**</td><td># The Motor System and Movement Disorders</td><td>**Kirsten Scott and Roger Barker**</td></tr>
</table>

OVERVIEW

The motor system is responsible for directing and controlling movement and ranges from simple reflex arcs (withdrawal of a limb from a painful stimulus) to highly sophisticated volitional motor acts (playing the piano). Historically, movements have been conceptualised as being either 'closed-loop' (directly guided and modified by sensory inputs providing feedback) or 'open-loop' (triggered by a decision to move which acts as the input, with no initial feedback). In reality, almost all movements rely on some degree of sensory feedback and there is also a degree of volition in some apparently 'closed-loop' movements, making this dichotomy an oversimplification.

Movement control can best be modelled using a hierarchy of different motor areas within the nervous system (see Figure 5.6.1), with spinal cord reflex arcs at the lowest level of the hierarchy and limbic and association cortical areas at the highest level. At every level, disease or lesions give a distinct clinical syndrome. Many psychiatric conditions are associated with subtle motor abnormalities on examination, which are difficult to assign to a particular level in the hierarchy and often confounded by the use of drugs for psychiatric illness that have motor features as part of their side-effect profile.

5.6.1 Neuroanatomy of the Motor System

At the highest level in the motor hierarchy are those structures involved with the planning and initiation of a movement. The origin of the desire to move is probably within the mesolimbic system, which has dopaminergic connections to the amygdala and nucleus accumbens, playing a complex role in seeking a particular (often emotional) 'reward'. The posterior parietal cortex is also involved at this level, providing inputs relating to visual processing or stimuli of interest, for example food or, in the case of substance dependence the opportunity for a 'hit'. The basal ganglia then translate this desire into a movement, providing the basis for initiation and planning of the movement required (reaching for food).

The basal ganglia have a number of cortical connections including to the supplementary motor area and the lateral premotor cortex (see Figure 5.6.2 for the neuroanatomy). The supplementary motor area is active when people are imagining a movement, suggesting it is involved in planning the specific sequence of movements required to achieve an end.

The lateral premotor cortex has connections to sensory areas as well as the cerebellum and is thought to play a greater role in 'closed-loop' movements.

Once the movement is initiated, projections from the cortex to descending motor pathways in the brainstem and spinal cord activate the final motor pathway of the motor neurons innervating the muscles.

Feedback from the periphery as well as from motor pathways within the central nervous system is then used to coordinate movement primarily through the cerebellum, which also has the capacity to learn and refine new movements.

5.6.2 Movement Disorders

The utility of this hierarchy in understanding motor control is by considering conditions that affect each level of it (see Figure 5.6.1). Starting at the highest level of the hierarchy (shown in purple), damage to these structures leads to either a problem of initiation of movement or an inability to suppress excess or involuntary movements.

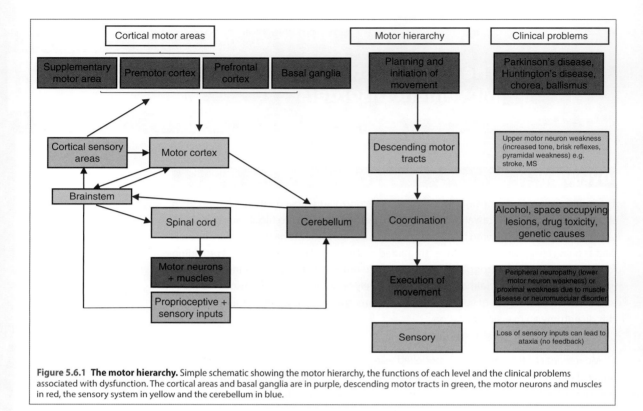

Figure 5.6.1 The motor hierarchy. Simple schematic showing the motor hierarchy, the functions of each level and the clinical problems associated with dysfunction. The cortical areas and basal ganglia are in purple, descending motor tracts in green, the motor neurons and muscles in red, the sensory system in yellow and the cerebellum in blue.

So, for example, the basal ganglia and their projections are affected in Parkinson's disease where the dopaminergic output from the substantia nigra to the striatum is decreased, resulting in a hypokinetic movement disorder with bradykinesia (slowed movement), rigidity, gait problems and a rest tremor (see Figure 5.6.2 and the more detailed schematic showing the connections within the basal ganglia in Figure 5.6.3). The motor features can be treated by the replacement of dopamine but this eventually leads to excessive movements in many patients as a result of the pathway being abnormally stimulated by oral dopaminergic drugs (so called levodopa-induced dyskinesias). Another disorder of the basal ganglia is Huntington's disease, where there is a loss of striatal outputs leading to overactivation of cortical motor areas and therefore hyperkinesia (seen as fidgety movements, chorea; see Figure 5.6.2 and Figure 5.6.3, showing how these arise). Treatment therefore relies on reducing the dopaminergic activity in the basal ganglia by using therapies for psychosis such as olanzapine or sulpiride

or dopamine-depleting agents such as tetrabenazine. Figure 5.6.3 shows a simplified overview of the basal ganglia circuitry underlying these disorders.

Psychomotor retardation is also a complex movement disorder caused by alterations in the limbic system at the very highest part of the hierarchy (resulting in decreased motivation) and also in changes in the frontostriatal pathways and cortical regions (supplementary motor area and premotor cortex) involved in the desire to move and the initiation of movement.

Finally, damage to cortical association areas, which provide inputs to the motor areas such as the posterior parietal cortex, can lead to problems in actually understanding how to perform a motor act (i.e. apraxia) or, in the case of the frontal cortex, motor sequencing.

At the next level of the hierarchy (shown in blue in Figure 5.6.1), cerebellar disorders result in problems relating to coordination and motor learning. This is commonly seen as a side effect of antiepileptic medications such as carbamazepine or phenytoin, alcohol use

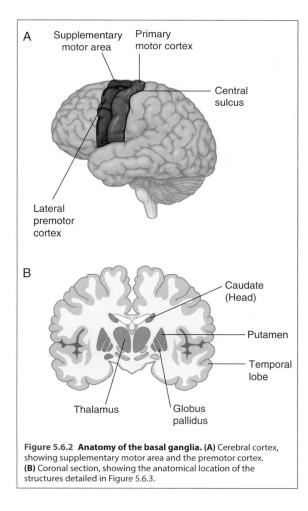

A Supplementary motor area | Primary motor cortex | Central sulcus | Lateral premotor cortex

B Caudate (Head) | Putamen | Temporal lobe | Globus pallidus | Thalamus

Figure 5.6.2 Anatomy of the basal ganglia. (A) Cerebral cortex, showing supplementary motor area and the premotor cortex. **(B)** Coronal section, showing the anatomical location of the structures detailed in Figure 5.6.3.

or infarcts affecting the cerebellum, as well as conditions such as multiple sclerosis and some inherited disorders of the brain.

Disorders affecting the primary motor cortex, premotor cortex and the associated descending tracts result in an 'upper motor neuron' lesion (shown in green in Figure 5.6.1). This is defined by increased tone and brisk reflexes in the affected limbs. The weakness is worst in the extensors in the arm and the flexor muscles in the legs. There is often an associated extensor plantar response. Conditions that typically cause this are strokes, multiple sclerosis or trauma. In contrast, lesions lower in the motor hierarchy targeting the final motor pathway result in a 'lower motor neuron' syndrome, with the affected muscles/limbs showing wasting, weakness with reduced tone and absent reflexes. This is commonly seen when nerves are trapped coming out of the spine (radiculopathies) as well as in inherited or acquired neuropathies and most forms of motor neuron disease.

5.6.3 Psychiatric Conditions and Movement Disorders

Movement disorders managed by neurologists are often complicated by psychiatric features and may also present to psychiatrists if behavioural disturbances are the major presenting feature. This probably reflects the somewhat arbitrary nature of the function of the higher levels of motor control and the fact that most diseases are not restricted to any one structure in the brain. A good example of this is Huntington's disease. This genetic disorder has early pathology within the basal ganglia but it is not restricted to this site and typically involves cortical areas as well. Most patients with Huntington's disease also have behavioural change, apathy and mood disturbance, which are often more disabling than the associated movement disorder and can be the major presenting feature. Other basal ganglia disorders such as Parkinson's disease can be complicated by major psychiatric problems that are either part of the condition (e.g. depression and anxiety, which may pre-date the onset of motor abnormalities) or a consequence of treatment. In the latter case, treatment with dopamine agonists (and to a lesser extent levodopa) can cause impulse control disorders or other neuropsychiatric problems such as paranoia and hallucinations. Other rarer basal ganglia disorders such as Wilson's disease (where damage results from copper deposition in the basal ganglia) may also present to psychiatrists, with behavioural disturbances being a more prominent feature than the movement disorder (asking about a family history and ensuring that testing for 24-hour urinary copper, caeruloplasmin and genetic screening has been considered are therefore important in this context).

Other neurodegenerative conditions such as frontotemporal dementia may also start with behavioural symptoms in the absence of any major motor deficits and thus first come to psychiatric clinics. In addition, some forms of inherited motorneuron disease also can present with frontotemporal dementia-like behavioural issues. This is most commonly seen in families with a hexanucleotide repeat in the *C9orf72* gene

In younger patients, subacute development of a movement disorder (and seizures) associated with psychiatric

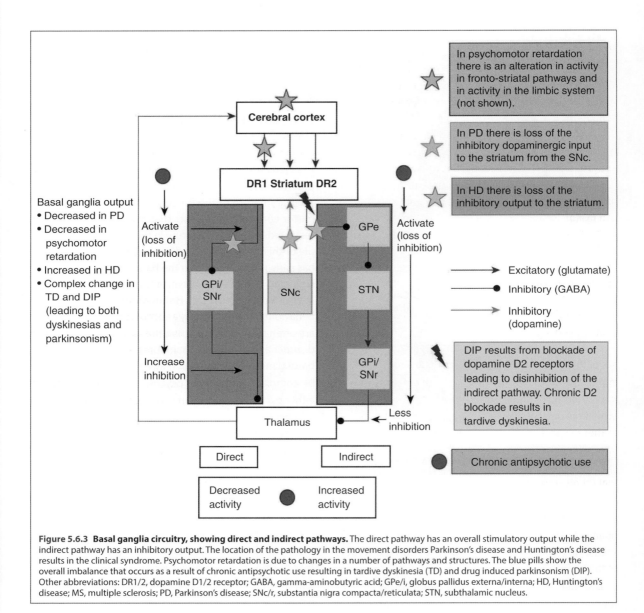

In psychomotor retardation there is an alteration in activity in fronto-striatal pathways and in activity in the limbic system (not shown).

In PD there is loss of the inhibitory dopaminergic input to the striatum from the SNc.

In HD there is loss of the inhibitory output to the striatum.

Cerebral cortex

DR1 Striatum DR2

Basal ganglia output
• Decreased in PD
• Decreased in psychomotor retardation
• Increased in HD
• Complex change in TD and DIP (leading to both dyskinesias and parkinsonism)

Activate (loss of inhibition)

Activate (loss of inhibition)

GPe

GPi/ SNr

SNc

STN

Increase inhibition

GPi/ SNr

Excitatory (glutamate)

Inhibitory (GABA)

Inhibitory (dopamine)

DIP results from blockade of dopamine D2 receptors leading to disinhibition of the indirect pathway. Chronic D2 blockade results in tardive dyskinesia.

Thalamus

Less inhibition

Direct

Indirect

Chronic antipsychotic use

Decreased activity

Increased activity

Figure 5.6.3 Basal ganglia circuitry, showing direct and indirect pathways. The direct pathway has an overall stimulatory output while the indirect pathway has an inhibitory output. The location of the pathology in the movement disorders Parkinson's disease and Huntington's disease results in the clinical syndrome. Psychomotor retardation is due to changes in a number of pathways and structures. The blue pills show the overall imbalance that occurs as a result of chronic antipsychotic use resulting in tardive dyskinesia (TD) and drug induced parkinsonism (DIP). Other abbreviations: DR1/2, dopamine D1/2 receptor; GABA, gamma-aminobutyric acid; GPe/i, globus pallidus externa/interna; HD, Huntington's disease; MS, multiple sclerosis; PD, Parkinson's disease; SNc/r, substantia nigra compacta/reticulata; STN, subthalamic nucleus.

symptoms such as depression or psychosis may be due to antibody-mediated limbic encephalitis (such as that caused by LG1 (leucine-rich glioma-inactivated 1) antibodies, resulting in very characteristic faciobrachial dystonic seizures, or the much more variable and difficult to describe movement disorder associated with anti-NMDA (*N*-methyl-D-aspartate) receptor antibody encephalitis). The mechanism is not entirely clear but the antibodies disrupt receptors involved in neurotransmission and so can disrupt relevant motor pathways at a number of sites. It is important to consider

these syndromes as they are potentially reversible with immunomodulation or may be associated with underlying malignancy, which is treatable if caught early.

Neurodevelopmental disorders such as Tourette syndrome are characterised by semi-involuntary movements (tics) but are also associated with a clinical syndrome including attention deficit hyperactivity disorder, obsessive–compulsive disorder, depression and behavioural disorders. Finally, it is worth remembering that some recreational drugs can produce involuntary movements, such as cocaine ('crack dancing') and Spice (synthetic marijuana).

Movement disorders have been described in schizophrenia and affective disorders. These include catatonia, waxy flexibility and even dyskinesias that pre-date the use of medication with antipsychotic action. The underlying mechanisms are not clear. Catatonia responds to benzodiazepines and it has therefore been proposed that it is due to dysfunction in the GABAergic pathways in the basal ganglia (see dark blue pathways in Figure 5.6.3), with some imaging studies showing abnormalities in frontal and motor cortical regions in these patients. Waxy flexibility (the maintenance of limbs in externally imposed positions) is often part of catatonia and is also poorly understood but may share a similar pathophysiology to catatonia. The presence of rigidity and dyskinesias in treatment naïve patients is also poorly understood. One could hypothesise that the dopaminergic abnormalities known to be associated with schizophrenia (see Section 9.10.5) also result in a change in the balance between the pathways in the basal ganglia and prefrontal cortex, important for control of movement (see Figure 5.6.3). Neurological conditions that may present in the psychiatry clinic are summarised in Table 5.6.1. In addition to these changes it is important to consider HIV in any unexplained neurological presentation as it may lead to infectious, inflammatory and even autoimmune lesions that mimic other conditions.

5.6.4 Extrapyramidal Side Effects

The most common movement disorder seen in psychiatric practice is extrapyramidal side effects (EPSE) of medication used for psychosis. These may appear acutely after treatment initiation, typically presenting with acute dystonia (sustained abnormal posturing or muscle spasms) in the first 7 days of treatment or a dose change. This is thought to be due to an imbalance between dopamine (in particular the D2 receptor) and acetylcholine receptor blockade in the basal ganglia. Drugs with the highest ratio of dopamine to acetylcholine binding carry the highest risk of EPSEs. Clozapine has the lowest risk followed by atypical drugs with antipsychotic action such as olanzapine, quetiapine and low doses of risperidone. The exact effect on the circuitry is unclear. Young men are at highest risk of this side effect. It is thought that this is because they have the greatest density and activity of D2 receptors and therefore that blockade has a greater effect. It is treated with acute administration of anticholinergic drugs such as procyclidine.

Akasthisia (pacing and a feeling of restlessness) may arise within the first three months of treatment and may be misdiagnosed as anxiety or agitation. The neurobiological basis of this is not clear but is thought to be due to an imbalance between dopaminergic and serotonergic/noradrenergic transmitter systems and in their connections. It remains a challenge to treat but is usually managed by reducing the dose of the medication

Table 5.6.1 Things not to miss in the psychiatry clinic

Clinical manifestation	Conditions to consider	Circuit abnormalities
Chorea (fidgety movements)	Huntington's disease, Sydenham's chorea (group A streptococcal infection), drug toxicity Wilson's disease, inflammatory problems such as systemic lupus erythematosus, syphilis as well as thyrotoxicosis and polycythaemia rubra vera	Disruption of balance between inhibitory and excitatory circuits in the basal ganglia (all of these conditions result in a degenerative, infectious or inflammatory lesions in the basal ganglia)
Hypokinetic disorder with tremor	Parkinson's disease, drug side effects	Loss of dopaminergic striatal input from the substantia nigra pars compacta
Seizures and a movement disorder	Limbic encephalitis, paraneoplastic syndrome, neurodevelopmental disorders	Antibody-mediated disruption of neurotransmitter signalling (exact circuitry is not clear)
Tics	Tourette syndrome	Involves basal ganglia circuitry, poorly defined
Stiff legs	Spinal-cord lesion causing stiffness (spasticity) Dystonia Parkinsonism Stiff person syndrome	Spastic legs are usually due to a lesion in the descending motor pathway (corticospinal tract), they are stiff with brisk reflexes and upgoing plantars Dystonia also manifests as 'stiffness' but may be variable, only affect certain muscle groups and won't be associated with brisk reflexes; this is due to alterations in pathways within the basal ganglia and/or cortex, causing agonist and antagonist muscles to be coactivated

used for the psychosis, along with the addition of beta blockers and benzodiazepines (which probably treat the consequences rather than the cause of the problem).

Drug-induced parkinsonism (tremor, rigidity and/or bradykinesia) induced by medications used to treat psychosis may occur within weeks or months of treatment initiation but is typically seen after years of treatment. This is thought to be a result of chronic D2 receptor blockade, which then leads to disinhibition of the inhibitory pathways at the beginning of the indirect pathway (see Figure 5.6.3), changing the balance between the indirect and direct pathways and leading to a clinical syndrome similar to Parkinson's disease (but usually symmetrical as opposed to the asymmetry that usually characterises idiopathic Parkinson's disease). While idiopathic Parkinson's disease is characterised by presynaptic dopamine loss (decreased production), drug-induced parkinsonism is characterised by a postsynaptic deficit (blockade of the D2 receptor) and won't respond to treatment with levodopa. Elderly patients with psychiatric disorders can therefore be easily misdiagnosed as having idiopathic Parkinson's disease and needlessly treated with levodopa. On the other hand, pre-existing idiopathic Parkinson's disease may be unmasked by the use of drugs with antipsychotic action in the elderly. Dopamine transporter (DAT) imaging can be useful for differentiating between these conditions as dopamine transporters are found on the presynaptic nerve terminals and thus remain unchanged in drug-induced parkinsonism.

Tardive dyskinesia often accompanies drug-induced parkinsonism but may also be seen on its own usually following years of drug treatment. The mechanism of this is unclear but is thought to be due to increased sensitivity to dopamine after chronic blockade: an increase in D2 receptor density in the striatum alters the balance between the indirect and direct pathways (as shown in Figure 5.6.3). As in Parkinson's disease this is also complicated by noradrenergic, serotonergic and cholinergic pathways and is therefore not as simple as the schematic suggests.

Other drugs that block central dopamine receptors have also been associated with EPSEs (including lithium,

sodium valproate, serotonin reuptake inhibitors and tricyclics, used to treat depression). All of the major EPSEs are more prevalent with typical (compared to atypical) antipsychotics, at least according to current follow-up data. The mechanism underlying this is thought to be due to receptor occupancy: typical drugs used for psychosis require 70–80% receptor occupancy to have a therapeutic effect while atypical medications are able to have a similar effect with lower receptor occupancy (possibly due to the additional blockade of serotonin 5-HT2A receptors). The treatment usually consists of withdrawal or decreased dosing of the drug. This is sometimes not possible if it is effectively controlling their psychosis.

5.6.5 Functional Movement Disorders

Many of the above disorders are hard to distinguish from functional movement disorders which are likely to have a different underlying neurobiology (see Section 9.13). These patients often have attentional problems (increased self-directed attention and abnormal expectations of movement), which then manifest as movement disorders that vary in their severity over short periods of time and can be successfully treated with specialised physiotherapy and cognitive behavioural therapy. They often have comorbid psychiatric disorders but this is not always the case.

Conclusions and Outstanding Questions

Subtle movement abnormalities are seen in many psychiatric conditions and can be due to drug side effects. Many neurological disorders can present with psychiatric problems in the first instance so they should be considered in the differential diagnosis.

Outstanding Questions

- How can we best avoid the long-term complications of drugs used in psychiatric practice?
- How can we improve the care for patients who have disorders with both psychiatric and neurological features?

FURTHER READING

Albin RL, Young AB, Penney JB. The functional anatomy of basal ganglia disorders. *Trends Neurosci* 1989; 12(10): 366–375.

Cotzias GC, Papavasiliou PS, Gellene R. Modification of Parkinsonism: chronic treatment with L-DOPA. *N Engl J Med* 1969; 280: 337–345.

Varley JA, Webb AJS, Balint B et al. The Movement disorder associated with NMDAR antibody-encephalitis is complex and characteristic: an expert video-rating study. *J Neurol Neurosurg Psychiatry* 2019; 90: 724–726.

5

<table>
<tr><td>**5.7**</td><td>**Computational Models of Learning**</td><td>Rebecca P. Lawson and Vincent Valton</td></tr>
</table>

OVERVIEW

The advent of neuroimaging techniques has driven advances in how we understand *where* in the brain different aspects of cognition are instantiated, and *how* this neural activity relates to behaviour. While the translation of this approach to studying neuropsychiatric disorders has had some successes, it could be argued that it fails to capture *what* the brain is doing. Computational models serve as a bridge from brain to behaviour (see Figure 5.7.1), permitting the formulation of mechanistic hypotheses about neural computations and how they might be different in clinical conditions. Most applications of computational models to psychiatric disorders concern altered learning about the world. While many formal models of learning exist, two have had widespread success in their application to psychiatry: reinforcement learning and Bayesian models. Both models are concerned with how we learn from past experiences to form expectations about the world around us.

5.7.1 Learning Models: The Basics

Imagine you are halfway through a gruelling shift at work. You stop by your usual vending machine, press the button for coffee, bring the cup to your lips and take a sip. Surprise! It's orange juice. In formal learning theory the discrepancy between what you expected (coffee) and what you received (orange juice) is said to generate a **prediction error**. Prediction errors challenge your expectations, which drives **new learning**. In some contexts, our expectations arise from the passive association of a cue and an outcome, such as feeling hungry when we are cued by an advert for our favourite restaurant, otherwise known as Pavlovian conditioning [2]. In instrumental contexts, we learn to associate a voluntary action with a particular outcome, such as pressing a button and receiving a coffee [3]. Whatever the form of learning, these systems allow organisms to adapt their behaviour according to the underlying predictive relationships in the environment.

Simple formulations of prediction-error-driven learning can be specified mathematically. For example, inspired by early behaviourist work on conditioning, Rescorla and

Wagner [4] described an error-driven learning algorithm which states that:

$$V\left(S^{t+1}\right)= V\left(S^t\right)+ \alpha\delta$$

where $V\left(S^{t+1}\right)$ represents the new expected value, V, of a given cue, S, in the future (i.e. time $t+1$), $V\left(S^t\right)$ is the value of that cue now, and δ is the prediction error, the difference between what is expected, $V\left(S^t\right)$, and the actual outcome received, R, so:

$$\delta= V\left(S^t\right)-R$$

The extent to which prediction error drives learning to update our expectations about the world is controlled by the learning rate, α. Someone with a high learning rate will update their expectations based on prediction errors very readily, whereas someone with a low learning rate will be relatively insensitive to prediction errors.

In 1997, seminal research in non-human primates demonstrated that the firing activity of midbrain dopamine neurons represents prediction errors exactly as formalised by this simple learning algorithm [5]; see Figure 5.7.2A. Subsequent studies in humans have used

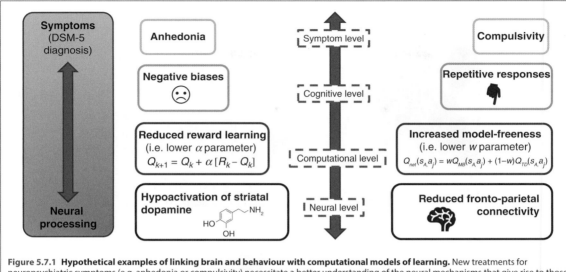

Figure 5.7.1 Hypothetical examples of linking brain and behaviour with computational models of learning. New treatments for neuropsychiatric symptoms (e.g. anhedonia or compulsivity) necessitate a better understanding of the neural mechanisms that give rise to those symptoms. Cognitive computational neuroscience tries to breakdown the symptoms underlying diagnosis into measurable behaviours (cognitive level) which can be described mathematically (computational level). These computational processes can then be linked to brain function (neural level) to gain insights into *how* the brain is functioning differently (both pre- and post-treatment), rather than just observing *that* the brain is functioning differently. DSM-5, *Diagnostic and Statistical Manual of Mental Disorders*, 5th edition [1].

computational models to estimate trial-by-trial prediction errors based on human behaviour in reward learning tasks. These computational indices of behaviour can be combined with concurrent neuroimaging methods, and this approach confirmed prediction-error responses in a network of regions extensively innervated by the monoamine system in humans [9].

By explicitly linking computation to brain function, we now understand many aspects of what dopamine neurons *actually do* and how their activity shapes normative and aberrant behaviour. However, most of the brain's neuromodulatory systems – which incidentally are the target of most psychotropic medication – likely play a role in neural computations (see Section 4.6). Understanding how these learning computations might be carried out differently in neuropsychiatric conditions is a major focus of computational psychiatry. This chapter serves as a brief review of some of the most fruitful applications of learning models in psychiatry to date.

5.7.2 Learning Models Applied to Compulsivity

Studies in humans and rodents suggest that, when we act on the world, our behaviour is mediated by two modes of control: fast, but inflexible 'habitual' control;

and slower, but flexible 'goal-directed' control. Habits form when rewarded or reinforced actions are more likely to be repeated. In contrast, 'goal-directed' behaviour is driven by a predictive model of maximising rewards. Computationally, this has been expressed as two different forms of reinforcement learning: model-free and model-based, respectively [10]). Model-free reinforcement learning relies on the integrity of the midbrain dopamine system and guides people to act based on the recent history of rewards (as described above), whereas model-based reinforcement learning calculates optimal actions by forward planning and depends on the prefrontal cortex [11].

The balance between these two systems is susceptible to disruption and has been studied extensively in neuropsychiatric disorders. For example, persistent drug-taking behaviour might reflect a failure to suppress drug-related stimulus–response habits. Indeed, it has been shown, using both cognitive tasks and computational models, that methamphetamine- and alcohol-dependant individuals exhibit more model-free behaviour than matched controls [12]. Similarly, binge eating and obsessive–compulsive disorder, both diagnosed on the basis of compulsive behaviours, present with marked increases in model-free control [12]. These

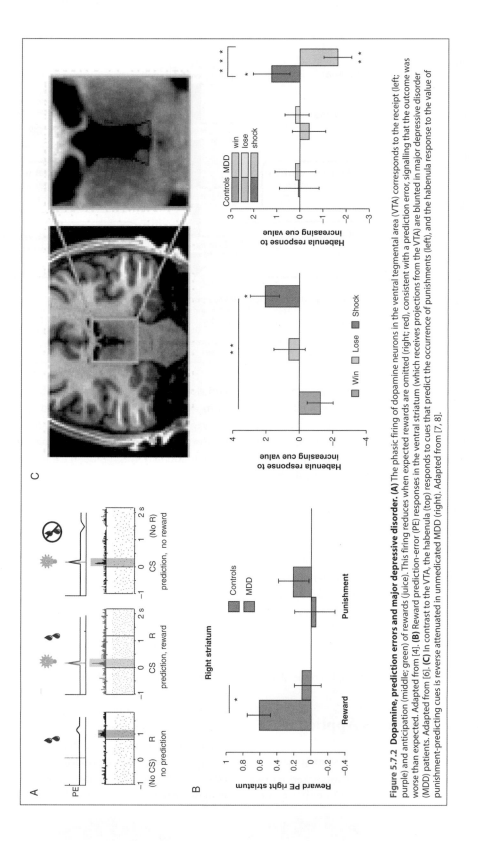

Figure 5.7.2 Dopamine, prediction errors and major depressive disorder. (A) The phasic firing of dopamine neurons in the ventral tegmental area (VTA) corresponds to the receipt (left; purple) and anticipation (middle; green) of rewards (juice). This firing reduces when expected rewards are omitted (right; red), consistent with a prediction error, signalling that the outcome was worse than expected. Adapted from [4]. **(B)** Reward prediction-error (PE) responses in the ventral striatum (which receives projections from the VTA) are blunted in major depressive disorder (MDD) patients. Adapted from [6]. **(C)** In contrast to the VTA, the habenula (top) responds to cues that predict the occurrence of punishments (left), and the habenula response to the value of punishment-predicting cues is reverse attenuated in unmedicated MDD (right). Adapted from [7, 8].

findings suggest that an increased propensity towards habit formation is characteristic of compulsive disorders. Indeed, a recent large-scale study showed that deficits in goal-directed control are strongly associated with a symptom dimension comprising 'compulsive behaviour and intrusive thoughts'[13]. See Section 5.8 for more on habits and compulsivity. Interestingly, transcranial magnetic stimulation of frontoparietal brain networks can shift decision making from habitual towards goal-directed [14], which may offer a promising non-invasive intervention to ameliorate deleterious habit-based behaviours.

5.7.3 Learning Models Applied to Mood

Anhedonia (hyposensitivity to rewards) and negative emotional biases (hypersensitivity to punishments) are core features of major depressive disorder (MDD), and both lend themselves to the application of reinforcement-learning models. In the context of reward learning, **blunted reward prediction errors** have been reported in key parts of the depression circuitry (e.g. ventral striatum, anterior cingulate cortex), and this blunting was more pronounced in the most severely depressed patients [15] . This is consistent with a prominent hypothesis that reduced dopamine signalling plays a role in the pathogenesis of depression. However, an important caveat is that the blunted reward prediction errors were also present in healthy participants taking an acute dose of selective serotonin reuptake inhibitors, which suggests that they might in part reflect effects of medication [15]. See Section 5.13 for more on anhedonia.

Another possibility is that MDD might be characterised by **enhanced learning from punishments** instantiated by brain regions that play a role in negatively motivated behaviour. The habenula, for example, is extensively connected with the dorsal and medial raphe nuclei and ventral tegmental area, the sources of the brain's serotonin and dopamine neurons, respectively. This unique position as a hub between corticolimbic networks and midbrain monoaminergic nuclei provides a means through which valenced stimuli can modulate motor output. Human neuroimaging studies applying reinforcement-learning models, have confirmed that the habenula tracks the value of cues predicting punishments such as painful electric shocks [16]. Interestingly, these negative-value responses are blunted in unmedicated patients during a major

depressive episode (Figure 5.7.2C). A blunted habenula response to punishments in MDD has been replicated in a number of studies, and restoration of habenula function is seen as a possible target for experimental treatments such as ketamine and deep brain stimulation [17].

Further work is needed to understand the complex interplay between the serotonin and dopamine systems in the context of prediction-error processing but, taken together, these studies underscore the utility of computational modelling in better understanding the causes of and treatments for depressive symptoms.

5.7.4 Learning Models Applied to Schizophrenia

Computational models of learning have also seen widespread application to understand the vagaries of schizophrenia and psychosis (see also Section 9.9). The negative symptoms (blunting of affect and anhedonia) have been described as reinforcement-learning-related reward impairments akin to MDD [18]. This suggests that dysregulation of a common computational process in the brain can result in similar symptoms across different diagnostic categories.

The positive symptoms (delusions and hallucinations) have also been modelled as failures of learning, specifically using Bayesian frameworks [19]. Here, sensory evidence (e.g. visual inputs, also referred to as the **likelihood**) and **prior knowledge** are defined as probability distributions (Figure 5.7.3A). The width of these distributions represents the confidence or reliability ascribed to each source of information and the discrepancy between them amounts to a prediction error. Bayes' rule tells us how to optimally combine these sources of information to arrive at our **posterior beliefs** according to the following equation, where A is some state of the world we want to estimate and B is the sensory data in front of us:

$$P(A|B) = \frac{\overbrace{P(B|A)}^{\text{likelihood}} * \overbrace{P(A)}^{\text{prior}}}{P(B)}$$

where the left side is labelled $\underbrace{P(A|B)}_{\text{posterior}}$

For example, in the hollow mask illusion (Figure 5.7.3A), the inside of a mask appears to us like a normal convex face. In Bayesian terms, this is due to the relative weighting of the imprecise sensory likelihood and strong confidence in our prior expectation about how faces typically appear. As a result, the combination of these two – our posterior belief – aligns with the precise prior, and

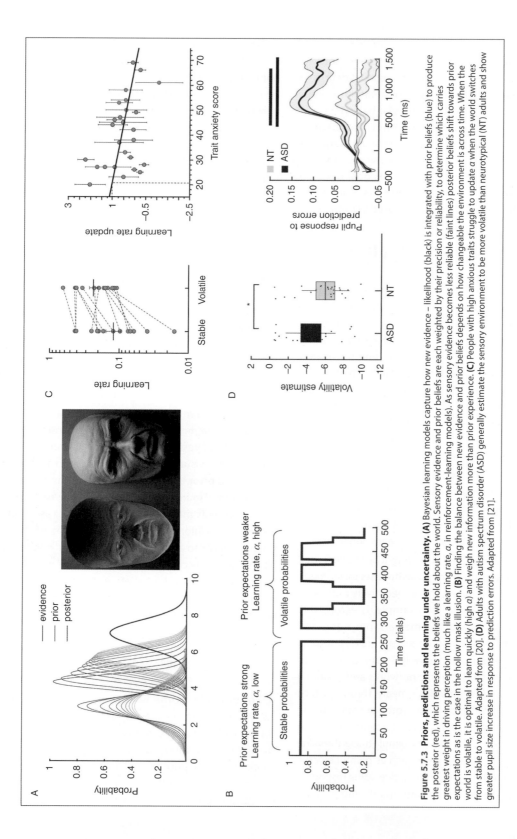

Figure 5.7.3 Priors, predictions and learning under uncertainty. (A) Bayesian learning models capture how new evidence – likelihood (black) is integrated with prior beliefs (blue) to produce the posterior (red), which represents the beliefs we hold about the world. Sensory evidence and prior beliefs are each weighted by their precision or reliability, to determine which carries greatest weight in driving perception (much like a learning rate, α, in reinforcement-learning models). As sensory evidence becomes less reliable (faint lines) posterior beliefs shift towards prior expectations as is the case in the hollow mask illusion. **(B)** Finding the balance between new evidence and prior beliefs depends on how changeable the environment is across time. When the world is volatile, it is optimal to learn quickly (high α) and weigh new information more than prior experience. **(C)** People with high anxious traits struggle to update α when the world switches from stable to volatile. Adapted from [20]. **(D)** Adults with autism spectrum disorder (ASD) generally estimate the sensory environment to be more volatile than neurotypical (NT) adults and show greater pupil size increase in response to prediction errors. Adapted from [21].

the inside of the mask appears convex. This framework can also be used to explain the acquisition of unusual expectations (e.g. delusions) or perceptual aberrations (e.g. hallucinations) in schizophrenia.

Psychosis has been partially explained as an *under*-weighting of prior expectations relative to sensory inputs, and consistent with this people with schizophrenia are less susceptible to the hollow mask illusion [19]. It has also been suggested that an *over*-weighting of prior expectations, at the expense of sensory reality, offers a compelling account of hallucinations [22]. Research is still ongoing at this stage, but it may be that both over- and under-weighting of prior expectations are present, either at different levels of abstraction (low level visual expectations vs. high level cognitive priors), or across the prodromal, acute or chronic stages of the disorder [23]. Interestingly, patients on medication for psychosis showed preserved influence of priors on early visual perception [24], suggesting that the computational pathology thought to underlie the schizophrenia state is possibly ameliorated when treatment is successful.

5.7.5 Hierarchical Learning Models Applied in Neuropsychiatry

A core aspect of the learning models described in this section is flexibility; prediction errors are not fixed stable quantities but need to be employed adaptively to adjust our best predictions about the world in proportion to how quickly the environment changes. This flexibility is controlled by the learning rate (α) and seminal studies have shown that humans can adjust their rate of learning in response to the changing statistics of the world: increasing α when learning is productive (such as when the world is volatile) and decreasing α when learning is less beneficial (such as when the world is stable; Figure 5.7.3B). These computational mechanisms have been linked to the function of the anterior cingulate cortex and the widespread cortical connections of the locus coeruleus–noradrenaline (LC–NA) system, which are well placed to enact rapid changes in neural processing. In humans, pupil size is often used as a non-invasive proxy for the activity of the system, and has been shown to encode both prediction errors and volatility [20, 21].

Difficulties estimating the volatility of the environment, and updating learning in response to volatility, have recently been demonstrated across a range of neuropsychiatric conditions. For example, anxiety proneness is associated with difficulties controlling the dynamic adjustment of α in response to volatility, and the pupil response to volatility is also reduced in high trait-anxious individuals [20]. In autistic adults, hierarchical learning models have been used to assess individual differences in how volatile the world is estimated to be. This work shows that autistic adults estimate the world to be more volatile than neurotypicals, which is linked to a heightened pupil response to prediction errors [21]. In contrast, a similar learning model was recently employed to understand auditory hallucinations – with hallucinators shown to weigh prior beliefs more over sensory inputs and estimate the world to be *less* volatile across time [22]. It seems then that it is not just the calculation of prediction error that is vulnerable in psychopathology, but the way in which those prediction errors are contextualised in relation to how changeable the environment is or is estimated to be. With the application of sophisticated models to quantify individual differences in learning at various levels of abstraction, this fundamental cognitive mechanism will likely be an important transdiagnostic construct in explaining (mal)adaptive behaviour [25].

Conclusions and Outstanding Questions

Computational psychiatry is an endeavour in its infancy – but important strides have been made in linking behavioural differences to brain function, via computational models that describe *how* the behaviour is generated and also *how* these computations are instantiated in the brain. The application of learning models has opened a new window of understanding for the mechanisms underlying a range of different psychopathologies. However, the next challenge for the field will be to translate these advances to the clinic [26].

Outstanding Questions

- Can computational models help predict individual treatment response and guide personalised interventions?
- Can computational psychiatry inform the development of novel interventions and therapies?
- How do we ensure that computational models are readily interpretable and provide meaningful insights to clinicians and researchers?
- How can we capture the dynamic nature of mental disorders using computational models?

REFERENCES

1. American Psychiatric Association. *Diagnostic and Statistical Manual of Mental Disorders*, 5th ed. (DSM-5). American Psychiatric Association, 2013.

2. Pavlov PI. Conditioned reflexes: an investigation of the physiological activity of the cerebral cortex. *Ann Neurosci* 2010; 17(3): 136–141.

3. Thorndike EL. Animal intelligence: an experimental study of the associative processes in animals. *Psychol Rev: Monogr Suppl* 1898; 2(4): i–190.

4. Rescorla RA, Wagner AR. A theory of Pavlovian conditioning: variations in the effectiveness of reinforcement. In *Classical Conditioning II: Current Research and Theory*. Appleton-Century-Crofts, 1972, pp. 64–99.

5. Schultz W, Dayan P, Montague PR. A neural substrate of prediction and reward. *Science* 1997; 275(5306): 1593–1599.

6. Kumar P, Waiter G, Ahearn T et al. Abnormal temporal difference reward-learning signals in major depression. *Brain* 2008; 131(8): 2084–93.

7. Lawson RP, Seymour B, Loh E et al. The habenula encodes negative motivational value associated with primary punishment in humans. *Proc Natl Acad Sci USA* 2014; 111(32): 11858–11863.

8. Lawson RP, Nord CL, Seymour B et al. Disrupted habenula function in major depression. *Mol Psychiatry* 2017; 22: 202–208.

9. O'Doherty JP, Dayan P, Friston K, Critchley H, Dolan RJ. Temporal difference models and reward-related learning in the human brain. *Neuron* 2003; 38(2): 329–337.

10. Daw ND, Niv Y, Dayan P. Uncertainty-based competition between prefrontal and dorsolateral striatal systems for behavioral control. *Nature Neurosci* 2005; 8(12): 1704–1711.

11. Smittenaar P, FitzGerald TH, Romei V, Wright ND, Dolan RJ. Disruption of dorsolateral prefrontal cortex decreases model-based in favor of model-free control in humans. *Neuron* 2013; 80(4): 914–919.

12. Voon V, Derbyshire K, Rück C et al. Disorders of compulsivity: a common bias towards learning habits. *Mol Psychiatry* 2015; 20(3): 345–352.

13. Gillan CM, Kosinski M, Whelan R, Phelps EA, Daw ND. Characterizing a psychiatric symptom dimension related to deficits in goal-directed control. *eLife* 2016; 5: e11305.

14. Nord CL, Popa T, Smith E et al. The effect of frontoparietal paired associative stimulation on decision-making and working memory. *Cortex* 2019; 117: 266–276.

15. Bromberg-Martin ES, Matsumoto M, Hikosaka O. Distinct tonic and phasic anticipatory activity in lateral habenula and dopamine neurons. *Neuron* 2010; 67(1): 144–155.

16. Yang Y, Wang H, Hu J, Hu H. Lateral habenula in the pathophysiology of depression. *Curr Opin Neurobiol* 2018; 48: 90–96.

17. Gold JM, Waltz JA, Matveeva TM et al. Negative symptoms and the failure to represent the expected reward value of actions: behavioral and computational modeling evidence. *Arch Gen Psychiatry* 2012; 69(2): 129–138.

18. Valton V, Romaniuk L, Douglas Steele J, Lawrie S, Seriès P. Comprehensive review: computational modelling of schizophrenia. *Neurosci Biobehav Rev* 2017; 83: 631–646.

19. Dima D, Roiser JP, Dietrich DE et al. Understanding why patients with schizophrenia do not perceive the hollow-mask illusion using dynamic causal modelling. *Neuroimage* 2009; 46(4): 1180–1186.

20. Browning M, Behrens TE, Jocham G, O'Reilly JX, Bishop SJ. Anxious individuals have difficulty learning the causal statistics of aversive environments. *Nature Neurosci* 2015; 18(4): 590–596.

21. Lawson RP, Mathys C, Rees G. Adults with autism overestimate the volatility of the sensory environment. *Nature Neurosci* 2017; 20(9): 1293.

22. Powers AR, Mathys C, Corlett PR. Pavlovian conditioning: induced hallucinations result from overweighting of perceptual priors. *Science* 2017; 357(6351): 596–600.

23. Corlett PR, Horga G, Fletcher PC et al. Hallucinations and strong priors. *Trends Cogn Sci* 2019; 23(2): 114–127.

24. Valton V, Karvelis P, Richards KL et al. Acquisition of visual priors and induced hallucinations in chronic schizophrenia. *Brain* 2019; 142(8): 2523–2537.

25. Sandhu TR, Xiao B, Lawson RP. Transdiagnostic computations of uncertainty: towards a new lens on intolerance of uncertainty. *Neurosci Behav Rev* 2023; 148: 105123.

26. Browning M, Carter CS, Chatham C et al. Realizing the clinical potential of computational psychiatry: report from the Banbury Center Meeting, February 2019. *Biol Psychiatry* 88(2): E5–E10, https://doi.org/10.1016/j.biopsych.2019.12.026

5

5.8	**Habit Formation**	**Claire M. Gillan**

OVERVIEW

To understand the most sophisticated human capacities, such as analytical inquiry, social interaction or creativity, it is important to first understand the most basic. This chapter aims to introduce one of the most fundamental brain processes there is – the ability to form habits, to automate the routine and to ignore things that have become predictable. Habits are brilliant in their simplicity and the poetic irony is that we notice least these behaviours that we know the best. If you take one thing away from this chapter, let it be this: without our ability to develop habits, to automate tasks we have performed 100 times or more, our brains would lack capacity to support any of the advanced functions that we prize as humans. At every level of complex thought, habits provide the essential scaffolding. Aside from the fundamental importance of understanding habits for gaining a broader concept of how the brain processes information and arrives at decisions, habits are of extra interest to those in the field of psychiatry. As you will learn, habits play a key role in a range of compulsive disorders, including obsessive–compulsive disorder and addiction.

5.8.1 Theoretical Foundations

Habits are behaviours that are elicited by stimuli; they are automatic and fast, rather than carefully selected to satisfy our current needs and wants ('goals') [1]. The kind of stimuli that can elicit a habitual response range from the sound of a foghorn blasting in your ear to contextual stimuli as subtle and diffuse as a place or time. Habits are thought to develop through practice, and as such they flourish within our **routines** – the often-repeated acts of everyday life, such as dressing, bathing, commuting or cooking. Thanks to our brain's habit system, these sorts of activities are performed fluidly, through the chaining of simple habits into more elaborate sequences, and without much in the way of concentration or mental effort. In describing habits, it is necessary to introduce another important term for this chapter: **goal-directed** processing. Goal-directed behaviours are the antithesis of habits; slow and considered, designed to meet our ever-changing needs, they require planning, simulation and reflection to achieve the best possible outcome.

5.8.2 Behavioural Experiments

The first experiments in this space were positioned to measure the relative contribution of goal-directed versus habitual associations to behaviour in the rodent. The most famous of these is the **outcome-devaluation test**. Adams [2] trained rats in an operant chamber (an experimental box where rodents complete behavioural tests) to perform an action that would yield some delicious food pellets (Figure 5.8.1A). Following training, he then reduced the value of the pellets by pairing their ingestion with nausea-inducing lithium chloride injections, thereby inducing a taste aversion (Figure 5.8.1B). Rats are good at learning what foods are dangerous to them and so pick this up fast and will no longer eat the pellets following this procedure. The principal question this allowed Adams to test was if the rats would rein in their lever pressing when returned to the operant chamber. Goal-directed actions are, by definition, intended to achieve a current goal. It follows that if the rats' lever pressing is a goal-directed act, when the outcome of an action is no longer desirable to

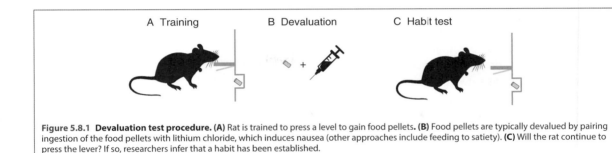

Figure 5.8.1 Devaluation test procedure. (A) Rat is trained to press a level to gain food pellets**. (B)** Food pellets are typically devalued by pairing ingestion of the food pellets with lithium chloride, which induces nausea (other approaches include feeding to satiety). **(C)** Will the rat continue to press the lever? If so, researchers infer that a habit has been established.

the rat, the lever pressing should terminate (Figure 5.8.1C). To the surprise of some, this newly acquired distaste for food pellets translated to a reduction in lever pressing in the rodent. This suggested that the rats were able to connect their level-pressing behaviour prospectively to the outcome it produces, and then 'decided' (if you will) not to respond in light of their newfound revulsion to food pellets, evidencing goal-directed control over their behaviour. Importantly, Adams found that goal-directed behaviour in the rodent was not always present – when a separate group of rats were *over*-trained (receiving five times the lever-press training in the operant chamber), sensitivity to devaluation was near abolished. The rats now appeared to perform the response automatically, without thought for the consequences.

Beyond devaluation, another popular and classic approach to quantifying habits is **contingency degradation**. Here, subjects' sensitivity to the causal relationship between action and outcome is tested. This is typically achieved by increasing the likelihood that an outcome is presented, absent of the action. For example, in the training phase of an experiment, the probability that a reward is presented might be 0 if the action is not performed and 0.5 if the action is performed. That means that the reward is never delivered if the subject does not respond, but it is delivered 50% of the time on trials where they do respond. When the experimenter seeks to degrade that contingency, they simply increase the former probability to 50% also. That means that reward is equally likely when the subject responds or does not respond – resulting in a state of no contingency between action and reward. Similar to the outcome-devaluation procedure, if the individual is behaving in a goal-directed manner, they should cease performing the action when it loses its causal relationship to reward [3]. These two

procedures are generally considered to be the foundation of modern research in habits and permitted the earliest neuroscientific investigations.

5.8.3 The Neuroanatomy of Habits and Goals

Devaluation and contingency degradation paradigms have been used extensively in lesion studies and other causal manipulations carried out in rodents; more recently, this work has been extended to humans using functional and structural imaging. Emerging from these cross-species investigations has been consensus that the putamen (dorsolateral striatum in the rodent brain) and its connection to the premotor and sensorimotor cortices are likely critical in the development and maintenance of stimulus–response habits (e.g. [4, 5]). Human neuroimaging has largely converged on these findings, showing increased putamen–premotor cortex connectivity in those who tend to depend the most on habits [6] and increasing involvement of the putamen with extended training [7]. In terms of goal-directed control, as a more multi-faceted and complex process, it is no surprise that a more distributed set of brain regions are thought to be necessary for successful execution. Of those most well studied, the orbitofrontal cortex is thought to play a central role in using motivation to drive flexible goal-directed actions (e.g. [8, 9]), and the caudate and hippocampus are thought to play a more targeted role in linking actions to their consequences and maintaining the cognitive map of a given decision space (e.g. [3, 10]). It is important to note however that, given the complex nature of planning, the importance of these regions depends critically on the methodology employed [11]. See Section 5.15 for more on the neurobiology of goal-directed action from the perspective of fronto-executive function.

5.8.4 Contemporary Issues

Although hugely influential, the devaluation test and contingency degradation paradigms suffer from the same limitation. They force one to conceptualise habits and goal-directed actions as two endpoints on a behavioural axis and, in doing so, it impedes our understanding of the underlying neural processes, which a wealth of data suggests are functionally separable and may even operate in a hierarchical manner [12]. If a rat continues to respond in a devaluation test, we can say he or she has developed a habit, but we do not know if that behavioural endpoint has arisen due to (1) a build-up of strong and forceful associative links between stimulus and response, (2) a decrement in cognitive control – in our ability to rein in even the most tenuous of stimulus–response associations or (3) indeed both. To address this gap, modern approaches have attempted to separate these processes and study them relatively independently.

5.8.4.1 Model-Based Planning

The vast majority of work in this area has centred on the study of (2) above, the brain processes that contribute to our ability to exert goal-directed control over actions. The most prominent approach has been the study of 'model-based planning', a formal definition of goal-directed control that is operationalised as the extent to which people use a cognitive map, or mental search, when making decisions [13]. The behavioural task used to measure this is called the '**two-step task**' and, in essence, it allows the neuroscientist to quantify the extent to which a player utilises a (model-based) mental search of the most probable consequences of each action and/ or uses a simpler strategy of (model-free) trial-and-error learning. Studies examining individual differences in model-based planning have confirmed that those who use the model-based strategy are less likely to display habits in a devaluation test [14]. Moreover, model-based planning is a characteristic of human decision making that develops throughout childhood and adolescence [15], but decreases with advancing age [16]. It relates to more general cognitive control abilities [17], intelligence quotient (IQ) [18] and working memory [16].

5.8.4.2 The Search for Habit

The other behavioural readout from this test, model-free learning, was intended to capture (and formalise) the fundamental reinforcement-learning processes that underpin the acquisition of stimulus–response linkages – the habit itself. But evidence that the sort of trial-and-error learning that subjects exhibit on this task relates to habits has been elusive. Particularly noteworthy is the observation that individual differences in model-free learning don't relate to one's success on a devaluation test [14]. Though initially considered a problem of the two-step task, recently researchers have begun to question if the behaviour seen in a devaluation test in humans is indicative of the strength of stimulus–response associations at all. The one observation of habits following over-training in humans was reported in 2009 [7], but a series of attempts to replicate this key finding have failed [19]. It has been speculated that individual differences in goal-directed decision making may have a substantially more prominent influence on human choice behaviour (at least in the laboratory) than the potentially more subtle influence of training duration. To address this, researchers have recently sought to leverage the fact that the goal-directed system needs more time and effort to be executed. For example, if the time pressure in a task is such that individuals *cannot* recruit the slower, goal-directed control system, over-training effects in humans can be revealed (i.e. habit expression) [20]. Similarly, the speed at which a response can be made might prove a more sensitive measure of the strength of stimulus–response links than actual choice behaviour [21]. In the next wave of research in this area, these methods will be crucial in understanding how habits and goals interact in real time.

5.8.5 Habits and Goals in OCD

It has long been observed that compulsive behaviours have a habit-like quality. They persist despite negative consequences, they are rigid and repetitive and they are experienced as automatic – the patient has a loss of control over their execution. This clinical observation fits quite remarkably with overlaps in the neurocircuitry of habit formation and quintessentially compulsive disorders like obsessive–compulsive disorder (OCD). For example, abnormal structure and function in frontostriatal circuitry have been consistently reported in OCD and it is these same circuits that are most associated with the balance between habit expression and goal-directed control [22]. First examined in 2011 using the devaluation test, patients with OCD were found to exhibit habits more than healthy controls, persisting in their button-press responding despite the fact that their actions no longer led to rewarding outcomes [23] (Figure 5.8.2A). Subsequent investigations revealed that this excess of habit expression in patients was not affected by training duration, suggesting that goal-directed brain systems might be responsible [24]. This notion has largely been supported by further experiments. For example, when goal-directed functions are probed independently in tasks that do not lend themselves to habit forming, patients continue to show deficits [25]. Moreover, imaging work has revealed abnormal patterns of activity in the orbitofrontal cortex and caudate – typically considered

goal-directed regions – as patients acquire and execute (respectively) their habits [26] (Figure 5.8.2B). The extent to which the acquisition of the habit plays a role in compulsivity remains largely an open question as an absence of evidence cannot be taken as evidence for absence. Serious limitations in our ability to study habits in a controlled laboratory setting in humans have been detailed above. Given this, it is entirely possible that only once those issues have been resolved can we fully understand how interactive these components might be. Hints that the story might not end here come from evidence of hyperactivity in the putamen in OCD patients during a 'compulsion provocation' study [27], which suggests that, even if not responsible for acquiring compulsions, the habit system likely plays a central role in maintaining them. Future work will be needed to fully address this limitation of the current state of the art. For more on the neurobiology of OCD, see Section 9.6.

5.8.6 Habits and Goals in Compulsivity

The extent to which these failures in goal-directed control are specific to OCD, or reflective of a broader class of compulsive disorders, has been the recent topic of debate. While early evidence from Voon and colleagues pointed to a shared pattern of model-based planning deficits across OCD, addiction and binge-eating disorder [25], there was no positive control group in this study; that is, another (non-compulsive) disorder where deficient behaviour on this task would not be expected. Subsequent studies in, for example, schizophrenia [28] and social anxiety disorder [29] revealed similar deficits when compared to control subjects, casting doubt on the notion that goal-directed planning deficits are specifically related to compulsivity at all. Interestingly, the issue has found recent resolution, and appears less about the specificity of this cognitive model, but more broadly about the issues that we face in research, using highly comorbid disorder categories as listed in the *Diagnostic and Statistical Manual of Mental Disorders*, 5th edition (DSM-5) [30]. The question was first addressed in a large cohort of the general population who self-reported the dimensional severity of several aspects of mental illness and completed the two-step task [18]. Goal-directed planning was found to be negatively correlated with various aspects of mental health, showing a pattern that was perhaps just as non-specific

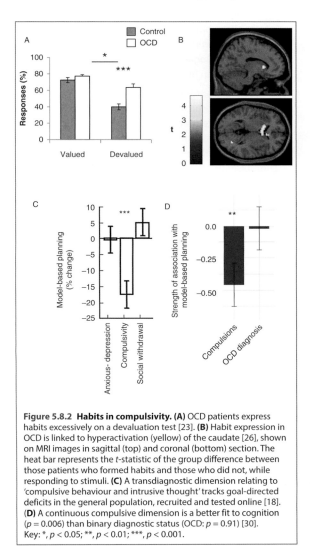

Figure 5.8.2 Habits in compulsivity. (A) OCD patients express habits excessively on a devaluation test [23]. **(B)** Habit expression in OCD is linked to hyperactivation (yellow) of the caudate [26], shown on MRI images in sagittal (top) and coronal (bottom) section. The heat bar represents the *t*-statistic of the group difference between those patients who formed habits and those who did not, while responding to stimuli. **(C)** A transdiagnostic dimension relating to 'compulsive behaviour and intrusive thought' tracks goal-directed deficits in the general population, recruited and tested online [18]. **(D)** A continuous compulsive dimension is a better fit to cognition ($p = 0.006$) than binary diagnostic status (OCD: $p = 0.91$) [30]. Key: *, $p < 0.05$; **, $p < 0.01$; ***, $p < 0.001$.

as the in-person case–control studies. Critically, the picture changes when the co-occurrence of symptoms within the same individual is taken into account. Using a data-reduction technique called factor analysis, three dimensions of mental health could be used to replace the nine 'disorder-relevant' questionnaire total scores, which probed eating disorders, apathy, impulsivity, alcohol addiction, OCD, depression, anxiety and schizotypy. The three dimensions that best explained the data were anxious depression, compulsivity and social withdrawal. Crucially, model-based planning deficits were found to be uniquely linked to the dimension of mental health pertaining to compulsivity (Figure 5.8.2C). This approach illustrates how there appears to be a specific link between compulsivity and goal-directed control, which standard diagnostic frameworks do not adequately capture. Indeed, subsequent work in patients showed that goal-directed deficits in diagnosed patients are more closely linked to their levels of self-reported compulsivity than the diagnosis they were assigned in a clinical interview [31] (Figure 5.8.2D). These papers highlight the limitations of research aimed at finding neat associations between DSM-5 diagnostic categories and brain changes, going beyond the scope of this chapter. Future work will need to take these issues seriously if observed associations between cognition and mental health phenomena are ever to see clinical practice.

Conclusions and Outstanding Questions

In conclusion, there exists a dichotomy between habits and goal-directed control. Contemporary research suggests these are parallel, interactive, functions of the brain – not all or nothing. In this section, we have seen how reinforcement-learning frameworks (e.g. model-based and model-free) have significantly enriched the field. Goal-directed/model-based forms of processing are deficient in compulsive disorders and along a spectrum of compulsivity in the general population.

Outstanding Questions

- Significant methodological gaps exist in research into habits in humans, making it difficult to evaluate their role in compulsive disorders. Can we develop new methodologies that can successfully and reliably induce habits in humans in a laboratory setting?

- Categorical disorder frameworks present problems for research because different disorders co-occur with high rates of frequency in the same individuals. Can we use dimensional and transdiagnostic approaches in mental health research to better understand compulsivity and deficits in goal-directed behaviour?

REFERENCES

1. Dickinson A. Actions and habits: the development of behavioural autonomy. *Philos Trans R Soc London B* 1985; 308(1135): 67–78.

2. Adams CD. Variations in the sensitivity of instrumental responding to reinforcer devaluation. *Q J Exp Psychol B* 1982; 34: 77–98.

3. Yin HH, Ostlund SB, Knowlton BJ, Balleine BW. The role of the dorsomedial striatum in instrumental conditioning. *Eur J Neurosci* 2005; 22(2): 513–523.

4. Yin HH, Knowlton BJ, Balleine BW. Lesions of dorsolateral striatum preserve outcome expectancy but disrupt habit formation in instrumental learning. *Eur J Neurosci* 2004; 19(1): 181–189.

5. Smith KS, Graybiel AM. Habit formation coincides with shifts in reinforcement representations in the sensorimotor striatum. *J Neurophysiol* 2016; 115(3): 1487–1498.

6. de Wit S, Watson P, Harsay HA et al. Corticostriatal connectivity underlies individual differences in the balance between habitual and goal-directed action control. *J Neurosci* 2012; 32(35): 12066–12075.

7. Tricomi E, Balleine BW, O'Doherty JP. A specific role for posterior dorsolateral striatum in human habit learning. *Eur J Neurosci* 2009; 29(11): 2225–2232.

8. Valentin VV, Dickinson A, O'Doherty JP. Determining the neural substrates of goal-directed learning in the human brain. *J Neurosci* 2007; 27(15): 4019–4026.

9. Killcross S, Coutureau E. Coordination of actions and habits in the medial prefrontal cortex of rats. *Cereb Cortex* 2003; 13(4): 400–408.

10. Vikbladh OM, Meager MR, King J et al. Hippocampal contributions to model-based planning and spatial memory. *Neuron* 2019; 102(3): 683–693.e4.

11. Schreiner DC, Renteria R, Gremel CM. Fractionating the all-or-nothing definition of goal-directed and habitual decision-making. *J Neurosci Res* 2020; 98(6): 998–1006.

12. Cushman F, Morris A. Habitual control of goal selection in humans. *Proc Natl Acad Sci USA* 2015; 112(45): 13817–13822.

13. Daw ND, Gershman SJ, Seymour B, Dayan P, Dolan RJ. Model-based influences on humans' choices and striatal prediction errors. *Neuron* 2011; 69(6): 1204–1215.

14. Gillan CM, Otto AR, Phelps EA, Daw ND. Model-based learning protects against forming habits. *Cogn Affect Behav Neurosci* 2015; 15(3): 523–536.

15. Decker JH, Otto AR, Daw ND, Hartley CA. From creatures of habit to goal-directed learners: tracking the developmental emergence of model-based reinforcement learning. *Psychol Sci* 2016; 27(6): 848–858.

16. Eppinger B, Walter M, Heekeren HR, Li SC. Of goals and habits: age-related and individual differences in goal-directed decision-making. *Front Neurosci* 2013; 7: 253.

17. Otto AR, Skatova A, Madlon-Kay S, Daw ND. Cognitive control predicts use of model-based reinforcement learning. *J Cogn Neurosci* 2015; 27(2): 319–333.

18. Gillan CM, Kosinski M, Whelan R, Phelps EA, Daw ND. Characterizing a psychiatric symptom dimension related to deficits in goal-directed control. *elife* 2016; 5.

19. de Wit S, Kindt M, Knot SL et al. Shifting the balance between goals and habits: five failures in experimental habit induction. *J Exp Psychol Gen* 2018; 147(7): 1043–1065.

20. Hardwick R, Forrence A, Krakauer J, Haith A. Time-dependent competition between habitual and goal-directed response preparation. *Nature Hum Behav* 2019; 3(12): 1252–1262.

21. Luque D, Molinero S, Watson P, López FJ, Le Pelley ME. Measuring habit formation through goal-directed response switching. *J Exp Psychol Gen* 2020; 149(8): 1449–1459.

22. Graybiel AM, Rauch SL. Toward a neurobiology of obsessive–compulsive disorder. *Neuron* 2000; 28(2): 343–347.

23. Gillan CM, Papmeyer M, Morein-Zamir S et al. Disruption in the balance between goal-directed behavior and habit learning in obsessive–compulsive disorder. *Am J Psychiatry* 2011; 168(7): 718–726.

24. Gillan CM, Morein-Zamir S, Urcelay GP et al. Enhanced avoidance habits in obsessive–compulsive disorder. *Biol Psychiatry* 2014; 75(8): 631–638.

25. Voon V, Derbyshire K, Rück C et al. Disorders of compulsivity: a common bias towards learning habits. *Mol Psychiatry* 2015; 20(3): 345–352.

26. Gillan CM, Apergis-Schoute AM, Morein-Zamir S et al. Functional neuroimaging of avoidance habits in obsessive–compulsive disorder. *Am J Psychiatry* 2015; 172(3): 284–293.

27. Banca P, Voon V, Vestergaard MD et al. Imbalance in habitual versus goal directed neural systems during symptom provocation in obsessive–compulsive disorder. *Brain* 2015; 138(Pt 3): 798–811.

28. Morris RW, Quail S, Griffiths KR, Green MJ, Balleine BW. Corticostriatal control of goal-directed action is impaired in schizophrenia. *Biol Psychiatry* 2015; 77(2), 187–195.

29. Alvares GA, Balleine BW, Guastella AJ. Impairments in goal-directed actions predict treatment response to cognitive–behavioral therapy in social anxiety disorder. *PLoS One* 2014; 9(4): e94778.

30. American Psychiatric Association. *Diagnostic and Statistical Manual of Mental Disorders*, 5th ed. (DSM-5). American Psychiatric Association, 2013.

31. Gillan C, Kalanthroff E, Evans M et al. Comparison of the association between goal-directed planning and self-reported compulsivity vs obsessive–compulsive disorder diagnosis. *JAMA Psychiatry* 2020; 77(1): 77–85.

Wolfram Schultz

5.9 Reward, Pleasure and Motivation

OVERVIEW

Rewards are crucial for individual and evolutionary survival and have three major functions: learning, approach (motivation, decision making) and emotion. Neurophysiological work in animals has elucidated neuronal mechanisms for learning and approach. Key brain centres for reward are dopamine neurons, the striatum, the orbitofrontal cortex and the amygdala, each of them interconnected and associated with other brain structures in which reward information is often processed in conjunction with sensory and motor mechanisms. Although it is difficult to make categorical functional distinctions between highly connected brain structures, some simplification is possible: dopamine neurons play a prime role in reinforcement learning and updating of economic decision variables; striatum neurons confer reward information to movements and decisions; the orbitofrontal cortex has a prime function in decisions; and the amygdala, classically known for fear processing, has a substantial role in reward processes suitable for economic decision making. Any disturbance in these crucial neuronal survival mechanisms has serious consequences for the welfare of individuals.

5.9.1 The Functions of Reward

Brain reward systems serve to acquire substances for individual survival and to propagate the genes via sexual reproduction. Although the term 'reward' is often meant as bonus or happiness, reward function extends to all substances and mating partners that are evolutionarily beneficial: genes for brains that maximise such rewards have the highest success in evolution (and genes for less optimal brains are less likely to be passed on).

The function of reward is to assure individual and evolutionary survival (proximal and distal functions). We die if we don't eat and drink, and our genes disappear if we don't mate. Rewards result in learning (coming back for more, conceptualised in reinforcement theory), elicit positive motivation and economic choice (maximising reward, conceptualised in economic theory) and make us happy (subjective feelings of pleasure, happiness and the desire for more). On the other hand, reward processing can go wrong in a large number of psychiatric and substance misuse disorders (Schultz, 2011).

Although rewards are detected by sensory systems, there are no specific receptors for reward. Rather, although being physical objects, events or situations, rewards have subjective value that reflect individual differences or needs. Such valuations may condense into a personal reward 'profile': some people or animals value some rewards more than others, like money vs adventure, or cocaine vs alcohol vs abstinence. In not being fully defined by physical characteristics, reward is made up by the brain. Subjective reward value is mathematically defined as economic utility. In times of scarcity, which is the default biological, and human, condition, we need more than just reward: we need to get the best available reward to compete for individual and evolutionary survival. We get that best reward by learning and by maximising utility in choices.

5.9.2 Learning

Learning by reinforcement serves to maximise reward intake (and avoid damage and aversive events). The most fundamental form of learning was proposed by Pavlov and conceptualised in Rescorla–Wagner and related reinforcement-learning models; it consists of conferring reward prediction to a neutral stimulus (Figure 5.9.1A). See Section 5.7 for more on models of learning. Learning is governed by prediction errors, defined as reward received minus reward predicted. In initial learning steps, there may be no prediction, and any reward elicits a positive prediction error. That error endows the stimulus with reward prediction, which may increase with repeated experience (Figure 5.9.1B). Pavlov's dog learns gradually, over repeated trials, that the bell, which intrinsically means nothing, comes to predict a sausage, and the dog starts salivating to the sound of the bell. Spoken more formally, the bell predicts nothing at the outset of learning, and the sausage elicits a positive prediction error. As the bell's prediction (of the sausage) grows, the prediction error decreases gradually to zero. However, when the reward is less than predicted, a negative prediction error occurs that reduces the prediction (Figure 5.9.1C).

What Pavlov, and common perceptions, did not know is that reinforcement learning requires more than stimulus–reward pairing: the reward needs to be contingent (depend) on a stimulus for the stimulus to become a reward predictor (Figure 5.9.1D) (Delamater, 1995). So, when a reward occurs as frequently during a stimulus as during its absence, the stimulus does not specifically predict the reward and hence is not learnt as a reward predictor, despite being paired with reward. Contingency is crucial for learning, and inadequate perception of background reward may compromise reward prediction.

This scenario describes learning from scratch, but in most cases some prediction already exists, and a reward elicits a positive or negative prediction error relative to that prediction. Learning then consists of updating existing predictions. And reinforcement learning is not restricted to the stimulus immediately preceding the reward: the reward-predicting stimulus acquires reward value itself and constitutes a higher-order reward, which

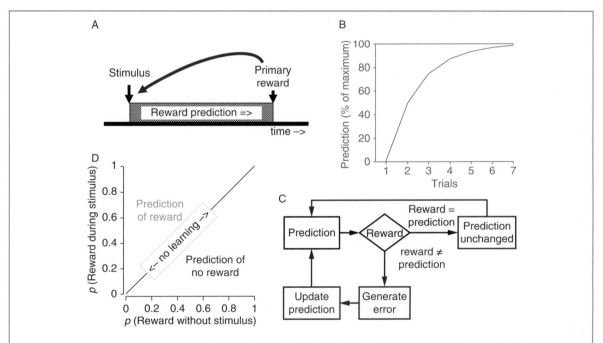

Figure 5.9.1 Basic principles of reinforcement learning. (A) Acquisition of reward prediction from primary reward. **(B)** Gradually flattening and plateauing learning curve driven by reward prediction error, with changing prediction over repeated trials. **(C)** Error-driven learning. Red: prediction error, blue: no prediction error. Behaviour is driven by prediction and results in reward. Depending on the reward being different from the prediction (red) or equal to the prediction (blue), a prediction error occurs (or not) that will change the prediction on the next trial (or not). **(D)** Reward contingency. Reward prediction, and hence learning, depends not only on how often the stimulus and reward are paired, but also how often the reward occurs in the absence of the stimulus. *p*: probability. Redrawn from Dickinson (1980).

itself can induce predictions of that stimulus. This may go on repeatedly and predict reward well before it actually occurs, thus contributing advance information for economic decisions (Sutton and Barto, 1998). It is like going through a city and following predictive pub signs and street names well before the drink is actually in your mouth.

5.9.3 Positive Motivation and Reward Choice

Besides maximising reward by reinforcement learning, humans and animals need to be motivated to acquire rewards. In doing so, they tend to maximise reward by choosing the best option that is available to them. Positive motivation is a manifestation of desire and can be measured as frequency and speed of reaction (reaction and movement time) and as preference between rewards. Better rewards elicit stronger motivation for these rewards. General preferences are difficult to assess in an objective manner because of potentially inaccurate report or memory. By contrast, observable choice reveals preference relationships at that moment. Such preference is defined as the probability of choosing one option over all available alternatives within a given option set. The most straightforward, and least confounded, preference test is binary choice in which two options are presented simultaneously, and the person or animal selects one of them (and forgoes the other). Consistent preference for the best option constitutes rational choice and results in reward maximisation. Rational choice is often violated in human and animal behaviour, which can be prevented by restricting choices with bounds that allow a person or animal to understand the choice options and the consequences of selecting them (bounded rationality).

The value of a reward for someone is determined by its usefulness (utility) and how frequently it occurs (expected utility). Being subjective, utility cannot be measured but is inferred from observable choice. The impact of reward frequency is often distorted; low frequencies often have an increased influence. Further factors influencing utility are subjective tendencies toward reward delay (temporal discounting, impatience), risk (variation of reward amount, chance of loss, or their combination), and many emotional, social and cultural factors. Utility applies to single choice options, and the decision maker behaves as if choosing the option with the higher expected

utility. By contrast, revealed preference is a relationship between all options and thus depends on the utility of every option. Reinforcement learning, through reward prediction errors, updates the utility of the just-experienced choice option, thus linking learning to choice.

5.9.4 Neuronal Reward Systems

Given the crucial role of reinforcement learning and choice for maximising reward, dedicated brain systems have evolved that support and control these processes. Processing of reward without other information is found in four prime structures, namely the midbrain dopamine system, striatum (putamen, caudate nucleus, ventral striatum), orbitofrontal cortex and amygdala (Figure 5.9.2) (Schultz, 2015). These structures are closely interconnected, with each one sending axons to the other three structures. Several closely connected structures also contain reward signals. Further cortical and subcortical brain regions process reward in association with sensory stimuli and movements, all of them being involved in identifying and choosing between rewards.

Information processing systems, including brains, use time-specific signals. Signals for reward and choice are measured in animals as action potentials that influence downstream neurons and ultimately lead to reward acquisition. In humans, typical reward signals are, for example, measured as blood oxygen level-dependent (BOLD) changes by functional MRI.

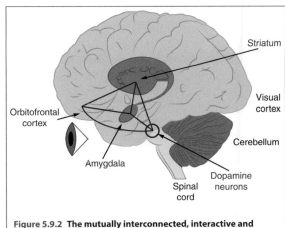

Figure 5.9.2 The mutually interconnected, interactive and cooperative reward circuit in the brain. Only the four most important reward structures are indicated. They are the orbitofrontal cortex (economic decision making), amygdala (reward detection and decision making), dopamine neurons (reinforcement learning) and striatum (reward processing for movements).

5.9.4.1 Dopamine Neurons

Dopamine neurons are not only crucially involved in Parkinson's disease but emit also, separately, one of the strongest reward signals of the brain. This is the brain system whose function is altered in, and responsible for, drug addiction, obesity and other reward dysfunctions. Most dopamine neurons in the ventral tegmental area and substantia nigra show a sharp response that reflects a reward prediction error, both at the time of the ultimate reward and with reward-predicting stimuli. A reward, or predictive stimulus, that is better than predicted (positive prediction error) elicits an increased response, a fully predicted reward elicits no response and a reward that is worse than predicted elicits a depression (negative error) (Schultz et al., 1997). Thus, during learning, the dopamine response to a reward transfers to the preceding reward-predicting stimulus (Figure 5.9.3). In fact, the response to each primary and higher-order reward depends on its prediction, thus dopamine neurons implement the teaching term of efficient reinforcement models (Rescorla and Wagner, 1972; Sutton and Barto, 1998), see Section 5.7. The dopamine reward signal has an initial component that reflects the attention a reward draws before it is properly identified, suggesting that dopamine responses are also involved in attention. Separate from this two-component reward signal, later, slower and more heterogeneous dopamine changes reflect behavioural activation and can merge with reward responses when temporal resolution between reward and movement is insufficient (which can be controlled in monkeys but is difficult in rodents and human neuroimaging).

The dopamine reward signal codes formal economic utility, rather than physical value (Stauffer et al., 2014). The signal has postsynaptic effects that are appropriate for updating neuronal value signals in the striatum, frontal cortex and amygdala after the reward has been encountered in previous choices. In this way, the dopamine signal helps people and animals to choose the best reward.

5.9.4.2 Striatum

The dorsal and ventral striatum are the recipients of the nigrostriatal dopamine system. This is where dopamine exerts its effects on reward and addiction (ventral striatum with nucleus accumbens) and on movement (dorsal striatum; with this pathway deficient in Parkinson's disease). But the majority of neurons in the striatum are themselves involved in their own reward processing, which is described here. Most neurons in the dorsal and ventral striatum respond to various reward-predicting stimuli and to reward itself (some of them coding a prediction error). Other striatal neurons show slow activations during reward expectation, often together with movement preparation, suggesting a role in goal-directed action in which the reward goal is represented while the animal prepares and executes the action. In social settings, striatal neurons distinguish between their own and others' reward and the action required to obtain it (Báez-Mendoza et al., 2013).

Striatal neurons signal separately the value of each reward irrespective of being chosen (action value), which is an input variable for competitive, winner-take-all decision models (Samejima et al., 2005). These neurons receive the dopamine reward signal and influence downstream neurons according to their dopamine receptor: D1-receptor-carrying neurons direct action choice to the contralateral body side via the direct basal ganglia pathway, whereas D2-carrying neurons promote ipsilateral choice via the indirect pathway (Tai et al., 2012). The dopamine influence updates the action value in striatum neurons after reception of the chosen reward: if a received reward is worse than predicted, the ensuing negative prediction-error response decreases the action value of the chosen option, and vice versa for a better-than-predicted reward.

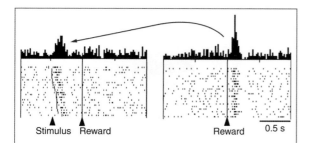

Stimulus Reward   Reward   0.5 s

Figure 5.9.3 How dopamine neurons respond to reward and reward prediction. Response transfer of dopamine neuron from primary reward to conditioned, reward-predicting stimulus. Each row of dots represents neuronal activity during a single experimental trial, with time along the x-axis. The top bar charts represent the sum of the neuronal responses over all trials shown below. The right-hand chart shows dopamine responses to a reward that is not predicted by any specific stimulus; the left-hand chart shows the responses to the reward-predicting stimulus but no response to the now-predicted reward itself. Redrawn from Romo and Schultz (1990).

5.9.4.3 Orbitofrontal Cortex

Orbitofrontal neurons carry distinct types of reward information for decision making. The neurons signal the value of choice objects (object value), predict the value of the reward the animal is choosing (chosen value) and code the risk of getting a small rather than a large reward (Figure 5.9.4) (Padoa-Schioppa and Assad, 2006; O'Neill and Schultz, 2010). The role in decision making is particularly apparent with signals that integrate reward value from multicomponent choice options in close correspondence to economic revealed preference theory (Pastor-Bernier et al., 2019). You may prefer a smaller sweeter apple to a larger less-sweet apple, and orbitofrontal neurons pick up the higher value of your preferred apple, even though sweetness and size are two entirely different characteristics. Some orbitofrontal signals adapt to the currently used reward distribution: a reward that is in the top range of a distribution elicits a large response but only a small response when the identical reward is in the bottom range of a distribution with higher mean (Tremblay and Schultz, 1999). Such adaptations assure efficient use of the limited neuronal coding range.

Neurons in the dorsolateral prefrontal cortex integrate reward information into movement-related activity, distinguish between their own reward and the reward for another monkey, and follow competitive social video games (Hosokawa and Watanabe, 2012). Thus, compatible with multiple lesion deficits, the frontal cortex shows a wide variety of functions that serve optimal reward acquisition.

5.9.4.4 Amygdala

This large and ancient group of subcortical nuclei in the medial temporal lobe is not only famously involved in memory and fear but has recently been recognised as a prime reward structure of the brain. This conceptual change requires reassessment of amygdala function in reward disorders like drug addiction and obesity. Thus, distinct from fear processing, neurons in several subnuclei of the amygdala respond to reward and conditioned, reward-predicting stimuli (Paton et al., 2006). The reward response implements reward contingency beyond stimulus–reward pairing (Bermudez and Schultz, 2010). The neurons respond to a stimulus during which the animal receives more reward compared to stimulus absence; however, the neurons stop responding when the reward is identical between stimulus presence and absence (where the stimulus loses its specific reward

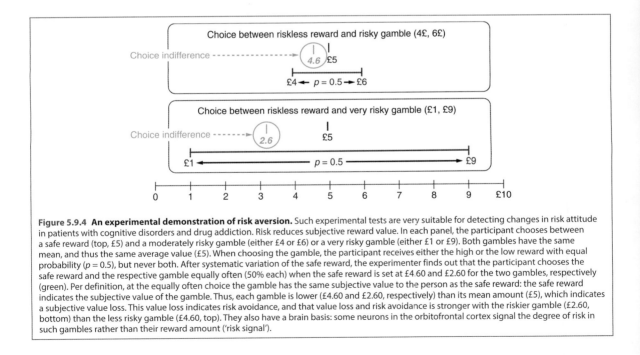

Figure 5.9.4 An experimental demonstration of risk aversion. Such experimental tests are very suitable for detecting changes in risk attitude in patients with cognitive disorders and drug addiction. Risk reduces subjective reward value. In each panel, the participant chooses between a safe reward (top, £5) and a moderately risky gamble (either £4 or £6) or a very risky gamble (either £1 or £9). Both gambles have the same mean, and thus the same average value (£5). When choosing the gamble, the participant receives either the high or the low reward with equal probability (p = 0.5), but never both. After systematic variation of the safe reward, the experimenter finds out that the participant chooses the safe reward and the respective gamble equally often (50% each) when the safe reward is set at £4.60 and £2.60 for the two gambles, respectively (green). Per definition, at the equally often choice the gamble has the same subjective value to the person as the safe reward: the safe reward indicates the subjective value of the gamble. Thus, each gamble is lower (£4.60 and £2.60, respectively) than its mean amount (£5), which indicates a subjective value loss. This value loss indicates risk avoidance, and that value loss and risk avoidance is stronger with the riskier gamble (£2.60, bottom) than the less risky gamble (£4.60, top). They also have a brain basis: some neurons in the orbitofrontal cortex signal the degree of risk in such gambles rather than their reward amount ('risk signal').

prediction), despite continuing stimulus–reward pairing. Although reward contingency has only been properly tested with amygdala neurons, it applies probably to other reward structures as well.

Amygdala neurons are also involved in economic decision making. Their reward signal transitions from reward value early in a trial to coding the ultimate choice. Other amygdala neurons predict reward save–spend choices or code social reward value during observational learning from a conspecific (Grabenhorst et al., 2019). Thus, amygdala neurons are involved in both fundamental reward processing and in sophisticated economic decision processes.

5.9.5 Human Imaging of Pleasure

While our behaviour tends to maximise reward via reinforcement learning and choice, the tangible feeling of seeking and obtaining reward is pleasure and euphoria. These processes are mediated by the dopamine system, which rounds up the role of this system in reward.

An objective assessment of emotional reward functions may be difficult in animals, but human imaging can help by assessing subjective feelings reported by test participants and relating them to measurable brain activity. A good case is amphetamine-induced euphoria that correlates with dopamine receptor stimulation in the human ventral striatum and demonstrates a role of dopamine in pleasure (Figure 5.9.5A) (Drevets et al., 2001). The experiment used positron emission tomography, which allows researchers to visualise dopamine activity via monitoring of radioactive raclopride binding to dopamine receptors. Raclopride binding competes with naturally released dopamine at the receptor, such that reduced raclopride binding indicates increased dopamine release. This is exactly what was observed when the indirect dopamine agonist amphetamine was injected (amphetamine increases extracellular dopamine by blocking reuptake). Importantly, the amphetamine-induced reduction of raclopride binding correlated with the euphoria induced by amphetamine, which indicates that dopamine receptor stimulation is involved in emotion. Correspondingly, functional MRI BOLD responses in human ventral striatum reflecting dopamine signals correlate with future reported happiness ratings about monetary outcomes

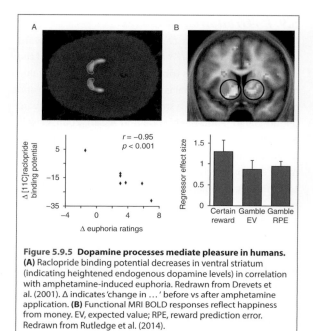

Figure 5.9.5 Dopamine processes mediate pleasure in humans. (A) Raclopride binding potential decreases in ventral striatum (indicating heightened endogenous dopamine levels) in correlation with amphetamine-induced euphoria. Redrawn from Drevets et al. (2001). Δ indicates 'change in ...' before vs after amphetamine application. **(B)** Functional MRI BOLD responses reflect happiness from money. EV, expected value; RPE, reward prediction error. Redrawn from Rutledge et al. (2014).

(Figure 5.9.5B) (Rutledge et al., 2014). Thus, although lacking the cellular resolution of neurophysiology, the third major reward function – pleasure – is associated with dopamine-mediated reward processes.

Conclusions and Outstanding Questions

The seemingly elusive concept of reward can be scientifically addressed in a way that allows accurate measurements of the value a reward has for the individual decision maker and to the measurement of neuronal reward signals. Neuronal signals serve the key reward functions in reinforcement leaning and decision making. These signals are distributed across different brain regions, which each contribute their own signature.

Outstanding Questions

- Can one imagine economic decision models without referring to the concept of value? Could such models explain the frequent 'irrational' (disadvantageous) choices of humans? Or can there be a variety of choice mechanisms that are recruited for different choices (and go wrong in different scenarios)?
- Are there different learning mechanisms in the brain that are recruited by different types of learning? The answer is most likely yes, as some forms of learning

are preserved in impaired dopamine neurotransmission, as seen in Parkinson's disease. So, what are these different learning systems, subcortical and cortical?

- When reward processing goes wrong in humans, like with drug addiction and obesity, we usually search for drug medication. But can we develop behavioural therapies for some suitable patients? What kind of knowledge from psychological and economic behavioural theory and from the neuroscience of reward should we choose to address such potential therapies?

REFERENCES

Báez-Mendoza R, Harris C, Schultz W (2013). Activity of striatal neurons reflects social action and own reward. *Proc Natl Acad Sci USA* 110: 16634–16639.

Bermudez MA, Schultz W (2010). Responses of amygdala neurons to positive reward predicting stimuli depend on background reward (contingency) rather than stimulus-reward pairing (contiguity). *J Neurophysiol* 103: 1158–1170.

Delamater AR (1995). Outcome selective effects of intertrial reinforcement in a Pavlovian appetitive conditioning paradigm with rats. *Anim Learn Behav* 23: 31–39.

Dickinson A (1980). *Contemporary Animal Learning Theory*. Cambridge University Press.

Drevets WC, Gautier C, Price JC et al. (2001). Amphetamine-induced dopamine release in human ventral striatum correlates with euphoria. *Biol Psychiatry* 49: 81–96.

Grabenhorst F, Báez-Mendoza R, Genest W, Deco G, Schultz W (2019). Primate amygdala neurons simulate decision processes of social partners. *Cell* 177: 986–998.

Hosokawa T, Watanabe M (2012). Prefrontal neurons represent winning and losing during competitive video shooting games between monkeys. *J Neurosci* 32: 7662–7671.

O'Neill M, Schultz W (2010). Coding of reward risk distinct from reward value by orbitofrontal neurons. *Neuron* 68: 789–800.

Padoa-Schioppa C, Assad JA (2006). Neurons in the orbitofrontal cortex encode economic value. *Nature* 441: 223–226.

Pastor-Bernier A, Stasiak A, Schultz W (2019). Orbitofrontal signals for two-component choice options comply with indifference curves of revealed preference theory. *Nat Comm* 10: 4885.

Paton JJ, Belova MA, Morrison SE, Salzman CD (2006). The primate amygdala represents the positive and negative value of visual stimuli during learning. *Nature* 439: 865–870.

Rescorla RA, Wagner AR (1972). A theory of Pavlovian conditioning: variations in the effectiveness of reinforcement and nonreinforcement. In Black AH, Prokasy WF (eds.), *Classical Conditioning II: Current Research and Theory*. Appleton Century Crofts, pp. 64–99.

Romo R, Schultz W (1990). Dopamine neurons of the monkey midbrain: contingencies of responses to active touch during self-initiated arm movements. *J Neurophysiol* 63: 592–606.

Rutledge RB, Skandalia N, Dayan P, Dolan RJ (2014). A computational and neural model of momentary subjective well-being. *Proc Natl Acad Sci USA* 111: 12252–12257.

Samejima K, Ueda Y, Doya K, Kimura M (2005). Representation of action-specific reward values in the striatum. *Science* 310: 1337–1340.

Schultz W (2011). Potential vulnerabilities of neuronal reward, risk, and decision mechanisms to addictive drugs. *Neuron* 69: 603–617.

Schultz W (2015). Neuronal reward and decision signals: from theories to data. *Physiol Rev* 95: 853–951.

Schultz W, Dayan P, Montague RR (1997). A neural substrate of prediction and reward. *Science* 275: 1593–1599.

Stauffer WR, Lak A, Schultz W (2014). Dopamine reward prediction error responses reflect marginal utility. *Curr Biol* 24: 2491–2500.

Sutton RS, Barto AG (1998). *Reinforcement Learning*. MIT Press.

Tai L-H, Lee AM, Benavidez N, Bonci A, Wilbrecht L (2012). Transient stimulation of distinct subpopulations of striatal neurons mimics changes in action value. *Nat Neurosci* 15: 1281–1289.

Tremblay L, Schultz, W (1999). Relative reward preference in primate orbitofrontal cortex. *Nature* 398: 704–708.

National Neuroscience Curriculum Initiative online resources

Creatures of Habit: The Neuroscience of Habit and Purposeful Behavior

Alana I. Mendelsohn

| 5.10 | Emotion | Angela C. Roberts and Hannah F. Clarke |

OVERVIEW

Emotions are powerful motivators of our behaviour, whether they be driving us to find food for survival, to avoid 'being food' for another predator or helping us to negotiate our way through the maze of social interactions critical for our ultimate success as individuals. Thus, ignoring our emotions is at our own peril. However, because of the central role they play in our decision making their regulation is paramount and, not surprisingly, failure to regulate effectively has a major deleterious impact on our mental health. Symptoms of emotion dysregulation, including anxiety and anhedonia, are widespread across psychiatric, neurological and neurodevelopmental disorders but whether they respond to any of the treatments currently available is unpredictable. For progress to be made we need a far better understanding of how the brain achieves emotion regulation. This chapter sets out our current knowledge of how the brain contributes to both regulation and dysregulation of emotion and highlights some of the outstanding questions in the field.

5.10.1 What Is Emotion?

Emotional behaviour in its simplest sense is behaviour driven by the need to fulfill goals, both internal and social. These goals preserve the individual and its reproductive success, such as feeding, social dominance, social bonding, sex, parental care and shelter. Given the importance of these goals, when emotional states are elicited they act as very powerful motivators of behaviour. Basic emotions include fear, sadness, anger, happiness and disgust. All of these emotions may be recognised in apes, some of them in lower species. More complex emotions that are more likely to be exclusive to humans are hypothesised to be derived from these basic ones. For example, embarrassment and worry may stem from fear (fear of looking stupid in front of peers); grief, from sadness; envy, jealousy and contempt from anger; joy, love and nostalgia, from happiness; guilt and shame, from disgust.

Emotions are generally positive or negative. One way of thinking about emotions, then, is that they stem from the presence or absence of positive and negative reinforcers (Rolls, 2013). A positive reinforcer is one that we and other animals will work to obtain, such as food or sex. A negative reinforcer is one that we and other animals will work to avoid, like loud noise. Thus, the presentation of a positive reinforcer may result in pleasure, elation and even ecstasy depending upon intensity. Likewise, presentation of a negative reinforcer may result in apprehension leading to fear or terror. Alternatively, loss/omission of a positive reinforcer could lead to frustration, anger, rage or sadness and grief, while omission of a negative reinforcer could result in relief.

Three obviously related, but nevertheless distinct dimensions of emotional responses are (1) **subjective** (i.e. verbal report about how an individual *feels*); (2) **behavioural** (i.e. what an individual *does*): this could include behaviour in social situations, changes in facial expression such as anger, running away from danger, seeking out reward; (3) **physiological**: this includes changes in heart rate and respiration (autonomic responses), and neuroendocrine responses such as adrenaline or corticosteroids secreted from the adrenals. While the word 'emotion' is often used in everyday parlance to refer to 'feelings' rather than the behaviour, it is behaviour and not personal experience that has consequences for survival and reproduction.

When studying emotions or emotional disorders, all three types of measure are important, but have their limitations. For example, human subjects find it very difficult to describe their emotional feelings, not only because this may be intrinsically difficult but also because of linguistic constraints. Behavioural indices of emotion can be measured precisely in animals, but in humans they consist mainly of self-report, questionnaires or observations of symptoms by human observers, often clinicians. Physiological responses can be measured effectively in humans and other animals, but it is known that physiological responses don't always correlate with subjective feelings. Recently, there has been a concerted effort to avoid using emotional words such as fear/anxiety or anhedonia (loss of pleasure) to describe the responses of animals to threatening stimuli or rewarding stimuli, respectively. Fear, anxiety and anhedonia are words commonly used to refer to feelings in humans but feelings are the one component of the emotional response that cannot be measured in animals, so whether manipulations in the brain of animals alter subjective feelings alongside physiological and behavioural responses cannot be ascertained (see LeDoux, 2015 for detailed discussion).

Why is emotion and its regulation important to the clinician? First, there are many brain disorders associated with dysregulated emotions: not only psychiatric disorders such as depression, mania, anxiety disorders and schizophrenia but also the developmental disorder of autism and neurodegenerative disorders such as frontotemporal dementia and Parkinson's disease. Second, emotions can have a powerful effect on our physiology and can influence our ability to get well after medical illness that doesn't have a primary effect on the brain. Third, emotions are an intrinsic part of human, and likely animal, experience.

5.10.2 Theories of Emotion

Controversy did, and still does, surround the roles of physiological responses associated with emotion. The major responses include changes in heart rate, blood pressure, galvanic skin resistance (a measure of the skin's electrical conductance – often called skin conductance response – as affected by sweating), muscle tension and arousal in the form of increases in adrenaline and cortisol. These changes can be linked with specific emotional experience. For example, an individual with spider phobia displays increases in heart rate, skin conductance, vasomotor activity and decreased respiration specifically in response to, even a picture of, a spider. These autonomic changes are therefore correlates of anxiety. Somewhat different patterns of bodily responses accompany the emotional feelings of sadness or anger, for example. However, just how separate the patterns are for different emotions is unclear. Equally important is whether such autonomic or visceral changes are merely adaptive responses to stress (i.e. the results of emotional experience, e.g. to facilitate flight or fight) or whether they also contribute to, or even form the basis of, emotional feelings.

William James (1884) appeared to reject the 'common sense' view that emotional expression results from emotional experience and reversed the causal relationships between the two. He stated: 'My thesis on the contrary is that the bodily changes follow directly the perception of the exciting fact, and that our feeling of the same changes as they occur IS the emotion'. Thus, we don't cry because we're sad – we're sad because we cry. At about the same time, Lange was promoting a related, but distinct idea that emotion could be experienced as organic symptoms (thus essentially introducing the notion of psychosomatic illness), so the idea that emotional experience derives from bodily experience is generally called the **James–Lange theory**. However, these words have been taken out of context because James also made it explicit that he was referring only to those emotions that have 'distinct bodily expression' and that he was only arguing that physiological expression was a necessary component, not that the physiological response *was* the emotion. Many researchers, but especially Walter Cannon in earlier times, argued strongly against the view that bodily feelings contributed to emotional experience. Along with a doctoral student, Philip Bard, who revealed the role of the hypothalamus in producing a coordinated emotional output, the **Cannon–Bard model** provided a neurobiological account of emotion, emphasising the importance of cortical and subcortical processing and cognitive appraisal. Their argument against visceral feedback was mainly on the grounds that, without feedback from the viscera, animals are still able to express emotions; that the same bodily responses occur across a range of emotions; that we are not aware enough of our visceral activity for this to be an important cue; and that visceral changes mediated by autonomic activity are too slow to be a source of emotional feelings, which can arise very rapidly. Importantly, it apparently was also shown that artificial induction of the visceral changes typical of strong emotions, for example by injecting adrenaline to produce tachycardia, did not actually produce emotional experiences.

However, over time, most of these objections have either garnered very weak evidence in their support or have been overturned. For example, Hohmann (1996) found that subjective feelings of anger and fear were diminished in subjects with spinal cord transection and that the effect was greater the higher the level of the transection. Importantly, the subjects could act *as if* they were angry in appropriate situations, but subjectively this 'anger' lacked emotional colouring and intensity. We also now know that there are major pathways innervating the brain from the viscera, including pathways carrying fine sympathetic afferents via the lamina I in the spinal cord and fine parasympathetic afferents via the nucleus of the solitary tract (Figure 5.10.1). These then project to the posterior/mid insula, anterior insula and right orbitofrontal cortex by way of the parabrachial nucleus and the ventromedial nucleus of the thalamus (Craig, 2002).

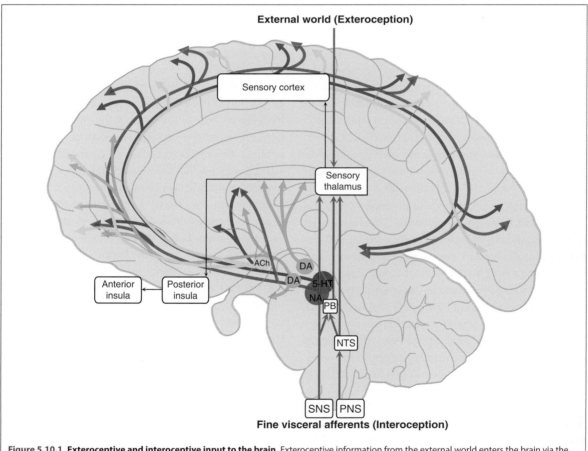

Figure 5.10.1 Exteroceptive and interoceptive input to the brain. Exteroceptive information from the external world enters the brain via the specific sensory organs and is relayed to the primary sensory cortices via the sensory thalamus (the exception being the olfactory pathway which excludes the thalamus). This information is combined with interoceptive information from the body in the form of fine visceral afferents of the autonomic system, which arise from both the sympathetic and parasympathetic nervous systems (SNS and PNS, respectively) and enter the brain via the spinal cord and the nucleus tractus solitaris (NTS) and parabrachial nucleus (PB) of the brainstem. They then route via the sensory thalamus to brain regions such as the posterior and anterior insula. These processes are also subject to modulation by the ascending monoaminergic neurotransmitter systems that include dopamine (DA, green), acetylcholine (ACh, yellow), serotonin (5-hydroxytryptamine; 5-HT, orange) and noradrenaline (NA, blue).

Indeed, the anterior insula has been proposed by Craig to contribute to emotional experience. We also know that some individuals can be remarkably sensitive to their visceral output while others are not (Critchley et al., 2004). Moreover, it has since been shown that different emotions can at least crudely be differentiated by considering the combinations of peripheral signals from multiple organs.

Finally, the classic study by Schachter and Singer (1962) provided evidence that artificially induced autonomic/visceral changes could elicit emotional experience. Although not always easily replicated, they demonstrated that peripherally injected adrenaline could elicit an emotional state if subjects were uninformed or misinformed as to the physiological consequences of the injections, but that the specificity of the state (quality of the emotion) induced was dependent upon cognitive interpretation of the context in which it was given. Together, these findings supported **Schachter and Singer's hypothesis** that without an immediate proximal explanation for body state, the peripheral changes would induce cognitive evaluation of a situation and elicit *different* emotions, depending on the external environmental context. Thus, it brought together theories stressing physiological arousal and those emphasising the neural underpinnings of cognitive appraisal.

Although still hotly debated many scientists would argue that 'hunger' is not an emotional state, but merely an internal sensation. To become an emotion, it is argued that the sensation of hunger must trigger cognitive appraisal of the situation that then elicits an emotional state. For example, 'anxiety' may be elicited if the prospect of getting food in the near future is unlikely because you are living in the wilderness and finding food is becoming increasingly difficult.

5.10.2.1 Pharmacological Treatments of Emotional Disorders and Their Relevance to Theories of Emotion

The importance of bodily feelings in emotional disorders is illustrated by considering **somatic anxiety and depression** and their treatment with drugs that target the gamma-aminobutyric acid (GABA), noradrenaline and serotonin systems. While the GABAergic benzodiazepines (e.g. diazepam) are successfully used to treat different types of anxiety, beta-adrenergic receptor blockers (e.g. propranolol) are effective specifically in treating 'somatic'

rather than 'psychic' forms of anxiety. Somatic anxiety results largely from bodily symptoms (e.g. palpitations, hyperventilation) as opposed to cases where anxiety results from external stressors ('psychic anxiety'). A study by Peter Tyrer used the Hamilton anxiety scale, subjective ratings and physiological measures, including pulse and respiratory rate, to compare the effects of placebo, diazepam and propranolol on groups of somatic and psychic anxious subjects (Tyrer and Lader, 1974). The results show that whereas diazepam is effective for treating both psychic and somatic anxiety, the beta blocker propranolol was effective only for treating somatic anxiety. Although psychic anxiety patients showed a greatly reduced pulse rate under propranolol, they reported no subjective reduction in their anxiety. Similar distinctions can also be seen after treatment with the selective serotonin reuptake inhibitors (SSRIs) – current-day common first-line treatments for both anxiety and depression. The SSRI paroxetine significantly outperformed placebo treatment in alleviating the psychological measures of depression and anxiety, but had little effect on the somatic symptoms (Schalet et al., 2016).

These clinical psychopharmacological data not only illustrate the fractionation of anxiety and depression into psychic (cognitive) and somatic components but also the importance of the cognitive interpretation of bodily feelings emphasised by Schachter. They also implicate separate neurobiological circuits in the expression of psychological versus somatic symptoms and emphasise the clinical importance of selecting the correct drug for a given symptom profile. Thus, SSRIs may be more beneficial for individuals with high measures of psychic symptoms, than those with a high somatic-symptom profile.

5.10.3 Aetiology of Disorders of Emotion

Many disorders of emotion, such as mood and anxiety disorders, have an onset during development, occurring before, during or post puberty (Kessler et al., 2005), which is strongly suggestive of developmental factors in the pathogenesis of these disorders. Adolescence is a particularly vulnerable period because the prefrontal cortex is showing its greatest maturational changes, which continue well on into early adulthood. Ultimately, developmental maturation of the brain is dependent upon an interaction between our genes and our childhood and adolescent experiences, and is highly sensitive to stress, either physical or psychological. Stress can impact on the endocrine system and the immune system, the results of which can have dramatic effects on the development of the neural circuits underlying cognition and emotion, increasing the likelihood of developing a mood or anxiety disorder (Heim and Binder, 2012). Stress can also influence our genome through epigenetic mechanisms, changes which may be passed on to subsequent generations. For a summary of all these influences see Figures 5.10.2 and 5.10.3. Many of these effects are now the focus of studies in adolescents, to identify those social and biological factors that make an individual more vulnerable to succumbing to stress-related disorders later in life, but also, conversely, those factors that can help protect an individual, making them more resilient. In parallel, studies of the effects of stress during development in animals are beginning to provide insight into the underlying molecular mechanisms (Kappeler and Meaney, 2010).

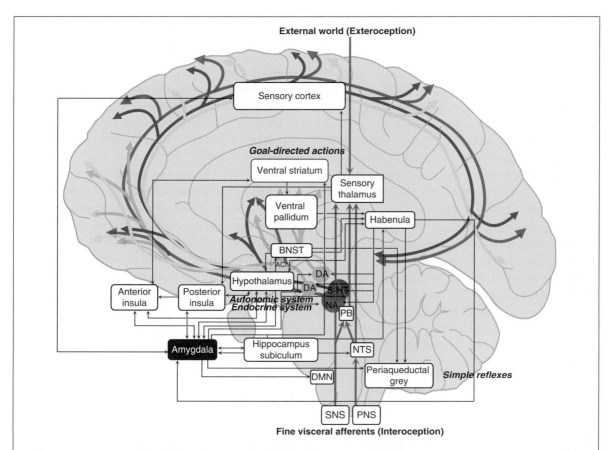

Figure 5.10.2 Subcortical processing of emotional information. Multiple subcortical structures in the brain contribute to the processing of emotional information and the responses that it generates. Many of these structures are part of the limbic system. These include medial temporal lobe structures such as the amygdala and anterior hippocampus, which are known to induce emotional responses via connections with structures including the hypothalamus, periaqueductal grey and deep mesencephalic nucleus (DMN), which regulate the endocrine and autonomic systems, and the ventral striatum, which coordinates goal-directed actions appropriate to emotional input. Modulation of neurotransmitter release across these regions, as well as in the cortex, affects processes such as arousal, attention and motivation. Together, this leads to behavioural and physiological changes such as freezing to a threatening stimulus or approaching a stimulus predicting reward, physiological responses including alterations in heart rate and respiration and ultimately subjective changes via projections to the association cortex. Importantly, the regulation of these responses is modulated by the individual's genetic variation and their historical experiences of the cognitive and physiological sequelae of stress. ACh, acetylcholine, yellow; BNST, bed nucleus of the stria terminalis; DA, dopamine, green; 5-HT, serotonin, orange; NA, noradrenaline, blue; NTS, nucleus tractus solitarius; PB, parabrachial nucleus; PNS, parasympathetic nervous system; SNS, sympathetic nervous system.

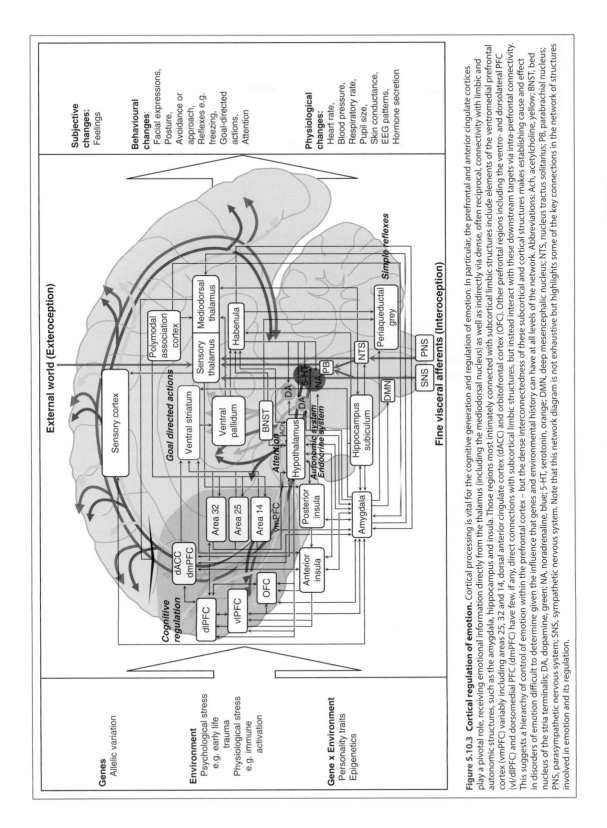

Figure 5.10.3 Cortical regulation of emotion. Cortical processing is vital for the cognitive generation and regulation of emotion. In particular, the prefrontal and anterior cingulate cortices play a pivotal role, receiving emotional information directly from the thalamus (including the mediodorsal nucleus) as well as indirectly via dense, often reciprocal, connectivity with limbic and autonomic structures, such as the amygdala, hippocampus and insula. Those regions most intimately connected with subcortical limbic structures include elements of the ventromedial prefrontal cortex (vmPFC) variably including areas 25, 32 and 14, dorsal anterior cingulate cortex (dACC) and orbitofrontal cortex (OFC). Other prefrontal regions including the ventro- or dorsolateral PFC (vl/dlPFC) and dorsomedial PFC (dmPFC) have few, if any, direct connections with subcortical limbic structures, but instead interact with these downstream targets via intra-prefrontal connectivity. This suggests a hierarchy of control of emotion within the prefrontal cortex – but the dense interconnectedness of these subcortical and cortical structures makes establishing cause and effect in disorders of emotion difficult to determine given the influence that genes and environmental history can have at all levels of the network. Abbreviations: Ach, acetylcholine, yellow; BNST, bed nucleus of the stria terminalis; DA, dopamine, green; NA, noradrenaline, blue; 5-HT, serotonin, orange; DMN, deep mesencephalic nucleus; NTS, nucleus tractus solitarius; PB, parabrachial nucleus; PNS, parasympathetic nervous system; SNS, sympathetic nervous system. Note that this network diagram is not exhaustive but highlights some of the key connections in the network of structures involved in emotion and its regulation.

5.10.4 Neuroanatomy of Emotion: A Focus on Subcortical Systems

Based upon a series of earlier discoveries by Broca ('*le grande lobe limbique*' or smell brain) and Papez (Papez's emotion circuit involving the hippocampus, hypothalamus and medial cortex), **Maclean** introduced the notion of the 'limbic system' mediating visceral functions and affective behaviours including feeding, defence, fighting and reproduction. The term 'limbic system' is still often used to refer to brain systems involved in emotions, but the structures comprising the limbic system have changed over the years, with additional structures being added and the relative importance of other structures, such as the hippocampus, being downplayed. We now know that the principal components of the neural circuit underpinning emotion are the hypothalamus, amygdala, orbitofrontal cortex, ventral striatum, cingulate cortex, insula, habenula and bed nucleus of the stria terminalis. While the hippocampus is primarily associated with the laying down of episodic memories, nevertheless, the anterior hippocampus (or ventral hippocampus in rodents) does appear to play a role in emotional processing. There is still an ongoing debate as to whether there is a common set of brain structures important for *all* emotional behaviour or whether different emotions, such as fear or disgust, use a different set of brain structures by virtue of the fact that different emotions evolved for different reasons.

The amygdala is buried in the anterior portion of the temporal lobes immediately anterior to the hippocampus. It is composed of a number of nuclei with distinct inputs and outputs, three of the most relevant being the central, basal and lateral nuclei. The amygdala plays an important role in learning about the emotional significance of stimuli in the environment and coordinating the expression of the physiological and behavioural responses that contribute to the induction of the emotional state. It is well placed to perform this function because it receives highly processed sensory information about stimuli in the outside world from all the unimodal association cortices (different regions of the association cortex that process information from just one modality, e.g. somatosensory or auditory) and also receives internal visceral signals from the periphery, informing it about the state of the body (Figure 5.10.2). In turn, the amygdala sends projections to the hypothalamus where it can control endocrine and autonomic responses, the brainstem where it can control autonomic and simple behavioural reflexes,

such as freezing, and the basal ganglia, orbitofrontal and cingulate cortices, where it can influence higher-order processing for controlling goal-directed actions. Rats with lesions to specific nuclei of the amygdala fail to acquire and express responses (called conditioned responses) to stimuli associated with threat, such as freezing and increases in heart rate to the presentation of a tone that the rat has learned predicts mild footshock. Similarly, the amygdala in humans has been shown to be important for the recognition of fearful faces and for developing conditioned responses to environmental stimuli that predict punishment. Damage to the amygdala, as occurs in Urbach–Wiethe disease and herpes simplex encephalitis, impairs fear recognition and development of conditioned responses. Moreover, functional MRI (fMRI) studies have shown that the amygdala is activated when presented with fearful faces (reviewed in LeDoux, 2007). More recently, the bed nucleus of the stria terminalis, which is intimately connected with the amygdala, has also been implicated in threat responses in humans and other animals, particularly in more uncertain contexts. Similar effects are seen with respect to rewarding stimuli. Rats and monkeys with damage to the amygdala fail to display positive arousal and acquire novel responses to stimuli in the environment associated with rewards such as sweet foods (Everitt et al., 2006). In humans, the amygdala is activated while we look for and select items from high-incentive restaurant menus (Arana et al., 2003).

5.10.5 Role of the Cortex and Cognition in the Generation and Regulation of Emotion

Ultimately, emotions are the product of activity across multiple networks (Figure 5.10.3). The amygdala can be activated by threats presented subliminally (not consciously perceived) and trigger physiological responses in the absence of feelings of fear. In contrast, conscious experience most likely arises from cortical processing, but this is the least well understood of the emotion circuitry. As already discussed, cognition, a product of cortical processing, is an integral part of the appraisal process for a given emotion, and emotions can have a profound influence on cognition (comprehensively reviewed in Joormann and Stanton, 2016). Moreover, cognition not only contributes to emotion generation but also emotion regulation. Emotion regulation is how emotions that are generated can be modulated. Regulation can occur relatively automatically, outside of the person's awareness, but it can also happen almost before the initial response has been generated, thus making it difficult to differentiate between emotion generation and regulation. Despite these issues there has been considerable progress in humans, characterising the different automatic and goal-directed strategies that influence emotional responding and the contribution of cognitive/executive mechanisms, all of which appear to involve the prefrontal cortex (Braunstein et al., 2017). Executive functions such as working memory, attentional set shifting (e.g. switching attention from one aspect of a stimulus, such as shape, to another, such as colour) and response inhibition have all been hypothesised to contribute to aspects of emotion regulation including cognitive reappraisal (reinterpreting the emotional significance of a stimulus), attentional disengagement (diverting attention away from a negative stimulus) and response suppression (suppressing outward observable emotional responses). The former two strategies are components of the range of cognitive and behavioural therapies that can be used to treat anxiety and mood disorders.

5.10.6 Neurobiological Insights into Emotional Disturbance from fMRI

Common findings emerging from an extensive neuro-imaging literature on patients with mood, anxiety and borderline personality disorders, are changes in grey matter density and, in particular, altered activity across a network of regions including the amygdala, insula, hippocampus, anterior cingulate, orbitofrontal and dorsolateral prefrontal cortices (for review of depression see Pizzagalli and Roberts, 2022). Hyperactivity of the amygdala and insula during task performance, as well as at rest, suggests that these changes may often act as a final common pathway in these disorders (Etkin and Wager, 2007). This is frequently accompanied by reduced activity in the rostral and subgenual anterior cingulate cortex and more extensively throughout the ventromedial prefrontal cortex (for review see Shin and Liberzon, 2010) and lateral prefrontal cortex. In contrast, in treatment-resistant depressed subjects, overactivity has been reported in the ventromedial prefrontal cortex, which is reduced following eventual successful treatment. Overactivity has also been reported in the dorsal anterior cingulate and dorsomedial prefrontal cortices and shown to be correlated with autonomic arousal and subjective anxiety.

Increasingly, investigations are focusing on functional networks as distinct from independent nodes (brain regions). Functional networks are collections of brain structures whose activity increases and/or decreases synchronously both at rest and during performance of cognitive and emotional tasks. It is hypothesised that the connectivity between these brain structures at rest may reflect the history of their correlated activity during goal-directed performance. Ultimately, cognitive and emotional behaviours emerge from the integration of activity across these networks. In mood and anxiety disorders, altered activity within and between salience, attentional and executive networks is found not only in adults but also in adolescents, with evidence that alterations within some of these networks may be predisposing. Many imaging studies are now adopting a transdiagnostic approach, determining changes in activity associated with a particular symptom, such as anxiety or anhedonia, across diagnoses. This will address the question, for example, as to whether there is a common set of circuit changes associated with anhedonia, regardless of whether the patient has schizophrenia, depression or Parkinson's disease. However, for this to be successful, a better characterisation of the symptom, per se, is needed as, for example, anhedonia could be a loss of pleasure at the level of consumption (drinking a glass of red wine), anticipation (thinking about that glass of red wine at the end of the day) or motivation (willingness to travel across town for that glass of red wine).

Thus, many questions are left unanswered. Which of these alterations in activity are directly causing the symptoms and which are compensatory? How do these alterations contribute to the different aspects of a symptom, such as the negative bias, failure to disengage from salient negative stimuli and enhanced reactivity to uncertainty which are associated with disorders of anxiety? Moreover, how do alterations in activity in one node of a network impact on activity in the rest of the network, or across networks, and which of these nodes have the greatest impact? It is difficult to address many of these questions without studying the effects of independent manipulations of these brain regions in animals and determining not only their effect on the range of physiological and behavioural responses associated with threat and reward, and their regulation, but also on activity across brain networks.

5.10.7 What Is Hampering Progress in Developing New Effective Treatments?

Despite the ever more sophisticated technology available to image the brains of patients and the advent of viral mediated techniques to identify brain circuits controlling behaviour in animals there has been a dearth of new treatment strategies. There are a number of factors that have slowed down progress. First, **characterisation of the disorders**. Until recently the focus has been on finding treatments for disorders per se, which has proven difficult, especially since in depression, for example, two patients can be diagnosed with the same disorder but have no overlapping symptoms. Even if they do have the same symptoms, the symptoms themselves are poorly characterised, often determined on the basis of a psychiatric consultation or on answers to questionnaires. Thus, the same symptom, for instance anxiety, may arise from a variety of distinct psychological/neurobiological causes. Second, the **correlational nature of fMRI**. This has made it difficult to determine whether observed changes in patients are causal or compensatory and, specifically, which symptoms they are related to. Third, a **lack of focus of animal studies on the cortical contribution to processing of threat and reward**, and fourth, **the reliance of such studies on a few simple laboratory tests** to measure defensive or reward-driven responses, which cannot dissect out the higher-order contributions of cortical processing (reviewed in Roberts, 2020). Finally, it is important to recognise that there are **marked differences in the overall cortical organisation between rodents and humans**, in particular the prefrontal cortex and anterior cingulate cortex. In contrast, the organisation of these frontal regions in non-human primates appears much more similar to that of humans, making the potential for translation that much more likely. Thus, studies in non-human primates are essential to bridge the current translational gap between humans and rodents and will play a pivotal role in both forward translation into the clinic but also back translation to rodents, in order to facilitate the development of a new generation of treatment strategies.

Conclusions and Outstanding Questions

This brief summary of the current state of our understanding of emotion regulation and dysregulation will hopefully have made clear the importance of an interdisciplinary approach to that understanding. Neurobiological investigations of emotional behaviour and cognition in animals provide a critical link to functional neuroimaging investigations in humans. Our ability to understand psychological processes at a neural level is increasing and with this should come further progress in our ability to diagnose and to effectively treat neuropsychiatric disorders.

Outstanding Questions

- What are the precise psychological mechanisms that underlie the contribution of the distinct regions of the prefrontal and anterior cingulate cortices to the processing of threat and reward in animals and how do they relate to strategies of cognitive regulation of emotion in humans?

- What is the nature of the hierarchical interactions within the prefrontal and anterior cingulate cortices in the regulation of threat and reward processing? For example, dorsolateral and ventrolateral prefrontal regions send efferents to ventromedial prefrontal regions, which in turn have direct access to the amygdala. How do these systems interact in the control of emotion?

- Are different neural circuits generating cognition and emotion differentially vulnerable to stress at different stages of development and, if so, how does that influence the somatic and psychological symptoms of the disorder that develops?

- How does psychological and/or physical stress impact on the body and brain during development to leave a person vulnerable to developing mental health problems later in life?

- Upon what neural circuits and neurochemical systems do existing therapies act to have their efficacious action?

Answers to these questions will help us to develop new therapies and to target existing therapies more effectively as we begin to fractionate out the distinct underlying causes of mood and anxiety disorders in individual patients.

REFERENCES

Arana FS, Parkinson JA, Hinton E et al. (2003). Dissociable contributions of the human amygdala and orbitofrontal cortex to incentive motivation and goal selection. *J Neurosci* 23: 9632–9638.

Braunstein LM, Gross JJ, Ochsner KN (2017). Explicit and implicit emotion regulation: a multi-level framework. *Soc Cogn Affect Neurosci* 12: 1545–1557.

Craig AD (2002). How do you feel? Interoception: the sense of the physiological condition of the body. *Nat Rev Neurosci* 3: 655–666.

Critchley HD, Wiens S, Rotshtein P, Ohman A, Dolan RJ (2004). Neural systems supporting interoceptive awareness. *Nat Neurosci* 7: 189–195.

Etkin A, Wager TD (2007). Functional neuroimaging of anxiety: a meta-analysis of emotional processing in PTSD, social anxiety disorder, and specific phobia. *Am J Psychiatry* 164: 1476–1488.

Everitt BJ, Cardinal RN, Parkinson JA, Robbins TW (2006). Appetitive behavior. *Ann NY Acad Sci* 985: 233–250.

Heim C, Binder EB (2012). Current research trends in early life stress and depression: review of human studies on sensitive periods, gene–environment interactions, and epigenetics. *Exp Neurol* 233: 102–111.

Hohmann GW (1996). Some effects of spinal cord lesions on experienced emotional feelings. *Psychophysiology* 3: 143–156.

James W (1884). What is an emotion? *Mind* 9: 188–205.

Joormann J, Stanton CH (2016). Examining emotion regulation in depression: a review and future directions. *Behav Res Ther* 86: 35–49.

Kappeler L, Meaney MJ (2010). Epigenetics and parental effects. *BioEssays* 32: 818–827.

Kessler RC, Berglund P, Demler O et al. (2005). Lifetime prevalence and age-of-onset distributions of DSM-IV disorders in the National Comorbidity Survey Replication. *Arch Gen Psychiatry* 62: 593.

LeDoux J (2007). The amygdala. *Curr Biol* 17: R868–R874.

LeDoux J (2015). *Anxious*. Oneworld Publications.

Pizzagalli DA, Roberts AC (2022). Prefrontal cortex and depression. *Neuropsychopharmacology* 47: 225–246.

Roberts AC (2020). Prefrontal regulation of threat-elicited behaviors: a pathway to translation. *Annu Rev Psychol* 71: 357–387.

Rolls ET (2013). *Emotion and Decision-making Explained*. Oxford University Press.

Schachter S, Singer J (1962). Cognitive, social, and physiological determinants of emotional state. *Psychol Rev* 69: 379–399.

Schalet BD, Tang TZ, DeRubeis RJ et al. (2016). Specific pharmacological effects of paroxetine comprise psychological but not somatic symptoms of depression. *PLoS One* 11: e0159647.

Shin LM, Liberzon I (2010). The neurocircuitry of fear, stress, and anxiety disorders. *Neuropsychopharmacology* 35: 169–191.

Tyrer PJ, Lader MH (1974). Response to propranolol and diazepam in somatic and psychic anxiety. *BMJ* 2: 14–16.

National Neuroscience Curriculum Initiative online resources

This "stuff" is really cool: Maria Pico-Perez, *"Feedback For Lisa"* on treating emotional *regulation with neurofeedback*

John D. Mollon

5.11 Perception

OVERVIEW

Many psychiatric conditions are characterised by hallucinations or by subtler alterations in perception [1–3]. To understand such symptoms, it is useful to have some understanding of normal perception. What are the intervening processes between an image falling on our retina and our recognition of a familiar face in a complex scene? Or between the variations in air pressure reaching our cochlea and our recognition of the specific words that are being spoken – as well as our recognition that they are being spoken by our youngest cousin?

5.11.1 Feature Analysis

5.11.1.1 The Visual System

The first stage in the remarkable train of processes involved in perception (and the best understood) is the extraction of particular features from the physical stimulus. The retina, for example, does not transmit a passive image to the brain, pixel by pixel. Within the retina, there are at least 19 different types of ganglion cell, which act as 'pre-processors', extracting different attributes from the ever-shifting pattern of light that falls on the rods and cones – attributes such as lightness, colour, temporal change, spatial detail, fine and coarse texture, and motion [4, 5]. The different types of ganglion cell are distinguished by their morphologies, by their immuno-chemistry (i.e. the proteins they express), by the strata of the retina in which their dendritic fields extend – and by the different sites within the visual brain to which their reports are delivered.

The main destination of signals from the retina (though certainly not the only one) is the primary visual cortex, the 'striate' cortex, which lies at the very back of the brain, in the occipital lobe. Here, the specialisations of individual neurons for particular features are maintained, but a new type of tuning famously emerges: many neurons are selective for edges of a particular orientation, and often this preference is combined with tuning for other attributes, such as colour or direction of motion [5–7]. Particular regions of 'pre-striate cortex' – the parts of the occipital lobe anterior to the primary visual cortex – appear to be specialised for the analysis of particular attributes, such as motion or colour or the disparities between the images on the retinas of the two eyes that give rise to stereoscopic perception of depth.

The cortical neurons that detect a particular visual feature (e.g. colour, orientation) typically have lateral, and mutually inhibitory, connections with nearby neurons that detect the same feature in adjacent areas of the field – an arrangement that is thought to allow our perceptual system to adjust to the current average value of a given attribute and to emphasise local departures from that average. Sometimes, however, this useful adjustment gives rise to the class of illusions called 'simultaneous contrast'. An example is given in Figure 5.11.1.

Another class of perceptual distortions arises from temporary miscalibrations in the arrays of feature-detecting neurons [7, 9]. For example, if we look fixedly for some minutes at a waterfall or at a moving flow of traffic, then – for a few moments afterwards – stationary objects may appear to move in the opposite direction. Such 'negative motion after-effects' are thought to arise from reductions in the sensitivity of a selective subset of the directionally selective neurons that are present at early stages of the visual system.

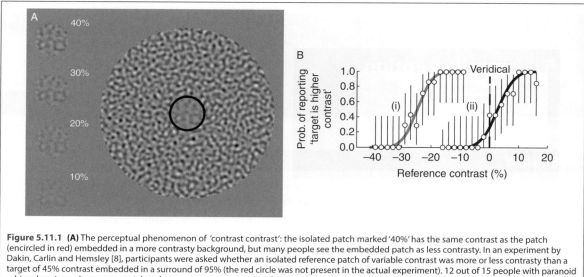

Figure 5.11.1 (A) The perceptual phenomenon of 'contrast contrast': the isolated patch marked '40%' has the same contrast as the patch (encircled in red) embedded in a more contrasty background, but many people see the embedded patch as less contrasty. In an experiment by Dakin, Carlin and Hemsley [8], participants were asked whether an isolated reference patch of variable contrast was more or less contrasty than a target of 45% contrast embedded in a surround of 95% (the red circle was not present in the actual experiment). 12 out of 15 people with paranoid schizophrenia made average matches that were more accurate (i.e. they experienced a weaker illusion) than the most accurate non-clinical control person. **(B)** The graph shows the probability of reporting that the embedded patch was more contrasty as a function of the actual contrast of the reference patch (at zero on the x-axis, the match would be veridical). The green (more leftward) curve is for a typical non-clinical control, and the red (rightward) curve is for typical participant with schizophrenia. Dakin and his colleagues suggest that in schizophrenia there may be an impairment of the normal processes that adjust sensitivity to contrast according to the average current level. Adapted from Dakin, Carlin and Hemsley [8].

Pathologies may affect one visual attribute more than another. Indeed, the first suggestion that the optic nerve might contain different fibres for different attributes came from the former Surgeon to the Confederate Army J. J. Chisholm, who observed in 1869 that spatial vision recovered before colour vision in a case of optic neuritis [10]. Conversely, colour recognition may be relatively preserved in cases where carbon monoxide poisoning leads to 'visual form agnosia', an inability to recognise objects by their shape [11].

5.11.1.2 The Auditory System

Neurons specific for particular features of the stimulus are also found in the auditory system. The individual fibres that leave the cochlea of the ear are tuned just to particular frequencies of sound, but at subsequent stages (including the cochlear nucleus, the inferior colliculus and the auditory cortex; Figure 5.11.2A) there are, for example, neurons that respond to a particular direction of change of frequency – to a rising pitch or to a falling one [12]. The response of such a cell is illustrated in Figure 5.11.2B. A change in the frequency of sound can be seen as analogous to motion across the visual field: in the one case there is motion along the basilar membrane of the ear's

cochlea and in the other there is motion across the retina. So is there an auditory analogue of the negative motion after-effect discussed above? Indeed there is: if listeners are exposed to a band of frequencies that repeatedly increase in a sawtooth fashion, then afterwards a steady sound appears to fall in pitch [13].

5.11.1.3 Beyond Feature Analysis

In sum, at early stages of our sensory systems there are many parallel neural channels, often morphologically or anatomically distinct, that identify particular features of the external stimulus. But there is much more to our perception than this. First, there is the large matter of 'perceptual organisation'. The brain must parse the visual or auditory scene into distinct objects (e.g. faces, words), deciding what elements of the scene belong together, distinguishing figure from ground and estimating the three-dimensional arrangement of the scene. Second, the *identity* of each object must be recognised. In addition, corrections must be made to the estimated size, shape, colour, loudness, etc. of objects according to the conditions of viewing or listening – a process often termed 'perceptual constancy'. These several processes, described in the sections that follow, are not independent

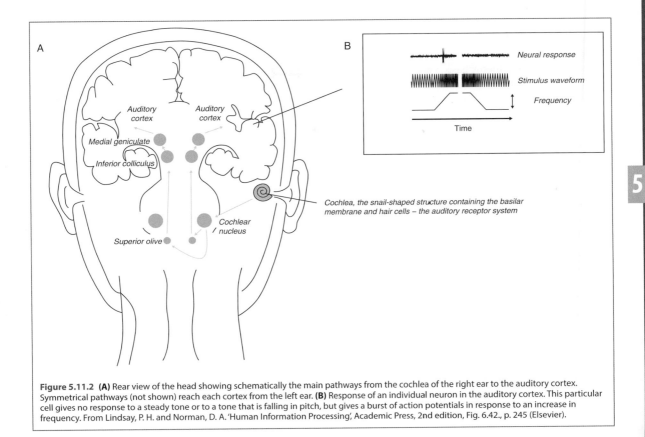

Figure 5.11.2 **(A)** Rear view of the head showing schematically the main pathways from the cochlea of the right ear to the auditory cortex. Symmetrical pathways (not shown) reach each cortex from the left ear. **(B)** Response of an individual neuron in the auditory cortex. This particular cell gives no response to a steady tone or to a tone that is falling in pitch, but gives a burst of action potentials in response to an increase in frequency. From Lindsay, P. H. and Norman, D. A. 'Human Information Processing', Academic Press, 2nd edition, Fig. 6.42., p. 245 (Elsevier).

and successive. For example, some independent cue or some sudden recollection may cause a switch in our identification of an ambiguous object; and then our entire three-dimensional interpretation of the scene may change. What we initially perceived as an object may be reinterpreted as a shadow, and then its apparent colour may change. If a sound is reinterpreted as coming from a nearby insect rather than from distant farm machinery, its apparent loudness may change.

5.11.2 Perceptual Organisation

In the first half of the twentieth century, the Gestalt psychologists identified several rules that describe how the elements of a visual or auditory scene will be perceptually organised, that is, how the elements will be grouped to form segregated objects [14]:

(1) **Proximity in space**. Our ability to localise sounds is valuable not only in itself, but also because it allows the segregation of one auditory stream from another. For example, it allows us to follow one source of speech out of several at a busy drinks party (and not necessarily the person we are nominally listening to!). Similarly, in binocular stereo vision, elements that lie in different planes are displaced relative to one another on the two retinas and so emerge as distinct objects at different depths – allowing us to penetrate camouflage that defeats the monocular eye.

(2) **Similarity**. The elements in an auditory or visual scene tend to be grouped, and perceived as one object or sound source, if they are similar in some quality. In vision, this might be similarity in size, in colour, in orientation of contour, in texture or in shape. In hearing, similarity of frequency in successive tones determines whether a sequence will be heard as two streams or one.

(3) **'Common fate'**. If a subset of elements in the scene change in a correlated way, they tend to be grouped. Thus, elements in a visual scene that move together are grouped together and are segregated from a background that is static or is moving in a

different way. For example, 'motion parallax' allows us to break camouflage by moving our head: elements in different planes move relative to one another (the geometric basis is formally the same as for as binocular stereo vision; see above). In hearing, shared onset times, or shared fluctuation in amplitude, or shared direction of change of frequency promote grouping of different components [14]. Note that the 'law of common fate' could often be taken as a special case of the law of similarity (2) – since nowadays we know that the visual and auditory systems contain detectors for dynamic features of the stimulus, such as direction of movement or direction of change of pitch (see above and Figure 5.11.2B).

(4) **Good continuation**. If a subset of elements in an auditory or visual scene form a simple pattern (e.g. if the elements in a visual scene fall on a straight line or a smooth curve), they tend to be perceived as one object. In hearing, smooth trajectories of frequency (glides) often lead to grouping.

It is often held that the universality of these rules implies that they are innate, inbuilt in our perceptual systems. However, this does not necessarily follow: the rules of organisation reflect the statistical properties of the physical world that we all share. Thus it is logically possible that the rules are learnt.

5.11.3 The Identification of Objects

What neural processes allow us to identify a stimulus as a member of the generic class of chairs or of faces or of voices? And do similar processes allow us to identify our favourite chair or the face or voice of our lover?

Many neuroscientists, implicitly or explicitly, subscribe to the doctrine of 'gnostic units', the hypothesis that words, objects, faces, voices are represented in the brain by the activity of individual neurons [14]. The doctrine was explicit in the writings of the eighteenth-century theorist Charles Bonnet [15], and was developed in the twentieth century by Jerzy Konorski [16] and by Horace Barlow [17]. To build a gnostic unit, outputs of feature detectors (see above) at earlier levels might be connected to ever-more specific neurons at successive levels, giving, at the apex of the pyramid, a 'grandmother cell', a cell that responds only when your grandmother is present. Closely linked to this hypothesis is the idea that such cells constitute the 'engram', the (still elusive) physical basis of memory (see Section 5.14).

The problem with the gnostic unit hypothesis is that it implies that the information is frozen in place. In order to distribute to other parts of the brain the information that your grandmother is present, many dedicated fibres would be required, adding to the bulk of the brain's white matter. A conventional alternative is 'ensemble coding', where a given object is represented by the pattern of activity in a population of neurons [14]; but then there is the problem of how that pattern is identified and how the information is distributed to other sites in the brain. What is needed is an abstract representation that can move freely over a 'cerebral bus', where the same neurons carry different information at different times, rather than being dedicated to a particular object or concept [18].

5.11.4 The Influence of Context and Experience: Illusions and Hallucinations

Consider the two spoken phrases 'I scream, I yell' and 'ice cream sundae'. The initial acoustic sequences are identical (or, at any rate, they could be made so in a computer-generated stimulus). Yet the after-coming information changes the way that we segment the stimulus (Subsection 5.11.2 above) and changes the words that we hear. In everyday life, in constructing our percepts, we unconsciously draw both on the current context and on our long experience of the physical and social worlds. And often the physical input is the minor contributor to our internal reconstruction of a spoken message or of a three-dimensional scene. Most of the time, our brain gets it right and we are blissfully unaware of the many unconscious assumptions that are being made. But occasionally our expectations mislead us, and we are suddenly aware of an illusion that arises from our mistaken interpretation of the visual or auditory input [19]. If our personal history is different from that of most people, we may perceive malevolence in a facial expression, or in spoken words, that seem neutral to others [3].

When the external contribution to visual analysis is badly degraded (e.g. in macular degeneration or in optic nerve disease) and central visual processes are unconstrained by the input, then vivid hallucinations of people, animals or objects may occur in the absence of psychosis or of cognitive impairment. Charles Bonnet, who first described this rare syndrome in his own grandfather [15], held that the hallucinations reflected activity in the same fibres in the brain that were normally dedicated to the corresponding percepts (see above, Subsection 5.11.3). Bonnet assures us that his grandfather was entertained by the hallucinations, recognising them to be no more than that: 'His brain is a theatre whose machines perform scenes that surprise the spectator all the more in that they are quite unforeseen'.

Conclusions and Outstanding Questions

The core processes of perception across the different senses include feature analysis, perceptual organisation and object recognition. These processes are highly interactive, rather than independent and successive. Our resulting percept of the outside world depends as much on context and on our experience as on the current input from our eyes and ears. Illusions and hallucinations may arise from errors at different stages of perceptual analysis, but what is remarkable is how efficiently our senses serve most of us most of the time.

Outstanding Questions

- What neural processes underlie the perceptual organisation of visual and auditory scenes?
- Are words, faces, objects and concepts represented in the brain by the activity of single neurons?
- In what format is information about perceptual objects transmitted to other parts of the brain?
- How are the normal processes of perception hijacked to generate hallucinations?

5

REFERENCES

1. Silverstein S, Keane BP, Blake R et al. (2015). Vision in schizophrenia: why it matters. *Front Psychol* 6: 41.

2. Dakin S, Frith U (2005). Vagaries of visual perception in autism. *Neuron* 48: 497–507.

3. Fletcher P (2021). Visions. In Fabian A, Gibson J, Sheppard M, Weyland S (eds.), *Vision*. Cambridge University Press.

4. Grunert U, Martin PR (2021). Morphology, molecular characterization, and connections of ganglion cells in primate retina. *Annu Rev Vis Sci* 7: 73–103.

5. Masland R (2020). *We Know It When We See It: What the Neurobiology of Vision Tells Us about How We Think*. Basic Books.

6. Snowden R, Thompson P, Troscianko T (2012). *Basic Vision: An Introduction to Visual Perception*, 2nd ed. Oxford University Press.

7. Mollon JD (1977). Neural analysis. In von Fieandt K, Moustgaard IK (eds.), *The Perceptual World*. Academic Press, pp. 71–97.

8. Dakin S, Carlin P, Hemsley D (2005). Weak suppression of visual context in chronic schizophrenia. *Curr Biol* 15: R822–R824.

9. Mollon JD (1974). After-effects and the brain. *New Scientist* 61: 479–482.

10. Chisholm JJ (1869). Colour blindness, an effect of neuritis. *Ophthalmic Hospital Reports*, 214–215.

11. Milner AD, Perrett DI, Johnston RS et al. (1991). Perception and action in 'visual form agnosia'. *Brain* 114 (Pt 1B): 405–428.

12. Paraouty N, Stasiak A, Lorenzi C, Varnet L, Winter IM (2018). Dual coding of frequency modulation in the ventral cochlear nucleus. *J Neurosci* 38: 4123–4137.

13. Shu ZJ, Swindale NV, Cynader MS (1993). Spectral motion produces an auditory after-effect. *Nature* 364: 721–723.

14. Bizley JK, Cohen YE (2013). The what, where and how of auditory-object perception. *Nat Rev Neurosci* 14: 693–707.

15. Bonnet C (1769). *Essai Analytique sur les Facultés de l'Ame*, Volume 2, 2nd ed, Cl. Philibert.

16. Konorski J (1967). Some new ideas concerning the physiological mechanisms of perception. *Acta Neurobiol Exp* 27: 147–161.

17. Barlow HB (1972). Single units and sensation: a neuron doctrine for perceptual psychology? *Perception* 1: 371–394.

18. Danilova MV, Takahashi C, Mollon JD (2020). How does the human visual system compare the speeds of spatially separated objects? *PLoS One* 15: e0231959.

19. Gregory RL (1973). The confounded eye. In Gregory RL Gombrich EH (eds.), *Illusion in Nature and Art*. Duckworth, pp. 49–95.

National Neuroscience Curriculum Initiative online resources

This "stuff" is really cool: Halide Bilge Turkozer, *"Windows to The Soul" on visual. perception and psychosis*

Trevor W. Robbins and
Barbara J. Sahakian

OVERVIEW

Attention is a key cognitive domain and without it we could not learn. Furthermore, getting distracted and losing the focus of our attention at critical times, such as attending to our mobile phones when a text arrives rather than attending to oncoming traffic in a busy street, could be life-threatening. Several psychiatric symptoms, across a range of mental health disorders, appear to involve problems in the regulation of attention.

5.12.1 What Is Attention?

Psychologists consider attention to be a construct that connotes an individual's active interaction with their environment, intervening between sensory input and perception to memory and higher-order cognition [1, 2]. Attention has different forms including selective attention (i.e. the ability to process one stimulus while ignoring other distractors) and sustained attention (i.e. the ability to monitor sensory input over prolonged periods despite fatigue). Vigilance is a related term, referring to the ability to maintain attention in order to detect rare target signals, for example stimuli in the environment such as potholes in the road or children running into the street. Vigilant attention is also engaged when monitoring threat and may be exacerbated in patients with anxiety. These brief definitions cover a range of tasks and situations. Thus, selective attention can be restricted to a single sensory modality, such as vision or hearing, or it can be focused onto particular features of a stimulus, such as its spatial position or colour, rather than its shape.

Bottom-up attention (sometimes called 'exogenous') is attracted by the sensory physical salience of a stimulus – that is, its intensity or prominence (e.g. its brightness or loudness). Exogenous attention can also be recruited by the motivational importance of a presented stimulus – that is, whether it is important for achieving one's goals. Such attention often appears to be automatic and is sometimes unconscious or implicit. For example,

the startle response to a loud stimulus can be reduced by presenting a much quieter stimulus (below the level of conscious detection) just before it (so-called pre-pulse inhibition). In contrast, top-down (or 'endogenous') attention is generally triggered by the absence of a stimulus such as a goal-object which is being searched for, like a lost mobile phone. The control of divided attention (important for multi-tasking) is also an important function of 'top-down' executive attentional processes. The focus and efficiency of attention often interacts with motivational and arousal states of the individual; obviously, inattention is a common consequence of drowsiness.

5.12.2 ADHD as a Prototypical Syndrome of Attentional Impairment

These different forms of attention and their interactions with other states are mediated by defined neural networks, impairments in which lead to numerous deficits, often present in a variety of psychiatric disorders including schizophrenia, depression and anxiety, but notably in both child and adult attention deficit hyperactivity disorder (ADHD). According to the American Psychiatric Association's *Diagnostic and Statistical Manual of Mental Disorders* (DSM-5), ADHD is characterised by a persistent pattern of inattention and/or hyperactivity that interferes with functioning or development [3]. The attentional impairments include deficits in both sustained and selective attention that are especially prominent in a so-called 'inattention' subgroup phenotype [4, 5]. These symptoms lead to functional impairments in everyday situations of poor attention to school work, difficulties in listening to to instructions even when given personally, distractibility, and more general problems of behavioural organisation, leading to impairments in working memory and planning [6].

5.12.3 Measurement of Attention

In the laboratory, attention is measured by a number of tasks [1]. Selective attention was most famously measured using the dichotic listening test, whereby subjects are required to shadow or repeat aloud the speech input from one auditory channel, while ignoring the other. When a significant stimulus such as your own name is suddenly introduced into the unattended channel you attend to it immediately. The flanker task explicitly requires the subject to ignore peripherally presented distractors. The Cambridge Neuropsychological Test Automated Battery (CANTAB) Intra–Extra Dimensional (ID/ED) Test (www.cambridgecognition.com/intra-extra-dimensional-set-shift-ied/) of extra-dimensional set shifting can be considered as a test of selective attention, requiring the subject to respond to one stimulus feature predicting reward and then to switch to another, previously irrelevant, stimulus feature when the feedback changes – thus exhibiting cognitive flexibility.

Sustained attention is usually measured by a so-called continuous performance task (CPT), in which target stimuli, often amongst distractors, have to be detected over a protracted period. Conner's CPT has been frequently employed to investigate ADHD. A related test is the CANTAB rapid visual information processing (RVIP) task where subjects have to detect target sequences of digits in a continuous stream presented at a rate of about 100 per minute [4]. In such tests, it is common to employ parameters derived from signal detection theory (see [1, 2] for more details):

- d' (pronounced 'd-prime') captures discriminability – how good or bad your ability is at detecting a target stimulus from other unimportant non-target stimuli (e.g. distractors)
- 'beta' measures overall motivational bias (such as the general tendency to respond to any stimulus whether target or non-target)

The effects of different psychiatric conditions or behavioural states on attention can then be captured by measuring how they affect these signal detection measures (see [1, 2] for more details).

Such tasks are used not only to help diagnose disorders and define impairments that need remediation, but also to test for efficacy of potential, often pharmacological, treatments. In the case of ADHD, there are efficacious medications including d-amphetamine (Adderall) or methylphenidate (Ritalin), which may also have specific effects to improve attention. These stimulant drugs enhance the activity of the central dopamine and noradrenaline neurotransmitter systems by a variety of mechanisms. While it is still not entirely clear which of the various drug actions is most responsible for the therapeutic (including attentional) benefits of these drugs, human and experimental animal research indicates that both dopamine and noradrenaline play modulatory roles by affecting the arousal and motivational states of forebrain attentional networks [7].

5.12.4 Neural Basis of Attention

Converging evidence from electrophysiological recording in non-human primates, studies with experimental animals and human neuroimaging using functional MRI (fMRI) together with EEG, as well as observations of brain-damaged patients, has helped to define several of the neural networks underlying the different forms of attention (see Figures 5.12.1 and 5.12.2). A seminal paper by Petersen and Posner [8] identified three main systems;

(1) A system mediating 'alerting': neurotransmitter projections from the brainstem and midbrain (including the dopaminergic, noradrenergic, serotoninergic and cholinergic systems) to the forebrain are hypothesised to have an especially profound effect on the right cerebral hemisphere and are implicated in tasks measuring sustained attention.

(2) Visual attention orientation can involve overt eye movements or can be uncoupled from eye movements, as in 'covert' attention to external cues (i.e. exogenous attention). This involves structures in the posterior cortex, especially regions of the parietal cortex such as in the lateral intraparietal cortex, as well as subcortical elements such as the thalamic pulvinar and the superior colliculus.

(3) 'Executive' (or endogenous) attention is when attention is governed by instructions, rules and motivational goals. This system is centred on the anterior cingulate and prefrontal cortices.

Subsequent work, mainly based on human neuroimaging and primate electrophysiology, has divided the neural system of attention into dorsal and ventral attentional networks. The dorsal network includes the dorsal frontoparietal cortex, premotor cortex and the frontal eye fields. Corbetta and colleagues [9] have proposed that the dorsal network specifically mediates top-down endogenous orienting to specific stimulus features in space.

Important nodes of the ventral network are the right lateralised temporoparietal lobe junction and right ventral prefrontal cortex (inferior frontal gyrus). Damage to the temporoparietal lobe junction in neurological cases or its experimental inactivation by transcranial magnetic stimulation causes a dramatic sensory neglect of stimuli in contralateral space. On the basis of functional neuroimaging evidence, Corbetta and colleagues [9] proposed that the ventral network mediates exogenous orienting, especially to stimulus targets in unexpected locations or to abrupt changes in stimuli or phases of tasks. However, it has also been suggested that the ventral attentional network has more complex roles than merely attentional orienting [10]. Furthermore, the temporoparietal lobe junction is an important area for social cognition, and therefore attention to social and emotional stimuli is likely to be of particular salience. The two attentional networks are coordinated by hitherto unknown mechanisms. Attention to different sensory modalities is mediated by similar regions and there is an important synergy of these systems to provide effective integration of attention across the different senses [11].

More recent work on the attentional systems in the anterior cortex has suggested the possibility of further network differentiation. Thus, there is a general executive network comprising lateral frontoparietal regions, which contrasts with a so-called default-mode network (DMN), which includes the medial prefrontal cortex and other cortical structures such as the posterior cingulate cortex and precuneus. The DMN is inactive in response to external stimuli and tasks, and most active when conscious attention is being directed to internal mental states [12]. The precise functions of the DMN, however, are controversial and recently a more central role for the DMN in higher cognitive processing has been proposed [13].

5.12.5 Mechanisms of Attentional Deficits in ADHD

5.12.5.1 Structural Imaging

There is substantial evidence of structural damage in the attentional networks shown in Figures 5.12.1 and 5.12.2 in child and adolescent ADHD, with rather less evidence available for adult ADHD [14–16]. Findings include grey matter loss in the inferior parietal lobule, anterior cingulate cortex and lateral prefrontal cortex (see Section 4.4 for frontal neuroanatomy). White matter abnormalities are found in the cingulum bundle and inferior and superior longitudinal fasciculi, which connect anterior and posterior cortical structures (see Section 4.5 for white matter tract anatomy). It should be noted that there are also significant reductions of volume in the basal ganglia

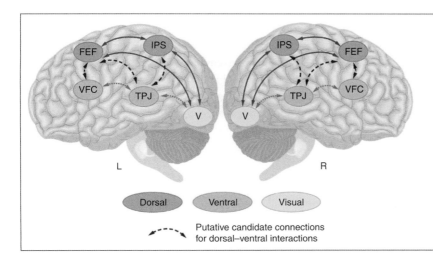

Figure 5.12.1 Schematic illustration of the components of the dorsal (blue) and ventral (orange) attention system in the human brain. Whereas there is evidence for a bilateral organisation of the dorsal system, the ventral system might be more lateralised to the right hemisphere, although this assumption is challenged by recent neuroimaging data. Putative intra- and internetwork connections are exemplarily depicted by bidirectional arrows. Interhemispheric connections between homologous areas are not shown. FEF, frontal eye fields; IPS, intraparietal sulcus; VFC, ventral frontal cortex; TPJ, temporoparietal junction; V, visual cortex.

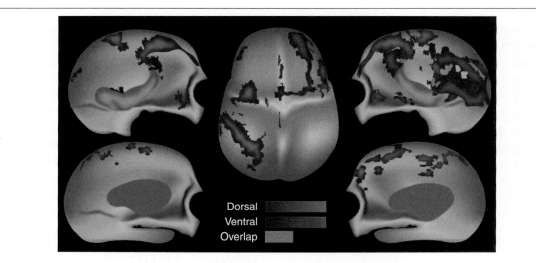

Figure 5.12.2 Anatomical basis of the dorsal and ventral attention systems and the overlap between them as shown by functional MRI. Voxels (three-dimensional pixels) in the dorsal system (blue scale) were significantly correlated ($p < 0.01$) with both the intraparietal sulcus and frontal eye field regions in all three resting-state conditions (fixation, eyes open and eyes closed). Voxels in the ventral system (red scale) were significantly correlated with both the temporoparietal junction and ventral frontal cortex regions in all three resting-state conditions. Voxels significantly correlated with all four regions in all three conditions are shown in orange. Data are displayed on the lateral and medial surfaces of the left hemisphere (left), the dorsal surface (centre), and the lateral and medial surfaces of the right hemisphere (right).

and the cerebellum, which are likely important for the behavioural symptoms of ADHD, but their precise roles in attentional function, although probable in terms of anatomical connectivity with the cortical structures of the attentional networks, remains fully to be elucidated.

In adult ADHD patients, neuroanatomical abnormalities have been found in grey matter volume in the right inferior frontal gyrus and white matter of the inferior longitudinal fasciculus. These abnormalities were also present in patients' first-degree relatives, who also showed deficits in the CANTAB RVIP test of sustained attention, suggesting a neurocognitive endophenotype for ADHD [4], showing a greater prevalence in unaffected relatives of patients than in the general population. Endophenotypes are quantitative biological traits present in the unaffected relatives of patients that are assumed to be closer to heritable factors (i.e. gene expression) than the clinical presentation per se. Such traits may thus indicate a possible neurobehavioural source of some of the symptoms expressed in ADHD.

5.12.5.2 Functional Imaging

A meta-analysis by Cortese et al. [17] of functional imaging studies showed that child and adolescent ADHD is associated with prominent hypoactivation in the ventral attentional system (comprising the temporoparietal junction, the supramarginal gyrus, frontal operculum and anterior insula) and the frontoparietal executive system (including the lateral frontal pole, dorsal anterior cingulate cortex, dorsolateral anterior prefrontal cortex, lateral cerebellum, anterior insula and inferior parietal lobe). The deficiencies in ventral attentional network activation have been postulated to underlie difficulties in ADHD individuals in orienting to salient external stimuli. On the other hand, hyperactivation of some nodes of this network may correspond to distractibility, but this needs further empirical support. There is also less evidence to date of dorsal attentional system underactivation but some evidence of hyperactivation in the DMN, consistent with a lack of attention to external tasks. Reductions of activity in the frontoparietal executive network are consistent with broad impairments in executive functioning present in ADHD, including attentional control and cognitive flexibility (attentional set shifting). For adult ADHD the most marked fMRI deficits have involved hypoactivation of the frontoparietal executive network and right inferior frontostriatal inactivation during a rewarded sustained attention task, similar to findings in child and adolescent ADHD.

5.12.6 Pharmacological Treatment of Attentional Deficits in ADHD

If psychological treatments are not sufficiently effective, medication with methylphenidate (Ritalin), various forms of amphetamine, or atomoxetine (Strattera) are recommended ADHD treatments for children (over 5) and adolescents, according to National Insitute for Health and Care Excellence guidelines in the United Kingdom. Although medication with these psychomotor stimulant drugs has confirmed efficacy in treating ADHD symptoms, effects on formal laboratory measures of attentional functioning have been both less well studied and weaker. Nevertheless, in placebo-controlled double-blind studies there is evidence of significant improvement in several aspects of attention, including divided attention and cognitive flexibility as well as the commonly used CPT for sustained attention [18]. A study comparing effects of methylphenidate and atomoxetine on a CPT found in child and adolescent ADHD that methylphenidate was superior to atomoxetine (an atypical stimulant drug which more selectively affects noradrenaline reuptake), particularly in reducing errors of omission [19]. The effects on CPT performance did not predict clinical reduction in symptoms, emphasising that there are other components of disturbed cognitive function in ADHD [20]. It is possible that atomoxetine may be more effective at ameliorating other aspects of executive function, such as response inhibition in control of impulsive symptoms.

It is not clear which precise neural loci stimulants are operating on to exert the attentional improvements. There is evidence that the improvements in sustained attention under methylphenidate are related to dopamine release in the caudate nucleus [21]. However, the cortex receives modulation from the locus coeruleus noradrenergic system and from the dopaminergic ventral tegmental area and it would appear likely from preclinical experimentation that some of the effects of stimulants and atomoxetine are mediated there also [7]. In a pharmacological fMRI study of child and adolescent ADHD, it has been shown that deficits in a CPT were remediated by methylphenidate in conjunction with normalised activation and connectivity of temporoparietal, frontostriatal and frontocerebellar networks [22]. Whether such effects are primarily mediated via dopamine at D1 or D2 receptors in the neocortex (D1 receptors greatly predominating at a ratio of 9:1) or via noradrenergic receptors

(or both) is unclear. The relative success of these drugs in ameliorating ADHD symptoms has been attributed in part to the involvement of genes affecting dopamine (e.g. the D4 receptor) and noradrenaline receptors in ADHD. However, inferring an aetiological role of these genes in attentional impairments in ADHD may be premature because the improvements seen in ADHD are often observed in healthy volunteers [21]. Because of the side effects associated with stimulant drug treatment there have been attempts to remediate attentional difficulties by suitable cognitive training methods, which may have promise, but their impact on the neural systems of attention is yet to be subject to major investigation.

5.12.7 Attention in Other Psychiatric Disorders

A multidisciplinary neuroscientific approach to understanding some of the symptoms and their treatment for ADHD has been described here. However, attentional impairments have also been implicated in several other psychiatric disorders, even appearing as DSM-5 criteria for major depressive disorder symptoms (for example, the 'diminished ability to concentrate') but these are generally less well understood, and certainly have not been successfully treated despite the recent recognition of their importance. Attentional deficits are an important component of the intellectual deterioration manifest in Alzheimer's disease and other dementias, and may be an important target for remediation by cholinergic drugs [23].

Attentional deficits that grossly resemble those observed in ADHD are also present in schizophrenia, and there is evidence of similar impairments in forebrain attentional systems such as the frontoparietal executive network and anterior cingulate cortex [24]. There are also some interesting differences. For example, patients with schizophrenia have deficits in pre-pulse inhibition (see Subsection 5.12.1) which is associated with dopamine-dependent mechanisms within frontostriatal circuitry [25]. ADHD is not associated with such impairments [26]. Moreover, distinct pathophysiological and aetiological factors may cause different types of malfunctioning of the same attentional networks and this may also be reflected in some differences in pharmacological treatment – which in the case of schizophrenia has focused thus far on drugs with cholinergic mechanisms, such as the alpha-7 nicotinic receptor agonists, or glutamatergic actions, such as D-cycloserine – without confirmed efficacy [27]. However, it is of interest to dimensional accounts of psychiatric disorders that both CPT performance and attentional set shifting have shown improvements in response to stimulant drug medication in laboratory studies, perhaps indicating some transdiagnostic commonalities in these attentional symptoms [28].

Conclusions and Outstanding Questions

Overall, it is apparent that problems in different aspects of attention are pervasive in psychiatric disorders and represent an important focus for treatment given that attention is essential for noticing changes in the environment that we live in, and to their importance. Attention is also required for effective communication with others, including interpersonal therapeutic relationships. For example, good attention is needed for successful engagement and psychological therapies, such as cognitive behavioural treatment.

Outstanding Questions

- Is ADHD on the increase or is it that general practitioners and other medical doctors have become more aware of the diagnosis?
- Do different psychiatric disorders exhibit different forms of attentional dysregulation?
- Can the various forms of attention be related to specific neural networks or neuromodulatory transmitters?
- How do drugs currently employed in the treatment of ADHD actually work in terms of neurochemical mechanism?

REFERENCES

1. R. Parasuraman, D. R. Davies, eds. *Varieties of Attention*. Academic Press, 1984.

2. A. C. Nobre, S. Kastner, eds. *The Oxford Handbook of Attention*. Oxford University Press, 2014.

3. American Psychiatric Association. *Diagnostic and Statistical Manual of Mental Disorders*, 5th ed. (DSM-5). American Psychiatric Association, 2013.

4. V. A. Pironti, M. C. Lai, U. Müller et al. Neuroanatomical abnormalities and cognitive impairments are shared by adults with attention-deficit/hyperactivity disorder and their unaffected first-degree relatives. *Biol Psychiatry* 2014; 76(8): 639–647.

5. G. Savulich, E. Thorp, T. Piercy et al. Improvements in attention following cognitive training with the novel "decoder" game on an iPad. *Front Behav Neurosci* 2019; 13: 2.

6. A. Mueller, D. S. Hong, S. Shepard, T. Moore. Linking ADHD to the neural circuitry of attention. *Trends Cogn Sci* 2017; 21: 471–488.

7. N. Del Campo, S. R. Chamberlain, B. J. Sahakian et al. The roles of dopamine and noradrenaline in the pathophysiology and treatment of attention-deficit hyperactivity disorder. *Biol Psychiatry* 2011; 69: 145–157.

8. S. E. Petersen, M. I. Posner. The attention system of the human brain. *Annu Rev Neurosci* 1990; 13: 25–42.

9. M. Corbetta, E. Akbudak, T. E. Conturo et al. A common network of functional areas for attention and eye movements. *Neuron* 1998; **21**: 761–773.

10. A. C. Nobre, M. M. Mesulam. Large scale networks for attention biases. In Nobre A. C. and Kastner S., eds. *The Oxford Handbook of Attention*. Oxford University Press, 2014, pp. 105–151.

11. S. Vossel, J. J. Geng, G. R. Fink. Dorsal and ventral attention systems: distinct neural circuits but collaborative roles. *Neuroscientist* 2014; 20: 150–159.

12. S. L. Bressler, V. Menon. Large-scale brain networks in cognition: emerging methods and principles. *Trends Cogn Sci* 2010; 14: 277–290.

13. D. Vatansever, D. Menon, A. Manktelow et al. Default mode dynamics for global functional integration. *J Neurosci* 2015; 35(46): 15254–15262.

14. F. X. Castellanos, P. P. Lee, W. Sharp et al. Developmental trajectories of brain volume abnormalities in children and adolescents with attention-deficit/hyperactivity disorder. *JAMA* 2002; 288: 1740–1748.

15. L. J. Seidman, E. M. Valera, N. Makris. Structural brain imaging of attention deficit/hyperactivity disorder. *Biol Psychiatry* 2005; 57: 1263–1272.

16. T. Frodl, N. Skokauskas. Meta-analysis of structural MRI studies in children and adults with attention deficit/hyperactivity disorder indicates treatment effects. *Acta Psychiatry Scand* 2012; 125: 114–126.

17. S. Cortese, C. Kelly, C. Chabernaud et al. Towards systems neuroscience of ADHD: a meta-analysis of 55 fMRI studies. *Am J Psychiatry* 2012; 169: 1038–1055.

18. O. Tucha, S. Prell, L Mecklinger et al. Effects of methylphenidate on multiple components of attention in children with attention deficit hyperactivity disorder. *Psychopharmacology* 2006; 185: 315–326.

19. A-C. V. Bédard, M. A. Stein, J. M. Halperin et al. Differential impact of methylphenidate and atomoxetine on sustained attention in youth with attention-deficit/hyperactivity disorder. *J Child Psychol Psychiatry* 2015; 56: 40–48.

20. E. E. DeVito, A. D. Blackwell, L. Kent et al. The effects of methylphenidate on decision making in attention-deficit/hyperactivity disorder. *Biol Psychiatry* 2008; 64: 636–639.

21. N. Del Campo, T. D. Fryer, Y. T. Hong et al. A positron emission tomography study of nigro-striatal dopaminergic mechanisms underlying attention: implications for ADHD and its treatment. *Brain* 2013; 136(11): 3252–70.

22. A. Cubillo, R. Halari, A. Smith et al. A review of fronto-striatal and fronto-cortical brain abnormalities in children and adults with attention deficit hyperactivity disorder (ADHD) and new evidence for dysfunction in adults with ADHD during motivation and attention. *Cortex* 2012; 48(2): 194–215.

23. A. D. Lawrence, B. J. Sahakian. Alzheimer disease, attention, and the cholinergic system. *Alzheimer Dis Assoc Disord* 1995; 9: 43–49.

24. S. J. Luck, J. M. Gold. The construct of attention in schizophrenia. *Biol Psychiat* 2008; 64: 34–39.

25. A. Mena, J. C. Ruiz-Salas, A. Puentes et al. Reduced prepulse inhibition as a biomarker of schizophrenia. *Front Behav Neurosci* 2016; 10: 202.

26. D. Fiefel, A. Minassian, W. Perry. Prepulse inhibition of startle in adults with ADHD. *J Psychiatry Res* 2009; 43: 484–489.

27. C. Lustig, M. Sarter. Attention and the cholinergic system: relevance to schizophrenia. *Curr Top Behav Neurosci* 2016; 28: 327–362.

28. T. W. Robbins. Pharmacological treatment of cognitive deficits in mental health disorders. *Dialogues Clin Neurosci* 2019; 21(3): 301–308.

<table>
<tr><td>**5.13**</td><td>**Apathy, Anhedonia and Fatigue**</td><td>Jonathan Roiser and Masud Husain</td></tr>
</table>

OVERVIEW

Motivation – the capacity to experience enthusiasm for achieving a goal, which helps to initiate, guide and maintain behaviour – is a fundamental psychological process that serves to enable both survival and thriving in the face of challenge. Loss of motivation can have a debilitating impact on everyday function, resulting in difficulty working, studying and taking care of responsibilities at home; and, in extreme cases, a total loss of motivation results in the absence of any behaviour at all. Disrupted motivation can be expressed through a variety of clinical symptoms, including apathy, anhedonia and fatigue, which tend to cluster together. These motivational symptoms are very common, occurring across a broad range of neuropsychiatric conditions, for example depression, schizophrenia and Parkinson's disease, but as yet we have no specific treatments for them. This chapter provides an introduction into research into the neuroscientific and psychological mechanisms underlying motivation, which has yielded important information regarding the key brain circuitry and cognitive operations involved. There are several key messages. (i) Motivation is a multifactorial construct, comprising several distinct cognitive operations, and dysfunction in any one of these has the potential to result in motivational symptoms. (ii) The brain regions underlying different components of motivation have been studied extensively in both animals and humans, and consistently converge on a relatively circumscribed circuit, often termed the brain's 'reward system'. (iii) This circuit is extensively innervated and modulated by monoamine neurotransmitters originating from the midbrain, especially dopamine. These insights are starting to be translated into the understanding of motivational symptoms, providing an important basis for the development of new treatments.

5.13.1 History and Definitions

Apathy, anhedonia and fatigue are observed across neurological and psychiatric disorders (Table 5.13.1). These syndromes were first reported in the nineteenth century, and although different terminologies were used for different patients, it is now recognised that they overlap greatly and relate to a loss of motivation (amotivation) [1], which occurs across a range of brain disorders.

The term apathy, largely used in neurology, is defined as amotivation for physical, cognitive or emotional activity, particularly related to the initiation of action. In psychiatry, amotivation is more often referred to as anhedonia, commonly occurring in depression and schizophrenia. Classically, anhedonia was defined by Ribot solely as an inability to experience **pleasure**. However, this definition was later broadened to include a motivational component, including a loss of **interest** in seeking pleasure or rewards, and the *Diagnostic and Statistical Manual of Mental Disorders* (DSM–5) accordingly defines anhedonia as 'Markedly diminished interest or pleasure in all, or almost all, activities' [2]. Apathy and anhedonia also relate to two other common symptoms: anergia and fatigue. The former refers to feeling drained even without exertion, whereas the latter refers to tiredness following

Table 5.13.1 Prevalence of apathy and anhedonia in different conditions

Disorder	Apathy in population (%)	Anhedonia in population (%)
Alzheimer's disease	49	61
Frontotemporal dementia	72	–
Huntington's disease	47	–
Major depressive disorder	38	37
Parkinson's disease	40	46
Schizophrenia	47	45
Stroke	36	–
Traumatic brain injury	61	22
Vascular dementia	65	–

'–' indicates when anhedonia has not been reliably estimated in a patient population. The reader is referred to Husain and Roiser's review [1] for citations to the corresponding studies.

activity. Many patients may articulate lack of motivation in terms of feeling fatigued.

Syndromes associated with amotivation are clinically very important and have a profound impact on quality of life. For example, in depression a constellation of interest/activity/fatigue symptoms robustly predicts poor response to antidepressant treatment. Amotivation can also occur in individuals without a mental disorder, for example in systemic illnesses or chronic fatigue syndrome. An important question is whether, in addition to peripheral factors, there might be central nervous system contributions to such symptoms.

5.13.2 Measurement

Anhedonia and apathy are typically measured using either questionnaires or structured interviews. The closeness of apathy and anhedonia as constructs is underscored by their co-occurrence: for example, in Parkinson's disease there are substantial correlations between scores on apathy and anhedonia scales; and in schizophrenia they typically cluster together as negative symptoms. Fatigue also correlates with apathy and anhedonia in several brain disorders.

These findings demonstrate the importance of deconstructing apathy, anhedonia and fatigue into component processes, rather than considering them as monolithic entities. Over the past 50 years neuroscience research has identified several brain mechanisms that may drive amotivation. These can be conceptualised within the framework of **effort-based decision making for rewards** – in other words, how the potential benefit of a desirable outcome is weighed up against the effort

required to attain it. These mechanisms appear to be affected in people with amotivation, regardless of their specific diagnosis.

5.13.3 Cognitive Components of Motivation

There exist several behavioural paradigms to examine amotivation in animals, and in many cases analogous tests for humans have been developed [3]. These typically examine one or more of the decision, appetitive, consummatory or learning phases of behaviour (see Figure 5.13.1).

Despite a lack of complete agreement, one area of consensus is that there might be separable mechanisms that underlie amotivation in different people. Some possible cognitive operations that could be involved include:

Option generation: Patients with amotivational syndromes can often perform behaviours when prompted by others but experience difficulty in initiating activities. While this is difficult to measure in animals, human participants can be tested for their ability to generate options for real-life scenarios (for example, 'It's a sunny day. What could you do?'), similar to cognitive flexibility. In schizophrenia, apathy correlates inversely with the ability to generate options.

Decision making and option selection: Individuals might experience difficulty in selecting between possible options, which requires integrating different types of information, for example: valuation of outcomes; probability of reward (or penalty); and the effort required to gain the reward (see Figures 5.13.2C–F). Apathetic Parkinson's disease

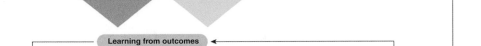

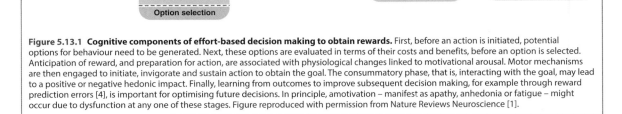

Figure 5.13.1 Cognitive components of effort-based decision making to obtain rewards. First, before an action is initiated, potential options for behaviour need to be generated. Next, these options are evaluated in terms of their costs and benefits, before an option is selected. Anticipation of reward, and preparation for action, are associated with physiological changes linked to motivational arousal. Motor mechanisms are then engaged to initiate, invigorate and sustain action to obtain the goal. The consummatory phase, that is, interacting with the goal, may lead to a positive or negative hedonic impact. Finally, learning from outcomes to improve subsequent decision making, for example through reward prediction errors [4], is important for optimising future decisions. In principle, amotivation – manifest as apathy, anhedonia or fatigue – might occur due to dysfunction at any one of these stages. Figure reproduced with permission from Nature Reviews Neuroscience [1].

patients show reduced inclination to exert physical effort for rewards. In extreme states of amotivation, any effort might be considered too costly, such that no actions are performed.

Anticipation: Once an option has been selected, anticipatory arousal typically occurs, reflected in physiological measures such as heart rate or pupil dilatation. For example, anticipatory pupil dilatation increases in proportion to potential reward magnitude before a speeded movement is made to obtain reward; this is blunted in apathetic patients [5] (see Figures 5.13.2A and 5.13.2B).

Action and effort: The initiation, maintenance and invigoration of action together constitute part of appetitive behaviour, often referred to as 'wanting' (distinct from 'liking', see below) [8]. Studies examining this process in rodents typically measure how much effort an animal is willing to exert to obtain reward. For example, in a variation of the T-maze, rodents decide between scaling a barrier to obtain highly rewarding food versus a low-effort, low-reward food option [6] (see Figure 5.13.2C), and the speed with which high-effort trials are completed can be measured; while in humans equivalent tasks assess speed of button pressing or grip strength (see Figure 5.13.2D and Figure 5.13.2E). Another task is Pavlovian–instrumental transfer, in which rodents initially learn associations through Pavlovian (passive) conditioning, and then perform a completely separate instrumental task in the presence of the Pavlovian conditioned stimulus, which results in an invigoration of instrumental responding. Human analogues of such tasks have been developed [7], and there is evidence of lower inclination to exert effort in both depression and psychosis [9].

Hedonic impact: Consummatory behaviour refers to the achievement of a goal, the subjective enjoyment of which is often referred to as 'liking' [8]. One probe in rodents is the sucrose preference test: given the choice between water and dilute sucrose solution, animals quickly develop a preference for the latter, and this is attenuated in some rodent models of depression. Pleasure can also be indexed in animals through measuring facial expressions during consumption of sweet substances [8]. In human studies, hedonic responses are usually measured through self-report; surprisingly, 'liking' may actually be intact in schizophrenia with pronounced negative symptoms, and in depression. Clinically, this could be potentially important, for example in the context of psychological treatments such as behavioural activation therapy, where the focus is on promoting recovery by encouraging patients to engage in activities they enjoy.

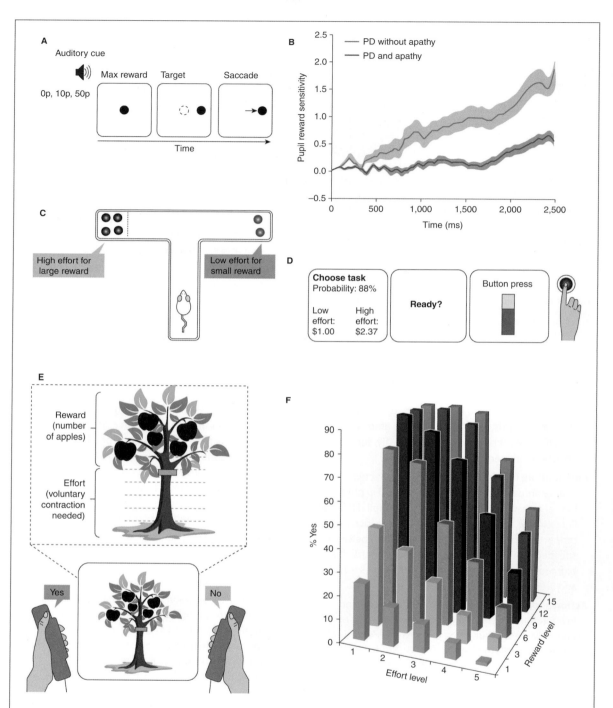

Figure 5.13.2 Behavioural paradigms for assessing motivation. (A) A speeded saccade for reward task, in which the monetary reward depends on the speed of response. The reward on offer is announced at the beginning of each trial, before the saccade target is presented. **(B)** On this task, participants' pupils normally dilate more with greater anticipated reward. Reward sensitivity of the pupils is blunted in individuals with Parkinson's disease (PD) and apathy, compared with individuals with PD but without apathy [5]. **(C)** Rodent T-maze experiments, where an animal must make a choice between easier and more effortful options, reveal that depletion of dopamine in the ventral striatum, or damage to the anterior cingulate cortex, shifts rats from a strategy of working hard for large rewards (scaling an obstacle, indicated by dashed line) to opting for a smaller reward that requires less effort [6]. **(D)** Effort task that requires human participants to select between low or high physical effort options (number of button presses) associated with different levels of reward [6]. **(E)** Effort task in which human participants decide to accept or reject offers in which different levels of reward are available for different levels of physical effort (grip force). The image on the screen displays the reward on offer (depicted as the number of apples on a tree) and the effort required to obtain it (indicated by the height of the yellow line on the tree trunk). **(F)** On the task in (E), the likelihood of accepting offers increases with reward on offer and decreases with increasing effort required [7]. Figure reproduced with permission from Nature Reviews Neuroscience [1].

Learning: Individuals need to learn from the outcomes of their actions to guide future choices. This is reinforcement learning [4], in other words how rewards or penalties associated with a stimulus or an action alter subsequent behaviour through updates to stimulus value. In early work, this was often achieved by analysing performance on early versus late trials in, for example, the Iowa Gambling Task (see Subsection 5.15.8). However, the interpretation of such differences is challenging, as several processes could potentially contribute to altered behaviour, including option valuation, hedonic impact and learning. A fruitful alternative approach that has gained popularity in recent years is to use computational modelling.

5.13.4 Brain Mechanisms of (A)Motivation

5.13.4.1 Lesion and Stimulation Approaches

Studies of amotivation following lesions (often strokes) in humans have identified a network of frontostriatal regions

crucial for motivation, often termed the 'reward circuit' [10]. This includes the basal ganglia (particularly globus pallidus and ventral striatum), anterior cingulate cortex and ventromedial prefrontal cortex (often referred to as medial orbitofrontal cortex). Complementary evidence comes from historical studies of patients institutionalised for psychiatric disorders, who were reported to gain pleasure from self-stimulation of electrodes implanted near the ventral striatum. However, this might in fact have led to patients simply *wanting* to engage in more pleasurable activities, rather than actually increasing *liking*. More recent studies found that anterior cingulate cortex stimulation induced the expectation of an imminent challenge to overcome, indicating a potential role for this region in representing effort.

Findings from investigations of effort-based decision making for reward in animals also implicate this circuit and regions projecting to it (see Figure 5.13.3), in particular the ventral tegmental area (part of the midbrain). The ventral tegmental area is a source of dopamine neurons

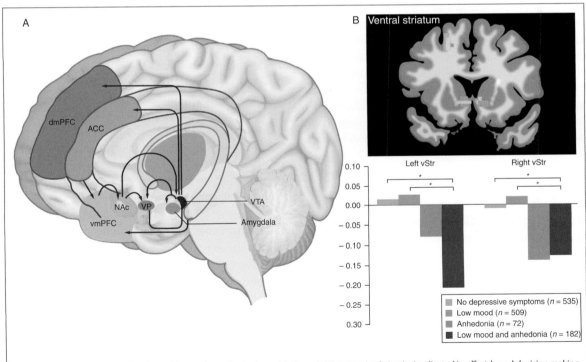

Figure 5.13.3 Brain regions implicated in apathy, anhedonia and fatigue. (A) Frontostriatal circuits implicated in effort-based decision making for rewards include the dopaminergic projection from the ventral tegmental area (VTA) to the basal ganglia, specifically the ventral striatum (vStr, which includes the nucleus accumbens (NAc)) and ventral pallidum (VP). These regions project, via the thalamus, to different parts of the prefrontal cortex, including the ventromedial prefrontal cortex (vmPFC), dorsomedial prefrontal cortex (dmPFC) and anterior cingulate cortex (ACC). These regions in turn project back to the basal ganglia. **(B)** Activation of the ventral striatum in response to anticipation of reward on a monetary incentive task is reduced in adolescents with depressive symptoms, especially anhedonia [11]. Figure reproduced with permission from Nature Reviews Neuroscience [1]; part B is reprinted with permission from the American Journal of Psychiatry [11].

(see Subsection 4.6.3 for background on dopaminergic pathways in the brain), which innervate and modulate the reward circuit (see below). In rodents, lesions or disconnections of the nucleus accumbens (part of the ventral striatum) or anterior cingulate cortex profoundly reduce willingness to allocate effort for rewards. Both classical intracranial self-stimulation studies and modern optogenetic methods (which use lasers to activate genetically modified neurons in a highly anatomically and temporally specific manner) have revealed that rodents will work to receive stimulation of the ventral tegmental area, supporting a central role for dopamine in motivation (see also Section 5.9).

5.13.4.2 Functional Neuroimaging Studies in Amotivational Syndromes

Neuroimaging studies in healthy humans examining effort-based decision making for rewards provide convergent results to the aforementioned lesion and stimulation approaches. A meta-analysis of fMRI studies suggested that, whereas the ventromedial prefrontal cortex, ventral striatum and ventral tegmental area preferentially signal reward, the anterior cingulate cortex and anterior insula appear to preferentially encode effort [12]. Studies across a variety of neurodegenerative conditions have revealed that apathy is associated with disruption to the anterior cingulate cortex, ventromedial prefrontal cortex, ventral striatum and ventral tegmental area [7]. Work examining the neural correlates of anhedonia in depression has implicated a similar network that shows blunted activation during motivational processing, although the precise pattern of results is not identical across studies. A large study of motivational processing in adolescents identified a robust inverse relationship between ventral striatum activation during reward anticipation and concurrent depressive symptoms (especially anhedonia: see Figure 5.13.3B), as well as future risk of depression [11].

5.13.4.3 The Role of Dopamine

While several neurotransmitters have been implicated in amotivation, including serotonin, noradrenaline and glutamate, the greatest body of evidence exists for dopamine. There is a large literature on the effect of pharmacological manipulations of dopamine on motivational processing in both humans and animals. Dopamine depletions lead to robust reductions in instrumental conditioned responding, an aspect of sustaining effort, as well as Pavlovian–instrumental transfer [8]. Direct microinjections of dopamine agonists and antagonists into the ventral striatum of rats reveal, respectively, increases and decreases in conditioned reinforcement. Importantly, hedonic ('liking') responses during the receipt of reward appear to be unaffected by dopamine manipulations [8].

Dopamine is also involved in reinforcement learning. A landmark study revealed that phasic dopamine neuron firing in the midbrain corresponds to the evolution of reward prediction errors [4], which has since been confirmed using optogenetic methods. Dopamine may also play a role in making actions to obtain reward. When rats navigate mazes to retrieve rewards, dopamine signals ramp up gradually as animals come closer to their goals [13]. These ramping signals may encode the expected value of reward, which is necessary to decide whether a reward is worth the effort. Intriguingly, dopamine release seems to be contingent on action: it is attenuated when animals must **inhibit** movement to obtain a reward.

Human psychopharmacology studies provide largely consistent evidence linking dopamine to effort-based decision making for reward [14]. Dietary depletion of dopamine precursors, which reduces dopamine synthesis, attenuates sensitivity to rewards during decision making. Levodopa (l-3,4-dihydroxyphenylalanine; a medication for Parkinson's disease, which increases dopamine synthesis), amphetamine and methylphenidate (which block dopamine reuptake), and dopamine D2/3 receptor agonists all enhance several of the cognitive components depicted in Figure 5.13.1, including: vigour of responses (that is, affecting action); choices of effortful and risky options (influencing cost–benefit decision making); and reward learning. Finally, in depression, striatal dopamine D2/3 receptor binding and dopamine transporter binding (measured using positron emission tomography), are both negatively correlated with anhedonia. Despite clear evidence for the importance of dopamine transmission in motivation, standard pharmacological treatments for depression generally do not target the dopamine system, which may be one reason that they are relatively ineffective at treating amotivational symptoms (although in the USA bupropion, which inhibits dopamine as well as noradrenaline reuptake and is used for smoking cessation in the UK, is licensed as an antidepressant).

Conclusions and Outstanding Questions

A variety of cognitive and neural mechanisms are potentially involved in the genesis of apathy, anhedonia and fatigue. An important take-home message is that surface manifestations (i.e. the clinical phenotype) might not be sufficient to capture these, as different constellations of disrupted mechanisms might occur in different individuals. Although these symptoms are clinically debilitating and have a profound impact on quality of life, to date there have been few attempts to develop specific treatments, either pharmacological or psychological, for amotivation. Therefore this is an important area for the development of new therapeutic interventions.

Outstanding Questions

- Are the same cognitive operations and brain circuits involved in similar motivational symptoms across different disorders? And if so, might transdiagnostic and dimensional formulations provide better insights than existing categorical approaches?

- To what extent are apathy and anhedonia expressions of dysfunction in the same underlying processes, and in what ways do they differ in terms of their cognitive architecture, brain circuitry and neuropharmacology?

- How could we better measure the cognitive operations of option generation, reward anticipation and hedonic impact behaviourally?

- Which of our existing treatments (whether pharmacological, psychological or direct brain interventions) are effective at treating motivational symptoms; and which might have the potential to exacerbate motivational impairment?

5

REFERENCES

1. Husain M, Roiser JP. Neuroscience of apathy and anhedonia: a transdiagnostic approach. *Nat Rev Neurosci* 2018; 19(8): 470–484.

2. American Psychiatric Association. *Diagnostic and Statistical Manual of Mental Disorders*, 5th ed. (DSM-5). American Psychiatric Association, 2013.

3. Der-Avakian A, Barnes SA, Markou A, Pizzagalli DA. Translational assessment of reward and motivational deficits in psychiatric disorders. *Curr Top Behav Neurosci* 2016; 28: 231–262.

4. Schultz W, Dayan P, Montague PR. A neural substrate of prediction and reward. *Science* 1997; 275(5306): 1593–1599.

5. Muhammed K, Manohar S, Ben Yehuda M et al. Reward sensitivity deficits modulated by dopamine are associated with apathy in Parkinson's disease. *Brain* 2016; 139(10): 2706–2721.

6. Salamone JD, Yohn SE, López-Cruz L, San Miguel N, Correa M. Activational and effort-related aspects of motivation: neural mechanisms and implications for psychopathology. *Brain* 2016; 139(5): 1325–1347.

7. Bonnelle V, Manohar S, Behrens T, Husain M. Individual differences in premotor brain systems underlie behavioral apathy. *Cereb Cortex* 2016; 26(2): bhv247.

8. Berridge KC, Robinson TE. What is the role of dopamine in reward: hedonic impact, reward learning, or incentive salience? *Brain Res Brain Res Rev* 1998; 28(3): 309–369.

9. Treadway MT, Bossaller NA, Shelton RC, Zald DH. Effort-based decision-making in major depressive disorder: a translational model of motivational anhedonia. *J Abnorm Psychol* 2012; 121(3): 553–558.

10. Levy R, Dubois B. Apathy and the functional anatomy of the prefrontal cortex–basal ganglia circuits. *Cereb Cortex* 2005; 16(7): 916–928.

11. Stringaris A, Vidal-Ribas Belil P, Artiges E et al. The brain's response to reward anticipation and depression in adolescence: dimensionality, specificity, and longitudinal predictions in a community-based sample. *Am J Psychiatry* 2015; 172(12): 1215–1223.

12. Pessiglione M, Vinckier F, Bouret S, Daunizeau J, Le Bouc R. Why not try harder? Computational approach to motivation deficits in neuro-psychiatric diseases. *Brain* 2018; 141(3): 629–650.

13. Hamid AA, Pettibone JR, Mabrouk OS et al. Mesolimbic dopamine signals the value of work. *Nat Neurosci* 2015; 19(1): 117–126.

14. Martins D, Mehta MA, Prata D. The "highs and lows" of the human brain on dopaminergics: evidence from neuropharmacology. *Neurosci Biobehav Rev* 2017; 80: 351–371.

5.14 **Memory**

Amy L. Milton and Jon S. Simons

OVERVIEW

The term memory, in its broadest sense, refers to the influence of prior experience on subsequent behaviour. Memory impacts everyday life in countless ways (e.g. recalling a past social occasion, producing factual information about an object, or knowing how to ride a bicycle). There is no universally accepted classification of human memory, but an appreciation of the way memory operates can be important for improving clinical outcomes. Alterations in memory are key features of multiple psychiatric disorders. In addition, patients' memory for medical information has a major influence on their adherence to recommended treatments [1]. Around 40–80% of medical information provided by healthcare practitioners is forgotten immediately, and much of what is remembered is recalled incorrectly. Thus, understanding how memory works can provide an appreciation of the obstacles patients face in remembering medical information and suggestions for helping to overcome them.

5.14.1 Cognitive and Psychological Divisions of Memory

Theorists have distinguished between shorter- and longer-term forms of memory for more than a century. For example, Francis Galton [2] described 'a presence chamber where full consciousness holds court, and an ante-chamber full of ideas, situated just beyond the ken of consciousness'. Similarly, William James [3] wrote of primary memory ('the specious present') and secondary memory ('the psychological past'). This distinction between short-term and long-term memory (as they are now termed) is a feature of almost all modern-day characterisations of memory, and considerable evidence indicates that each type of memory comprises several separate systems (Figure 5.14.1).

5.14.1.1 Short-Term and Long-Term Memory
Short-term memory is the name given to the limited capacity system used to temporarily hold information in mind, whereas long-term memory stores information over extended periods of time, with essentially unlimited capacity. Evidence for the separation of short-term and

long-term memory comes from many sources. One example is the 'serial position curve', a U-shaped function typically observed when participants are asked to recall a list of previously studied words. Better recall is usually seen of the first few words in the list (the 'primacy' effect) and the last few words (the 'recency' effect). Atkinson and Shiffrin [4] attributed the primacy effect to long-term memory, because when only a few words have been presented there is time to repeat them to oneself before the next item appears, whereas the recency effect was attributed to the last few items in the list still being present in short-term memory at the time of recall. Consistent with this interpretation, a distracting task, such as counting backwards for a few seconds between list learning and recall, displaces the last few list items from short-term memory, eliminating the recency effect, but leaves the primacy effect intact.

Studies of patients with brain lesions also support a separation between short-term and long-term memory. Patients with amnesia, such as Henry Molaison (known in the medical literature as HM until his death in 2008), typically exhibit impaired long-term memory but relatively preserved short-term memory. HM became amnesic in

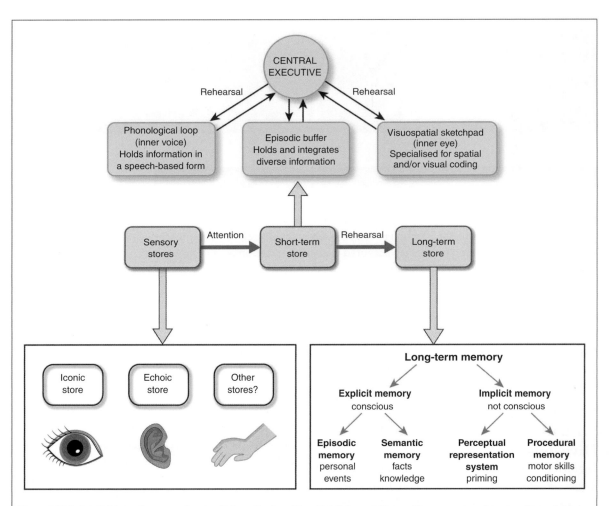

Figure 5.14.1 Subdivisions of memory. Perceived information is registered briefly in modality-specific sensory stores (visual, auditory, etc.) but is rapidly lost unless we pay attention to it, in which case it can be processed in a limited-capacity short-term store. Baddeley's working memory model is a widely accepted characterisation of short-term memory, with distinct roles for a phonological loop, visuospatial sketchpad, episodic buffer and central executive. If information is rehearsed or processed further, it can transfer into a long-term store of essentially unlimited capacity capable of holding information over time. Numerous divisions of long-term memory have been proposed, differentiating particularly between explicit and implicit forms of memory.

his mid-20s after an operation to relieve symptoms of severe epilepsy that involved surgery to the hippocampus and surrounding structures in the medial temporal lobe. Although the surgery was an effective treatment for HM's epilepsy, he was left with a catastrophic memory deficit, almost completely unable to retain any memory of events that happened after his operation [5]. However, HM's ability to complete tasks that required recall from short-term memory suggests that short-term and long-term memory have at least partly separable neuroanatomical bases. Patients with damage to other areas, such

as the parietal regions, show disproportionate deficits to short-term memory, while sparing performance on many long-term memory tasks [6]. More recent functional neuroimaging studies support the view that different brain areas are involved in short-term and long-term memory. Activity in medial temporal lobe regions such as the hippocampus is often observed when participants encode or retrieve information from long-term memory [7], whereas asking participants to retain information in short-term storage tends to be associated with activity in inferior frontal and parietal areas [8].

5.14.1.2 Divisions of Short-Term Memory

The most widely accepted characterisation of short-term memory is Baddeley and Hitch's (1974) [9] working memory model (as depicted in blue on Figure 5.14.1). The revised version of their model [10] comprises four components: a phonological loop, responsible for temporary retention of spoken verbal material; a visuospatial sketchpad, involved in temporary storage and manipulation of spatial and visual information; an episodic buffer, which holds and integrates information from the phonological loop, visuospatial sketchpad and long-term memory; and the central executive, a processing system that coordinates operation of the other systems for performing demanding cognitive tasks (Figure 5.14.1).

Numerous empirical findings provide insights into the structure of the **phonological loop**. One is the phonological similarity effect, in which recall of a list of words that sound similar is significantly worse than recall of a list of words with distinct sounds, whereas visual or meaning-based similarity has little effect on recall [11]. This suggests that speech-based representations are used in storing the words, and that recall requires discrimination between memory traces, which is more difficult for similar phonological representations. Another finding is the word-length effect, in which recall of a list of long words is worse than recall of a list of short words [12], suggesting that phonological loop capacity might be determined by the time required to pronounce words. Based on these findings, Baddeley [13] divided the phonological loop into a phonological store and an articulatory control process. The phonological store is concerned with speech perception, whereas the articulatory control process is linked to speech production that gives access to the phonological store. By this account, the phonological similarity effect can be attributed to confusions between similar representations in the phonological store, and the word-length effect can be attributed to the time taken to repeat longer words to oneself via the articulatory control process.

It has been argued that the **visuospatial sketchpad** can also be divided into two components [14]. The visual cache passively stores information about visual form and colour and is subject to decay and interference by new visual information. The inner scribe processes spatial information and allows information in the visual cache to be refreshed, maintaining it for longer. This distinction is supported by evidence from patients with brain lesions involving temporal and occipital regions, including patients who perform better on spatial processing tasks than on visual imagery tasks.

Evidence for a distinct, multimodal short-term store, the **episodic buffer**, comes from neuroimaging research [15]. When participants were asked to perform a working memory task that required the temporary retention of integrated verbal and spatial information, activation in the right frontal cortex was greater for retention of integrated rather than modality-specific information, consistent with an episodic buffer. By contrast, posterior brain regions exhibited modality-specific working memory effects, with activity in the left hemisphere consistent with the phonological loop and right hemisphere activity associated with the visuospatial sketchpad.

5.14.1.3 Moving Information to Long-Term Memory: Consolidation and Reconsolidation

The transition from short- to long-term memory, or 'consolidation', is widely accepted as requiring changes in the efficiency of synaptic signalling between the neurons that constitute the memory trace, or 'engram'. The engram can be defined as a network of neurons that fires during a particular experience, and that is also activated when the memory is subsequently recalled. The notion that the functional changes produced by past experiences (i.e. memory) are reflected in structural changes in the brain was popularised by Donald Hebb [16] and is consequently known as 'Hebbian plasticity'. This theoretical position gained support with the discovery of the physiological process of 'long-term potentiation' by Tim Bliss and Terje Lømo [17] (see Section 2.4.6) and subsequent demonstrations that long-term potentiation and 'cellular-level' consolidation depend on common molecular mechanisms (Figure 5.14.2). While the newly forming engram can be sustained for a few hours by changes in intracellular signalling and receptor function (e.g. phosphorylation of receptors to increase their efficiency), these changes cannot persist beyond 3–4 hours without structural changes in the synapse, involving the production of new proteins. This 'cellular-level consolidation' occurs within 4–6 hours of an experience. In the longer term, explicit memories (see Figure 5.14.1 and Subsection 5.14.1.4) undergo 'systems-level consolidation', during which the engram appears to transfer from the hippocampus to the

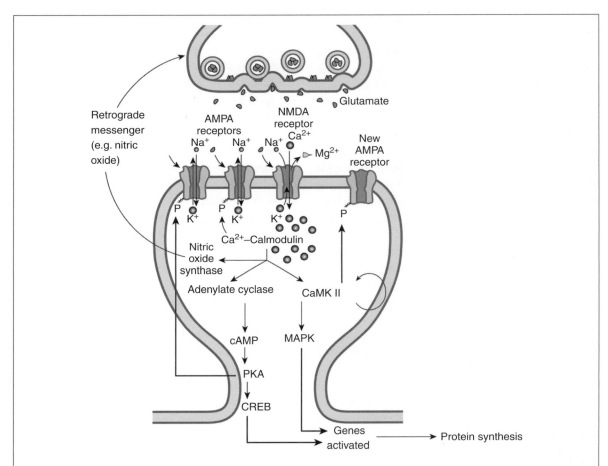

Figure 5.14.2 Research investigating the molecular mechanisms of memory has been strongly guided by the mechanisms reported to underlie the synaptic plasticity process of long-term potentiation. This is widely accepted as depending upon the NMDA subtype of glutamate receptor, which requires both activation of the neuron and binding of glutamate to the receptor to allow the entry of calcium into the neuron. Calcium activates protein kinases that can mediate short-term increases in signalling efficiency (e.g. through phosphorylation of receptors to modulate their sensitivity to stimulation) and, in the longer term, can translocate to the nucleus to stimulate gene transcription and protein synthesis. Neuromodulators, such as noradrenaline and acetylcholine, can modulate this canonical pathway, making changes in synaptic efficacy more or less likely depending on the subtypes of receptors activated. Abbreviations: AMPA, alpha-amino-3-hydroxy-5-methyl-4-isoxazole-propionic acid; CaMK II, calcium/calmodulin-dependent protein kinase II; cAMP; cyclic adenosine 3,5-monophosphate; CREB, cAMP-response element binding protein; MAPK, mitogen-activated protein kinase; NMDA, N-methyl-D-aspartate; PKA, protein kinase A.

neocortex [18], most likely involving additional rounds of synaptic plasticity in which the information encoded in the hippocampal engram becomes represented by another set of neurons within the cortex. Systems-level consolidation was originally proposed to account for the graded pattern of retrograde amnesia shown by patients such as HM (namely, memories further in the past were more preserved than memories from the years leading up to his surgery) though this explanation is not universally accepted [19, 20].

Memories were traditionally thought to be stored permanently within the brain following their initial consolidation, but recent evidence indicates that memories instead undergo repeated cycles of 'reconsolidation' [21, 22]. When what is predicted to happen based on past experience does not actually occur, this produces a 'violation of expectations' or 'prediction error', which destabilises the engram and allows it to be updated with new information [23] (see Section 5.7 for an explanation of prediction error). This updating requires similar, though not identical, molecular mechanisms to initial memory storage processes. Reconsolidation has been most extensively demonstrated for implicit memories (see Figure 5.14.1 and below), where there has been interest in exploiting the process to develop new treatments for mental health disorders such as post-traumatic stress disorder (PTSD) and drug addiction [24]. It is worth noting that although prolonged exposure therapy (see Subsection 5.14.3.2) also depends upon violating a patient's expectations, this type of therapy engages the process of extinction learning, which is a psychologically and neurobiologically distinct process [25].

5.14.1.4 Explicit and Implicit Long-Term Memories

Within long-term memory, one influential distinction is between implicit and explicit memory. Whereas the contents of explicit memory are accessible to conscious awareness, and can be talked about, implicit memories are less consciously accessible [26]. For example, you may know how to ride a bike, but if you had to describe exactly how you balance to stay upright when riding you would probably be at a loss. Studies in patients with amnesia also make the distinction clear: implicit memory is typically preserved whereas explicit memory is not [27]. Such individuals may have little or no conscious recollection of a particular study episode and yet show evidence that their subsequent behaviour has been 'implicitly' influenced by that prior episode. For example, they may not recall having previously read a list of words, and yet subsequently show increased accuracy in identifying the words when only their first few letters are now presented. Patients exhibiting a disproportionate deficit in implicit memory are rarer. However, patient MS [28], whose lesion affected the occipital cortex, performed as well as controls at explicit memory, but was severely impaired on implicit memory tasks.

5.14.1.5 Episodic and Semantic Explicit Memories

A further important distinction is between episodic and semantic memory [29]. Episodic memory involves recollection of specific events or episodes occurring in a particular time and place (e.g. remembering what you had for breakfast this morning). Semantic memory, by contrast, comprises general knowledge about objects, people, facts, concepts and the meanings of words,

without awareness of where or when the information was learned (e.g. knowing that breakfast is a meal eaten in the morning). Episodic memory is specific to each person, whereas semantic memory can be culturally shared. Episodic memory often involves 'mental time travel', thinking back to a specific moment in one's personal past and consciously 'reliving' a prior episode as it was previously experienced. Much of the evidence supporting the separation of episodic and semantic memory comes from patients with amnesia, such as HM, who exhibited profound impairment on episodic memory tasks, but was able to name pictures of everyday objects, define concepts, etc.

5.14.2 Neuroanatomical Divisions of Memory

5.14.2.1 The Medial Temporal Lobe

The medial temporal lobe consists of the hippocampus, fornix and amygdala, as well as surrounding structures, the entorhinal, perirhinal and parahippocampal cortices (Figure 5.14.3). Numerous studies indicate that different regions within the medial temporal lobe may support functionally distinct memory systems. According to this view, a system involving the hippocampus supports the recollection of stored memories with their associated spatiotemporal context or narrative, whereas an anatomically separate system that includes the perirhinal cortex is thought to underlie familiarity-based recognition of prior occurrence. Several studies have documented amnesic patients with selective damage to the hippocampus or connecting structures such as the fornix who show impaired recollection in the context of preserved familiarity-based memory performance [30]. Selective lesions of the perirhinal cortex in humans are rarer, but patients with damage that included the perirhinal cortex have been reported to show impaired familiarity-based recognition memory [31].

Importantly, the structure of the hippocampus allows it to act as a computational 'autoassociator', which automatically encodes experiences without requiring an explicit 'teaching signal' or conscious effort. Computational models of the hippocampus show that its structure can support phenomena such as retrieving a full engram from a partial input (known as 'pattern completion') and distinguishing between distinct episodes (known as

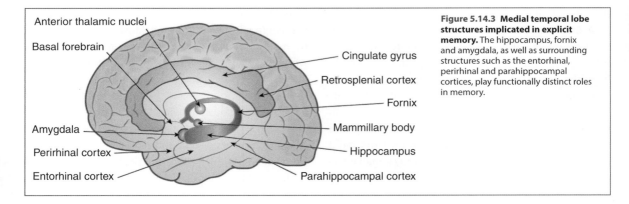

Figure 5.14.3 Medial temporal lobe structures implicated in explicit memory. The hippocampus, fornix and amygdala, as well as surrounding structures such as the entorhinal, perirhinal and parahippocampal cortices, play functionally distinct roles in memory.

'pattern separation'). Furthermore, with time the explicit (episodic) memory is thought to become independent of the hippocampus, though this account is not unanimously accepted [19, 20]. There remains debate within the field as to whether the memory becomes 'semanticised' [20] as it transfers from the hippocampus to the cortex, with some arguing that the mental time travel associated with the recall of episodic memories always depends upon the hippocampus [19]. Despite these unresolved issues within the literature, the fact that this 'systems-level consolidation' process occurs is not disputed. Systems-level consolidation depends critically upon hippocampal levels of the neurotransmitter acetylcholine, with higher levels supporting encoding in the hippocampus, and lower levels supporting consolidation of the memory in the cortex [32]. Dysregulation of cholinergic signalling following neurodegeneration may give rise to some symptoms of dementia (see Section 5.14.3.1).

The amygdala, which lies rostral to the hippocampus, has been particularly implicated in implicit emotional memory, associating cues in the environment with their emotional and motivational relevance (e.g. spiders with fear, or a £20 note with joy). Through its connections with the hippocampus, the amygdala also mediates the influence of emotion on episodic memory (e.g. 'flashbulb' memories). The amygdala receives a wide range of sensory inputs, including those from external and internal (bodily) environments, and contextual information provided by the hippocampus. Through connections to the hypothalamus, brainstem and the nucleus accumbens, the amygdala can coordinate neuroendocrine, autonomic and both simple reflexive and complex voluntary behavioural responses.

5.14.2.2 Cortical Regions

With the advent of functional neuroimaging, roles in explicit memory have also been discovered for regions of prefrontal and parietal cortices. Distinct contributions have been proposed for three main prefrontal regions (Figure 5.14.4) in the cognitive control of encoding and retrieving hippocampally-stored information: the ventrolateral prefrontal cortex, dorsolateral prefrontal cortex and anterior prefrontal cortex. Parietal regions such as angular gyrus are thought to form key parts of a 'core recollection network' [33]. The prefrontal cortex is also implicated in the expression of implicit memories. In particular, the rodent equivalent of the ventromedial prefrontal cortex can inhibit amygdala activity and so the expression of emotional memories such as fear [34]. The engagement of the ventromedial prefrontal cortex appears to be critical for successful prolonged exposure therapy.

Neuropsychological evidence on the role of the parietal lobe in memory is more recent, and surprising because studies of patients with parietal lobe damage have traditionally focused on their problems with visuospatial attention and/or visually guided action. Patients whose parietal lesions overlapped closely with the areas activated in healthy volunteers during performance of an episodic memory task nevertheless performed as well on the task as the healthy controls [35]. However, when patients were asked to rate how *confident* they were in each of their accurate memory responses, they exhibited reduced confidence in each accurate memory [36]. Patients with parietal lesions are also impaired at freely recalling events from their lifetimes, but unimpaired when answering specific questions about the same

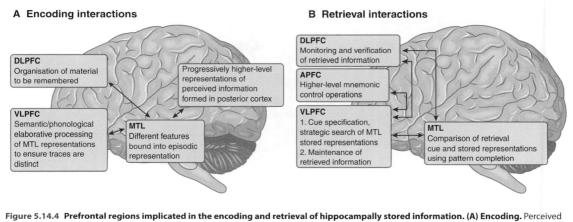

Figure 5.14.4 Prefrontal regions implicated in the encoding and retrieval of hippocampally stored information. (A) Encoding. Perceived information is processed in hierarchical cortical areas, resulting in progressively higher-level representations that are integrated and associated into a bound memory trace in the medial temporal lobe (MTL). Top-down control of encoding is provided by the prefrontal cortex, involving elaborative semantic and/or phonological processing of the MTL representation in the ventrolateral prefrontal cortex (VLPFC). Material is selected, manipulated and organised in the dorsolateral prefrontal cortex (DLPFC). These control processes ensure the separation of traces so as to reduce interference between them. **(B) Retrieval.** Retrieval cues are specified and elaborated in the VLPFC, before being used to strategically search stored representations in the MTL. Using a process of pattern completion, the retrieval cue is iteratively compared with stored representations until correspondence is achieved and a candidate memory identified. This memory representation is retrieved and maintained online by the VLPFC while various monitoring and verification processes are undertaken in the DLPFC. Higher-level mnemonic control processes, should they be required, are supported by anterior prefrontal cortex (APFC).

events [37]. Such patients exhibit normal source memory but produce reduced subjective 'remember' judgements [38]. These findings suggest that the parietal lobes might contribute to the subjective experience of remembering.

One suggestion has been that parietal regions such as the angular gyrus are involved in integrating multimodal memory features into a conscious representation that enables the subjective 'reliving' of an event. Anatomical connectivity data indicate that the angular gyrus has rich interactivity with the frontal, temporal and hippocampal systems, among other areas [39]. It is thus plausible that it might act as a cross-modal hub where converging multisensory information is combined and integrated. Consistent with this proposal, the angular gyrus displays greater activity during retrieval of integrated audiovisual compared to unimodal auditory or visual information [40]. Moreover, classifier analysis indicated that specific individual multimodal episodic memories, but not unimodal memories, could be decoded from patterns of activity in the angular gyrus, and that classifier accuracy tracked the trial-by-trial subjective vividness with which participants rated their memories.

5.14.3 Disorders of Memory

5.14.3.1 Dementia

Memory can be affected in different ways by a variety of neurological and psychiatric disorders. One of the most well known is dementia, which affects more than 7% of people over the age of 65 (see also Chapter 10 for more on neurodegeneration). Patients with early progression of different forms of dementia can show evidence of the distinction between episodic and semantic memory. Compared to the brains of healthy older adults (Figure 5.14.5A), in the early stages of Alzheimer's disease, patients can have atrophy that disproportionately affects the medial temporal lobe areas (Figure 5.14.5B) and is also associated with a loss of the neurotransmitter acetylcholine. By contrast, patients with early semantic dementia often have atrophy that is most apparent in the lateral temporal lobe areas (Figure 5.14.5C). With progression of the disease, both kinds of patients eventually have atrophy of the temporal lobes, and exhibit impairment in both forms of memory (and many other cognitive functions), but in their very early stages, selective impairments can

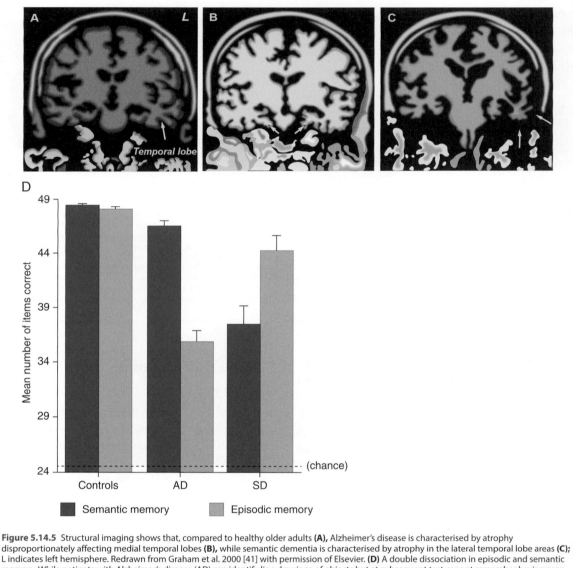

Figure 5.14.5 Structural imaging shows that, compared to healthy older adults **(A),** Alzheimer's disease is characterised by atrophy disproportionately affecting medial temporal lobes **(B),** while semantic dementia is characterised by atrophy in the lateral temporal lobe areas **(C);** L indicates left hemisphere. Redrawn from Graham et al. 2000 [41] with permission of Elsevier. **(D)** A double dissociation in episodic and semantic memory. While patients with Alzheimer's disease (AD) can identify line drawings of objects but at subsequent test cannot remember having seen them before, patients with semantic dementia (SD) cannot identify the drawings but do remember which they have seen previously. Redrawn from Simons et al. 2002 [43], with permission from Elsevier.

be seen. Patients with early Alzheimer's disease resemble amnesic patients, with impaired episodic memory and preserved semantic knowledge. Patients with semantic dementia suffer profound degradation of semantic knowledge [42] but less apparent episodic memory impairment. For example, Simons and colleagues [43] asked patients to perform a semantic task that involved identifying drawings that are associated with each other (e.g. a pyramid is associated with a palm-tree rather than a fir-tree). The patients' episodic memory was later tested for the same drawings. A distinction was observed between impaired episodic and preserved semantic memory in Alzheimer's disease, and impaired semantic and preserved episodic memory in semantic dementia (Figure 5.14.5D).

TREATMENTS FOR DEMENTIA

The National Institute for Health and Care Excellence (NICE) in the UK recommends pharmacological treatments for dementia as part of a programme of person-centred care and support. Two major classes of drugs are used to manage to the symptoms of dementia – acetylcholinesterase (AChE) inhibitors (donepezil, galantamine and rivastigmine) and the NMDA receptor antagonist memantine. AChE inhibitors promote cholinergic signalling by preventing AChE from breaking down acetylcholine, enhancing the cholinergic signalling that remains in the brains of patients with dementia and so improving memory. Memantine works by directly blocking the NMDA subtype of glutamate receptor, preventing further atrophy caused by the excessive neurotoxic release of glutamate in the brains of Alzheimer's disease patients.

5.14.3.2 Post-Traumatic Stress Disorder

Memory deficits can also be observed in psychiatric disorders such as PTSD and depression. PTSD is often considered as a disorder of aberrantly strong and over-generalised implicit memory, but it is often associated with a 'paradoxical' amnesia for explicit memories of the traumatic event. This is due to high levels of stress hormones producing different effects on the neural circuitry supporting explicit and implicit memories. While high levels of noradrenaline and glucocorticoids (such as cortisol) impair the function of the hippocampus, they promote plasticity within the amygdala [44]. This dual effect leads to an overly strong implicit fear memory, without the spatiotemporal context, or continuous narrative, provided by hippocampal-dependent explicit memory. Furthermore, high levels of stress also impair explicit memory retrieval while having less of an effect on implicit memories [45]. Hippocampal volume is reduced in PTSD patients compared to trauma-exposed controls without PTSD [46] though it has been difficult to establish conclusively whether reduced hippocampal volume is a cause or consequence of PTSD. In addition to differences in hippocampal volume, there are also reductions in the volume of prefrontal areas.

The formation of 'maladaptive' trauma memories – often modelled using Pavlovian conditioning in animals and healthy human volunteers – has been a major focus for theories of PTSD [47] and for the development of treatments to manage symptoms caused by these memories.

Recently, there has been much interest in understanding other learning processes, such as sensitisation of fear learning, in PTSD populations [48].

TREATMENTS FOR PTSD

NICE primarily recommends behavioural therapies for PTSD, including cognitive behavioural therapy and, if this is ineffective, eye-movement desensitisation and reprocessing (EMDR). These treatments are primarily based upon fear extinction learning, in which exposure to a fearful or threatening stimulus (whether real or imaginal) is combined with the teaching of relaxation techniques and coping strategies. In EMDR, this approach is augmented by asking patients to perform a concurrent sensory task, such as moving their eyes back and forth. In this way, the patient is exposed to the traumatic stimuli in the absence of the fear response, leading to the formation of a new, prefrontal-dependent 'extinction' memory that inhibits the expression of the original fear memory. This process appears to be enhanced through the concurrent performance of sensory tasks in EMDR. Recent research has begun to reveal the neural circuitry underlying this enhancement, which appears to depend upon a circuit between the superior colliculus, mediodorsal thalamus and basolateral amygdala [49].

Conclusions and Outstanding Questions

Memory can be studied at multiple levels, with the basic mechanisms of memory storage appearing to be largely conserved across different memory types, relying on distinct networks of brain regions. Understanding the mechanisms by which memories are stored and retrieved gives rise to the possibility of developing new treatments for memory disorders, including dementia and neuropsychiatric conditions.

Outstanding Questions

- How does activity within specific networks of neurons with a brain region relate to memory storage? Might it ever be possible to visualise 'memory traces' in humans?

- How does the brain give rise to the subjective experience of remembering?

- Can we use our knowledge of fundamental memory mechanisms to improve patient care in the case of neurodegenerative and neuropsychiatric conditions?

REFERENCES

1. P. Ley. *Communicating with Patients: Improving Communication, Satisfaction and Compliance*. Croom Helm, 1988.

2. F. Galton. *Inquiries into Human Faculty and Its Development*. Macmillan, 1883.

3. W. James. *Principles of Psychology*. Holt, 1890.

4. R. C. Atkinson, R. M. Shiffrin. Human memory: a proposed system and its control processes. In K. W. Spence, J. T, Spence (eds.), *The Psychology of Learning and Motivation*, volume 2. Academic Press, 1968, 89–195.

5. W. B. Scoville, B. Milner. Loss of recent memory after bilateral hippocampal lesions. *J Neurol Neurosurg Psychiatry* 1957; 20: 11–21.

6. T. Shallice, E. K. Warrington. Independent functioning of verbal memory stores: a neuropsychological study. *Q J Exp Psychol* 1970; 22(2): 261–273.

7. D. L. Schacter, A. D. Wagner. Medial temporal lobe activations in fMRI and PET studies of episodic encoding and retrieval. *Hippocampus* 1999; 9: 7–24.

8. R. N. A. Henson, N. Burgess, C. D. Frith. Recoding, storage, rehearsal and grouping in verbal short-term memory: an fMRI study. *Neuropsychologia* 2000; 38: 426–440.

9. A. D. Baddeley, G. Hitch. Working memory. In G. H. Bower (ed.), *Psychology of Learning and Motivation*, volume 8. Academic Press, 1974, pp. 47–89.

10. A. D. Baddeley. The episodic buffer: a new component of working memory? *Trends Cogn Sci* 2000; 4: 417–423.

11. A. D. Baddeley. Short-term memory for word sequences as a function of acoustic, semantic and formal similarity. *Q J Exp Psychol* 1966; 18(4): 362–365.

12. A. D. Baddeley, N. Thomson, M. Buchanan. Word length and the structure of short-term memory. *J Verb Learn Verb Behav* 1975; 14(6): 575–589.

13. A. D. Baddeley. *Human Memory: Theory and Practice*. Psychology Press, 1990.

14. R. H. Logie. *Visuo-spatial Working Memory*. Psychology Press, 1995.

15. V. Prabhakaran, K. Narayanan, Z. Zhao, J. D. E. Gabrieli. Integration of diverse information in working memory within the frontal lobe. *Nat Neurosci* 2000; 3: 85–90.

16. D. O. Hebb. *The Organization of Behavior: A Neuropsychological Theory*. Wiley, 1949.

17. T. V. P. Bliss, T. Lømo. Long-lasting potentiation of synaptic transmission in the dentate area of the anaesthetized rabbit following stimulation of the perforant path. *J Physiol* 1973; 232: 331–356.

18. L. R. Squire. Memory and the hippocampus: a synthesis from findings with rats, monkeys, and humans. *Psychol Rev* 1992; 99(2): 195–231.

19. L. Nadel, M. Moscovitch. Memory consolidation, retrograde amnesia and the hippocampal complex. *Curr Opin Neurobiol* 1997; 7: 217–227.

20. G. Winocur, M. Moscovitch, B. Bontempi. Memory formation and long-term retention in humans and animals: convergence towards a transformation account of hippocampal–neocortical interactions. *Neuropsychologia* 2010; 48: 2339–2356.

21. D. J. Lewis. Psychobiology of active and inactive memory. *Psychol Bull* 1979; 86: 1054–1083.

22. K. Nader. Memory traces unbound. *Trends Neurosci* 2003; 26: 65–72.

23. R. S. Fernández, M. M. Boccia, M. E. Pedreira. The fate of memory: reconsolidation and the case of prediction error. *Neurosci Biobehav Rev* 2016; 68: 423–441.

24. A. L. Milton, B. J. Everitt. The psychological and neurochemical mechanisms of drug memory reconsolidation: implications for the treatment of addiction. *Eur J Neurosci* 2010; 31: 2308–2319.

25. E. Merlo, A. L. Milton, Z. Y. Goozée, D. E. H. Theobald, B. J. Everitt. Reconsolidation and extinction are dissociable and mutually exclusive processes: behavioral and molecular evidence. *J Neurosci* 2014; 34(7): 2422–2431.

26. D. L. Schacter. Implicit memory: history and current status. *J Exp Psychol Learn Mem Cogn* 1987; 13: 501–518.

27. P. Graf, L. R. Squire, G. Mandler. The information that amnesic patients do not forget. *J Exp Psychol Learn Mem Cogn* 1984; 10 : 164–178.

28. J. D. E. Gabrieli, D. A. Fleischman, M. M. Keane, S. L. Reminger, F. Morrell. Double dissociation between memory systems underlying explicit and implicit memory in the human brain. *Psychol Sci* 1995; 6: 76–82.

29. E. Tulving. Episodic and semantic memory. In E. Tulving, W. Donaldson (eds.), *Organization of Memory*. Academic Press, 1972, pp. 381–403.

30. A. P. Yonelinas, N. E. Kroll, J. R. Quamme et al. Effects of extensive temporal lobe damage or mild hypoxia on recollection and familiarity. *Nat Neurosci* 2002; 5(11): 1236–4121.

31. E. A. Buffalo, P. J. Reber, L. R. Squire. The human perirhinal cortex and recognition memory. *Hippocampus* 1998; 8: 330–339.

32. M. E. Hasselmo. The role of acetylcholine in learning and memory. *Curr Opin Neurobiol* 2006; 16(6): 710–715.

33. M. D. Rugg, K. L. Vilberg. Brain networks underlying episodic memory retrieval. *Curr Opin Neurobiol* 2013; 23(2): 255–260.

34. M. R. Milad, G. J. Quirk. Fear extinction as a model for translational neuroscience: ten years of progress. *Annu Rev Psychol* 2012; 63: 129–151.

35. J. S. Simons, P. V. Peers, D. Y. Hwang et al. Is the parietal lobe necessary for recollection in humans? *Neuropsychologia* 2008; 46(4): 1185–1191.

36. J. S. Simons, P. V. Peers, Y. S. Mazuz, M. E. Berryhill, I. R. Olson. Dissociation between memory accuracy and memory confidence following bilateral parietal lesions. *Cereb Cortex* 2010; 20(2): 479–485.

37. M. E. Berryhill, L. Phuong, L. Picasso, R. Cabeza, I. R. Olson. Parietal lobe and episodic memory: bilateral damage causes impaired free recall of autobiographical memory. *J Neurosci* 2007; 27: 14415–14423.

38. P. S. R. Davidson, D. Anaki, E. Ciaramelli et al. Does lateral parietal cortex support episodic memory? Evidence from focal lesion patients. *Neuropsychologia* 2008; 46: 1743–1755.

39. M. L. Seghier. The angular gyrus: multiple functions and multiple subdivisions. *Neuroscientist* 2013; 19(1): 43–61.

40. H. M. Bonnici, F. R. Richter, Y. Yazar, J. S. Simons. Multimodal feature integration in the angular gyrus during episodic and semantic retrieval. *J Neurosci* 2016; 36(20): 5462–1571.

41. K. S. Graham, J. S. Simons, K. H. Pratt, K. Patterson, J. R. Hodges. Insights from semantic dementia on the relationship between episodic and semantic memory. *Neuropsychologia* 2000; 38: 313–324.

42. J. R. Hodges, K. Patterson, S. Oxbury, E. Funnell. Semantic dementia. Progressive fluent aphasia with temporal lobe atrophy. *Brain* 1992; 115: 1783–1806.

43. J. S. Simons, K. S. Graham, J. R. Hodges. Perceptual and semantic contributions to episodic memory: evidence from semantic dementia and Alzheimer's disease. *J Mem Lang* 2002; 47: 197–213.

44. B. Layton, R. Krikorian. Memory mechanisms of posttraumatic stress disorder. *J Neuropsychiatry Clin Neurosci* 2002; 14: 254–261.

45. D. de Quervain, L. Schwabe, B. Roozendaal. Stress, glucocorticoids and memory: implications for treating fear-related disorders. *Nat Rev Neurosci* 2017; 18: 7–19.

5

46. D. C. M. O'Doherty, K. M. Chitty, S. Saddiqui, M. R. Bennett, J. Lagopoulos. A systematic review and meta-analysis of magnetic resonance imaging measurement of structural volumes in posttraumatic stress disorder. *Psychiatry Res Neuroim* 2015; 232: 1–33.

47. T. M. Keane, R. T. Zimering, R. T. Caddell. A behavioral formulation of PTSD in Vietnam veterans. *Behav Ther (N Y)* 1985; 8: 9–12.

48. V. Rau, J. P. DeCola, M. S. Fanselow. Stress-induced enhancement of fear learning: an animal model of posttraumatic stress disorder. *Neurosci Biobehav Rev* 2005; 29: 1207–1223.

49. J. Baek, S. Lee, T. Cho et al. Neural circuits underlying a psychotherapeutic regimen for fear disorders. *Nature* 2019; 556(7744): 339–343.

National Neuroscience Curriculum Initiative online resources

This "stuff" is really cool: Mudit Kumar, *"A Journey Through Memories"*

<table>
<tr><td>**5.15**</td><td>**Fronto-Executive Functions**</td><td>**Angela C. Roberts and**
Trevor W. Robbins</td></tr>
</table>

OVERVIEW

The frontal lobes of the brain have often been associated with rather vague conclusions about their functions in both the healthy and diseased brain. However, recent research that utilises neuropsychological assessment of patients as well as functional neuroimaging in humans, and experimental studies of other mammalian species, has begun to elucidate their roles in what has been termed 'executive function' or 'cognitive control'. They have evolved in humans to occupy about a third of the entire cerebral cortex and are reciprocally connected to much of the rest of the brain. Their importance to psychiatry is that they have been implicated in virtually all forms of psychiatric disorder. The exact nature of their contribution to specific symptoms, however, is still to be determined.

5.15.1 What Is Executive Function?

Executive function is an umbrella term that encompasses the set of higher-order cognitive control processes which are necessary for optimal scheduling of complex sequences of behaviour, including attentional selection and resistance to interference, monitoring, behavioural inhibition, task switching, planning and decision making. It has been proposed that the construct of executive function should be considered as a multi-operational process by which multiple executive subprocesses work together to solve complex problems in an optimal manner (for review see Friedman and Miyake, 2017). Executive functions are important for navigating through nearly all of our daily activities. Individual differences in executive functions are associated with our academic and occupational functioning, interpersonal problems, substance use, physical health and mental health. Poor executive functioning predicts worry, rumination and poor use of adaptive emotion regulation, which are potent risk factors for psychopathology. Thus, not surprisingly, impairments in executive functioning (a 'dysexecutive syndrome') have been identified in most forms of psychopathology (for review see Snyder et al., 2015). Most disorders are associated with fairly uniform deficits across the different subprocesses of executive function, with

the largest effects being seen in schizophrenia, where it is associated with so-called 'hypofrontality'. Deficits are also seen however in depression, bipolar disorder, obsessive–compulsive disorder (OCD) and attention deficit hyperactivity disorder (ADHD). Effects are less clear in anxiety disorders but executive function deficits, specifically deficits in inhibiting competing responses (see Section 5.15.7), have been described in individuals with high trait anxiety and anxious worry, which is a risk factor for developing anxiety disorders and depression.

Executive dysfunction is generally linked to disorders of the frontal lobes, resulting for example from traumatic injury or stroke or from surgical removal of tumours or neurodegenerative diseases (e.g. Pick's disease, dementia with Lewy bodies and frontotemporal dementia). The classic frontal lobe injury case was that of the railway worker Phineas Gage who suffered an accident that destroyed part of his frontal lobes and changed his personality. However, many psychiatric disorders, including those mentioned above, also have more subtle pathologies of frontal lobe structures, which may be evident from neuroimaging as well as post-mortem studies.

This approximate correlation of executive functioning and the frontal lobes can lead to notions almost akin to phrenology, that this structure is a sort of 'centre' that mediates higher-order control over behaviour, but this would be a grossly oversimplified perspective. First of all, the frontal lobe and in particular the prefrontal cortex, the polymodal association cortex within the frontal lobes, is heterogeneous in structure (Figure 5.15.1). Traditionally, the prefrontal cortex has been divided into four main subregions, the dorsolateral, ventrolateral and ventromedial prefrontal cortex and the orbitofrontal cortex. Each of these subregions still contains a number of different areas with different cytoarchitectonic features, characterised by the shape, size and density of the neurons. These different areas almost certainly have different

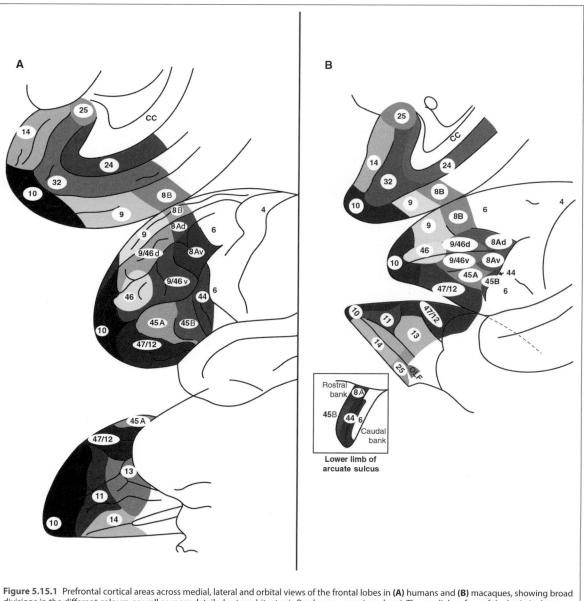

Figure 5.15.1 Prefrontal cortical areas across medial, lateral and orbital views of the frontal lobes in **(A)** humans and **(B)** macaques, showing broad divisions in the different colours, as well as more detailed cytoarchitectonic Brodmann areas (numbers). The medial surface of the brain is shown by upwards reflection. Abbreviations: CC, corpus callosum; OLF, olfactory sulcus. https://doi.org/10.1016/j.cortex.2011.07.002 with permission from Elsevier. Reproduced from Petrides et al. 2012. The prefrontal cortex: Comparative architectonic organization in the human and the macaque monkey brains. *Cortex* 48, 46–57.

functions and also work together in different ways via their distinct patterns of interconnections. The functions of some of these regions are described below. These regions also connect anatomically to many other brain regions and thus participate in many different networks. Some of these networks can be identified in functional imaging studies, such as the 'executive network', the 'default mode network' and the 'attention networks'. Finally, although it has been suggested that executive functioning corresponds simply to 'intelligence' as measured by standard intelligence quotient (IQ) tests, it appears that some aspects of executive functioning are more related to IQ than others and so it seems likely that there is diversity as well as unity in the executive function construct.

5.15.2 Measuring Executive Function and Issues of Diversity and Unity

The three most frequently studied executive functions are **response inhibition** (the ability to inhibit dominant, automatic or prepotent responses), **updating working memory representations** (the ability to monitor incoming information for relevance to the task at hand and then appropriately update by replacing old, no longer relevant information with newer, more relevant information) and **cognitive flexibility** (the ability to switch back and forth between tasks or mental sets).

To measure these functions, a number of different experimental tasks have been used, most commonly the n-back working memory task, verbal fluency, Stroop and Go–NoGo tasks (such as the stop-signal reaction time (SSRT) task), Trail Making Test, Wisconsin Card Sorting Test, Tower of London test of planning and the Iowa Gambling Task. Each of these tasks probably measures more than one component of executive functioning. The n-back task measures working memory and inhibition, the Stroop and the Go–NoGo tasks typically measure response inhibition and cognitive flexibility, the Trail Making Test measures set shifting and attentional monitoring and the Wisconsin Card Sorting Test taps particularly into cognitive flexibility as well as inhibition and basic learning and working memory functions.

Friedman et al. (2006) explored the interrelationships between three fundamental building blocks of executive function, updating working memory, response inhibition and cognitive flexibility using a set of nine tests (three for each function) in a large sample of monozygotic and dizygotic adult twins. They found that performance on the nine tests overall was significantly correlated, thus providing some evidence for unity of executive function (Figure 5.15.2). However, the intercorrelations were often quite small, although larger for those subgroups of tests measuring the same function, highlighting the diversity of executive functions and suggesting that they cannot be subsumed simply under one category. Furthermore, the different functions had different relationships with IQ test performance. Updating working memory was most related to IQ performance while cognitive flexibility and response inhibition were far less related. Additionally, while executive function shows high levels of heritability, cognitive flexibility is the only component that has significant relationships with environmental variance (Friedman and Miyake, 2017).

5.15.3 Prefrontal Cortex and Executive Function

In order to understand the role of the prefrontal cortex in executive control it is necessary to take account of its interactions with the rest of the brain (Figure 5.15.3), in particular the specialised processing modules of (i) the posterior cortex, including parietal (spatial attention) and inferotemporal (feature attention) areas, where it helps to mediate such functions as top-down control over attention; (ii) the language processing modules such as Wernicke's area, specialised in the comprehension of speech, interacting with Broca's speech and production area, which lies within the posterior ventrolateral region;

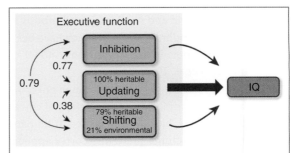

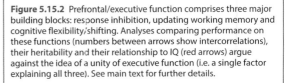

Figure 5.15.2 Prefrontal/executive function comprises three major building blocks: response inhibition, updating working memory and cognitive flexibility/shifting. Analyses comparing performance on these functions (numbers between arrows show intercorrelations), their heritability and their relationship to IQ (red arrows) argue against the idea of a unity of executive function (i.e. a single factor explaining all three). See main text for further details.

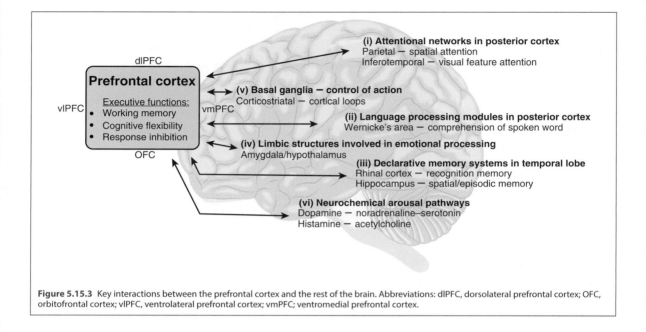

Figure 5.15.3 Key interactions between the prefrontal cortex and the rest of the brain. Abbreviations: dlPFC, dorsolateral prefrontal cortex; OFC, orbitofrontal cortex; vlPFC, ventrolateral prefrontal cortex; vmPFC; ventromedial prefrontal cortex.

(iii) the declarative memory systems in the temporal lobes including the rhinal cortex (recognition memory) and hippocampus (scene/episodic memory), especially implicated in memory retrieval. In addition, the prefrontal cortex interacts with subcortical structures such as (iv) the limbic structures involved in emotional processing, including the amygdala and hypothalamus (and brainstem centres of autonomic control) – this is where emotion regulation takes place (see also Section 5.10 on emotion); (v) the basal ganglia, which are involved in the higher-order control of action; and (vi) the neurochemical 'arousal' systems of the reticular core of the brain, including monoamine and cholinergic cell groups in the midbrain and hindbrain, some of which have been implicated for example in the 'helplessness model' of depression (Maier et al., 2006).

The following subsections provide examples of some of the major processes in which the prefrontal cortex has been implicated, based on evidence in humans and monkeys in which the prefrontal cortex appears similarly organised. Rodents (rats and mice) have been much used in experimental studies, especially in terms of genetic and disease models. However, the organisation of the prefrontal cortex in rodents is markedly different from that of humans and non-human primates, and thus interpreting the relevance of rodent functional studies of

the prefrontal cortex for humans needs care. For the sake of brevity, we focus on studies in monkeys and humans. The reader is referred to Dalley et al. (2004) for a review of evidence from studies of prefrontal cortical function in rodents and to Stuss and Knight (2013) for a comprehensive review of prefrontal cortical function.

5.15.4 Working Memory

Lesions of various regions of the dorsal and lateral prefrontal cortex impair delayed response tasks that require monkeys to remember, over a brief delay, spatial, object or proprioceptive information (Figure 5.15.4). In all cases there is a **sample** stage during which the monkey is (i) shown a peanut being hidden in one of two locations (spatial version), (ii) shown a peanut being hidden under one of two objects (object version) or (iii) required to press a lever one or five times (proprioceptive version). After a brief delay of a few seconds, in the **choice** stage of the task, monkeys have to (i) choose the spatial location of the food reward that they have just seen hidden, (ii) choose the object under which the food is hidden or (iii) make the same response that they have just made, that is, one or five lever presses. (There is some evidence that different regions of the prefrontal cortex impair different sensory versions of the delayed response task, but this remains controversial.) Prefrontal cortical lesions do not impair the

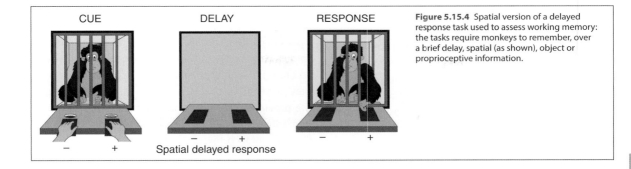

CUE   DELAY   RESPONSE

Spatial delayed response

Figure 5.15.4 Spatial version of a delayed response task used to assess working memory: the tasks require monkeys to remember, over a brief delay, spatial (as shown), object or proprioceptive information.

ability of the monkey to choose the correct response if there is no delay. Similar impairments in spatial delayed response (and n-back) performance have been seen in humans with damage to the dorsal prefrontal cortex and brain functional imaging studies have highlighted the dorsolateral prefrontal cortex as a significant node in the executive network of structures supporting spatial and verbal working memory.

Recording of neurons in dorsal and lateral regions of the prefrontal cortex in monkeys while they perform variations of these working memory tasks has shown some neurons are active during the delay period of the spatial and object versions of the delayed response task, as if they are keeping information about the spatial location or object 'on line' or 'in mind' when it is no longer present in the external environment. Different neurons show spatial and object selectivity. Other neurons are active specifically during the presentation of the specific cue, such as a specific spatial location or object, but not during the delay when the cue is no longer present. Still others become active towards the end of the delay period in advance of the action and are related to the specifics of the action. In the case of spatial delayed response, this activity is related to a response towards a specific location in space. It has been shown that cue-specific, delay-specific and response-specific neurons, which are all coding for the same location in space, reside in a single column of neurons running across the different layers of the cortex, from layer 1 superficially to the deepest layer 6, with adjacent columns containing neurons coding for a slightly different spatial location (Goldman-Rakic, 2002).

Subsequently it has been shown that neurons which can 'hold' information on line during a delayed response task can also be found in other association regions, including the posterior parietal and inferotemporal cortex. However, in the case of the inferotemporal cortex it has been shown that neurons only hold object information on line as long as there are no intervening distracting stimuli, whereas neurons in the PFC can hold information on line in the presence of distracting information. These findings have led to the proposal that the activity in neurons in the prefrontal cortex during the delay period could be thought of as representing active attention.

Human theories of working memory include the components of the 'articulatory loop' (short-term verbal memory rehearsal buffer), the visuospatial scratchpad (short-term visual memory) and a central executive (Baddeley and Hitch, 2007), which coordinates these buffers and serves to guide goal-directed behaviours and planning. Typical tests in humans include the n-back task whereby subjects have to keep on line items occurring several 'n' presentations back, the Cambridge Neuropsychological Test Automated Battery (CANTAB) spatial working memory task, where subjects have to search for reward tokens in an array of boxes on a touch-sensitive screen, and the Tower of London planning task, in which subjects have to reach a goal arrangement of discs from an initial starting position, in a minimum number of moves.

Patients with schizophrenia are especially impaired on working memory tasks and this has been related to underactivity and pathology of the dorsolateral prefrontal cortex. This deficit usually becomes apparent when the difficulty or 'load' of the working memory task is enhanced. Thus, patients may exhibit increased activity of the prefrontal cortex during performance of easier versions of the task in relation to controls, but hypoactivity when the task is made more difficult, perhaps because they cannot engage with it.

5.15.5 Attention

The prefrontal cortex has also been shown to be part of a distributed neuronal network involved in spatial and feature attention (see also Section 5.12). This was illustrated nicely in a positron emission tomography study in which subjects were required to attend to one of three different perceptual features – colour, form or movement (selective attention conditions) or all three (divided attention) – of a series of visual images that were presented consecutively, each one for a very short period of time (Figure 5.15.5). The ventrolateral prefrontal cortex was activated more in the selective, compared to the divided-attention condition, alongside increased activity in the visuocortical region involved in processing that specific visual information, for example the inferotemporal cortex for form or area V4 for colour. In contrast, the dorsolateral prefrontal cortex was activated most when subjects attended to all three features in the divided-attention condition (Corbetta et al., 1991).

Thus, the prefrontal cortex appears necessary for attending selectively to stimuli in the external world. In this sense it exerts executive control over the sensory input to posterior cortical regions and participates in the attentional networks. This capacity of the prefrontal cortex to direct attention externally may be related to working memory, which can be thought of as internalised attention to memory representations. For possible applications to ADHD see Section 5.12.5.

5.15.6 Cognitive Flexibility

A classic deficit in cognitive flexibility associated with damage to the prefrontal cortex is the failure to inhibit previously relevant rules (or attentional sets) governing behaviour, shown by frontal lesioned patients on the Wisconsin Card Sorting Test, who, having learned to sort a pack of cards according to a particular dimension (e.g. colour), are unable to then switch to sorting the cards according to a different dimension (e.g. shape). Instead, they perseverate, that is, persist in sorting according to the previously correct dimension. This impairment is primarily associated with damage to lateral regions of the prefrontal cortex. Monkeys (New World marmosets) with localised lesions of the cell bodies of neurons in the ventrolateral prefrontal cortex are also impaired at set shifting between two arbitrary visual form dimensions, 'shapes' and 'lines' (Dias et al., 1996). Here, animals have to learn which of two compound stimuli, composed of white lines superimposed over blue shapes, is associated with reward, a task derived from the animal-learning literature and which is presented on a touch-sensitive computer screen (Figure 5.15.6A). Over a series of discriminations involving new compound stimuli, composed of shapes and lines, they learn to always select a white line, regardless of the blue shape it is paired with (intradimensional shifts). At the time of the attentional shift, however, blue shapes become relevant, and the animal must learn to shift attention towards blue shapes (extradimensional shift) and learn which blue shape is rewarded, thus requiring a shift of attentional set. This version of attentional set shifting has been used successfully in humans and identifies activity in the ventrolateral prefrontal cortex associated with the shift. It has also been used to identify set-shifting impairments in a range of patients with neurodegenerative as well as psychiatric disorders. Moreover, resting-state activity in specific neural connections

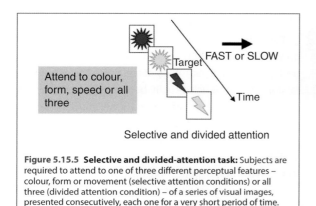

Selective and divided attention

Figure 5.15.5 Selective and divided-attention task: Subjects are required to attend to one of three different perceptual features – colour, form or movement (selective attention conditions) or all three (divided attention condition) – of a series of visual images, presented consecutively, each one for a very short period of time.

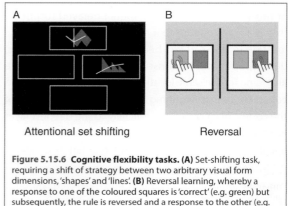

Attentional set shifting   Reversal

Figure 5.15.6 Cognitive flexibility tasks. (A) Set-shifting task, requiring a shift of strategy between two arbitrary visual form dimensions, 'shapes' and 'lines'. **(B)** Reversal learning, whereby a response to one of the coloured squares is 'correct' (e.g. green) but subsequently, the rule is reversed and a response to the other (e.g. purple) is correct.

between the ventrolateral prefrontal cortex and the caudate nucleus has been shown to correlate positively with performance on the extradimensional shift in human patients with OCD and controls (Vaghi et al., 2017).

The impairment in attentional set shifting is to be contrasted with that in reversal learning (Figure 5.15.6B), where the same visual objects are presented to the marmoset, but their reward status shifts; thus, following a period where stimulus A is rewarded and B punished, stimulus B suddenly becomes the consistently rewarded stimulus and A is now punished. The ability to exhibit cognitive flexibility and shift in this reversal-learning task is not dependent on the ventrolateral prefrontal cortex, but the orbitofrontal cortex. Patients with frontal lobe dementia, where the initial pathology can include hypoperfusion of the orbitofrontal cortex, are impaired in reversal learning. Moreover, patients with OCD, as well as their first-degree relatives who do not have a clinical diagnosis, have reduced activity in an orbitofrontoparietal cortex network (Chamberlain et al., 2008). This is termed an endophenotype, as it implies that deficient activity in this region, leading to cognitive inflexibility, may contribute to OCD symptoms (see Section 9.6 for more on OCD).

5.15.7 Cognitive Control (Including Inhibitory Control)

The Stroop task (naming the actual colour of ink a word is presented in when the word itself may connote a different colour) is a classic test of conflict which requires suppression of the automatic tendency to read the word in order for its (conflicting) colour to be named instead (Figure 5.15.7A). Experiments in healthy human volunteers have shown that efficient performance of this task involves an interaction between the anterior cingulate cortex and dorsolateral prefrontal cortex. Using various neuroimaging methods it has been shown that the anterior cingulate cortex becomes active during task performance and signals to other areas, such as the dorsolateral prefrontal cortex, the existence of conflict, which is then resolved by top-down activation of the latter in order to guide behaviour according to the rules of the task – in this case, reporting the colour of the ink. To do this, the dorsolateral prefrontal cortex presumably exerts a relative weakening or inhibition of the prepotent reading tendency, which allows facilitation of the correct alternative response strategy (reviewed in Miller and Cohen, 2001).

Other examples of such cognitive control can be observed in the classic delayed-gratification, Go–NoGo and SSRT tasks, which are often used to quantify impulsivity in psychiatric disorders such as ADHD, OCD and drug addiction. Impulsivity can be defined simply as the uncontrolled urge to respond prematurely without foresight. However, it has several different manifestations, including impulsive action and impulsive choice. The latter is measured in a classic delayed-gratification paradigm in which subjects are given the choice between small immediate rewards and large delayed rewards, impulsive choice being reflected in the choice of the small immediate reward. For impulsive action, the SSRT task requires inhibition of an action that has already been initiated. Briefly, subjects are encouraged to respond as quickly as possible in a choice reaction time task but then have to inhibit responding on certain trials when a warning 'beep' sound is presented (Figure 5.15.7B). Measures can be obtained not only of the 'Go' reaction time but also of the 'Stop' reaction time, the latter measuring behavioural inhibition and becoming longer the more impulsive the subject.

Patients with damage to the frontal lobes exhibit specific problems in the SSRT measure; the greater the volume of damage to the right inferior frontal cortex, the longer is their SSRT – although they have no impairments in 'Go' reaction time. Further work using functional neuroimaging has defined a network including this region and other cortical areas such as the anterior cingulate and presupplementary cortex as well as the basal ganglia, which mediate control over actions (Aron et al., 2014).

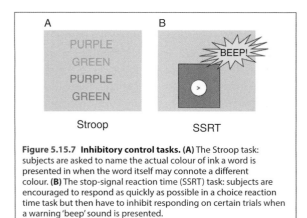

Figure 5.15.7 Inhibitory control tasks. (A) The Stroop task: subjects are asked to name the actual colour of ink a word is presented in when the word itself may connote a different colour. **(B)** The stop-signal reaction time (SSRT) task: subjects are encouraged to respond as quickly as possible in a choice reaction time task but then have to inhibit responding on certain trials when a warning 'beep' sound is presented.

Recent work has shown that some drugs that are used in the treatment of ADHD modulate activity in this pathway, alongside improvement in performance of the SSRT task.

5.15.8 Decision Making

Decision making is a complex form of cognition that involves several executive components including working memory, cognitive flexibility and inhibitory control – and is markedly impaired in most severe psychiatric disorders, including depression, bipolar disorder and schizophrenia, as well as in drug addiction. The importance of the frontal lobes in decision making was first emphasised by the work of Damasio and colleagues (Bechara et al., 2000) using the Iowa Gambling Task, in which volunteers are asked to select from four packs of cards in order to maximise the amount of money they can win (Figure 5.15.8). This task was invented to capture real-life decision making in the laboratory, after Damasio's observation of the disastrous consequences (e.g. bankruptcy, gambling, addiction and divorce) that large frontal lesions (that included the ventromedial prefrontal and orbitofrontal cortices) had on everyday decision making for patients (such as the patient 'EVR').

The packs of cards are associated with different reward–punishment payoffs such that some packs lead to large rewards but occasionally very large punishments whereas other packs result in moderate rewards and only occasional small punishments. Hence, after sampling the contingencies on the basis of trial-and-error learning, the most profitable outcomes are to play with the 'safer' cards. Patients with large frontal lesions, however, fail to use this strategy and persist with choosing the 'risky' packs – an impairment also seen in patients with drug addiction. They do not seem to develop 'hunches' about which packs are risky, and Damasio has related this to their inability to make contact with their 'feelings' associated with the cards through bodily feedback via cortical structures such as the insula (Bechara et al., 2000).

There has been a good deal of interest in determining the precise neuroanatomical substrates of decision making within the frontal lobes, as performance of the Iowa Gambling Task has been shown to recruit other regions besides the ventromedial prefrontal and orbitofrontal cortices, including dorsolateral prefrontal cortex. This may represent the additional functions of learning and memory that are required to perform the task effectively. In another test (the Cambridge Gambling Task), the odds of reward and punishment are presented more explicitly without the need for learning, and performance has been shown to depend quite specifically on the ventromedial prefrontal and orbitofrontal cortices, as well as on input structures, such as the insula.

5.15.9 Social and 'Hot' Cognition

Whereas many of the building blocks of executive functions such as working memory and cognitive control can be seen as relatively abstract ('cold') abilities devoid of the stresses of everyday life, it is apparent from the previous subsection that complex tasks such as decision making, with contingencies of rewards and punishments, are subject to much greater motivational demands.

This is also of course true of the even more complex processes involved in social interactions, including moral decision making, empathising and the reading of other's intentions ('Theory of Mind'). These functions are also the province of prefrontal cortex networks with other structures comprising the 'social brain' (such as the paracingulate cortex (area 32), the temporal pole and the superior temporal sulcus). It is still a matter of controversy as to whether new principles of function may be required to explain these social capacities over and above core executive abilities. However, there is some evidence that social functions are mediated by specific regions of the

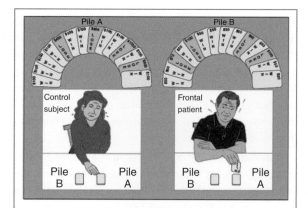

Figure 5.15.8 Decision making: the Iowa Gambling Task. Subjects are presented with four piles of cards, two of which are associated with varying probabilities of low rewards and punishments, represented by Pile B, and two piles with varying levels of high rewards but also high punishments, represented by Pile A. Controls develop hunches about the riskiness of choosing Pile A whilst patients with frontal lobe damage do not.

prefrontal cortex, especially the medial prefrontal cortex, which has been, for example, implicated in 'mentalising' functions, such as thinking about the self. Understanding in more detail the neural networks underlying social functions may be a major goal of the next period of research (for a review of current understanding see Rilling and Sanfey, 2011). These networks can include interactions between different regions of the prefrontal cortex, as in the interactions between the orbitofrontal and dorsolateral prefrontal cortices involved in moral dilemmas, in which utilitarian decision making is pitted against moral decision making. This is tested in the so-called 'trolley task', where one has to decide actively whether to sacrifice one life in order to save five lives. The complexities of social decision making have been shown to be relevant to such disorders as autism (with hypothetical deficits in the Theory of Mind) and depression (pathological ruminations about social relationships) as well as psychopathy and borderline personality disorders (e.g. failures in empathising).

5.15.10 Translating Neuroscience to New Treatments

The frontal lobes exert profound influences over cognition and behaviour through a variety of psychological processes. They are implicated in virtually every form of mental illness and so a major goal of future research is to identify suitable forms of treatment. These may include pharmacological, surgical and cognitive–behavioural therapy (CBT). Current drug therapies include methylphenidate as used in ADHD, which affects executive function by boosting catecholaminergic modulation of frontostriatal function. Another neuromodulatory form of treatment is via repetitive transcranial magnetic stimulation, which has been applied to the dorsolateral prefrontal cortex in patients with treatment-resistant depression.

Although training to enhance working memory has not yet been shown definitively to have beneficial effects, for example in schizophrenia, it is possible that future cognitive training methods will eventually be successful. Furthermore, it has been shown that when CBT has been successful in depression it has restored activity in the dorsolateral prefrontal cortex.

Conclusions and Outstanding Questions

The role of different regions of the prefrontal cortex in a range of key cognitive abilities and their integration with emotional and motivational processes that enable adaptive decision making is gradually becoming determined from multidisciplinary and also cross-species studies. These abilities become impaired in many psychiatric and neurological disorders and these impairments probably contribute directly to their symptomology. Hence, the prefrontal cortex is one of the most important brain regions for understanding mental health disorders.

Outstanding Questions

- We need to better understand the precise evolutionary and functional relationships of the human prefrontal cortex with that of other animals.

- We need to better understand how the prefrontal cortex contributes to the workings of discrete functional neural networks involving other brain regions.

- We need to better understand how the functions of prefrontal cortex are affected by such factors as stress, mediated by neurochemical modulatory systems such as provided by the monoamines (dopamine, serotonin and noradrenaline) as well as acetylcholine and histamine.

- We need a greater understanding of how existing treatments affect frontal functioning, so that better ones may be developed.

REFERENCES

Aron AR, Robbins TW, Poldrack RA (2014). Inhibition and the right inferior frontal cortex: one decade on. *Trends Cogn Sci* 18: 177–185.

Baddeley A, Hitch G (2007). The past, present and future of working memory. In Osaka N, Robert H, Logie RH, D'Esposito M (eds.), *The Cognitive Neuroscience of Working Memory*. Oxford University Press.

Bechara A, Damasio H, Damasio AR (2000). Emotion, decision making and the orbitofrontal cortex. *Cereb Cortex* 10: 295–307.

Chamberlain SR, Menzies L, Hampshire A et al. (2008). Orbitofrontal dysfunction in patients with obsessive–compulsive disorder and their unaffected relatives. *Science* 321: 421–422.

Corbetta M, Miezin FM, Dobmeyer S, Shulman GL, Petersen SE (1991). Selective and divided attention during visual discriminations of shape, color, and speed: functional anatomy by positron emission tomography. *J Neurosci* 11: 2383–2402

Dalley JW, Cardinal RN, Robbins TW (2004). Prefrontal executive and cognitive functions in rodents: neural and neurochemical substrates. *Neurosci Biobehav Rev* 28: 771–784.

Dias R, Robbins TW, Roberts AC (1996). Dissociation in prefrontal cortex of affective and attentional shifts. *Nature* 380: 69–72.

Friedman NP, Miyake A (2017). Unity and diversity of executive functions: individual differences as a window on cognitive structure. *Cortex* 86: 186–204.

Friedman NP, Miyake A, Corley RP et al. (2006). Not all executive functions are related to intelligence. *Psychol Sci* 17: 172–179.

Goldman-Rakic PS (2002). Chapter 33 The "psychic cell" of Ramón y Cajal. *Prog Brain Res* 136: 427–434.

Maier SF, Amat J, Baratta MV, Paul E, Watkins LR (2006). Behavioral control, the medial prefrontal cortex, and resilience. *Dialogues Clin Neurosci* 8: 397–406.

Miller EK, Cohen JD (2001). An integrative theory of prefrontal cortex function. *Annu Rev Neurosci* 24: 167–202.

Rilling JK, Sanfey AG (2011). The neuroscience of social decision-making. *Annu Rev Psychol* 62: 23–48.

Snyder HR, Miyake A, Hankin BL (2015). Advancing understanding of executive function impairments and psychopathology: bridging the gap between clinical and cognitive approaches. *Front Psychol* 6: 328.

Stuss D, Knight R, eds. (2013). *Principles of Frontal Lobe Function*, 2nd ed. Oxford University Press.

Vaghi MM, Vértes PE, Kitzbichler MG, Apergis-Schoute AM, et al. (2017) Specific frontostriatal circuits for impaired cognitive flexibility and goal-directed planning in obsessive–compulsive disorder: evidence from resting-state functional connectivity. *Biol psychiatry*, 81: 708–717.

National Neuroscience Curriculum Initiative online resources

This "stuff" is really cool: Austin Blum, *"Why I Can't Stop"* on impulsivity

Markus Boeckle and Nicola S. Clayton

5.16 Empathy and Theory of Mind

OVERVIEW

In order to comprehend the intricacies of human cognition and social interaction, it is crucial to explore the underlying cognitive processes that support them. This chapter delves into one of the core cognitive abilities – the 'theory of mind' (ToM), which allows individuals to infer the thoughts, beliefs and intentions of others. ToM plays a vital role in understanding the complexities of social interaction and contributes to our ability to empathise and communicate effectively. Within the context of psychiatry, investigating ToM impairments is particularly important as they are associated with several mental disorders, such as autism spectrum and schizophrenia. By examining these impairments, researchers aim to uncover the specific neuronal networks and cognitive mechanisms that underlie social cognitive abilities, as well as identifying commonalities and differences between patient groups. Gaining a deeper understanding of ToM and its role in various disorders will not only provide valuable insight into the complexities of human cognition but also guide the development of more effective interventions and treatments for affected individuals.

5.16.1 The Evolution of Social Intelligence

Many animals and most primates live in social groups. According to Jolly [1], it is the ability to survive the dynamics of a complex social world that has shaped primate intelligence. Dunbar [2] has further suggested that these cognitive affordances of living in groups lead to an increase in relative brain size of the neocortex. Presumably, it is a critical aspect of complex social life to keep track of who did what to you, where and when; and even more so to use this information to predict the actions and intentions of other individuals in your social network. The complexities of social life in some primates have led to the ability to understand and reason about the minds of other individuals, which is called 'theory of mind' (ToM). This ability enables some animal species and humans to understand and manipulate their conspecifics with their so-called Machiavellian intelligence [3].

Deceiving, manipulating and other forms of complex social interactions pose high cognitive demands. To use these abilities, it is important to differentiate between groups of individuals that differ in aspects of social relationships, including friend versus foe, kin versus non-kin, dominants versus subordinates and young versus old. Furthermore, it is not only necessary to remember and keep track of the dynamics between yourself and your relationship with others but also other individuals' social relationships (third-party relationships). Memorising and acting upon social dynamics between individuals does not necessarily require an ability to understand and reason about the minds of other individuals. It might be sufficient to rely on behavioural cues to cope with these social dynamics. For instance, it might be enough for another individual to respond to a conspecific's change of gaze direction up into the air without having a concept of the mental state of the other individual. It suffices to run to safety merely because of the change of gaze without mentalising that the content of the other's mind might be a 'predator flying above'. But a number of researchers, including Whiten and Byrne, have argued that primates living in complex societies have exactly this ToM ability [3]. Clayton and colleagues have argued that selective pressures of complex social life also apply to other animals that form social networks, such as different species of crows [4].

5.16.2 Theory of Mind

In 1978, Premack and Woodruff [5] coined the term theory of mind to refer to the ability to ascribe mental states to other individuals. The authors described an experiment in which a language-trained chimpanzee attributed and acted upon intentions of a human experimenter. The main difficulty with research and theories on ToM is differentiating it from simpler explanations based on associative learning and stimulus generalisation alone [6]. Additionally, ToM is a concept that is based on unobservable mental states, which themselves are inferred from behaviour. Humans do not know what other individuals think but by rule of similarity can infer similar mental states in other humans and verbally communicate about these. When researchers have to reason about mental states of preverbal kids or other species, it is not possible to infer these mental states via language. For this reason, it is essential to establish scientific methods that can distinguish between responses to behaviours of others and responses to mental states. It has been argued [7] that mental states intervene between cause and effect on a cognitive level. An illustrative example of such mental states in animals is tool use. New Caledonian crows have been shown to select and use tools to retrieve food. In order to do so, it is essential for crows to hold and use information on what kind of tools are currently available, what kind of tools they will need in the future and what kind of tool was previously helpful in the specific situation in the past. When interacting with another animal, an animal will respond to mental states rather than simpler non-cognitive mechanisms when it is more economic and effective. In the example of running for cover, it might be more economic and effective to respond to the slightest movement of a conspecific's head. In more complex behaviours like tactical deception, however, it will be

more economic and effective to reason about the mental states and intentions of the other individual.

It was proposed by Premack [8] that three levels of ToM can be discerned with increasing complexity:

- perceptual ToM
- motivational ToM
- informational ToM.

Perceptual ToM is related to the ability to follow the direction of another individual's gaze, potentially gaining knowledge about the attentional state of the other, or what the other is seeing. To follow and understand gaze directions may be particularly important for individuals living in social groups. While directing the gaze somewhere might potentially convey information about the internal state of the looking individual, it does not necessarily imply that the observer gains knowledge about the internal state of the looker. A number of different species are sensitive to gaze direction of other individuals and this might hint that ToM is utilised in these species. Still, gaze following might have simpler underlying mechanisms than ToM-like associative learning. For example, Povinelli and colleagues [9] conducted an experiment with chimpanzees that involved an experimenter holding a food treat. The chimpanzees were able to beg the experimenter for food, when he was looking at them, but knew not to beg him for food when his back was turned away from them. However, the chimpanzees were not able to inhibit begging when a blindfold covered the experimenter's eyes compared to a blindfold covering his mouth. Thus, they were not able to functionally differentiate between the trainer seeing and not seeing, based on whether or not the eyes were covered.

Motivational ToM is the ability to understand the desires, goals and intentions of the other individual. For example, Premack and Woodruff [5] conducted an experiment in which Sarah the chimpanzee was presented with a series of pictures depicting a human experimenter encountering a problem; for instance, opening a door. Sarah had to point to the correct picture containing the object that would be needed to solve the problem. The authors argued that this provided evidence for the chimpanzee's understanding of the intention of the human experimenter and thus his motivation. At issue here is whether simpler explanations are more parsimonious, namely that Sarah could have been reading changes in behaviour directly rather than needing to account for changes in the human's motivation and mind [10], a point which we will come back to a little later in this discussion.

Informational ToM is the ability to understand the beliefs and knowledge of others. Being able to differentiate between individuals who guess where some food might be hidden and those that know where it is actually hidden might prove important for various animals in their social life. Povinelli and colleagues [11] tested this concept when they presented chimpanzees with two human experimenters, a 'Guesser' and a 'Knower'. In the training sessions, the Knower was actively baiting (putting food into) containers in an experimental room, while the Guesser was not in the room. Screens were used to ensure the chimpanzees could see who was doing the baiting, but not which containers they baited. After all the containers were baited, the Guesser re-entered the room and both Knower and Guesser pointed to one of the containers. The chimpanzees received a reward only if they pointed towards the container the Knower pointed towards. In contrast to training sessions, the Guesser was left in the same room as the Knower during testing sessions, but had a bucket placed over their head. After the first testing trials, almost all the chimpanzees chose the Knower over the Guesser. In the first two test trials, however, they chose randomly. The fact that the chimpanzees failed to immediately transfer their predictions from the training to the testing conditions is critical. It suggests that the animals learned to choose the trainer without the bucket over his/her head instead of attributing knowledge to the Knower, an ability that should be spontaneous, not learned over time.

5.16.3 Development of Theory of Mind in Human Children

It has been shown that 13-month-old children, when presented with interactions between individuals on screen, respond to **violations of expectancy** (where what they expect to happen next does not happen) [12]. Typically, this is measured by using eye trackers to record direction of gaze and duration of looking at specific areas of the screen. At 18 months, children respond to false beliefs of interaction partners with anticipatory gaze direction [13]; for instance, when interaction partners search in the wrong place infants show a different gaze

pattern than during trials when they search in the right place. It is unclear, though, whether these early responses to ToM tasks are proof of a full development of socio-cognitive ability. At roughly 2 years of age, children start recognising themselves in the mirror [14] and, at the same time, begin to establish an understanding of emotions in others [15]. Ascribing mental states to one's self and others is not only related to actual situations, like thinking that someone is angry or happy, but can also be about beliefs about other persons' beliefs (second-order beliefs). An example of this is used in the well-known false-belief task, in which Sally stores her marble in the basket (see Figure 5.16.1). Later Anne comes and takes it out of the basket and puts it into the box. If children above the age of 3 years are then asked where Sally thinks the marble is, they will respond correctly that she will search at the place she left them – namely in the basket – thus ascribing to Sally a false belief [16] (Figure 5.16.2). Children under 3 years old cannot differentiate between their own knowledge and the knowledge of Sally and respond incorrectly that she will search at the place where Anne put it (where they themselves know it is). Even more complex intention and belief inferences are developed later in life at around 7–8 years, such as interpreting faux pas [17] (see Figure 5.16.2).

5.16.4 Theory of Mind in Patients with Autism Spectrum Disorder

Not all children develop the social and cognitive abilities needed for different aspects of ToM. Patients with autism show significant difficulties during social interactions, impaired verbal and non-verbal communicative abilities, reduced imagination and restricted interests and repetitive behaviour. Typically, these symptoms develop in the first 2 years but can already be present within the first 2 days after birth. The symptom onset thus coincides with the developmental stages when certain abilities necessary for ToM usually develop. Individuals with autism show reduced anticipatory behaviour during early development. There is a large body of literature that shows deficits in various abilities, including gaze following and gaze interpretation as well as joint attention – shared focus of two individuals on the same object [18]. Symptom severity differs considerably between individuals, which is why it is classed as a spectrum disorder. See Section 9.1.2 for more on the neurocognitive basis of autism.

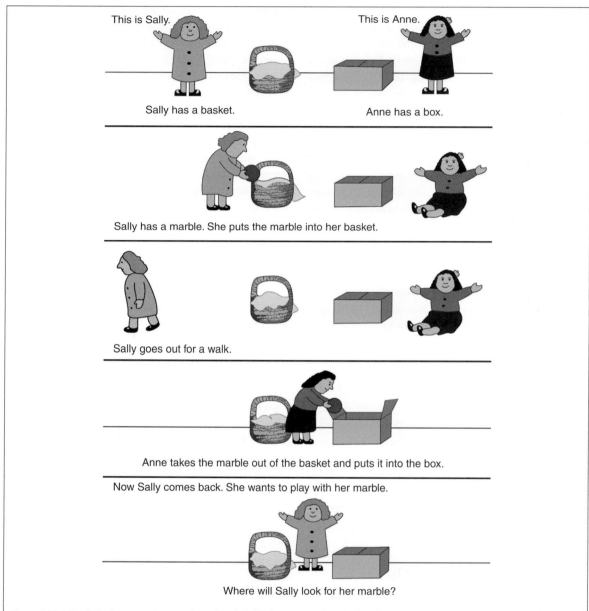

This is Sally.   This is Anne.

Sally has a basket.   Anne has a box.

Sally has a marble. She puts the marble into her basket.

Sally goes out for a walk.

Anne takes the marble out of the basket and puts it into the box.

Now Sally comes back. She wants to play with her marble.

Where will Sally look for her marble?

Figure 5.16.1 The Sally–Anne experiment, a classic false-belief task, is commonly used to assess the theory of mind development in children. In this task, Sally, one of the characters in the experiment, is shown placing a marble in a basket and then leaving the room. Meanwhile, Anne, another character, moves the marble from the basket to a box. The crucial point is that Sally is unaware of this change in the marble's location. Children participating in the experiment are then asked a critical question: 'Where will Sally look for her marble when she comes back?' The response options typically include the correct answer (the box, where the marble is actually located) and the false-belief answer (the basket, where Sally last saw the marble). By examining the children's responses, researchers can gain insights into their understanding of false beliefs and their ability to attribute mental states to others. The Sally–Anne experiment has been instrumental in advancing our understanding of the theory of mind development and the cognitive processes involved in recognising and reasoning about others' false beliefs.

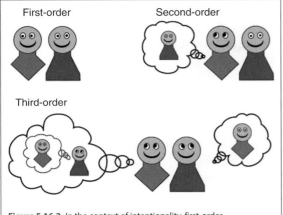

First-order   Second-order

Third-order

Figure 5.16.2 In the context of intentionality, first-order intentionality refers to an individual's ability to understand oneself as a distinct individual with beliefs, desires and intentions. It encompasses self-awareness and self-referential cognition. Second-order intentionality takes intentionality a step further by involving beliefs about others, recognising that others also possess beliefs, desires and intentions. This level of intentionality allows for the understanding of other minds and the ability to attribute mental states to others. Third-order intentionality builds upon second-order intentionality and involves having beliefs about the beliefs of others. It entails recognising that individuals not only have beliefs but also have beliefs about the beliefs of others. This higher level of intentionality enables individuals to engage in metacognitive processes, such as thinking about others' thoughts and intentions and taking perspective. Understanding these different levels of intentionality provides insights into the complex nature of human cognition, social interactions and the capacity for mental state attribution.

5.16.5 Theory of Mind in Patients with Schizophrenia

Studies demonstrating social cognitive impairments in patients with autism have led to the hypothesis that there are specific neuronal networks, which underlie cognitive abilities and processes supporting social interactions. Important mental illnesses with demonstrated impairments in ToM, for instance, include schizophrenia. ToM abnormalities can lead to positive and negative symptoms in the domains of willed action, self-monitoring and monitoring the intentions of others [19] but can also lead to over-mentalising [20]. In a meta-analysis Sprong and colleagues [21] showed that ToM performance across various tasks in patients with schizophrenia is below that of healthy controls (effect size: Cohen's $d = -1.1255$) with no other moderating effects like age, gender or intelligence quotient (IQ). Patients with schizophrenia in remission are less impaired than those currently undergoing an episode, compared to the control group (Cohen's $d = -0.692$). It remains unclear whether ToM impairments in patients with schizophrenia are caused by the symptoms of the disorder or are based on general impairments in cognitive abilities [21]. It appears that social cognitive impairments in schizophrenia can have state and trait-like components, which might explain the incomplete remission of ToM abilities during symptom-free periods [22]. Furthermore, mentalising as a more general ability under which ToM is categorised is ranked fourth within 22 cognitive impairments listed as affected by schizophrenia [23]. This would support the interpretation that schizophrenia does not afflict ToM specifically but cognitive abilities in general. In comparison, Brüne and Bodenstein [24] support the idea that there seems to be a specific ToM impairment in schizophrenia patients. Individuals with high genetic risk of developing schizophrenia as well as schizotypal individuals (i.e. people with

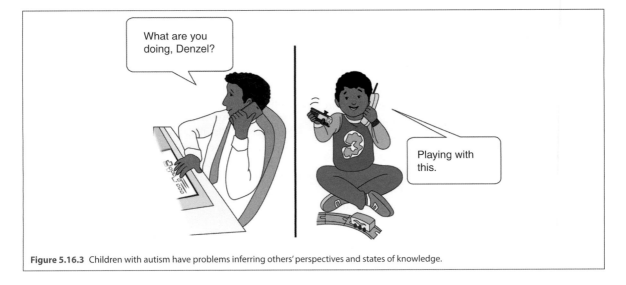

Figure 5.16.3 Children with autism have problems inferring others' perspectives and states of knowledge.

positive schizophrenia symptoms but not the severity of schizophrenia) show smaller but still observable deficits in mentalising and ToM [25, 26]. Interestingly, no differences between task presentation or presentation mode (verbal or non-verbal test) were found in individuals with schizophrenia according to the meta-analysis of Sprong and colleagues [21]. All these studies indicate that some symptoms in schizophrenia correlate with and are potentially caused by ToM deficits hampering social cognition. The underlying impaired cognitive mechanisms might specifically be a ToM-related neuronal network or a more general disruption of meta-cognitive abilities. In addition, impaired ToM may cause dysregulated views of the self, emotions and third-party-attributions as secondary effects or sequelae.

A meta-analysis [27] comparing adults with autism and schizophrenia found no difference between mentalising impairments in several cognitive–linguistic tasks including the Strange Stories and the Faux Pas tests (see the glossary), and in emotional tasks such as the Emotion Recognition from the Eyes test. Individuals with ToM deficits struggle to interpret double bluffs, figures of speech, jokes, lies, misunderstandings, persuading, pretending, sarcasm and white lies, but have less difficulty in the physical stories that do not need any understanding of second-order intentions. Similarly, recognising emotions based on facial expressions and understanding faux pas is hampered with ToM deficits. The lack of difference between autism and schizophrenia on these tasks suggests a partial, common deficit in both patient groups. Still, the psychometric tools might not be sensitive enough to differentiate genuine differences in the impairments in these two patient groups and might not evaluate the underlying neurocognitive networks. While symptoms might appear similar, autism is associated with problems in eye and gaze capabilities, and thus ToM deficits, in the first years of life. In schizophrenia, symptom onset, and thus changes in ToM capabilities, typically start later in life (roughly at the age of 20) and seem to relate to more general cognitive deficits. It is hypothesised that the visual–emotional and verbal–cognitive mentalising tasks might not sufficiently distinguish between these different kinds of mentalising processes, and/or how they are manifested in terms of performance on these tasks within each patient group.

> **GLOSSARY: TESTING IMPAIRMENTS IN MENTALISATION**
>
> **Strange Stories Test**: This test presents mentalistic stories with lies, jokes, etc. versus (the control condition) physical stories.
>
> **Faux Pas Test:** This test compares the ability of participants to understand and interpret stories with a faux pas and control stories without a faux pas.
>
> **Emotion Recognition from the Eyes Test:** In this test participants are asked to identify the six basic emotions from facial pictures.

Conclusions and Outstanding Questions

In conclusion, the study of ToM reveals significant insights into the cognitive processes underlying social interactions and their association with various mental disorders, such as autism and schizophrenia. Current research highlights the complex nature of ToM impairments, suggesting that these deficits may arise from either specific neuronal networks or more general disruptions in cognitive abilities. Furthermore, similarities and differences observed between autism and schizophrenia in terms of mentalising abilities call for a deeper investigation of the underlying neurocognitive mechanisms.

Outstanding Questions

- Current research into ToM impairments in autism and schizophrenia faces methodological limitations, making it challenging to accurately evaluate the underlying cognitive mechanisms. How can we develop new methodologies that can successfully and reliably assess ToM deficits in these populations within a laboratory setting?

- The co-occurrence of various mental disorders in the same individuals presents challenges in understanding the unique contributions of ToM impairments to each condition. Can we adopt dimensional and transdiagnostic approaches in mental health research to gain a more comprehensive understanding of ToM deficits and their relationship to social cognition across different disorders?

REFERENCES

1. Jolly A. Lemur social behavior and primate intelligence. *Science* 1966; 153(735): 501–506.

2. Dunbar RIM. Neocortex size as a constraint on group-size in primates. *J Hum Evol* 1992; 22(6): 469–493.

3. Whiten A, Byrne RW. *Machiavellian Intelligence II: Extensions and Evaluations*. Cambridge University Press, 1997.

4. Clayton NS, Dally JM, Emery NJ. Social cognition by food-caching corvids. The western scrub-jay as a natural psychologist. *Philos Trans R Soc London B* 2007; 362(1480): 507–522.

5. Premack D, Woodruff G. Does the chimpanzee have a theory of mind? *Behav Brain Sci* 1978; 1(4): 515–526.

6. Heyes CM. Theory of mind in nonhuman primates. *Behav Brain Sci* 1998; 21(1): 101–114.

7. Whiten A. When does smart behaviour-reading become mind-reading? In Carruthers P, Smith P, (eds.). *Theories of Theories of Mind*. Cambridge University Press; 1996, pp. 277–292.

8. Premack D. Does the chimpanzee have a theory of mind? Revisited, Machiavellian intelligence: social expertise and the evolution of intellect in monkeys, apes, and humans. In Byrne RW, Whiten A (eds.), *Machiavellian Intelligence: Social Expertise and the Evolution of Intellect in Monkeys, Apes, and Humans*. Clarendon Press, 1988, pp. 160–179.

9. Povinelli DJ, Eddy TJ, Hobson RP, Tomasello M. What young chimpanzees know about seeing. *Monogr Soc Res Child Dev* 1996: i–189.

10. Povinelli DJ, Vonk J. Chimpanzee minds: suspiciously human? *Trends Cogn Sci* 2003; 7(4): 157–160.

11. Povinelli DJ, Perilloux HK, Reaux JE, Bierschwale DT. Young and juvenile chimpanzees (*Pan troglodytes*) reactions to intentional versus accidental and inadvertent actions. *Behav Processes* 1998; 42(2): 205–218.

12. Surian L, Caldi S, Sperber D. Attribution of beliefs by 13-month-old infants. *Psychol Sci* 2007; 18(7): 580–586.

13. Neumann A, Thoermer C, Sodian B (eds.). *Belief-Based Action Anticipation in 18-Month-Old Infants*. International Congress of Psychology, 2008.

14. Suddendorf T, Simcock G, Nielsen M. Visual self-recognition in mirrors and live videos: evidence for a developmental asynchrony. *Cogn Devel* 2007; 22(2): 185–196.

15. Bischof-Kohler D. Empathy and self-recognition in phylogenetic and ontogenetic perspective. *Emotion Rev* 2012; 4(1): 40–48.

16. Baron-Cohen S, Leslie AM, Frith U. Does the autistic child have a "theory of mind"? *Cognition* 1985; 21(1): 37–46.

17. Baron-Cohen S, O'riordan M, Stone V, Jones R, Plaisted K. Recognition of faux pas by normally developing children and children with Asperger syndrome or high-functioning autism. *J Autism Dev Disord* 1999; 29(5): 407–418.

18. Baron-Cohen S, Wheelwright S, Jolliffe T. Is there a "language of the eyes"? Evidence from normal adults, and adults with autism or Asperger syndrome. *Visual Cogn* 1997; 4(3): 311–331.

19. Frith CD. *The Cognitive Neuropsychology of Schizophrenia*. Psychology Press, 2014.

20. Frith CD. Schizophrenia and theory of mind. *Psychol Med* 2004; 34(3): 385–389.

21. Sprong M, Schothorst P, Vos E, Hox J, Van Engeland H. Theory of mind in schizophrenia: meta-analysis. *Br J Psychiatry* 2007; 191(1): 5–13.

22. Balogh N, Égerházi A, Berecz R, Csukly G. Investigating the state-like and trait-like characters of social cognition in schizophrenia: a short term follow-up study. *Schizophr Res* 2014; 159(2–3): 499–505.

23. Heinrichs RW, Zakzanis KK. Neurocognitive deficit in schizophrenia: a quantitative review of the evidence. *Neuropsychology* 1998; 12(3): 426.

5

24. Brüne M, Bodenstein L. Proverb comprehension reconsidered – 'theory of mind' and the pragmatic use of language in schizophrenia. *Schizophr Res* 2005; 75(2–3): 233–239.

25. Cella M, Hamid S, Butt K, Wykes T. Cognition and social cognition in non-psychotic siblings of patients with schizophrenia. *Cogn Neuropsychiatry* 2015; 20(3): 232–242.

26. Ventura J, Wood RC, Hellemann GS. Symptom domains and neurocognitive functioning can help differentiate social cognitive processes in schizophrenia: a meta-analysis. *Schizophr Bull* 2011; 39(1): 102–111.

27. Chung YS, Barch D, Strube M. A meta-analysis of mentalizing impairments in adults with schizophrenia and autism spectrum disorder. *Schizophr Bull* 2013; 40(3): 602–616.

National Neuroscience Curriculum Initiative online resources

Oxytocin and the Social Brain

Sarah K. Fineberg and David A. Ross

5.17 Language

Matthew A. Lambon Ralph

OVERVIEW

Language and communication in all its forms is fundamental to our everyday and professional lives, as well as the success of the human species over generations. This chapter considers the multifaceted nature of language including its spoken and written forms. Having considered healthy language function, the chapter sets out how different facets of language can break down independently after damage to different brain areas, giving rise to some of the famous types of aphasia (acquired language impairments) and how these can be captured in simple computational models of language. The chapter then goes on to contrast the patterns observed after stroke with those that arise in the context of neurodegenerative diseases.

5.17.1 What Is Language?

Language is one of the fundamental higher cortical functions. While researchers sometimes debate how much of language and communication is unique to humans, there is little doubt that some of the success of the human species relies on our ability to communicate and thus organise our collective behaviour in sophisticated ways. With the advent of writing systems, we also have a way to store and transmit information over long periods of time, thus allowing the accumulation of knowledge and communication across generations. A second striking demonstration of the importance of language comes from the disability in professional activities and everyday life that results from acquired language impairments, or the challenges that follow from developmental language disorders. One can even make the case that our reliance on language continues to grow; the ability to generate and comprehend spoken language has always been present, while our reliance on written forms of language has grown as literacy has become ubiquitous in modern societies and has been accelerated through the advent of the internet and social media. In our contemporary lives, both the spoken and written word are central to knowledge transfer and also to the formation and binding of social groups and behaviours.

Language is often used as a singular term. Likewise, acquired disorders of language – aphasia – are also referred to as one unified disorder. Both are incorrect. Our language and communication abilities are very diverse, and these can break down in at least semi-discrete ways (see below). At the broadest levels, language can be split into spoken and written forms for both reception (i.e. comprehension) and expression. Language uses different organs (ears, eyes, mouth, hands) and relies on different parts of the brain to decode sensory inputs, control motor outputs and also encode internal representations for language-specific representations (e.g. the sounds of words – phonology) and meaning (semantic representations). While some cognitive behaviours always link stimulation to response, language need not do so. We can listen or read, decoding the meaning of language to build up internal models and memories without there being an external response. Correspondingly, we can use these internal long-term language representations and memories to initiate responses (e.g. speech or writing) in the absence of external stimulation.

5.17.2 A Very Brief History of Language in Neuroscience

Given the paradigmatic exemplar of language as human higher cortical function, it is perhaps not surprising that the study of language and its impairments has been prominent throughout cognitive and clinical neuroscience. Indeed, some language studies have taught us things about cognitive and brain functions more generally. Thus, among the prominent neurologists and neuropsychiatrists of the late-nineteenth century, many of them are remembered for their pioneering studies of language impairments, the implications these had for brain function and the discipline of neuroscience. Thus, Broca, Wernicke, Meynert, Dejerine (Eggert, 1977) and others are known for their first descriptions of selective language impairments following brain damage (so much so that the left inferior prefrontal cortex and the posterior superior and middle temporal gyri are still referred to as Broca and Wernicke's areas, respectively). These reports were important for multiple reasons: (i) they demonstrated that different aspects of language (e.g. speech production – Broca, spoken comprehension – Wernicke, reading – Dejerine) could break down selectively; (ii) they showed that that each was associated with damage to a different brain region – thus starting the ubiquitous goal of cognitive/clinical neuroscience to localise cognitive/sensory/affective functions to brain regions; (iii) they also quickly fathomed that not only regions but also the connections between them were important, such that language disorders might follow from disconnections (e.g. an inability to repeat might follow from a disconnection of the arcuate fasciculus, which connects posterior temporal areas to inferior frontal regions); and (iv) by putting these patterns together they proposed diagrams of language function in terms of multiple brain areas and their connections (Eggert, 1977). Although these early 'diagram-makers' drew important criticisms and challenges (Head, 1926), it is striking that many of the goals and targets of contemporary cognitive/clinical neuroscience (localisation of functions, brain networks, computational models, etc.) trace their roots back to these seminal studies of aphasia.

Over the next century, the tradition of studying language impairments that result from brain damage continued with an accumulation of detailed case studies and group studies. Although there were important contributions gleaned from patients with penetrative missile wounds from the First and Second World Wars (which proffered some clues about the location of damage without post-mortem (Head, 1926; Luria, 1976)), the most dominant aetiology has been patients with aphasia (disorders of language), very typically following left middle cerebral artery stroke (for aphasia) or posterior cerebral artery stroke (for pure alexia – impaired reading with preserved writing). During the 1960s and 1970s, these studies included the seminal work of Geschwind and the Boston group (Geschwind, 1972), and a little later Kertesz and colleagues, who developed formal assessment batteries to characterise the differences between patients (Shewan and Kertesz, 1980; Goodglass and Kaplan, 1983). In parallel, there was a rise in experimental psycholinguistic studies of language function in healthy participants. Both forms of investigation advanced our understanding of language functions and the underlying cognitive representations. In the 1980s and beyond, studies of language impairment – dominated by stroke – were joined by investigations of patients with neurodegenerative disorders (see below).

Until the last quarter of the twentieth century, there were limited advances in the localisation of function given that, before that time, post-mortem examination was the only method of relating impaired performance to underlying brain damage. Of course, the big innovation came with the advent of *in vivo* neuroimaging, initially through computerised tomography (CT), positron emission tomography (PET) and then magnetic resonance imaging (MRI). This allowed clinicians and researchers to relate the pattern of language impairments to the location and distribution of brain damage and, by repeating paired behavioural assessment and neuroimaging, it became possible to explore changes in language functions (e.g. during recovery or decline). The introduction of functional neuroimaging (initially through oxygen-15 water PET and then functional MRI (fMRI)), combined with experimental psycholinguistics, allowed exploration of the regions and networks implicated in language functions in health and in disease (Price, 2012). In more contemporary times, these techniques have been joined by brain stimulation methods (e.g. transcranial magnetic stimulation (TMS) and transcranial electrical stimulation (TES)) to explore the impact of transient, local disruption on behavioural function in patients and healthy participants (Pobric et al.,

2007; Hartwigsen et al., 2016), as well as invasive depth and cortical electrode neurophysiological investigations in neurosurgical patients (Lüders et al., 1986). Finally, the rise of advanced computing (also crucial for neuroimaging data processing and analysis) has allowed researchers to build formal computational models of language functions and hypothesize how these might relate to underlying brain networks (Ueno et al., 2011; Chen et al., 2017).

5.17.3 Aphasias, Dyslexias and Dysgraphias Post Stroke

One only needs to spend a short while in the clinical arena to realise that there are many different types and variations of language impairment (aphasia, alexia, etc.). As noted above, language comprises many different types of language activities supported by different senses, motor systems and brain regions, thus it is not surprising that the exact pattern of impaired and preserved abilities varies across patients. There are at least five sources of variation:

(1) Different language functions, or more likely different neurocomputations that support language (Patterson and Lambon Ralph, 1999), are localised in different brain regions. The exact pattern of impairment will, therefore, reflect the location and distribution of damage. Indeed, the clinical neuroscience of aphasiology attempts the reverse inference: comparing behavioural presentation and brain damage across a large enough sample of individuals in order to infer the localisation of language computations.

(2) The pattern of language impairment will change with the severity of damage to one or more underpinning brain systems.

(3) Patients' presentations will change during recovery (typically for at least 9 months or more after stroke or other forms of acute brain damage (Corbetta et al., 2015)) or during neurodegeneration.

(4) Premorbid individual differences can influence the pattern of impairment observed after brain damage, such that an inherently stronger system will be more robust to damage (Woollams et al., 2007). This is, of course, difficult to investigate given that, by definition, one cannot go back in time to assess someone, *pre ictus* (Hoffman et al., 2015; Woollams et al., 2017).

(5) Random variations including variations from day to day, noise in test measures, etc.

Various broad distinctions are firmly recognised. Some of these relate to absolute categorical differences between brain systems and others to more graded, dimensional variations between patient types (Butler et al., 2014). First, at the broadest level, we can relate impaired language functions to the primary sensory or motor systems involved: **aphasia** typically refers to receptive and/or expressive disorders of spoken language; **alexia** or **acquired dyslexia** to disorders of reading; and **dysgraphia** to deficits in spelling and writing. Each of these can then be split down into more specific subtypes. Most commonly, the labels used for these subtypes refer to the superficial patterns of impairments and preserved skills rather than to an underlying mechanistic account. Although the nomenclature for the subtypes of aphasia, alexia and agraphia has changed over time, some of the recognised subtypes include the following. **Global aphasia**, involving severe deficits in both receptive and expressive language function, is typically the most severe and all-encompassing type of aphasia (often following a large middle cerebral artery stroke, affecting subcortical, prefrontal, parietal and temporal lobe regions). The opposite, mildest example is **anomic aphasia** in which patients have word-finding difficulties without major deficits in comprehension, repetition or reading. Other patients have severe non-fluent and agrammatical speech, impaired ability to repeat or name yet better-preserved comprehension, at least at the single word level, which is referred to as **Broca's aphasia**. More selective speech production deficits are found in patients with **apraxia of speech** or **dysarthria** in which the motor planning and/or execution of motor-speech plans are disrupted. All these output-related deficits are classically associated with damage to left 'anterior regions' including the prefrontal cortex, premotor regions and the underpinning white matter (see Figure 5.17.1). In terms of receptive impairments, its purest albeit rarest form comes in patients with **transcortical sensory aphasia** (TSA; which follows damage to left lateral posterior temporo-parietal or prefrontal regions) who present with impaired comprehension and word-finding difficulties but have fluent speech and preserved repetition (Berthier, 2001). Patients with **Wernicke's aphasia** (typically associated with lesions of the left posterior superior and middle temporal gyri and temporoparietal junction) also have

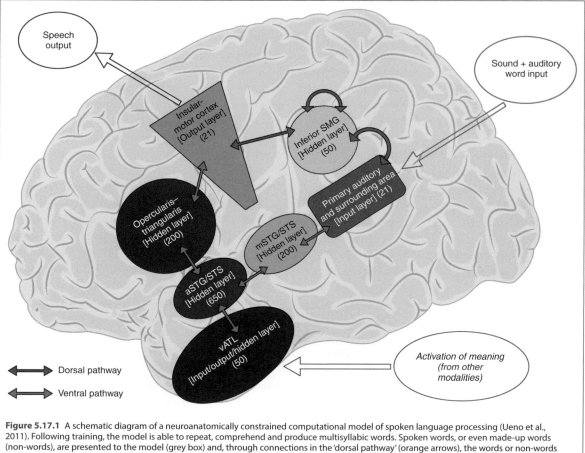

Figure 5.17.1 A schematic diagram of a neuroanatomically constrained computational model of spoken language processing (Ueno et al., 2011). Following training, the model is able to repeat, comprehend and produce multisyllabic words. Spoken words, or even made-up words (non-words), are presented to the model (grey box) and, through connections in the 'dorsal pathway' (orange arrows), the words or non-words can be spoken (cf. repetition). Connections in the 'ventral' pathway (green arrows) allow the model to transform the sequential spoken input into a stable semantic representation (i.e. comprehend spoken words). The model is also able to use these semantic representations to innervate speech output (i.e. as we do when speaking spontaneously or when naming visually presented items). The model also generates some of the classical types of aphasia after damage, including Broca's aphasia after damage to the prefrontal areas, conduction aphasia after lesioning of the dorsal pathway and transcortical sensory aphasia after damage to the ventral pathway. This computational model necessarily simplifies both the neuroanatomy and the target language phenomena. For example, it does not deal with sentence-level materials (cf. syntax) or implement other brain areas that have been implicated in other aspects of language processing (e.g. subcortical regions, angular gyrus, posterior middle temporal gyrus, etc.). Abbreviations: SMG, supramarginal gyrus; aSTG/STS, anterior superior temporal gyrus/superior temporal sulcus; mSTG/STS, middle superior temporal gyrus/superior temporal sulcus; vATL, ventral anterior temporal lobe.

impaired comprehension but, unlike those with TSA, they also have severely impaired receptive phonological skills, poor verbal short-term memory and repetition (Robson et al., 2012). Patients with Wernicke's aphasia will often produce fluent but phonologically disordered speech (neologisms). Finally, conduction aphasia (typically following damage to the posterior superior temporal gyrus, inferior supramarginal gyrus and the arcuate fasciculus) reflects a more selective impairment of repetition, phonological short-term memory and naming,

again with phonologically disordered speech output (Fridriksson et al., 2010). Indeed, during recovery, many patients with Wernicke's aphasia in the acute phase will partially recover into a conduction aphasic pattern. This point raises the important issues of recovery and rehabilitation, which are too large and complex to cover in this section (recent detailed reviews can be found elsewhere (Stefaniak et al., 2020)).

Sometimes, each language impairment can occur in isolation. Thus, for example, 'pure alexia' (Leff and Starrfelt,

2014) (typically after damage to the left ventral occipitotemporal region, e.g. after a posterior cerebral artery stroke) refers to a reading impairment without aphasia or agraphia (indeed, it is sometime known as 'alexia without agraphia', referring to the fact that such patients sometimes report being unable to read their own writing, after a delay). More commonly, patients will have a mixture of aphasia, alexia and agraphia which reflects either co-occurring damage to more than one relevant brain region or the fact that many of the language-related representations (e.g. the sound structure of words – phonology – or their meaning – semantics) are shared by different language tasks. Thus, when one of these 'primary systems' is impaired, a set of language activities are simultaneously impaired and in a predictable manner (Patterson and Lambon Ralph, 1999; Woollams et al., 2007; Ueno et al., 2011). The primary systems hypothesis makes a potentially important claim about the organisation of cognitive brain functions: that brain regions support different primary systems (e.g. phonology, semantics) rather than brain regions being designed and dedicated to different language tasks (e.g. naming, reading, repeating). In this formulation, each language activity requires a concerted effort across these primary systems, reflected in brain networks. A simple cooking analogy would be the relationship of ingredients to culinary dishes; the kitchen (cf. brain) is designed to store ingredients (cf. primary brain systems) and to allow for them to be combined (cf. network interactions) in order to produce a wide array of dishes. Thus, if a particular ingredient becomes scarce (e.g. yeast), a variety of different dishes (cf. breads) are compromised while others (cf. cakes) are unaffected.

5.17.4 Language Dysfunctions in Neurodegenerative Disease

Beyond stroke and other forms of acute brain damage, language impairments are a common and disabling symptom in various forms of dementia and other neurodegenerative diseases. Thus, in Alzheimer's disease, as well as the diagnostic features of amnesia, spatial disorientation and poor attention, most patients will complain of poor memory for the names of objects and people (**anomia**) and often go on to develop impairments in comprehension, repetition and phonological, short-term memory (Lambon et al., 2003).

Contemporary with the famous nineteenth-century descriptions of Broca's and Wernicke's aphasias, descriptions of progressive language impairments were also noted (Spatt, 2003). Unlike their stroke counterparts, these progressive forms of aphasia did not come to research prominence until the latter part of the twentieth century. Seminal studies included early descriptions of patients with a selective multimodal comprehension disorder which would come to be known as **semantic dementia** (Hodges et al., 1992) and also the recognition of **primary progressive aphasia** (PPA) in which the first and prominent presentation symptom was one of language (Mesulam, 2001). Contemporary classification systems (Gorno-Tempini et al., 2011) recognise three main subtypes of PPA: non-fluent PPA, logopenic-variant PPA and semantic-variant PPA (an alternative term for semantic dementia).

- **Non-fluent PPA** (which follows from atrophy centred on the left prefrontal and insular cortices) is characterised by relative preservation of comprehension but increasingly non-fluent speech production, which is often agrammatical in form and contains phonological distortions and features of apraxia of speech.

- **Logopenic-variant PPA** (associated with left hemisphere atrophy centred on the temporoparietal junction) is characterised by phonological short-term memory deficits and difficulties in producing connected speech though, when it is produced, it is typically fluent and grammatically well formed.

- **Semantic dementia/semantic variant PPA**: (associated with atrophy centred on the ventrolateral anterior temporal lobes bilaterally) is characterised by verbal and non-verbal semantic deficits, profound word-finding difficulties but striking preservation of other aspects of language (e.g. excellent phonological skills, repetition, etc.) and higher cognition (e.g. excellent memory for recent events, spatial orientation, visuospatial and problem-solving skills).

Conclusions and Outstanding Questions

The ability to process and produce spoken and written language is central to almost every aspect of our lives. When it breaks down after brain damage then patients are left with significant challenges. Different patterns of contrastive language impairment reflect damage to different cortical regions. These can be observed not only in stroke but also in neurodegenerative disorders.

Outstanding Questions

- While much has been discovered about the neural bases of language and its impairments (both acute and progressive), there are important developments and challenges for future research. As reflected in the structure of this chapter, language impairments are often studied in aetiological silos. Thus, until very recently, post-stroke aphasia and PPA were rarely directly compared (for a recent full-scale counter-example, see Ingram et al. (2020)). This makes it hard to understand where there are true similarities (which might point to common brain mechanisms) or deviations (which might reflect divergent functions of different brain regions or the contrastive effects of acute versus progressive brain disease (Welbourne et al., 2011)). Thus, for example, semantic problems after stroke are very different to those found in semantic dementia (Jefferies and Lambon Ralph, 2006), which probably reflects the different brain regions implicated in each disease.

- A second area for integration is the convergence of neuroscience explorations of healthy language functions with the clinical findings to generate unified neuroscientific models of healthy and impaired language function.

- Finally, there is a need to go beyond descriptive accounts of language impairments and towards formal computational models of healthy and language-impaired states (Ueno et al., 2011), which might also provide a formal basis for considering recovery of function, progressive deterioration and the mechanisms that lead to effective rehabilitation.

REFERENCES

Berthier, M. L. (2001). Unexpected brain-language relationships in aphasia: Evidence from transcortical sensory aphasia associated with frontal lobe lesions. *Aphasiology* 15(2): 99–130.

Butler, R. A., Lambon Ralph, M. A., Woollams, A. M. (2014). Capturing multidimensionality in stroke aphasia: mapping principal behavioural components to neural structures. *Brain* 137(12): 3248–3266.

Chen, L., Lambon Ralph, M. A., Rogers, T. T. (2017). A unified model of human semantic knowledge and its disorders. *Nat Hum Behav* 1(3): 0039.

Corbetta, M., Ramsey, L., Callejas, A. et al. (2015). Common behavioral clusters and subcortical anatomy in stroke. *Neuron* 85(5): 927–941.

Eggert, G. H. (1977). *Wernicke's Works on Aphasia: A Source-Book and Review*. Mouton.

Fridriksson, J., Kjartansson, O., Morgan, P. S. et al. (2010). Impaired speech repetition and left parietal lobe damage. *J Neurosci* 30(33): 11057–11061.

Geschwind, N. (1972). Language and the brain. *Sci Am* 226: 76–83.

Goodglass, H., Kaplan, E. (1983). *The Assessment of Aphasia and Related Disorders*. Lea & Febiger.

Gorno-Tempini, M. L., Hillis, A. E., Weintraub, S. et al. (2011). Classification of primary progressive aphasia and its variants. *Neurology* 76(11): 1006.

Hartwigsen, G., Weigel, A., Schuschan, P. et al. (2016). Dissociating parieto-frontal networks for phonological and semantic word decisions: a condition-and-perturb TMS study. *Cerebral Cortex* 26(6): 2590–2601.

Head, H. (1926). *Aphasia and Kindred Disorders of Speech*. Cambridge University Press.

Hodges, J. R., Patterson, K., Oxbury, S., Funnell, E. (1992). Semantic dementia: progressive fluent aphasia with temporal lobe atrophy. *Brain* 115(Pt6): 1783–1806.

Hoffman, P., Lambon Ralph, M. A., Woollams, A. M. (2015). Triangulation of the neurocomputational architecture underpinning reading aloud. *Proc Ntl Acad Sci USA* 112(28): E3719–E3728.

Ingram, R., Halai, A., Pobric, G. et al. (2020). Graded, multidimensional intragroup and intergroup variations in primary progressive aphasia and post-stroke aphasia. *Brain* 43(10): 3121–3135.

Jefferies, E., Lambon Ralph, M. A. (2006). Semantic impairment in stroke aphasia vs. semantic dementia: a case-series comparison. *Brain* 129: 2132–2147.

Lambon Ralph, M. A., Patterson, K., Graham, N., Dawson, K., Hodges, J. R. (2003). Homogeneity and heterogeneity in mild cognitive impairment and Alzheimer's disease: a cross-sectional and longitudinal study of 55 cases. *Brain* 126: 2350–2362.

Leff, A., Starrfelt, R. (2014). *Alexia: Diagnosis, Treatment and Theory*. Springer Verlag.

Lüders, H., Lesser, R. P., Hahn, J. et al. (1986). Basal temporal language area demonstrated by electrical stimulation. *Neurology* 36(4): 505–510.

Luria, A. R. (1976). *The Working Brain: An Introduction to Neuropsychology*. Penguin.

Mesulam, M. M. (2001). Primary progressive aphasia. *Ann Neurol* 49(4): 425–432.

Patterson, K., Lambon Ralph, M. A. (1999). Selective disorders of reading? *Curr Opin Neurobiol* 9(2): 235–239.

Pobric, G. G., Jefferies, E., Lambon Ralph, M. A. (2007). Anterior temporal lobes mediate semantic representation: mimicking semantic dementia by using rTMS in normal participants. *Proc Ntl Acad Sci USA* 104: 20137–20141.

Price, C. J. (2012). A review and synthesis of the first 20 years of PET and fMRI studies of heard speech, spoken language and reading. *NeuroImage* 62(2): 816–847.

5

Robson, H., Sage, K., Lambon Ralph, M. A. (2012). Wernicke's aphasia reflects a combination of acoustic–phonological and semantic control deficits: a case-series comparison of Wernicke's aphasia, semantic dementia and semantic aphasia. *Neuropsychologia* 50(2): 266–275.

Shewan, C. M., Kertesz, A. (1980). Reliability and validity characteristics of the Western Aphasia Battery (WAB). *J Speech Hear Disord* 45(3): 308–324.

Spatt, J. (2003). Arnold Pick's concept of dementia. *Cortex* 39(3): 525–531.

Stefaniak, J. D., Halai, A. D., Lambon Ralph, M. A. (2020). The neural and neurocomputational bases of recovery from post-stroke aphasia. *Nat Rev Neurol* 16(1): 43–55.

Ueno, T., Saito, S., Rogers, T. T., Lambon Ralph, M. A. (2011). Lichtheim 2: synthesizing aphasia and the neural basis of language in a neurocomputational model of the dual dorsal–ventral language pathways. *Neuron* 72(2): 385–396.

Welbourne, S. R., Woollams, A. M., Crisp, J., Lambon Ralph, M. A. (2011). The role of plasticity-related functional reorganization in the explanation of central dyslexias. *Cogn Neuropsychol* 28(2): 65–108.

Woollams, A. M., Lambon Ralph, M. A., Plaut, D. C., Patterson, K. (2007). SD-squared: on the association between semantic dementia and surface dyslexia. *Psychol Rev* 114(2): 316–339.

Woollams, A. M., Madrid, G., Lambon Ralph, M. A. (2017). Using neurostimulation to understand the impact of pre-morbid individual differences on post-lesion outcomes. *Proc Ntl Acad Sci USA* 114(46): 12279–12284.

National Neuroscience Curriculum Initiative online resources

This "stuff" is really cool: Amy Margolis, *"Spoken Word" on dyslexia and socioeconomic status*

| **5.18** | **Brain Networks and Dysconnectivity** | **Sarah E. Morgan and Ed Bullmore** |

OVERVIEW

The first clear vision of the brain as a network stemmed from the extraordinary work by Ramón y Cajal, the Nobel Laureate (1916) who defined the neuron and conceived of synaptic connections between neurons to form a cellular or microscopic network (see Figure 5.18.1A) on a spatial scale of micrometres to nanometres (i.e. 10^{-6}–10^{-9} metres). The mammalian brain also has a network organisation at a larger, mesoscopic scale (i.e. 10^{-4}–10^{-6} m), with cortical areas or subcortical nuclei connecting to each other via bundles or tracts of long-distance axonal projections (see Figure 5.18.1B), and at the macroscopic scale (i.e. centimetres to millimetres, or 10^{-2}–10^{-4} m), as can be measured using brain MRI (see Figure 5.18.1C). Increasingly detailed maps and technically dazzling images of micro, meso and macro brain network organisation are being produced across a range of species, from the nematode *Caenorhabditis elegans*, through *Drosophila* species, to rodents and monkeys. Several books and reviews provide more detail and scope on the flourishing field of connectomics or network neuroscience [1–5]; here we focus on a few high-level principles.

GLOSSARY

Connectome or brain graph: A model of brain network organisation where nodes, representing individual neurons or larger cortical areas, are connected by edges, representing the strength and direction of anatomical or functional connectivity between nodes.

Topology: Mathematical analysis of the pattern of connections in a network, regardless of the scale of the network or the physical distance between nodes. Modelling brain networks as graphs has focused increasing attention on their topology, to complement the traditional focus on their topography, or anatomical layout in physical space.

Degree: A topological measure of the centrality or 'hubness' of each node in the network. Most simply, degree is the sum of the weights of the edges that connect each node to all the other nodes. The hubs can then be defined as the nodes, with many strong connections throughout the network or high-degree centrality. There are many other metrics of centrality besides degree but they all capture some aspect of nodal hubness.

Module: A subset of nodes that are densely connected to each other and sparsely connected to nodes in other modules. Whole-brain networks can be decomposed into a set of modules, each typically comprising anatomically co-located or symmetrical cortical areas with a shared functional specialisation. Connectivity between modules is mediated by long-distance connections, or inter-modular edges, concentrated on a subset of so-called connector hubs.

Rich club: A subset of highly connected hub nodes that are more densely connected to each other than expected by chance. Rich-club organisation has been demonstrated from *Caenorhabditis elegans* to *Homo sapiens* and is likely an important topological feature for propagating information quickly and accurately across brain networks. Other topological features – like hub nodes and inter-modular edges – are also important in mediating global integration of brain networks.

Small-worldness: A small-world network, like the brain, has a topological pattern that is neither random nor regular. Segregated cliques of nodes are densely interconnected and spatially co-located to form non-random clusters with low wiring cost, like a regular lattice. Yet the network is topologically integrated, like a random graph, so there is a short path length (minimum number of edges) between any two nodes in the network, albeit with a higher wiring cost than a lower cost, but a more topologically segregated network.

5.18.1 Human MRI for Brain Network Mapping

MRI stands out as the most versatile, accessible, safe and useful technique for human brain network mapping. It can be used to measure two types of brain networks – structural and functional. Structural brain networks are based on statistical estimates of anatomical connectivity between brain regions; in other words, structural edges represent probable white matter tracts in the brain. In contrast, in functional brain networks, edges connect regions that show similar patterns of activity over time (Figure 5.18.1C). The regions are therefore functionally related to each other, even though they may not be monosynaptically connected in an anatomical network.

Once we have constructed a brain network, we can use tools from network science to characterise its connectivity; see Figures 5.18.1D and 5.18.2 and the glossary. Nodes (e.g. brain regions) that are highly connected are described as 'hubs' and play an important role in communicating information between different nodes and modules of the network. This integrative topological role of network hubs is reflected in their association with higher-order cognitive functions. For example, between-person variation in the degree of connectivity of hubs of structural brain networks explained a significant amount of between-subject variability in intelligence quotient (IQ), in around 300 healthy young people [8]: higher IQ was associated with higher-degree hubs (Figure 5.18.2). Another key observation is that brain networks are organised in modules, with dense connections within modules and weaker connections between modules. These modules tend to be spatially co-localised and are often specialised for particular motor or sensory functions.

5.18.2 Dysconnectivity and Mental Health Disorders

Given the importance of brain network connectivity for the normal information-processing functions of the brain, it is perhaps not surprising that neuropsychiatric disorders, defined by symptoms of cognitive and emotional disturbance, are associated with disorganisation of brain networks or dysconnectivity; see Figure 5.18.3.

Schizophrenia has emerged as a canonical example of a brain network disorder, as understood in the contemporary framework of network science and connectomics [13]. For example, the cortical hubs in multisensory association areas of structural MRI brain networks had abnormal degree in three independent case–control studies of psychosis [14]; see Figure 5.18.4. Functional brain networks have been shown to inform machine-learning-based detection of psychotic disorders with high accuracy (75–85%), again based on a highly reproducible cortical pattern of case–control differences in connectivity [15].

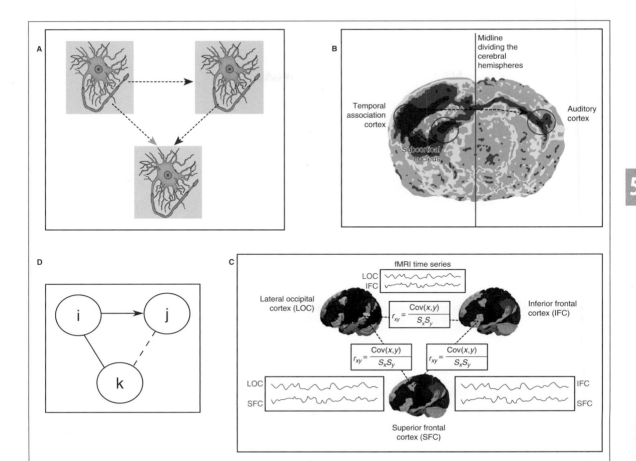

Figure 5.18.1 Brain networks, from micro to meso to macro, can generally be conceived as graphs. (A) Diagram of a microscopic cellular network (~10^{-6} m): three neurons are connected by axons and separated by synaptic gaps [6]; each node in the diagram represents a nerve cell (here assumed to be the same kind of nerve cell); the edges are synaptic connections, which are directed, weighted and signed (inhibitory (green) or excitatory (red)). **(B)** A mammalian brain mesoscopic network (~10^{-4} m): two cortical areas of grey matter, and a subcortical nucleus, each comprising large populations of neurons, are connected by white matter tracts that are precisely measurable by tract-tracing experiments [7]. Here, a tracer (coloured red) was injected into a source region of the mouse brain, in the temporal association cortex, and then propagated by axonal transport to contralateral cortical areas and subcortical nuclei (target regions) that are thus shown to be directly, anatomically connected to the source region. Compiling multiple such tract-tracing experiments, after injections into all cortical areas, the mouse brain connectome can be modelled as a set of cortical nodes with directed, weighted edges representing axonal projections between them. **(C)** Human brain macroscopic network (~10^{-2} m): three cortical areas of grey matter, defined by parcellation of functional (fMRI) (or structural) MRI data, are statistically related to each other. Here, the nodes are three cortical regions (LOC, lateral occipital cortex; IFC, inferior frontal cortex; SFC, superior frontal cortex) selected from the ~300 cortical and subcortical regions defined by contemporary whole human brain atlases or templates. The edges or lines drawn between nodes represent the strength of association, or functional connectivity, between regional mean fMRI time series measured in the resting state, while the participant lies quietly in the scanner, for 10–20 minutes. The edges are shown without arrowheads to indicate that functional connectivity metrics are symmetric or undirected, and don't tell us anything about the directed or causal relationships between regional nodes. Here, the metric used to estimate functional connectivity between each pair of regional nodes is Pearson's correlation coefficient (r), for which the formula is shown; Cov indicates covariance of low frequency oscillations in the two regional fMRI time series and s indicates the standard deviation of each time series. **(D)** Graph theory and topological analysis can be used across all spatial scales, to represent brain networks generally as a set of nodes {i, j, k} connected by edges that may be directed (arrowhead) or undirected (no arrowhead), variably weighted (broken lines) or binary (solid line). (A reproduced from Celula del lobulo cerebral electrico del torpedo. Coloracion por el liquido de boberi. Credit: Wellcome Collection (CC BY). B adapted with permission from [7].)

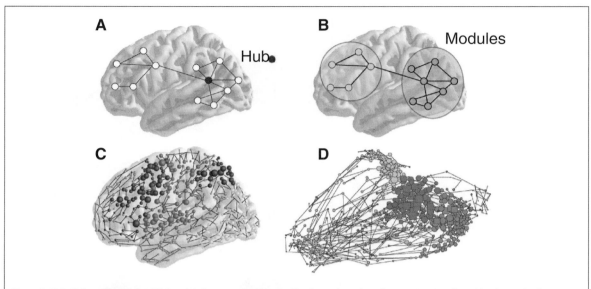

Figure 5.18.2 Hubs and modules. (A) A node's degree can be measured by the total number of connections it makes with other nodes, for example the red node has degree = 6. Nodes with a high degree relative to other nodes in the network are termed hubs. **(B)** Brain networks have a modular community structure, whereby they comprise several subsets of highly interconnected nodes called modules. Many of these features are highlighted in a brain functional network shown in both **(C)** anatomical space and **(D)** topological space. Panel D shows the same network as panel C, but the layout of cortical nodes has been organised by their topological proximity to each other, so that strongly interconnected nodes are close to each other in D, whereas the nodes have been organised by anatomical proximity, so that spatially neighbouring nodes are close to each other in C. Node size is proportional to degree in C and D and rich-club nodes are highlighted as squares in D. The modular organisation in both displays is highlighted by assigning different colours to nodes of different modules. We can see, for example, that nodes in the frontal and parietal cortices are spatially distributed or distant from each other, but topologically close, constituting the same (red) module and also often belonging to the rich club of interconnected hubs. (Reproduced with permission from [9–11]).

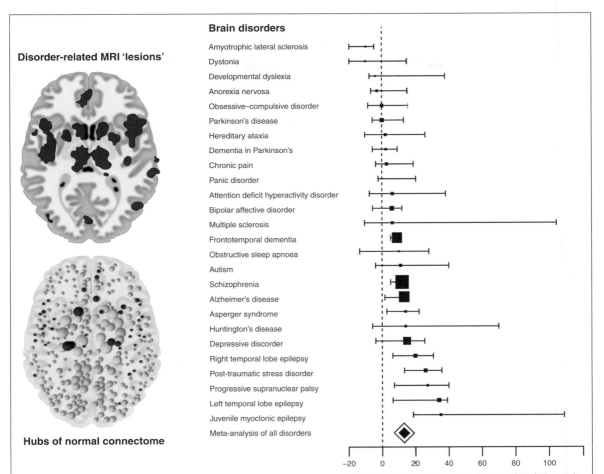

Disorder-related MRI 'lesions'

Hubs of normal connectome

Brain disorders

Amyotrophic lateral sclerosis
Dystonia
Developmental dyslexia
Anorexia nervosa
Obsessive–compulsive disorder
Parkinson's disease
Hereditary ataxia
Dementia in Parkinson's
Chronic pain
Panic disorder
Attention deficit hyperactivity disorder
Bipolar affective disorder
Multiple sclerosis
Frontotemporal dementia
Obstructive sleep apnoea
Autism
Schizophrenia
Alzheimer's disease
Asperger syndrome
Huntington's disease
Depressive discorder
Right temporal lobe epilepsy
Post-traumatic stress disorder
Progressive supranuclear palsy
Left temporal lobe epilepsy
Juvenile myoclonic epilepsy
Meta-analysis of all disorders

Difference between median degree of lesion and non-lesion voxels

Figure 5.18.3 Structural brain network hubs are disrupted in many brain disorders [12]. By meta-analytically combining results from multiple prior case–control MRI studies of various brain disorders, collectively representing data on more than 20,000 participants, we can produce MRI 'lesion' maps demonstrating areas of grey matter signal deficit (blue) in large numbers of cases of disorder compared to healthy controls. Brain regions that are lesioned by disorders often correspond to the hub regions of the healthy human connectome. For each of 26 disorders, the forest plot shows the difference in median degree or 'hubness' of lesioned nodes compared to non-lesioned nodes. The size of each box is proportional to the number of primary studies per disorder and the error bar is the 95% confidence interval. Results for all disorders are summarised by the diamond in the bottom row. We can see that the cortical nodes lesioned by several disorders, including schizophrenia and Alzheimer's disease, have significantly higher degree centrality than non-lesioned nodes. These results are consistent with the pathogenic hypothesis that high-degree network hubs are especially vulnerable to diverse pathological processes across many neuropsychiatric disorders. (Reproduced with permission from [12].)

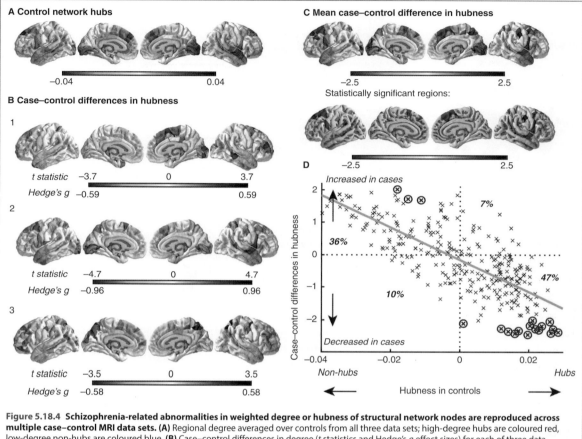

Figure 5.18.4 Schizophrenia-related abnormalities in weighted degree or hubness of structural network nodes are reproduced across multiple case–control MRI data sets. (A) Regional degree averaged over controls from all three data sets; high-degree hubs are coloured red, low-degree non-hubs are coloured blue. **(B)** Case–control differences in degree (*t* statistics and Hedge's *g* effect sizes) for each of three data sets. **(C)** Mean case–control difference in degree, on average over all data sets, for all nodes. A subset of 18 nodes had statistically significant abnormalities of degree – either decreased (blue) or increased (red) in cases of schizophrenia compared to healthy controls. **(D)** Scatterplot showing the mean degree of each regional node in the control network (*x*-axis) versus the case–control difference in degree (*y*-axis). Nodes with significantly decreased degree in schizophrenia (blue) are typically high-degree hubs of the control network; whereas nodes with significantly increased degree in schizophrenia (red) are non-hubs of the control brain network (Pearson's *r* = −0.76, *P* < 0.001). (Reproduced with permission from [14].)

Conclusions and Outstanding Questions

Brain networks can be measured across multiple scales and species. Mathematical tools drawn from graph theory can measure topological properties, like hubs and modules, that are relevant to normal cognitive function and to neuropsychiatric disorders including schizophrenia.

Outstanding Questions

- Can we develop non-invasive MRI markers which relate more precisely to known microscopic features of brain connectivity, such as myelination?

- How can we relate brain dysconnectivity to genetic and genomic data, to better understand the molecular mechanisms underlying MRI network changes?

- Can biomarkers based on brain connectivity be used to diagnose and predict outcome of mental health disorders in a clinical setting?

REFERENCES

1. Sporns O. *Networks of the Brain*. MIT Press, 2011.

2. Fornito A, Zalesky A, Bullmore ET. *Fundamentals of Brain Network Analysis*. Academic Press, 2016.

3. Fornito A, Zalesky A, Breakspear M. The connectomics of brain disorders. *Nat Rev Neurosci* 2015; 16: 159–172.

4. Bullmore E, Sporns O. Complex brain networks: graph theoretical analysis of structural and functional systems. *Nat Rev Neurosci* 2009; 10: 186–198.

5. Lynn CW, Bassett DS. The physics of brain network structure, function and control. *Nat Rev Phys* 2019; 1: 318–332.

6. Swanson LW, Lichtman JW. From Cajal to connectome and beyond. *Annu Rev Neurosci* 2016; 39: 197–216.

7. Rubinov M*, Ypma RJF*, Watson C, Bullmore ET. Wiring cost and topological participation of the mouse brain conenctome. *Proc Natl Acad Sci* 2015; 112: 10032–10037.

8. Seidlitz J, Váša F, Shinn M et al. Morphometric similarity networks detect microscale cortical organization and predict inter-individual cognitive variation. *Neuron* 2018; 97: 231–247.

9. Crossley NA, Mechelli A, Vértes PE et al. Cognitive relevance of the community structure of the human brain functional coactivation network. *Proc Natl Acad Sci USA* 2013; 110: 11583–11588.

10. Vértes PE, Bullmore ET. Annual research review: growth connectomics – the organization and reorganization of brain networks during normal and abnormal development. *J Child Psychol Psychiatry* 2015; 56: 299–320.

11. Bullmore E, Sporns O. The economy of brain network organization. *Nat Rev Neurosci* 2012; 13: 336–349.

12. Crossley NA, Mechelli A, Scott J et al. The hubs of the human connectome are generally implicated in the anatomy of brain disorders. *Brain* 2014; 137: 2382–2395.

13. Friston KJ, Frith CD. Schizophrenia: a disconnection syndrome? *Clin Neurosci* 1995; 3: 89–97.

14. Morgan SE, Seidlitz J, Whitaker KJ et al. Cortical patterning of abnormal morphometric similarity in psychosis is associated with brain expression of schizophrenia-related genes. *Proc Natl Acad Sci USA* 2019; 116: 9604–9609.

15. Morgan SE*, Young J*, Patel AX et al. Functional MRI connectivity accurately distinguishes cases with psychotic disorders from healthy controls, based on cortical features associated with neurodevelopment. *Biol Psychiatry Cogn Neurosci Neuroimag* 2021; 6: 1125–1134.

National Neuroscience Curriculum Initiative online resources

Missed Connections: A Network Approach to Understanding Psychiatric Illness

Aaron F. Alexander-Bloch, Danielle S. Bassett and David A. Ross

6

Modulators

6.1 The Hypothalamic–Pituitary (Neuroendocrine) Axis

Russell Senanayake, James MacFarlane, Merel van der Meulen, Waiel A. Bashari and Mark Gurnell

OVERVIEW

Although the term **neuroendocrine** is now applied to many different contexts in which the nervous system interacts with the endocrine system to regulate hormone release and bring about important changes in physiology, the hypothalamic–pituitary axis remains the best known and most well-characterised example of a neuroendocrine system. Here, the hypothalamus acts as the major coordinating centre, integrating a diverse array of intrinsic (e.g. higher cortical, autonomic, endocrine) and extrinsic (e.g. environmental) signals to direct the function of multiple different target cells/tissues within the central nervous system, pituitary gland and peripheral sites. Hypothalamic regulation of pituitary function has far-reaching consequences, governing the release of hormones from other key endocrine glands (e.g. adrenal, thyroid, gonad), which, in turn, regulate the function of many physiological pathways with important consequences for energy balance and metabolism, osmo- and thermo-regulation, heart rate and blood pressure control, central nervous system function, growth and reproduction.

6.1.1 Neuroanatomy of the Hypothalamus and Pituitary Gland

The hypothalamus is located at the base of the brain, below the third ventricle and in close proximity to the optic chiasm. It comprises a number of distinct nuclei, with discrete cell populations that have both neuronal and endocrine features. Similar to other neurons, these cells express neural markers and release a peptide or neurotransmitter following depolarisation; however, unlike most other neurons, the neurotransmitter is released directly into the bloodstream. The hypothalamus secretes both stimulatory and inhibitory factors to control hormone release from five major cell types in the anterior pituitary gland (corticotroph, gonadotroph, lactotroph, somatotroph and thyrotroph). Several hypothalamic hormones are released directly (from parvocellular neurons) into a primary capillary plexus at the level of the median eminence (Figure 6.1.1). These hormones then travel down hypophyseal portal veins in the pituitary stalk (infundibulum), to reach a secondary capillary plexus, which surrounds and supplies cells of the anterior pituitary gland – thus allowing relatively high hormone concentrations to reach their target cells rapidly. In contrast, axonal projections from magnocellular neurons in the hypothalamic paraventricular and supraoptic nuclei extend down the infundibulum to reach the posterior pituitary gland (Figure 6.1.1). Here, the axon terminals contain neurosecretory granules, which are stored for subsequent release. The anterior pituitary gland is therefore a site of independent hormone synthesis (in effect an 'endocrine factory'), while the posterior pituitary gland comprises mainly neural tissue (and functions as an 'endocrine storage depot').

6.1.2 The Hypothalamic–Pituitary–Adrenal (HPA) Axis

Corticotropin-releasing hormone (CRH, also known as corticotropin-releasing factor (CRF)) is secreted from the hypothalamus (medial parvocellular paraventricular nucleus) in response to various stimuli, including physical

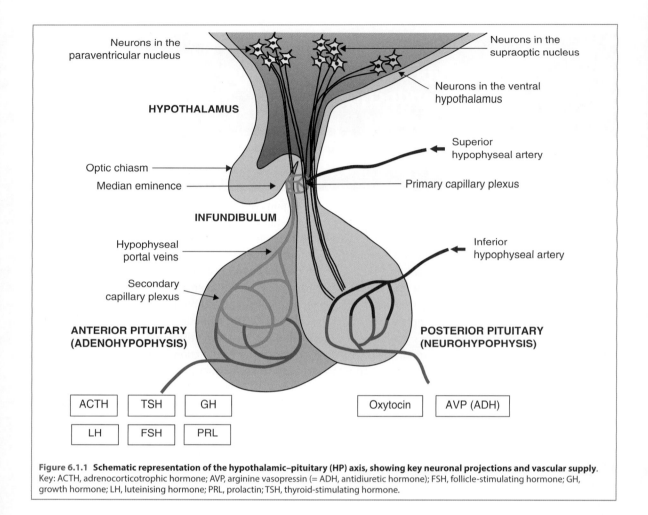

Figure 6.1.1 Schematic representation of the hypothalamic–pituitary (HP) axis, showing key neuronal projections and vascular supply. Key: ACTH, adrenocorticotrophic hormone; AVP, arginine vasopressin (= ADH, antidiuretic hormone); FSH, follicle-stimulating hormone; GH, growth hormone; LH, luteinising hormone; PRL, prolactin; TSH, thyroid-stimulating hormone.

and emotional stress and other triggers (e.g. hypoglycaemia). Binding to CRH receptors expressed on corticotroph cells in the anterior pituitary gland results in the secretion of adrenocorticotrophic hormone (ACTH, corticotropin) into the peripheral circulation. ACTH release is also augmented by arginine vasopressin (antidiuretic hormone), which is produced in adjacent nuclei of the paraventricular nucleus and is also increased following psychological stress (as well as other triggers). Binding of ACTH to the melanocortin 2 receptor expressed on cells of the zona fasciculata and zona reticularis of the adrenal cortex stimulates the synthesis and secretion of glucocorticoids (e.g. cortisol) and adrenal sex steroids (e.g. dehydroepiandrosterone), respectively (Figure 6.1.2). Importantly, this pathway is largely distinct from that governing synthesis and secretion of mineralocorticoids (e.g. aldosterone), which are

under independent control by the renin–angiotensin (–aldosterone) system (Figure 6.1.2). Cortisol has multiple effects (including regulation of metabolism, vascular tone and immune function), which are primarily mediated through the glucocorticoid receptor, a member of the steroid nuclear receptor superfamily of transcription factors. The glucocorticoid receptor is widely distributed in the central nervous system, including in the hippocampus, amygdala, cerebral cortex, midbrain and brainstem. Cortisol is also able to bind with high affinity to the mineralocorticoid receptor (another steroid nuclear receptor), which partly mediates its effects in the brain. See Subsection 6.3.3 for more on the effects of cortisol on the brain.

In normal physiology, CRH and ACTH are secreted in a pulsatile manner (including in response to stressful stimuli), with an underlying circadian (diurnal) rhythm,

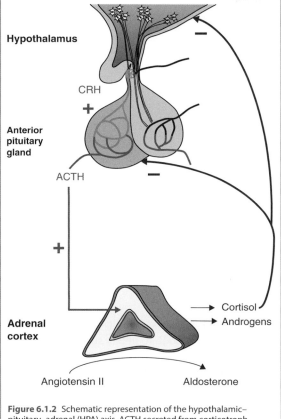

Figure 6.1.2 Schematic representation of the hypothalamic–pituitary–adrenal (HPA) axis. ACTH secreted from corticotroph cells in the anterior pituitary gland directs the synthesis and release of cortisol and androgens from the zona fasciculata and zona reticularis, respectively, in the adrenal cortex. Cortisol exerts negative feedback to inhibit CRH and ACTH release. Aldosterone production is largely independent of ACTH, and regulated by angiotensin II as part of the renin–angiotensin–aldosterone system. Key: ACTH, adrenocorticotrophic hormone; CRH, corticotropin-releasing hormone.

which is entrained by the activity of the suprachiasmatic nucleus. Hence, cortisol levels tend to be highest in the early morning on waking and decline during the course of the day to reach a nadir at midnight (Figure 6.1.3).

The HPA axis also exhibits classical negative feedback properties, with cortisol suppressing hypothalamic CRH and pituitary ACTH release (Figure 6.1.2). Exogenous corticosteroids (glucocorticoids, e.g. prednisolone/prednisone, dexamethasone) exert similar effects and, if high dosages are used for anything other than the shortest duration, can result in persistent suppression of HPA function. As ACTH has a trophic (sustaining) effect on the adrenal cortex, long-term exogenous glucocorticoid use can lead to adrenal atrophy, with the risk of precipitating an adrenal crisis if suddenly discontinued.

6.1.2.1 Psychological Manifestations of HPA Axis Dysfunction

In this subsection we explore the psychological manifestations of intrinsic disorders of the endocrine system. These may be less commonly seen in psychiatry than idiopathic disorders, but are important differential diagnoses for a range of psychiatric symptoms including depression, anxiety and psychosis. Scientifically, the underlying pathology means that these disorders can act as experimental models to elucidate more general principles of how hormones can contribute to brain symptoms. For discussion of the HPA axis in idiopathic psychiatric disorders, see Section 6.3.

HYPOADRENALISM (ADRENAL INSUFFICIENCY)

Adrenal insufficiency may be primary or secondary in origin. As in several other endocrine disorders, 'primary' means that the underlying dysfunction is at the level of the hormone-secreting (in this case adrenal) gland, while 'secondary' refers to abnormal stimulation of an otherwise normal gland. Primary adrenal insufficiency (often referred to as Addison's disease) is characterised by complete adrenocortical failure (with loss of glucocorticoids, mineralocorticoids and sex steroids) and is rapidly life-threatening if not promptly diagnosed and treated with adrenal replacement therapy [1–3]. A number of different causes are recognised (online appendix, Table S1; available at www.cambridge.org/CTNP). Secondary (central) adrenal insufficiency is a consequence of pituitary and/or hypothalamic dysfunction (with the latter sometimes referred to as tertiary adrenal insufficiency) (online appendix, Table S1). Adrenal insufficiency following cessation of exogenous glucocorticoids is common (reflecting the widespread use of corticosteroid therapy to treat an array of inflammatory, immune and neoplastic disorders). Preservation of mineralocorticoid secretion (reflecting normal renin–angiotensin–aldosterone function) in secondary/tertiary adrenal insufficiency may lead to a delay in diagnosis. Patients with central hypocortisolism are also at risk of life-threatening crises, especially during intercurrent illness. ACTH levels are elevated in primary adrenal insufficiency, but low or inappropriately normal in secondary/tertiary adrenal insufficiency.

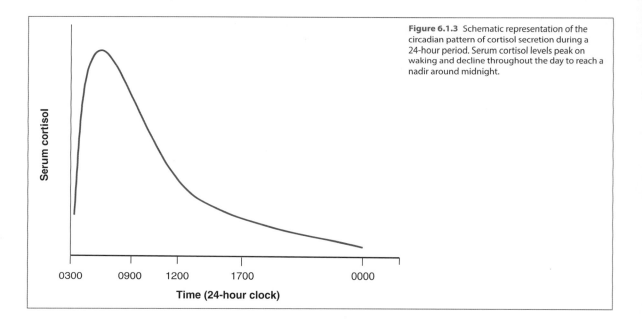

Figure 6.1.3 Schematic representation of the circadian pattern of cortisol secretion during a 24-hour period. Serum cortisol levels peak on waking and decline throughout the day to reach a nadir around midnight.

A major challenge with adrenal insufficiency is recognising its presence. A high index of suspicion is required because it frequently manifests in a non-specific manner; hence, adrenal insufficiency is known as the 'master of disguise'. Symptoms include tiredness, fatigue, anorexia, generalised weakness, aches and pains, weight loss, gastrointestinal upset, hypotension (especially postural) and hypoglycaemia. Electrolyte disturbance (hyponatraemia (with hyperkalaemia if primary adrenal insufficiency)) may provide an important clue to the presence of hypoadrenalism [3].

Not surprisingly, there is often a significant delay before the diagnosis is considered, and some patients are mistakenly deemed to have a primary depressive illness in the absence of any other physical explanation for their miscellaneous symptoms.

Even when the diagnosis has been made and appropriate hormone replacement therapy instituted, quality of life in patients with adrenal insufficiency may be significantly impaired. Indeed, a disease-specific questionnaire (AddiQoL) has been developed for patients with Addison's disease [4].

In recent years, the concept of 'adrenal fatigue' has been advanced as a condition caused by chronic exposure to stressful situations and manifesting with symptoms which overlap those of adrenal insufficiency.

Proponents argue that standard clinical investigations are not sensitive enough to detect subtle limitations of adrenal function and clinicians are therefore failing to recognise its presence. However, a recent systematic review was unable to find any evidence for the existence of adrenal fatigue as a nosological entity (see Table S1 legend).

HYPERCORTISOLISM (CUSHING SYNDROME)

Cushing syndrome, due to sustained exposure to supraphysiologic levels of glucocorticoid, may be ACTH-dependent (e.g. due to a pituitary adenoma or ectopic ACTH secretion syndrome) or ACTH-independent (e.g. during supraphysiologic exogenous corticosteroid therapy or due to an adrenal adenoma or carcinoma). Although Cushing syndrome in its most florid form is easily recognised, as with adrenal insufficiency the diagnosis is often delayed as several features overlap those seen in the general population (central obesity, hypertension, type 2 diabetes mellitus, osteoporosis). Hypercortisolism may be associated with various neuropsychiatric manifestations, including cognitive impairment, anxiety, emotional lability, depression, and even overt psychosis [5–7]. Glucocorticoid excess has been shown to inhibit long-term strengthening of synaptic connections (potentiation), which play a key role in memory formation and learning. Glucocorticoids also enhance the release of excitatory amino acids, which may explain hyperstimulatory neuropsychiatric manifestations. Psychiatric and neurocognitive features generally improve with treatment of hypercortisolism but may not resolve fully [8]. The impact of Cushing syndrome on quality of life can be assessed using disease-specific questionnaires [9, 10].

PSEUDO-CUSHING SYNDROME (NON-TUMORAL HYPERCORTISOLISM)

Certain clinical states can mimic Cushing syndrome, both symptomatically and on laboratory testing, including alcoholism, obesity and severe depression, but are not related to autonomous gland hyperfunction. However, investigation is fraught with pitfalls and early referral to a specialist centre is advised.

6.1.2.2 Investigation of the HPA Axis

Table 6.1.1 highlights the most commonly used screening tests for the investigation of suspected HPA dysfunction.

Table 6.1.1 Screening for HPA axis dysfunction

Suspected hypocortisolism
• 9 a.m.[a] serum cortisol[b] and serum electrolytes • Corticotropin (250 mcg synthetic ACTH$_{1-24}$ (tetracosactide = Synacthen®) stimulation test[b,c] • Plasma ACTH if adrenal insufficiency confirmed

Suspected Cushing syndrome
One or more of: • 1 mg overnight dexamethasone suppression test (DST)[b,d] • Late night[a] serum[b] or salivary[e] cortisol (minimum two samples) • 24 h urinary free cortisol estimation (ideally three collections)

[a]Random measurements of serum cortisol are generally best avoided because of the pulsatile and diurnal nature of CRH and ACTH release. Therefore, timed measurement (e.g. at 9 a.m. to exclude hypoadrenalism, or late in the evening/midnight to exclude hypercortisolism) is preferred. [b]Most clinical laboratories measure total (i.e. free and protein-bound) serum cortisol and, therefore, if cortisol binding globulin levels are raised (e.g. in the context of pregnancy or in a woman receiving oral oestrogen therapy), the measured serum cortisol will appear to be higher, which in turn may: (i) mask true hypoadrenalism; or (ii) falsely suggest hypercortisolism (e.g. with failure of adequate cortisol suppression during DST). [c]Where possible, corticotropin stimulation should be performed at 9 a.m., as this provides additional information by combining an unstimulated early morning measurement prior to injection (basal sample) with the peak response following supraphysiologic ACTH stimulation; this has particular value if using the test to screen for secondary adrenal insufficiency. [d]False positive DSTs may be seen in subjects with enhanced corticosteroid metabolism (either intrinsic fast metabolisers or during treatment with enzyme-inducing agents, e.g. carbamazepine, phenytoin, rifampicin). [e]Salivary (unlike serum) cortisol measurements involve estimation of free hormone levels; however, false elevations may be seen in cigarette smokers, those with poor dentition, and in diabetes mellitus.

6.1.3 The Hypothalamic–Pituitary–Thyroid (HPT) Axis

Thyrotropin-releasing hormone (TRH) is secreted from the hypothalamus (by parvocellular neurons in the paraventricular nucleus) in response to low circulating levels of thyroid hormones and other factors (e.g. environmental cold exposure). Binding to the TRH receptor on thyrotroph cells in the anterior pituitary gland stimulates the synthesis and secretion of thyroid-stimulating hormone (TSH). TSH then binds to the TSH receptor on thyroid follicular cells. TSH exhibits both a circadian and pulsatile pattern of secretion, peaking during the evening and early hours of the morning (nocturnal TSH surge).

In the thyroid gland, TSH stimulates the production of two main hormones: thyroxine (T4), which is produced in greater abundance (14:1) compared to triiodothyronine (T3), the biologically active form of thyroid hormone (Figure 6.1.4). Iodine, which is incorporated onto tyrosyl residues in thyroglobulin to yield mono- and di-iodotyrosines (which are then coupled to produce T4 and T3), is a key determinant of thyroid hormone biosynthesis. Conversion of T4 to T3 in peripheral tissues (in particular the liver) is facilitated by the type 1 deiodinase, a member of a family of deiodinases which also metabolise T4 and T3 to inactive forms. Type 2 deiodinase expression in the hypothalamus and pituitary gland regulates local T3 production to facilitate inhibition of TRH and TSH production as part of a classical negative feedback loop (Figure 6.1.4).

Thyroid hormone action in target tissues is mediated by two major receptor subtypes – alpha and beta and their splice variants – which are members of the steroid nuclear receptor superfamily. Thyroid hormones are critical regulators of a diverse array of physiological processes, including central nervous system development and function, metabolism, reproduction, bone turnover and cardiovascular function.

6.1.3.1 Psychological Manifestations of HPT Axis Dysfunction

HYPERTHYROIDISM

The term hyperthyroidism signifies a state of excess circulating thyroid hormones derived from the thyroid gland (as opposed to thyrotoxicosis, which also includes other sources, e.g. exogenous administration) (online appendix,

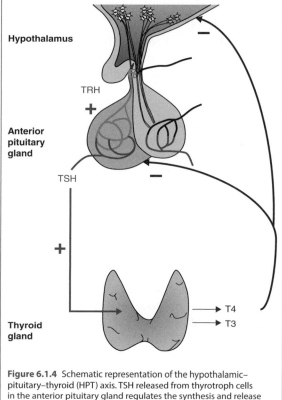

Figure 6.1.4 Schematic representation of the hypothalamic–pituitary–thyroid (HPT) axis. TSH released from thyrotroph cells in the anterior pituitary gland regulates the synthesis and release of thyroid hormones (T3 and T4) from the thyroid gland. Thyroid hormones (specifically T3) exert negative feedback to inhibit TRH and TSH release. Key: T3, triiodothyronine; T4, thyroxine; TRH, thyrotropin-releasing hormone; TSH, thyroid-stimulating hormone.

Table S2). Common symptoms include weight loss despite increased appetite, tremor, palpitations, heat intolerance, disturbed sleep and impaired memory and concentration. Clinical signs mirror symptoms (e.g. fine resting tremor, resting tachycardia and atrial fibrillation), with goitre and disease-specific manifestations (e.g. Graves' ophthalmopathy and dermopathy). Hyperthyroidism can be associated with psychological manifestations, including irritability, anxiety and depression, which are reported in up to 40% of patients [11–13]. Rarely, acute psychosis may be a presenting feature of hyperthyroidism and can complicate the management of thyroid storm: severe uncontrolled and life-threatening thyrotoxicosis. Several mechanisms have been proposed to explain the development of neuropsychiatric manifestations in thyrotoxicosis, including augmented beta-adrenoceptor-mediated adrenergic activity, stimulation of TSH receptors in the

hippocampus and cortex by TSH receptor autoantibodies in Graves' disease, and altered glucose metabolism in the limbic system.

APATHETIC HYPERTHYROIDISM

In apathetic hyperthyroidism, patients lack typical hyperthyroid symptoms; instead, neurobehavioural and psychological features predominate, with anxiety, lethargy and depression common presentations [14]. It is most frequently seen in elderly patients in whom the absence of classical features of thyroid hormone excess can contribute to significant delays in diagnosis. It is unclear whether the phenomenon is due to autonomic dysfunction associated with ageing.

HYPOTHYROIDISM

Hypothyroidism is characterised by low circulating thyroid hormone levels and, as with hyperthyroidism, may be primary or secondary in origin (online appendix, Table S3). Clinical manifestations include fatigue, weight gain despite reduced appetite, bradycardia, cold intolerance, constipation, hair loss and puffy facial appearance (myxoedema). The combination of cognitive impairment (forgetfulness, mental slowness, inattention), emotional lability and physical symptoms may be mistaken for a primary psychiatric disorder, and hypothyroidism can go unrecognised in patients presenting with affective disorders or overt psychosis. Once hypothyroidism is identified, symptoms usually respond to appropriate thyroid hormone supplementation [15, 16].

The combination of free T4 and TSH measurements allows the exclusion or confirmation of thyroid dysfunction in most patients.

6.1.3.2 Thyroid Hormone Therapy in Unipolar Depressive Disorder and Bipolar Depression

Both T4 and T3 therapy have been used in the management of non-psychotic major depression in otherwise biochemically euthyroid individuals. Most commonly, thyroid hormone therapy is added to ongoing antidepressant monotherapy when the patient has not responded adequately, although it may be started simultaneously to accelerate response. In a study using ^{18}F-fluorodeoxyglucose positron emission tomography, high-dose T4 therapy was associated with altered glucose metabolism in the anterior limbic network, with concomitant improvement of depression scores [17]. However, in a previous prospective, randomised, double-blind, placebo-controlled study, the same workers were unable to demonstrate a statistically significant improvement in symptoms with T4 therapy [18]. Others have advanced the case for T3 therapy in preference to T4, although its more rapid onset of action may predispose to unwelcome adverse effects (e.g. palpitations, sweating), and care must be exercised when considering any form of thyroid hormone therapy because of the risks of triggering known or occult cardiac disorders. Adverse effects on bone density may also occur with intermediate- to longer-term use.

6.1.4 The Hypothalamic–Pituitary– Gonadal (HPG) Axis

Gonadotropin-releasing hormone (GnRH), secreted from the hypothalamus (preoptic area and medial basal hypothalamus), binds to the GnRH receptor expressed on gonadotroph cells in the anterior pituitary gland to stimulate the synthesis and release of luteinising hormone (LH) and follicle-stimulating hormone (FSH) (Figure 6.1.5). Control of LH and FSH release is unique in that it relies on pulsatile GnRH secretion to upregulate release, whereas sustained (non-pulsatile) GnRH exposure (e.g. during exogenous GnRH agonist therapy) downregulates release. The pulse frequency also determines whether LH or FSH is produced in greater abundance, with more rapid pulse frequencies favouring LH release and vice versa for FSH. The pulsatile release of GnRH is relatively constant in males (every 1–2 hours) but varies across the menstrual cycle in females. GnRH neurons receive inputs from many other sensory and neuroendocrine cells which provide information about general health and fitness and external conditions – important prerequisites for future reproduction.

The actions of the gonadotropins are determined by the sex of the individual. Their primary target in females is the ovaries: FSH promotes follicular maturation, and LH is the major stimulator of ovulation; both are involved in ovarian steroidogenesis (i.e. production of oestradiol and progesterone). In males, LH drives Leydig cells to secrete testosterone which, together with FSH, stimulates spermatogenesis in Sertoli cells. The sex steroid hormones bind to their respective receptors (oestrogen, progesterone and androgen receptors – members of the steroid

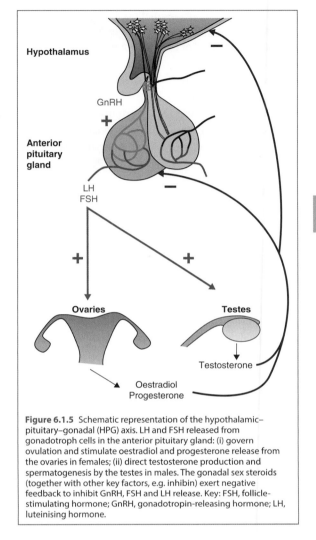

Figure 6.1.5 Schematic representation of the hypothalamic–pituitary–gonadal (HPG) axis. LH and FSH released from gonadotroph cells in the anterior pituitary gland: (i) govern ovulation and stimulate oestradiol and progesterone release from the ovaries in females; (ii) direct testosterone production and spermatogenesis by the testes in males. The gonadal sex steroids (together with other key factors, e.g. inhibin) exert negative feedback to inhibit GnRH, FSH and LH release. Key: FSH, follicle-stimulating hormone; GnRH, gonadotropin-releasing hormone; LH, luteinising hormone.

nuclear receptor superfamily) and exert widespread effects on sexual development and function, and other aspects of physiology (e.g. metabolism).

In males, testosterone exerts negative feedback on the anterior pituitary gland and hypothalamus (Figure 6.1.5). In females, oestradiol and progesterone suppress the release of GnRH and gonadotropins (the effects on GnRH may be mediated through neural pathways with afferent inputs to GnRH neurons rather than directly) (Figure 6.1.5); however, at the midpoint of the menstrual cycle the feedback effects of oestradiol on the hypothalamus become transiently positive, stimulating the preovulatory GnRH surge, which in turn triggers the preovulatory

LH surge. Other factors regulating the HPG axis include activin and inhibin, which have opposing effects on FSH secretion at the level of the anterior pituitary gland.

6.1.4.1 Psychological Manifestations of HPG Axis Dysfunction

For more on the role of sex hormones in idiopathic psychiatric disorders and in neurodegenerative diseases, see Section 5.3. Here, we explore the psychological manifestations of intrinsic disorders of the HPG axis.

HYPOGONADISM

Hypogonadism is characterised by low testosterone in males, low oestrogen in females and impaired fertility in both sexes. It can be classified as either primary (due to testicular or ovarian pathology) or secondary (due to pituitary or hypothalamic dysfunction). Primary gonadal failure in males may be a consequence of trauma, mumps, iatrogenic causes (e.g. chemotherapy, radiotherapy), or genetic conditions (e.g. Klinefelter syndrome). Causes of secondary hypogonadism include congenital (e.g. Kallmann syndrome and other inherited forms of hypogonadotropic hypogonadism) and acquired (e.g. pituitary adenoma, surgery, radiotherapy) disorders. In adult males, clinical manifestations include tiredness/fatigue, sexual dysfunction (with or without infertility), altered body composition (with reduced muscle mass and bone mineral density) and cognitive impairment. Both aromatase and androgen receptors are found in key regions of the brain involved in memory and learning, including the hippocampus and amygdala. Testosterone has been shown to increase concentrations of nerve growth factor (NGF) and upregulates NGF receptors in the forebrain. Androgens also attenuate N-methyl-D-aspartate (NMDA) receptor excitotoxicity in the hippocampus and protect against oxidative stress.

Adult females may experience menstrual dysfunction (with impaired fertility), mood change(s), lethargy and other features suggestive of premature menopause (e.g. vasomotor symptoms such as facial flushing and night sweats).

Patients with hypogonadotropic hypogonadism can experience psychological manifestations including anxiety and depression associated with reduced quality of life. If the onset is before puberty, affected individuals may experience problems with personality development, including altered perceptions of their body image and abnormal social adjustment [19].

6.1.4.2 Investigating the HPG Axis

In males, testosterone secretion shows a diurnal pattern and levels should ideally be measured in the morning (8–9 a.m.) to coincide with the natural peak. Testosterone levels decline with age and, where possible, levels should be compared with age-specific reference ranges. In females with a spontaneous normal regular menstrual cycle, there is usually little to be gained from laboratory measurement outside the context of investigation for infertility. When indicated, measurement of LH, FSH, oestradiol (± progesterone) should be referenced to the current phase of the menstrual cycle.

6.1.5 The Hypothalamic–Pituitary–Somatotropic (HPS) Axis

Growth hormone-releasing hormone (GHRH) is secreted from the arcuate nucleus of the hypothalamus and binds to the GHRH receptor on somatotroph cells in the anterior pituitary gland to stimulate growth hormone (GH) production and release. In contrast, somatostatin (SS), released from the anterior hypothalamus, directly inhibits pituitary somatotroph function. In this way, the synthesis and release of GH is tightly regulated by opposing hypothalamic signals. GH is secreted in a pulsatile manner and has a circadian rhythm. Under normal physiological conditions, GH secretion is maximal during the night, coinciding with the onset of slow-wave sleep. Levels also vary with the stage of development, being markedly higher during puberty, and followed by a sharp decline after the transition to young adulthood. Environmental triggers may also influence GH release: for example, exercise, trauma and hypoglycaemia serve as positive stimuli.

GH plays critical roles in neonatal and postnatal growth (particularly in the pubertal growth spurt), and regulates lipid (lipolytic), protein (anabolic) and carbohydrate (glucose) metabolism. GH exerts direct effects in some target tissues (e.g., adipocytes) through binding to the GH receptor (a transmembrane cytokine receptor), and indirect effects in others mediated by insulin-like growth factor 1 (IGF-1), which is produced principally in the liver in response to GH stimulation of hepatic GH receptor (Figure 6.1.6).

Synthesis and secretion of GHRH are inhibited by GH and IGF-1 while, in contrast, expression of SS is stimulated

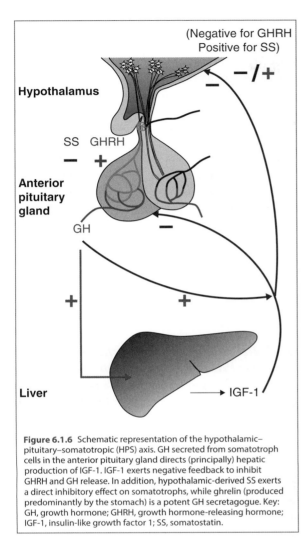

(Negative for GHRH
Positive for SS)

Figure 6.1.6 Schematic representation of the hypothalamic–pituitary–somatotropic (HPS) axis. GH secreted from somatotroph cells in the anterior pituitary gland directs (principally) hepatic production of IGF-1. IGF-1 exerts negative feedback to inhibit GHRH and GH release. In addition, hypothalamic-derived SS exerts a direct inhibitory effect on somatotrophs, while ghrelin (produced predominantly by the stomach) is a potent GH secretagogue. Key: GH, growth hormone; GHRH, growth hormone-releasing hormone; IGF-1, insulin-like growth factor 1; SS, somatostatin.

by the same hormones (Figure 6.1.6). Other factors that can downregulate the HPS axis include hyperglycaemia, glucocorticoids and leptin, while hypoglycaemia, high protein intake, fasting state and the potent GH secretagogue ghrelin (released from the stomach) all stimulate the HPS axis.

6.1.5.1 Psychological Manifestations of HPS Axis Dysfunction

GROWTH HORMONE DEFICIENCY

GH deficiency may be congenital or acquired (e.g. in the context of pituitary adenoma, intracranial radiotherapy, traumatic brain injury). The psychological manifestations of GH deficiency may be subtle and non-specific. Compared to matched controls, individuals with GH deficiency have lower self-esteem, increased difficulties with sexual relationships, a feeling of social isolation, inability to concentrate, increased anxiety and lower mood [20, 21]. GH replacement therapy has been shown to mitigate many, if not all, of these symptoms [22, 23].

ACROMEGALY

Acromegaly is a disorder of GH excess and is most commonly due to a somatotroph pituitary adenoma. It typically has an insidious onset. Clinical manifestations include enlarged hands and feet, enlarged tongue (macroglossia), prominent jaw (prognathism), frontal bossing and coarsening of facial features. Living with acromegaly can have a significant impact on quality of life [24], with many patients reporting social isolation, anxiety and depression, often linked to their change in appearance and the delay in diagnosis [25–27]. Reassuringly, an improvement in psychological well-being is observed in the majority of patients following commencement of appropriate treatment [28].

6.1.6 The Hypothalamic–Prolactin Axis

The regulation of prolactin secretion is largely governed by the inhibitory action of dopamine released from cells in the arcuate nucleus. Unique to the hypothalamic–prolactin axis is the absence of a primary hypothalamic-releasing hormone, although thyrotropin-releasing hormone (TRH) is able to stimulate prolactin secretion. Following release into the hypophyseal portal circulation, dopamine binds to dopamine D2 receptors (G-protein-coupled receptor family) expressed on anterior pituitary lactotroph cells to inhibit prolactin secretion. Lactotrophs undergo significant hypertrophy during pregnancy and lactation, and increased prolactin secretion may also occur with stress, exercise and sexual intercourse.

The prolactin receptor (cytokine receptor) is expressed primarily in the mammary glands and, at relatively lower levels, within the ovaries. In addition to its central roles in reproduction, prolactin has also been implicated in regulation of adipocyte function, islet differentiation [29] and immunomodulation [30].

Prolactin has a direct inhibitory action on pituitary lactotrophs, and glucocorticoids and somatostatin have also been shown to suppress prolactin secretion. Conversely, hormones such as TRH, oestrogen, GnRH and oxytocin may have a stimulatory effect.

6.1.6.1 Psychological Manifestations of Hypothalamic–Prolactin Axis Dysfunction

HYPERPROLACTINAEMIA

Numerous conditions and medications may cause hyperprolactinaemia, mainly by interfering with dopaminergic inhibition of anterior pituitary lactotroph function (online appendix, Table S5). Sustained elevation of prolactin can result in hypogonadism, galactorrhoea and, in some cases, infertility.

A possible role for hyperprolactinaemia in mediating anxiety, depression and increased hostility has been advanced [31]. However, the pathophysiological basis for such effects remains unclear, and others have postulated that the development of hyperprolactinaemia may simply be a marker of a primary psychological disturbance (i.e. effect rather than cause). Similarly, the potential impact of medication-induced hyperprolactinaemia on pre-existing psychiatric conditions remains uncertain, although previous data evaluating severity and disease course in schizophrenia did not show a correlation with elevation in prolactin levels [32].

Management of hyperprolactinaemia is largely tailored to the aetiology. However, when a pharmacological cause is suspected this may present a challenge, particularly for patients on medications to treat psychosis in whom withdrawal of the offending drug is not always feasible. Changing to (or adding) an agent with less propensity to cause hyperprolactinaemia, such as aripiprazole, may resolve the issue but, if in doubt, close liaison with the endocrine team is advised and allows exclusion of coincidental pathology (e.g. pituitary adenoma).

In patients with a prolactinoma, dopamine agonist therapy (e.g. cabergoline, quinagolide) is usually recommended as first-line management; however, there is increasing recognition of potentially serious adverse psychological effects of treatment in some patients: specifically, severe depression, manic episodes, psychosis [33] and profound impulsivity [34]. Patients (and where possible their relatives) should be advised of potential side effects of treatment and the need to seek early help if there are any concerns.

6.1.7 The Posterior Pituitary Gland

Release of stored hormones from the posterior pituitary gland is under direct control of hypothalamic neurons (paraventricular and supraoptic nuclei), which project to the posterior lobe (see Figure 6.1.1). Arginine vasopressin (antidiuretic hormone) is synthesised predominantly by neurons in the supraoptic nucleus, and oxytocin is produced by the magnocellular neurons of the paraventricular nucleus. Arginine vasopressin binds to specific receptors that are expressed in the vascular endothelium, where the hormone exerts its vasoconstrictor properties, and the renal collecting ducts, where it regulates water reabsorption. Oxytocin promotes uterine contraction during pregnancy and lactation during the postpartum period. It has also been shown to have a number of neurobehavioural effects, for example influencing mood, reducing fear/anxiety and promoting bonding and social interaction. See Section 8.3 for more on oxytocin and its role in attachment.

6.1.7.1 Psychological Manifestations of Posterior Pituitary Dysfunction

Abnormalities in arginine vasopressin release or action are associated with disordered salt and water balance. For example, excess secretion of arginine vasopressin leads to the syndrome of inappropriate antidiuretic hormone (SIADH); in contrast, impaired secretion (arginine vasopressin deficiency (AVP-D), also known as cranial diabetes insipidus (CDI)) or action (arginine vasopressin resistance (AVP-R), also known as nephrogenic diabetes insipidus (NDI)) of arginine vasopressin is associated with impaired ability to concentrate urine, with resultant polyuria.

SIADH

SIADH is an important cause of hypo-osmolar hyponatraemia. Clinical features vary depending on the speed of onset and severity of hyponatraemia, but include headache, nausea, fatigue, myalgia and confusion, and may progress to seizures and coma if not appropriately managed. Patients with SIADH are broadly clinically euvolaemic. Laboratory findings include: low serum sodium (<135 mmol/L), low serum osmolality (<270 mOsmol/kg), inappropriately elevated urinary osmolality (>100 mOsmol/kg) and inappropriate urinary sodium excretion (>30 mmol/L). The primary treatment is fluid restriction with close monitoring of the serum sodium to avoid unduly rapid correction (and the risk of pontine and extrapontine myelinolysis). Alterative treatment options include demeclocycline (inhibits renal response to arginine vasopressin) and vaptan therapy (inhibits arginine vasopressin binding to the vasopressin 2 receptor); however, their use requires specialist supervision.

Hyponatraemia is well recognised in patients with psychiatric illness, especially in the elderly [35]. Although certain medications predispose to the development of SIADH (e.g. selective serotonin reuptake inhibitors), other causes (e.g. excessive drinking (primary polydipsia)) should also be considered.

AVP-D AND AVP-R

AVP-D (CDI) and AVP-R (NDI) are characterised by absolute or relative deficiency of arginine vasopressin, respectively, and are associated with excess urine output and the development of hypernatraemia due to loss of free water. AVP-R may complicate other electrolyte disturbance (e.g. hypercalcaemia, hypokalaemia) and is linked to certain medications, including lithium (NB: discontinuation of lithium does not always reverse the condition).

Confirmatory testing requires formal water deprivation or hypertonic sodium chloride infusion, both of which should only be undertaken in a specialist endocrine unit.

Patients with AVP-D have a high incidence of neurocognitive dysfunction consequent on common underlying pathology (e.g. traumatic brain injury or surgery for a locally invasive lesion). A subgroup of patients with hypothalamic injury also lack normal thirst sensation, leading to so-called adipsic AVP-D (adipsic diabetes insipidus), which can be particularly challenging to manage. There is some evidence from animal models that arginine vasopressin itself may be required to potentiate higher brain function, with deficiency leading to impaired social recognition and anxiety-like behaviour [36].

Conclusions and Outstanding Questions

Disruption of the hypothalamic–pituitary neuroendocrine system can give rise to profound physical, cognitive and psychological manifestations. Therefore, just as the physician should keep a weather eye to the possibility of primary psychiatric disease in a patient with unexplained physical symptoms, similarly the psychiatrist must remain vigilant to the possibility of an unrecognised primary neuroendocrine disorder in a patient presenting with significant mental health issues. As we improve our understanding of how changes in neuroendocrine function impact cognitive and psychological processes, we open the door to potential novel approaches to the diagnosis and treatment of psychiatric disorders.

Outstanding Questions

- How do hormonal changes act on the brain to lead to specific psychological symptoms, and what determines which symptoms patients experience?

- Why do some of the psychological symptoms associated with endocrine abnormalities persist even when the underlying endocrine dysfunction has been corrected?

- Beyond treating the underlying endocrine disorder, should we treat psychological symptoms secondary to endocrine dysfunction in the same way as idiopathic psychiatric symptoms? Can we use our understanding of the pathophysiology to develop more tailored, more effective treatments?

- While cortisol levels and responses have been extensively investigated in the context of psychiatric disorders, the role of other neuroendocrine systems in idiopathic psychiatric disorders remains underexplored.

REFERENCES

1. Bergthorsdottir R, Leonsson-Zachrisson M, Odén A, Johannsson G. Premature mortality in patients with Addison's disease: a population-based study. *J Clin Endocrinol Metab* 2006; 91(12): 4849–4853.

2. Simpson H, Tomlinson J, Wass J, Dean J, Arlt W. Guidance for the prevention and emergency management of adult patients with adrenal insufficiency. *Clin Med* 2020; 20(4): 371.

3. Gurnell M, Heaney LG, Price D, Menzies-Gow A. Long-term corticosteroid use, adrenal insufficiency, and the need for steroid-sparing treatment in adult severe asthma. *J Intern Med* 2021; 290(2): 240–256.

4. Øksnes M, Bensing S, Hulting A-L et al. Quality of life in European patients with Addison's disease: validity of the disease-specific questionnaire AddiQoL. *J Clin Endocrinol Metab* 2012; 97(2): 568–576.

5. Kelly W. Psychiatric aspects of Cushing's syndrome. *QJM Int J Med* 1996; 89(7): 543–552.

6. Starkman MN, Schteingart DE. Neuropsychiatric manifestations of patients with Cushing's syndrome: relationship to cortisol and adrenocorticotropic hormone levels. *Arch Intern Med* 1981;141(2): 215–219.

7. Starkman MN, Gebarski SS, Berent S, Schteingart DE. Hippocampal formation volume, memory dysfunction, and cortisol levels in patients with Cushing's syndrome. *Biol Psychiatry* 1992; 32(9): 756–765.

8. Pivonello R, Simeoli C, De Martino MC et al. Neuropsychiatric disorders in Cushing's syndrome. *Front Neurosci* 2015; 9: 129.

9. Milian M, Teufel P, Honegger J. The development of the Tuebingen Cushing's disease quality of life inventory (Tuebingen CD-25). Part I: construction and psychometric properties. *Clin Endocrinol (Oxf)* 2012; 76(6): 851–860.

10. Cusimano MD, Huang TQ, Marchie A, Smyth HS, Kovacs K. Development and validation of the disease-specific QOL-CD quality of life questionnaire for patients with Cushing's disease. *Neurosurg Focus* 2020; 48(6): E4.

11. Demet MM, Özmen B, Deveci A et al. Depression and anxiety in hyperthyroidism. *Arch Med Res* 2002; 33(6): 552–556.

12. Suwalska A, Lacka K, Lojko D, Rybakowski J. Quality of life, depressive symptoms and anxiety in hyperthyroid patients. *Rocz Akad Med W Bialymstoku* 2005; 50: 61–63.

13. Bunevicius R, Prange AJ. Psychiatric manifestations of Graves' hyperthyroidism. *CNS Drugs* 2006; 20(11): 897–909.

14. Trivalle C, Doucet J, Chassagne P et al. Differences in the signs and symptoms of hyperthyroidism in older and younger patients. *J Am Geriatr Soc* 1996; 44(1): 50–53.

15. Samuels MH, Schuff KG, Carlson NE, Carello P, Janowsky JS. Health status, psychological symptoms, mood, and cognition in L-thyroxine-treated hypothyroid subjects. *Thyroid* 2007; 17(3): 249–258.

16. Samuels MH. Psychiatric and cognitive manifestations of hypothyroidism. *Curr Opin Endocrinol Diabetes Obes* 2014; 21(5): 377.

17. Bauer M, Berman S, Stamm T et al. Levothyroxine effects on depressive symptoms and limbic glucose metabolism in bipolar disorder: a randomized, placebo-controlled positron emission tomography study. *Mol Psychiatry* 2016; 21(2): 229–236.

18. Stamm TJ, Lewitzka U, Sauer C et al. Supraphysiologic doses of levothyroxine as adjunctive therapy in bipolar depression: a randomized, double-blind, placebo-controlled study. *J Clin Psychiatry* 2014; 75(2): 162–168.

19. Huisman J, Bosch J, Waal HD-V. Personality development of adolescents with hypogonadotropic hypogonadism. *Psychol Rep* 1996; 79(3_suppl): 1123–1126.

20. Degerblad M, Almkvist O, Grunditz R et al. Physical and psychological capabilities during substitution therapy with recombinant growth hormone in adults with growth hormone deficiency. *Eur J Endocrinol* 1990; 123(2): 185–193.

21. McKenna SP, Doward LC, Alonso J et al. The QoL-AGHDA: an instrument for the assessment of quality of life in adults with growth hormone deficiency. *Qual Life Res* 1999; 8(4): 373–383.

22. Sartorio A, Molinari E, Riva G et al. Growth hormone treatment in adults with childhood onset growth hormone deficiency: effects on psychological capabilities. *Horm Res Paediatr* 1995; 44(1): 6–11.

23. McMillan C, Bradley C, Gibney J, Healy M, Russell-Jones D, Sönksen P. Psychological effects of withdrawal of growth hormone therapy from adults with growth hormone deficiency. *Clin Endocrinol (Oxf)* 2003; 59(4): 467–475.

24. Webb S, Prieto L, Badia X et al. Acromegaly Quality of Life Questionnaire (ACROQOL), a new health-related quality of life questionnaire for patients with acromegaly: development and psychometric properties. *Clin Endocrinol (Oxf)* 2002; 57(2): 251–258.

25. Sievers C, Dimopoulou C, Pfister H et al. Prevalence of mental disorders in acromegaly: a cross-sectional study in 81 acromegalic patients. *Clin Endocrinol (Oxf)* 2009; 71(5): 691–701.

26. Szcześniak D, Jawiarczyk-Przybyłowska A, Rymaszewska J. The quality of life and psychological, social and cognitive functioning of patients with acromegaly. *Adv Clin Exp Med Off Organ Wroclaw Med Univ* 2015; 24(1): 167.

27. Sibeoni J, Manolios E, Verneuil L, Chanson P, Revah-Levy A. Patients' perspectives on acromegaly diagnostic delay: a qualitative study. *Eur J Endocrinol* 2019; 180(6): 339–352.

28. Wolters TLC, Roerink SH, Sterenborg R et al. The effect of treatment on quality of life in patients with acromegaly: a prospective study. *Eur J Endocrinol* 2020; 182(3): 319–331.

29. Gorvin CM. The prolactin receptor: diverse and emerging roles in pathophysiology. *J Clin Transl Endocrinol* 2015; 2(3): 85–91.

30. De Bellis A, Bizzarro A, Pivonello R, Lombardi G, Bellastella A. Prolactin and autoimmunity. *Pituitary* 2005; 8(1): 25–30.

31. Gomes J, Sousa A, Lima G. Hyperprolactinemia: effect on mood? *Eur Psychiatry* 2015; 30(S1): 1–1.

32. Meaney AM, O'Keane V. Prolactin and schizophrenia: clinical consequences of hyperprolactinaemia. *Life Sci* 2002; 71(9): 979–92.

33. Ioachimescu AG, Fleseriu M, Hoffman AR, Vaughan Iii TB, Katznelson L. Psychological effects of dopamine agonist treatment in patients with hyperprolactinemia and prolactin-secreting adenomas. *Eur J Endocrinol* 2019; 180(1): 31–40.

34. Barake M, Evins AE, Stoeckel L et al. Investigation of impulsivity in patients on dopamine agonist therapy for hyperprolactinemia: a pilot study. *Pituitary* 2014; 17(2): 150–156.

35. Siegler EL, Tamres D, Berlin JA, Allen-Taylor L, Strom BL. Risk factors for the development of hyponatremia in psychiatric inpatients. *Arch Intern Med* 1995; 155(9): 953–957.

36. Albers HE. The regulation of social recognition, social communication and aggression: vasopressin in the social behavior neural network. *Horm Behav* 2012; 61(3): 283–292.

6

<table>
<tr><td>**6.2**</td><td>**The Stress Response and Glucocorticoids**</td><td>Jeffrey W. Dalley and Joe Herbert</td></tr>
</table>

OVERVIEW

This section summarises the psychology and neurobiology of stress responses in humans. It considers the adaptive value of stress in enabling humans to detect real or perceived threats in the environment and, through learning, to build resilience through helpful coping responses. The conditions that favour 'toxic' forms of stress to prevail and so cause chronic metabolic, inflammatory and cognitive disorders are highlighted and discussed from the perspective of dysregulated cortisol signalling.

6.2.1 The Nature of Stress

Stress is a wide-ranging term that implies an undue or unusual demand on the individual that requires an adaptive or coping response. This response can be either beneficial, in the sense that the stressful event is overcome successfully, or damaging, since the adaptive response may incur either physical or psychological costs. Indeed, Hans Selye (1907–1982) first realised that stress was the cause of many non-specific symptoms associated with illnesses of the body and mind (Selye, 1955). This pioneering analysis led to the 'general adaptation syndrome' as a way to understand why individuals vary in their response to stress (see Figure 6.2.1).

Stressors themselves may be either physical (e.g. cold or heat, food or water deprivation, physical injury, etc.) or psychological (e.g. threat of aggression, a loss of relationship, employment, money, abuse, high workload, being a carer, etc.). The two categories are not clearly separable; for example, food shortages may lead to aggressive interactions and loss of employment can restrain food choice and availability. Stress may be acute and short-lasting, or persistent and repetitive; each engaging distinct brain and psychological mechanisms. However, a distinction should be made between 'stressors' (the event) and the 'stress response' (the reaction to that event), but this is not always made, and both are often subsumed under the rubric of 'stress'.

Not only the type of stress and its duration but the point in the life cycle at which it occurs is significant for altered brain function. In general, early-life adversity can have greater detrimental and long-lasting effects than that occurring later in life. This is reflected in abnormal patterns of brain connectivity in adulthood. But a major moderating factor at all ages is the context in which the stress occurs, the perception and assessment of the nature of the stress and the assets available for coping

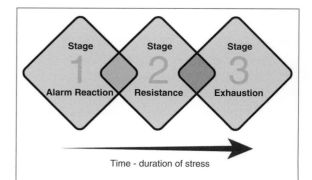

Time - duration of stress

Figure 6.2.1 Selye's three stages of stress. Stage 1 is the initial alarm stage where individuals organise an adaptive 'fight-or-flight' response. Stage 2 describes attempts by the individual to resist or compensate for the stressor to which it is exposed over a longer time scale. Stage 3 is the end stage of exhaustion when the impact of the stressor overwhelms the individual's capacity to deal with the stress. The final stage is reached when compensatory mechanisms are depleted, making individuals susceptible to disease.

with it. The individual quality of stress coping styles probably explains why some, but not all, people become susceptible to stress-related harms (de Kloet et al., 2019).

6.2.2 Endocrine Responses to Stress

Although stressors are varied, the endocrine response to them is a common one. Acute stressors, such as an argument or an accident, are characterised initially by activation of the autonomic system, including the secretion of adrenaline and noradrenaline from the adrenal medulla, usually for a few minutes or hours. Here we are concerned with more prolonged responses to persistent or repetitive stress, which results in elevated secretion of glucocorticoids, primarily cortisol, from the adrenal cortex. This can last for weeks or months or more. This is the final stage of a cascade of events, originating from the brain, that involves the recognition of the presence and nature of the stressor, its likely effect on individual well-being, the availability of means to counter or cope with that stress and the estimated likelihood of being able to do so (Figure 6.2.2). Stressors that are severe, involve loss or threat to well-being, and are seen as being either unpredictable or difficult to counter are those that are particularly liable to result in increased

release of corticotropin-releasing hormone (CRH) from the paraventricular nucleus of the hypothalamus, release of adrenocorticotropic hormone (ACTH) from the anterior pituitary gland, and subsequent heightened production of cortisol from the adrenal glands – the so-called hypothalamic–pituitary–adrenal (HPA) response. Release of cortisol is thus the final endpoint of a complex sequence of neural events that includes recognition and categorisation of the event (largely cortical), assessment of its significance (includes memory), emotional response (amygdala and hippocampus) and neuroendocrine reaction (hypothalamus).

There are two important elements of the cortisol response to stress: elevated levels and disruption of the daily cortisol rhythm. Both have significant, but different, effects on brain function. The first will increase the overall exposure of the brain to corticoids; the second will alter the daily pattern of cortisol, disrupting in particular the 'time-off' period during which the brain has little exposure to cortisol. But interpreting 'stress' simply by a neuroendocrine response should be hedged with caution as many non-stressful activities (e.g. sexually motivated behaviours) can result in dramatically raised corticoid levels (Koolhaas et al., 2011). Stressors that are chronic,

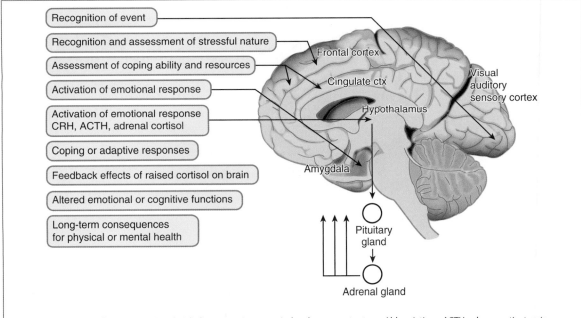

Figure 6.2.2 The neural events associated with the perception, appraisal and response to stress. Abbreviations: ACTH, adrenocorticotropic hormone; CRH, corticotropin-releasing hormone.

unpredictable and uncontrollable are those that dele-teriously impact the regulation of the HPA axis and are therefore relevant to disease.

6.2.3 Actions of Glucocorticoids on the Brain

Tissues only respond to steroids if they have the necessary receptors, and the brain is not an exception. The classic glucocorticoid receptor is a large cytoplasmic protein. This has various domains, to one of which cortisol binds. Once activated, the glucocorticoid receptor sheds some associated proteins (including heat shock proteins 70 and 90, and FKBP51, which is replaced by FKBP52) and travels into the cell nucleus. Here it binds to a DNA motif, which is present in a large number of genes, including brain-derived neurotrophic factor (BDNF). The result is either activation or suppression of these genes (see Figure 6.2.3).

The glucocorticoid receptor has a limited capacity, like all receptors. Under normal, basal, conditions, this recep-tor is not fully occupied, thus leaving room for detecting additional cortisol released during stress. Genetic variants

of the glucocorticoid receptor will alter this capacity, as well as its ability to bind to DNA, thus accounting for some of the individual variability in the response to stress. Another source of variation is epigenetic meth-ylation of DNA, which alters gene expression. This can occur in response to adverse effects in early life (e.g. poor parenting). Increased methylation of CpG sites in the DNA glucocorticoid-response element can have long-standing or even permanent effects on subsequent responses to stress during adulthood (Argentieri et al., 2017).

Most of the cells of the brain, both neurons and glia, express the glucocorticoid receptor. However, there are notably high concentrations in the hippocampus, amyg-dala and hypothalamus (i.e. the limbic system). There is also a second, membrane-bound, glucocorticoid recep-tor, which has a much faster response time than the cyto-plasmic one. Unlike the latter, membrane receptors act through classic cell signalling pathways, including protein kinases, cation channels and G-protein-coupled recep-tors. They are less well understood than the cytoplasmic receptors but seem to have similar downstream effects

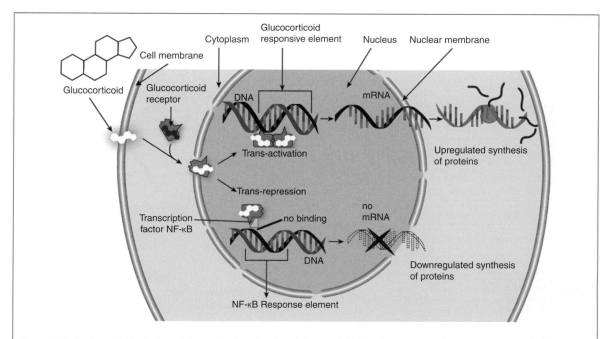

Figure 6.2.3 A schematic illustration of the mechanism of action of glucocorticoids on the genome. Following glucocorticoid binding, the glucocorticoid receptor complex moves to the nucleus where it influences the production of a number of proteins involved in immunological, metabolic and inflammatory processes. Such diverse outcomes are mediated by direct interactions with glucocorticoid response elements leading to trans-activation and trans-repression. Whereas trans-activation upregulates proteins involved in immune and metabolic processes, trans-repression downregulates immunosuppressive and pro-inflammatory proteins (adapted with permission from van der Goes et al. (2014)).

and are primary candidates for mediating stress-induced plasticity and, specifically, the 'wear and tear' (or allostatic load) of chronic stress (McEwen and Gianaros, 2011).

6.2.4 Neuronal and Behavioural Consequences of Raised Corticoids

Persistently raised cortisol levels or altered cortisol rhythms are known to have both neurological and behavioural effects. Currently, there are severe limitations in our ability to relate neural events to behavioural ones. This restricts interpreting the exact manner in which corticoids influence behaviour at a neural level.

6.2.4.1 Effects on Neurons

Increased cortisol levels have effects on both the morphology and biochemistry of neurons. Excess corticoids damage neurons but also make them more susceptible to other damaging agents. In the hippocampus, heightened corticoids diminish branching of dendrites in CA1 and CA3 (regions of the hippocampal pyramidal layer), and thus alter the number and morphology of the principal neurons (Uno et al., 1989). The hippocampus is one of the few sites in the adult brain that continues to make new neurons during adult life (neurogenesis) in humans as well as other species. Raised corticoids powerfully reduce the activity of progenitor cells in the dentate gyrus, which develop into new neurons. They also increase the rate of apoptosis (programmed cell death) and reduce the ability of these new neurons to make new connections to CA3. There is an associated suppression of BDNF, essential for synaptogenesis, and reduced neuronal number in chronically stressed rodents and primates (Uno et al., 1989). The associated behavioural effects include reduction in hippocampal-dependent memory, though there is still uncertainty about the functional consequences of reduced neurogenesis. One notion is that new neurons are involved in pattern recognition – the ability to detect novel sets of stimuli. Experimentally, raised corticoids have been found to have long-lasting effects on subsequent cognitive performance, and patients with Cushing's disease have deficits in attention, executive function and non-verbal memory. Disruption of the circadian corticoid rhythm has similar effects, but may also alter the expression of many genes, mostly those that control transcription.

These effects are not limited to the hippocampus. Dendritic spine density in the amygdala is also sensitive to raised glucocorticoids, and this may impact anxiety responses and associative learning. Chronic stress induces remodelling of synapses in the prefrontal and orbitofrontal cortex, as well as the striatum (Dias-Ferreira et al., 2009). This has implications for responses to rewards and punishments, decision making, as well as vigilance for new stressors, and there are close associations between these parts of the frontal lobe and the amygdala, and hence emotionality, such as anxiety and fear.

Raised glucocorticoids increase the vulnerability of neurons to other toxic agents, such as excess glutamate (e.g. released after a stroke). In contrast to their anti-inflammatory actions in the periphery, corticoids in the brain can be pro-inflammatory, and promote the release of cytokines including interleukins 1 and 6 from astrocytes and microglia. These pro-inflammatory interleukins represent a low-grade inflammatory state. This is one avenue whereby they may alter mood and memory.

6.2.4.2 Effects on Glia

The significance of glucocorticoids and their response to stress for brain function is not limited to neurons. There is increasing evidence that glia (see Section 1.4) are also very sensitive to their action. Astrocytes play major roles in maintaining the blood–brain barrier, in synaptic plasticity, in the constitution of the brain's extracellular matrix, in neuronal survival and in the generation of circadian rhythms. The effects that glucocorticoids have on them will therefore have correspondingly widespread consequences for brain function. Microglia are the primary immunologically responsive cells in the brain, and their activation by glucocorticoids probably underlies much of the pro-inflammatory action they have on the brain.

6.2.4.3 Effects on Mood and Cognition in Humans

Cushing's disease, in which cortisol is chronically raised, is associated with marked changes of mood, mostly depression, and difficulties with aspects of cognition such as short-term memory (see Section 6.1.2). Treatment relieves the changes in mood, but alterations in cognition tend to persist. Therapeutic glucocorticoids (e.g. prednisolone, dexamethasone) given in higher doses and for longer periods increase the rate of affective disorders and impairments of memory. Cortisol levels tend to rise with age in humans, and this has been associated with increasing difficulty with recent memory. Glucocorticoids have been shown in both animals and humans to consolidate memories of adverse or threatening (i.e. stressful) events, a function that is thought to occur in the amygdala and be enabled by coincident activation of the neural noradrenergic system. This has relevance to conditions such as post-traumatic stress disorder (PTSD). For the contribution of glucocorticoids to psychiatric disorders including depression and PTSD, see Section 6.3.

Conclusions and Outstanding Questions

Stress has diverse impacts on humans. Although it is universal, what is defined as a stress, and how the response to it is formulated is highly individual and modulated by many factors, including genetic variations, early adversities, social and financial resources and previous experience. The balance between stress resilience and stress vulnerability depends on the intensity, chronicity and controllability of stressors, with early life stress often having the most profound and persistent effects on the bodily systems.

Outstanding Questions

- What is the biological nature of so-called 'stress memories' encoded in early life?
- How can we harness knowledge of early stress impacts for treatment intervention in adults with refractory stress-related disorders?
- Will new therapeutic targets emerge for stress management from a deeper understanding of the immune and brain microglial systems?
- What is the nature of interactions between cognitive and emotional processes in coping with stress?

REFERENCES

Argentieri MA, Nagarajan S, Seddighzadeh B, Baccarelli AA, Shields AE (2017). Epigenetic pathways in human disease: the impact of DNA methylation on stress-related pathogenesis and current challenges in biomarker development. *EBioMedicine* 18: 327–350.

de Kloet ER, de Kloet SF, de Kloet CS, de Kloet AD (2019). Top-down and bottom-up control of stress-coping. *J Neuroendocrinol* 31: e12675.

Dias-Ferreira E, Sousa JC, Melo I et al. (2009). Chronic stress causes frontostriatal reorganization and affects decision-making. *Science* 325: 621–625.

Koolhaas JM, Bartolomucci A, Buwalda B et al. (2011). Stress revisited: a critical evaluation of the stress concept. *Neurosci Biobehav Rev* 35: 1291–1301.

McEwen BS, Gianaros PJ (2011). Stress- and allostasis-induced brain plasticity. *Annu Rev Med* 62: 431–445.

Selye H (1955). Stress and disease. *Science* 122: 625–631.

Uno H, Tarara R, Else JG, Suleman MA, Sapolsky RM (1989). Hippocampal damage associated with prolonged and fatal stress in primates. *J Neurosci* 9: 1705–1711.

van der Goes MC, Jacobs JW, Bijlsma JW (2014). The value of glucocorticoid co-therapy in different rheumatic diseases: positive and adverse effects. *Arthritis Res Ther* 16: S2.

6

National Neuroscience Curriculum Initiative online resources

To Bend and Not Break: The Neurobiology of Stress, Resilience, and Recovery

Erik A. Levinsohn and David A. Ross

Telomeres, Trauma, and Training

Ashley E. Walker, Elizabeth Fenstermacher and David A. Ross

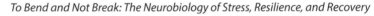

What to Say: *To Bend and Not Break: The Neurobiology of Stress, Resilience, and Recovery*

Jane Eisen

Clinical neuroscience conversations: *Translational Neuroscience and Stress Adaptation*

This "stuff" is really cool: Joseph Taylor, *"The Neuroscience of Kafka"* on stress and *perceived control*

Expert video: *Rachel Yehuda on Trauma and Resiliency*

Expert video: *Carlos Bolaños on Stress*

6.3 **Adrenal Steroids**   **Joe Herbert and**
Ian M. Goodyer

OVERVIEW

This chapter focuses on the observations that variations in adrenal steroid levels, particularly cortisol, contribute to psychopathology and major depression in particular. The associations are complex due to clinical heterogeneity together with physiological and genetic variations, influencing corticoid production, function and activation by environmental adversities. There is evidence that genetic differences in adrenal function, the impact of chronic early adversity, excess corticoid production or exogenous corticoids each contribute to the risk of depression, delay in clinical recovery and relapse. Further, psychiatric illnesses, mainly but not exclusively depression, may induce changes in corticoid activity. Elevated corticoids can affect psychological function, in particular reduced memory acuity for recall of and emotional responses to life experiences.

There is a suggestion that evening cortisol hypersecretion is associated with longer time to treatment response but not treatment insensitivity per se. Elevated cortisol levels may act as a moderator for choosing therapy or treatment response but this remains to be fully explicated. Providing anti-glucocorticoid medication to alter adrenal function in depressed patients has also been suggested but insufficiently evaluated. Although this chapter focuses primarily on major depression, altered corticoids have been implicated in other disorders, including post-traumatic stress disorder and conduct disorder. Cortisol itself may be moderated by other steroids, including dehydroepiandrosterone (DHEA), whose levels are highest in young people; reductions in DHEA will amplify the actions of cortisol. Finally, there are potentially important associations between corticoid activity and immune responses that remain markedly underspecified in depression and other mental illnesses.

6.3.1 Hormones and Psychological Symptoms

The list of symptoms of practically every endocrine disorder includes one or more abnormal changes in behaviour and many alterations in moods, thoughts and sensations consistent with those found in psychiatric disorders. This includes abnormalities in hormones from the gonads, thyroid, adrenal cortex and medulla, parathyroid, pituitary gland, gastrointestinal tract, pancreas and even those secreted by adipose tissue. In most cases, mental symptoms and their behavioural correlates are subsumed by more prominent physical signs and symptoms of the primary endocrine abnormality. However, any of these hormone-driven conditions may present with mental and/or behavioural symptoms and, on occasion, as a formal psychiatric disorder. These mental phenomena and their associated behaviours can be the result of either low or excess hormone secretion (see Section 6.1 for more on psychological features of endocrine disorders). Importantly, the converse of these observations is not true: most mental illnesses are not associated with overt endocrine disturbances, though some forms of major depressive disorder (MDD) are an exception.

Like all mental illnesses, MDD is clinically defined by observable signs and symptoms whose relationship with each other also occurs in the population at large to a greater extent than expected by chance alone. Descriptive clinical definitions of illnesses such as MDD are highly reliable and have resulted in considerable advances in our understanding of their prevalence and natural history. However, it has become apparent that there is clinical heterogeneity in MDD and that this is associated with corresponding aetiological (causal) and therapeutic heterogeneity in almost all clinical psychiatry disorders. MDD is therefore a syndrome, with moderate to low causal and prognostic validity and uncertain therapeutic responses across the life course. MDD has been particularly associated with alterations in circulating peripheral glucocorticoids at the extreme end of the normal physiological range.

6.3.2 The Hypothalamic–Pituitary–Adrenal Axis and the Early Social Environment

Everyday life involves managing stressors of varying degrees of severity, and the body must respond to these environmental stressors with physiological adaptations to restore homeostasis. The hypothalamic–pituitary–adrenal (HPA) system constitutes one of the principal pathways of the mammalian stress response, in which a cascade of events leads to elevations in glucocorticoid hormones. In response to a stressor, the hypothalamus increases the amount of corticotropin-releasing hormone (CRH) and arginine vasopressin that it produces and releases into the anterior pituitary gland, which responds by producing and releasing adrenocorticotropic hormone (ACTH). ACTH stimulates the adrenal gland to produce cortisol, a steroid hormone for which the brain is the principal target organ. Cortisol is necessary for survival, but when cortisol is chronically elevated or poorly regulated, it can have deleterious impacts on health. The basic physiology of the HPA axis and its response to stress are described further in Sections 6.1 and 6.2.

The HPA system is not fully mature at birth. There are manifest developmental changes throughout infancy in both basal HPA activity and cortisol reactivity. The system begins to show stable diurnal characteristics by 3 years of age but may not be fully mature until middle

childhood years. The developing HPA axis is under strong social regulation in infancy and early childhood and is vulnerable to perturbation in the absence of sensitive, responsive caregiving. This may include cortisol hypersecretion at times of increased environmental demands or hyposecretion if exposed to frequent and long-term childhood maltreatment characterised by passive emotional indifference, active personal criticism (e.g. 'You are useless'), physical or sexual abuse.

Different characteristics of the cortisol output may be associated with distinct patterns of behaviour. For example, persistently elevated morning cortisol is a hormonal risk for the emergence of depression whereas acute evening elevations indicating a loss of diurnal rhythm are correlates of current mental illness. Exposure to acute stressful environments that become chronic may be associated with high cortisol output switching to persistently reduced cortisol output that shows little subsequent reactivity to new stressors; this can occur in individuals with antisocial behaviour and psychopathic traits.

6.3.3 Individual Differences in Glucocorticoid Function

There are marked individual differences in levels of cortisol within the normal physiological range. The brain's exposure to cortisol depends on several factors: blood cortisol levels; blood levels of the transport protein cortisol binding protein (CBG); conversion of cortisol to inactive metabolites in the brain (e.g. by the enzyme 11-beta-hydroxysteroid dehydrogenase type 2 (11β-HSD2)); and export of cortisol from the brain by efflux transporters (Figure 6.3.1). A second, equally important feature is the marked daily rhythm in cortisol, which can vary several-fold from the early morning peak to the evening trough. This rhythm is itself made up of circa-horal (~ hourly) pulses, and the shape and frequency of these have marked effects on gene expression in the brain. There are many factors underlying individual differences, including gender (morning basal levels: females > males), genetic variants (including those in genes coding for the glucocorticoid receptor, 11β-HSD2, CBG and FKBP5), early adversity (altered responses to stress), current stress (work, relationships, finance, etc.) and as part of a physiological response to novel and potentially threatening events in the current environment. Cortisol levels may also alter as a consequence of the metabolic and psychological effects of mental illness itself.

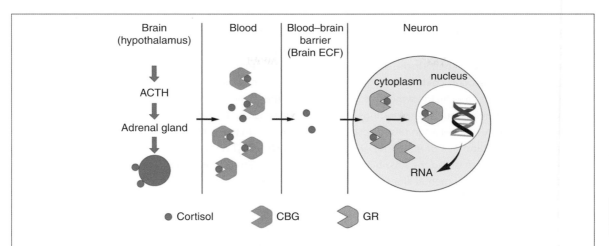

Figure 6.3.1 The process of transporting cortisol from blood to brain. Cortisol binds to plasma protein (CBG), but a fraction remains free. This crosses the blood–brain barrier and binds to another protein inside the cell (GR). This complex is transported to the cell nucleus, binds to a specific part of DNA and activates a set of genes. CBG, corticoid-binding globulin; GR, glucocorticoid receptor; ECF, extracellular fluid.

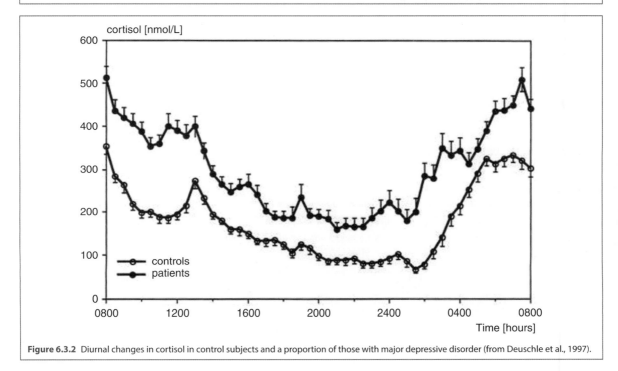

Figure 6.3.2 Diurnal changes in cortisol in control subjects and a proportion of those with major depressive disorder (from Deuschle et al., 1997).

6.3.4 Glucocorticoids as a Risk Factor for MDD

The earliest suggestions that glucocorticoids are potential causal factors in the emergence of psychiatric disorders came from observations of medical patients with disorders of the HPA axis or who were prescribed exogenous steroids. Psychological changes in such conditions are invariably associated with non-physiological elevated levels of circulating cortisol or related therapeutic steroids. For example, Cushing's disease is commonly associated with psychiatric syndromes of which MDD is common. These syndromes often resolve after the hypercortisolaemia is corrected although more persistent impairments in executive function, cognition and memory have been observed. Prolonged treatment with higher doses of glucocorticoid-like compounds (e.g. prednisolone) has also been associated with an increased risk of mental illnesses including MDD: a large-scale study of National Health Service patients in the UK showed that those treated with glucocorticoids had a higher prevalence of MDD and other psychiatric symptoms including mania and suicidal behaviour. These findings suggest there may be a causal link between raised cortisol and subsequent mental illnesses of which MDD appears the best candidate. There is also the possibility that the metabolic consequences of mental illnesses contribute to neuropathology. Major depression impedes efficient brain function and increases energy requirements. There are consequential increases in activity in the molecular, cellular and physiological systems involved in maintaining homeostasis. This elevated activity may potentially increase glucocorticoid output and thereby increase future neuroendangerment to the brain (Herbert, 2013).

Altered glucocorticoids have been implicated both as a risk for MDD (i.e. present before the emergence of the psychiatric disorder) and as an endocrine disturbance accompanying it (Figures 6.3.2 and 6.3.3). Higher morning waking cortisol levels increase the risk for subsequent MDD in adolescents of both sexes and in adult women. The risk is particularly marked in adolescent males with elevated but non-clinical levels of depressive symptoms (Owens et al., 2014). There is a surge of cortisol 30–60 minutes after wakening (cortisol awakening response) whose function is unknown. The cortisol awakening response can be increased by early childhood adversity, which may depend on the nature and duration of the adversity exposure. The effects of cortisol may also be sensitive to genetic variants, such as the number of repeats in the promotor of the serotonin (5-HT) transporter (5-HTTLPR) or the common Val/66/Met variant in the gene for BDNF (Goodyer et al., 2010). Individuals with these genetic variants appear to be at greater risk of MDD if they also have cortisol hypersecretion.

FKBP5 is a gene that produces proteins which can regulate the activity of the glucocorticoid receptor. Expression of *FKBP5* is regulated by corticosteroids at the transcriptional level through the DNA glucocorticoid response element. It can alter the affinity of the glucocorticoid receptor to corticosteroids, thus resulting in impaired glucocorticoid receptor signalling and feedback. These associations suggest that *FKBP5* variants might represent additional risk factors for MDD (Rao et al., 2016). However, results from studies across a range of countries have been somewhat inconsistent, so whether common variants in *FKBP5* are associated with MDD susceptibility in currently well individuals remains inconclusive.

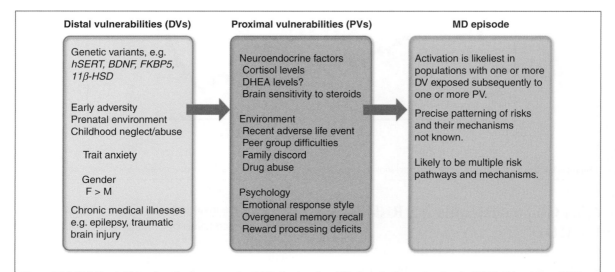

Figure 6.3.3 Distal (early-life) and proximal components contributing to vulnerability to major depressive disorder (MDD). Abbreviations: BDNF, brain-derived neurotrophic factor; DHEA, dehydroepiandrosterone; GR, glucocorticoid receptor; 11β-HSD, 11-beta-hydroxysteroid dehydrogenase; hSERT, serotonin transporter.

6.3.5 Possible Causal Mechanisms Associated with Glucocorticoids

Lack of understanding of the neurobiological basis of MDD, a clinically, aetiologically and therapeutically heterogeneous disorder, limits interpretation of the results described above (Herbert, 2013). There has been a neurobiological focus on BDNF, a growth factor that has been implicated in MDD, and which is very sensitive to glucocorticoids (Goodyer et al., 2010). Genetic variants associated with increased risk for MDD and other mood disorders in genome-wide association studies (GWAS) do not, however, include growth-factor genes. Meta-analysis of over 800,000 participants (including >240,00 depressed patients) from published GWAS studies has advanced our understanding of the complex genetic architecture of depression and provided several future avenues for understanding aetiology and potentially developing new treatment approaches (Howard et al., 2019). Combining GWAS with environmental risk and resilience factors is a logical next step. Fundamental genetic vulnerabilities in brain structure development may accompany the corticoid-mediated risks associated with *5-HTTLPR* (genetic variations in the serotonin transporter), *BDNF* and *FKBP5*

gene variants. Reduced hippocampal neurogenesis which continues into adult life is another candidate. Neurogenesis is very sensitive to both corticoids and BDNF. It is repressed by glucocorticoids and stimulated by selective serotonin reuptake inhibitors (SSRIs) in animal models. However, whether neurogenesis in the hippocampus is actually lowered in some forms of MDD, and whether increases occur in those who respond to treatment including psychotherapies and/or medicines for depression, is still uncertain, though hippocampal neurogenesis is reduced in post-mortem samples from depressed subjects. The role of hippocampal neurogenesis in depression has still to be clarified, though it may contribute to dysfunctional mnemonic recall of autobiographical events. Chronically elevated corticoids can activate microglia and be pro-inflammatory in the brain. Raised levels of cytokines, such as interleukins 1 and 6, have been postulated as contributing to the onset of MDD (Pariante, 2017) (see Section 6.4).

Disordered hormones are only one risk factor for MDD, and combine with others such as early adversity, trait anxiety, adventitious life events and the emergence of puberty (Figure 6.3.4). Genetic susceptibility factors,

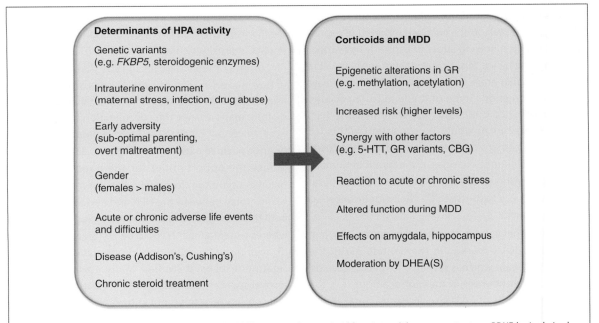

Figure 6.3.4 Determinants and moderators of individual differences in glucocorticoid function and the response to stress. BDNF, brain-derived neurotrophic factor; CBG, corticosteroid-binding globulin; DHEA(S), dehydroepiandrosterone (sulphate); GR, glucocorticoid receptor; 11β-HSD, 11-beta-hydroxysteroid dehydrogenase; 5-HTT, serotonin transporter.

which may include propensities for endocrine disruption (e.g. variants in the glucocorticoid receptor gene or *FKBP5*), have still to be clearly defined.

6.3.6 Changes in Glucocorticoids During an Episode of MDD

There is a long-standing interest in disturbances of cortisol during MDD. In a proportion of cases (30–50%), evening cortisol levels increase so the daily rhythm is flattened. Morning levels may or may not also increase. Whether this contributes to symptoms or helps define a clinical subtype has still not been established. There is some preliminary evidence that, in severely depressed patients, elevated evening cortisol is associated with current MDD symptoms while elevated morning cortisol is associated with childhood adversities. During depressive episodes, there is also increased resistance to negative feedback, such that an overnight dose of dexamethasone no longer suppresses morning levels of cortisol to those expected (the dexamethasone suppression test). The cortisol awakening response is reduced in some patients. These measures recover as psychiatric symptoms resolve, and in longitudinal studies their persistence or return is associated with recurrence or non-recovery of MDD.

Epigenetic changes in the glucocorticoid receptor gene (hypermethylation) have been reported in experimental animals following stress or early adversity (poor parenting), but since this is currently not measurable in the living human brain, it is not known whether it plays a part in depression. Some of the features associated with glucocorticoid receptor hypermethylation (e.g. feedback resistance) would be consistent with such changes and perhaps occur in humans. There have been reports of epigenetic changes in the blood in humans following childhood adversity, but since these alterations can be very tissue-specific, their significance has been questioned.

Hippocampal volume is reduced in depression, and this is particularly marked in the dentate gyrus, the neurogenic region which is sensitive to glucocorticoids. However, other neurons in the hippocampus (e.g. the pyramidal neurons of CA1) also show structural abnormalities in experimental animals treated with excess corticoids. Whether hippocampal volume is also a marker

for susceptibility to depression has not been reliably established, though reduced volumes (but with lowered cortisol) have been associated with vulnerability to PTSD.

6.3.7 Cortisol Hypersecretion, Cognition and Depression

Cortisol is known to affect memory processes. Stress- or pharmacologically induced elevations of cortisol levels enhance memory consolidation, particularly for negative events. Experimentally induced elevations of cortisol levels have also been shown to impair memory retrieval. Higher morning cortisol levels are associated with impaired recall of autobiographical memories, characterised by non-specific low detail and poor temporal precision of a prior experience (Owens et al., 2014). These observations are not influenced by the emotional valence of the recalled experience, suggesting a pervasive mnemonic deficit. In contrast, decreases in cortisol levels during retrieval of memory are associated with better quality of recall, and this is also regardless of emotional valence or length of the retention interval. Individuals with good autobiographical recall for past events with hedonic emotional qualities (specific positive recall of events), show lowered morning cortisol levels up to 3 years later (Askelund et al., 2019). This suggests a potential psychophysiological mechanism by which HPA axis function may lower the impact of proximal stress.

Currently the evidence suggests that, in situations of proximal environmental risk, raised cortisol levels (in association with activation of the central noradrenergic system) may enhance the consolidation of undesirable experiences but block the restorative properties of recall of prior positive experiences (Figure 6.3.5). This would reduce the opportunities for spontaneous recovery following symptom formation. Such psychophysiological interplay between the HPA and hedonic memory in both the emergence of mental illnesses and the processes whereby mental health could be restored would benefit from more investigation in population-based and treatment-focused studies. Many episodes of MDD recover spontaneously, but whether cortisol or variations in it contribute to this is not known. Neither do we know whether individual differences in cortisol contribute to patterns of recurrent depression.

Development	Childhood	Adolescence and adulthood	Episode of MDD
Glucocorticoids			
GR genetic variants 11β-HSD2	Epigenetic alterations (methylation reducing GR sensitivity/output)	Individual differences Levels and/or metabolism, awakening response Pathological elevation	Reduced feedback sensitivity Disrupted diurnal rhythm
Other events and factors			
Genetic variants e.g. *BDNF*, *FKBP5*, 5-HTT	Early adversity	Recent life events Puberty Gender Trait anxiety Autobiographical memory, rumination	Symptom pattern Impairment/severity Social and personal consequences Relapse, recurrence comorbidities

years →

Figure 6.3.5 Hormonal, genetic and environmental risk factors for the onset of an episode of major depression. GR, glucocorticoid receptor; 5-HTT, serotonin transporter.

6.3.8 Therapeutics of MDD and Glucocorticoids

Given the postulated causal effects of HPA dysregulation in MDD there is growing interest in using medications that inhibit cortisol secretion and/or increase glucocorticoid feedback sensitivity (Fischer et al., 2017). So far, studies are at proof-of-concept stage in many respects and there is insufficient information to form conclusive advice to healthcare organisations and practitioners. Manipulation of the HPA axis is currently not part of routine treatment for MDD or any mental disorder other than where symptoms are secondary to primary adrenal malfunction.

The potential use of glucocorticoid-related biomarkers as predictors of response to antidepressant or psychological treatments (which arguably operate on the same neurocognitive substrates as glucocorticoids) has yet to be adequately investigated. Longitudinal studies of moderate to severe MDD in adolescents treated as outpatients suggest that evening cortisol hypersecretion at baseline before treatment is associated with impaired social cognition, a greater number of subsequent personal negative life events and slower response to any psychological treatment. Severely ill hospitalised depressed adults show that better treatment response to antidepressant medication is predicted (in the short

term) by changes in the expression of blood FKBP51 (a protein produced by *FKBP5*) (Ising et al., 2019). This effect appears moderated by the genotype of the *FKBP5* variant rs1360780, with carriers of the minor (less common) allele showing the most pronounced association.

A number of studies have examined the efficacy of metyrapone (a drug that inhibits the synthesis of cortisol) as a direct and/or an augmenting agent in treatment-resistant cases but none have reported clinically meaningful effect sizes (McAllister-Williams et al., 2013). Mifepristone (a medication that is an anti-glucocorticoid by acting competitively on the glucocorticoid receptor) is also being trialled in mood disorders and psychosis but as yet results have not reported efficacy of clinical value (McAllister-Williams et al., 2013). Studies using these medications have not stratified patients at baseline by glucocorticoid parameters or other measures such as cytokine levels. Patient stratification is probably essential to detect an anti-glucocorticoid effect in depressed patients as theoretically only cortisol hypersecretors, or those carrying treatment-sensitivity gene variants for cortisol, are likely to show a clinically relevant response.

Both psychological therapy and SSRIs (such as fluoxetine) are known to have meaningful treatment effects and are recommended by the National Institute for Health and Care Excellence in the UK but we do not yet know what treatment works for which patient (Goodyer et al., 2017; Goodyer and Wilkinson, 2019). Overall, there is now sufficient evidence to undertake more scientifically rigorous studies of HPA axis activity in MDD. Epidemiologically principled studies should recruit adolescents and young adults in sufficient numbers (>2,000) to examine a range of glucocorticoid parameters, inflammatory markers and gene variants to map the characteristics of glucocorticoid function over time, in both sexes, across adolescent development and early adulthood. Clinical studies should undertake formal adaptive randomised controlled trial designs with sufficient patients (at least 1,000) to ensure sufficient power for valid results, with glucocorticoid characteristics and related key parameters (listed above) to improve detection of moderators of treatment response. An appropriate design would be taking patients through distinct therapy phases and noting what treatment works for whom and what glucocorticoid characteristic (if any) predicts treatment response. Such studies would provide much needed definitive information about the value of the HPA axis in predicting risk and as a therapeutic decision-making parameter, as well as revealing with greater clarity the underlying pathophysiological mechanisms involved in these clinically and aetiologically heterogeneous disorders.

6.3.9 Other Disorders, Other Steroids

Although the focus has been on disordered cortisol in depression, corticoids have been implicated in other psychiatric disorders. Lowered cortisol has been associated both with current PTSD and as a risk factor for developing it after a traumatic stressful event, but the literature is not unanimous, and cortisol assays are not currently part of clinical diagnosis or management of PTSD. There are scattered reports of cortisol dysregulation in conduct disorder and in psychotic states, but these are far from established. See Section 9.11.2 for a discussion of HPA axis responses in borderline personality disorder. Since cortisol responds to stressful events or emotional states, it would not be surprising if cortisol were to reflect this in a proportion of cases. There is also the considerable problem of symptom overlap, leading to blurred boundaries between psychiatric diagnoses.

DHEA is secreted from the adrenal gland in high amounts during fetal development and forms the basis for steroidogenesis by the placenta. At birth, levels fall dramatically, but rise again in adrenarche (around 8 years). Peaking in early adulthood, DHEA levels then fall progressively to about a quarter of those at the maximum by late 60s onwards. There is considerable evidence that DHEA moderates the actions of cortisol, so the effects of cortisol may be accentuated by decreased levels of DHEA. DHEA also has activating actions on the immune system and may be part of the process of immunosenescence. DHEA has been found to be reduced in episodes of depression, and the cortisol/DHEA ratio has been proposed as a useful index of endocrine function in depression but these observations have yet to be replicated. Further, reduced DHEA will amplify the neural actions of cortisol and the molar ratio may give a more accurate estimate of their combined action on the brain. Finally, there are early reports of DHEA being useful as an adjunctive treatment of MDD but no definitive trials have yet been carried out.

Conclusions and Outstanding Questions

The contribution of altered adrenal steroids, particularly cortisol, to mental disorder and, mostly, major depression, is evident from the current literature, but requires more investigation. Revealing how cortisol levels interact with genetic and experiential factors, influence neural and psychological functions, and also affect treatment choice and hence therapeutic response are all key questions for future basic and clinical research.

Outstanding Questions

- Should assessment of adrenal function be part of clinical assessment of depression and other psychiatric disorders?
- What neural and psychological mechanisms are responsible for corticoid contribution to the emergence and treatment of mood-related psychiatric disorders?
- Are there subtypes of psychiatric disorder that are particularly associated with different forms of altered adrenal function, and does this have therapeutic implications?

REFERENCES

Askelund AD, Schweizer S, Goodyer IM, van Harmelen AL (2019). Positive memory specificity is associated with reduced vulnerability to depression. *Nat Hum Behav* 3(3): 265–273.

Deuschle M, Schweiger U, Weber B et al. (1997). Diurnal activity and pulsatility of the hypothalamus-pituitary-adrenal system in male depressed patients and healthy controls. *J Clin Endocrinol Metab* 82: 234–238.

Fischer S, Strawbridge R, Vives AH, Cleare AJ (2017). Cortisol as a predictor of psychological therapy response in depressive disorders: systematic review and meta-analysis. *Br J Psychiatry* 210(2): 105–109.

Goodyer IM, Wilkinson PO. (2019). Practitioner review: therapeutics of unipolar major depressions in adolescents. *J Child Psychol Psychiatry*; 60(3): 232–243.

Goodyer IM, Croudace T, Dudbridge F, Ban M, Herbert J (2010). Polymorphisms in *BDNF* (Val66Met) and *5-HTTLPR*, morning cortisol and subsequent depression in at-risk adolescents. *Br J Psychiatry* 197(5): 365–371.

Goodyer IM, Reynolds S, Barrett B et al. (2017). Cognitive behavioural therapy and short-term psychoanalytical psychotherapy versus a brief psychosocial intervention in adolescents with unipolar major depressive disorder (IMPACT): a multicentre, pragmatic, observer-blind, randomised controlled superiority trial. *Lancet Psychiatry* 4(2): 109–119.

Herbert J (2013). Cortisol and depression: three questions for psychiatry. *Psychol Med* 43(3): 449–69.

Howard DM, Adams MJ, Clarke TK et al. (2019). Genome-wide meta-analysis of depression identifies 102 independent variants and highlights the importance of the prefrontal brain regions. *Nat Neurosci* 22(3): 343–352.

Ising M, Maccarrone G, Brückl T et al. (2019). *FKBP5* gene expression predicts antidepressant treatment outcome in depression. *Int J Mol Sci* 20(3): 485.

McAllister-Williams RH, Smith E, Anderson IM (2013). Study protocol for the randomised controlled trial: antiglucocorticoid augmentation of anti-depressants in depression (the ADD study). *BMC Psychiatry* 13: 205.

Owens M, Herbert J, Jones PB et al. (2014). Elevated morning cortisol is a stratified population-level biomarker for major depression in boys only with high depressive symptoms. *Proc Natl Acad Sci USA* 111(9): 3638–3643.

Pariante CM (2017). Why are depressed patients inflamed? A reflection on 20 years of research on depression, glucocorticoid resistance and inflammation. *Eur Neuropsychopharmacol* 27(6): 554–559.

Rao S, Yao Y, Ryan J et al. (2016). Common variants in *FKBP5* gene and major depressive disorder (MDD) susceptibility: a comprehensive meta-analysis. *Sci Rep* 6: 32687.

6

<table>
<tr><td>**6.4**</td><td>**Inflammation and Immune Responses**</td><td>**Mary-Ellen Lynall**</td></tr>
</table>

OVERVIEW

Multiple psychiatric disorders have been associated with abnormalities in the immune system and evidence from human and animal studies suggests that the immune system is likely to be implicated in the pathogenesis of these disorders, at least in a subset of patients. However, our understanding of *how* the immune system contributes to symptoms in humans is in its infancy. Moreover, translating this new understanding to improved clinical care will require biomarkers of immune dysfunction that allow us to identify which patients might benefit from alternative immunomodulatory treatment approaches. Following a brief primer on the immune system and its relationship to the brain, this chapter summarises the immune abnormalities associated with psychiatric disorders in case–control studies, outlines the evidence for a causal contribution of immunopathology to psychiatric conditions and considers possible sources of the observed inflammation.

6.4.1 Background

To begin, let's recap the principal functions and features of the immune system, and our current understanding of the relationship between the immune system and the brain. The function of the immune system is to protect the body from pathogens (organisms that cause disease) and tissue damage (e.g. injury or cancer). The immune system generates inflammatory responses to pathogens and tissue damage, but also plays a critical role in the regulation and resolution of inflammation. Cells in the immune system can circulate in the blood or reside in tissues or lymphoid organs (including the thymus, spleen, bone marrow and lymph nodes).

The immune system is composed of an innate and an adaptive arm. The innate system provides the initial response to injury – this response is rapid, and is not specific to any particular pathogen, instead triggered by generic classes of molecules present on pathogens – pathogen-associated molecular patterns (PAMPs) – or molecules released by damaged or dying cells following tissue injury – damage-associated molecular patterns (DAMPs). The innate immune system includes phagocytic cells such

as neutrophils and monocytes, as well as soluble factors such as the complement system, acute phase proteins and cytokines. Cytokines can have different roles in different contexts; some are predominantly pro-inflammatory, such as interleukin 6 (IL-6) while others are anti-inflammatory, like interleukin 10 (IL-10). Monocytes develop in the bone marrow, circulate and mature in the blood, and can travel to tissues where they mature into macrophages. Tissue macrophages can be derived from circulating monocytes or, alternatively, seeded into tissues prenatally. Neutrophils are short-lived cells (several days) and are normally found in the blood. They are some of the first responders to an insult: signals from a tissue indicating damage or the presence of pathogens cause neutrophils to migrate to the site of injury. Acute phase proteins are markers of inflammation that are increased in blood during acute inflammation and include C-reactive protein (CRP). Acute phase proteins have many and varied functions, which include tagging microbes for destruction, altering blood clotting and mediating negative feedback on the inflammatory response.

The adaptive system, which includes T and B cells, provides a delayed but specific response to infection or damage by recognising and targeting particular molecules. When the immune system responds to a molecule with a targeted response, such as by the production of antibodies (immunoglobulins) directed against the molecule, this inciting molecule is called an antigen. Pathogens generally possess multiple antigens (often proteins on their surface) that can elicit a specific immune response. Chemicals, pollens and (under pathological circumstances such as autoimmune disease) one's own cellular proteins can also act as antigens. A key benefit of the adaptive system is that responses to pathogenic antigens generate highly specific memory of previous infections, based in part on gene rearrangements in B and T cells, so that subsequent encounters with a previously seen pathogen generate a stronger and more rapid response; this is the basis of vaccination.

There are some cross-overs between the innate and adaptive immune systems. The innate system also has memory, but this is based on epigenetic changes rather than on gene rearrangement. This memory is less specific than adaptive memory in that an initial immune challenge can alter the innate response to subsequent, unrelated challenges. Adaptive immune cells can also communicate by secreting cytokines, often the same ones as those secreted by innate immune cells, including IL-6 and IL-10.

Traditionally, the immune system and the brain/mind were considered distinct systems, separated by the blood–brain barrier. There are myeloid immune cells resident in the brain, microglia. However, unlike most immune cells, which are produced in the bone marrow from late embryogenesis onwards and replenished from the bone marrow throughout the lifespan, microglia are instead derived from embryonic yolk sac primitive macrophages. These cells invade the brain in early embryogenesis and proliferate *in situ*. It is unclear whether peripheral myeloid cells can enter the brain to contribute to this microglial pool in humans. Moreover, until recently, the brain was also thought to lack a lymphatic system (the drainage system by which tissue fluid is monitored by lymph nodes, a key part of the immune system). All this seemed to reinforce the idea that the brain is segregated from the peripheral immune system. It makes sense that the brain is protected from inflammation to a degree. Neurons do not, for the most part, regenerate, so the collateral damage and cell death that accompany inflammation are particularly problematic in the brain. Moreover, the

brain sits in an enclosed box (the skull), so the oedema that usually accompanies inflammation could cause dangerous compression. However, it is increasingly clear that the immune system and brain are deeply entwined: immune cells regulate the development and activity of the nervous system, and the nervous system regulates immune responses throughout the body [1]. Some key recent discoveries have radically altered our understanding of immune–brain interactions:

- In addition to microglia and perivascular macrophages, the brain has its own local immune system in the meninges, the lining of the brain, comprising a broad range of adaptive and innate immune cells [2].
- The brain does have its own lymphatic drainage system, externalised to the meninges [3, 4].
- Immune cells migrate to the meninges and brain both from the peripheral bone marrow (via blood) and directly from the skull bone marrow, via microscopic channels in the skull [5].

These meningeal immune and lymphatic systems provide additional mechanisms by which the body's immune system can affect and be affected by the brain.

6.4.2 How Can the Immune System and Brain Interact to Alter Mental States and Behaviour?

Mechanistic studies, primarily in rodents, have revealed that there are multiple pathways by which the immune system can act on the brain to induce behavioural change (see Figure 6.4.1). These include:

(1) **Cytokines acting on the brain endothelium or cytokines crossing the blood–brain barrier to act directly in the brain.** For example, one study in mice showed that peripheral blood IL-6 crossing a damaged blood–brain barrier contributes to the behavioural response to stress [6].

(2) **Effects of inflammation on metabolism.** Inflammation induces enzymes which alter metabolism, including indoleamine 2,3-dioxygenase (IDO). Increased IDO reduces the availability of neurotransmitter precursors (e.g. tryptophan, a precursor to serotonin), and causes the production of neurotoxic metabolites [7].

(3) **Infiltration of peripheral immune cells into the brain.** For example, repeated social defeat stress in mice causes monocytes to migrate from the periphery

to the brain, where some (but not all) studies have found they contribute to anxiety-like behaviour [8].

(4) **The effects of antibodies on the brain.** This is suggested by associations between autoantibodies and psychosis – especially antibodies against the *N*-methyl-D-aspartate (NMDA) receptor, and against components of the voltage-gated potassium-channel complex (LGI1, leucine-rich glioma inactivated 1 and CASPR2, contactin-associated protein 2) [9, 10]. Experiments delivering patient-derived antibodies to rodents ('passive transfer') and examining the effects of antibodies on cell cultures and live brain slices support a causal role for these antibodies in symptoms. For example purified antibodies derived from the blood of patients with NMDA receptor antibodies and psychosis were shown to alter NMDA receptor function and long-term potentiation at glutamatergic synapses [11].

(5) **Effects of immune cells in the meninges.** For example, CD4+ (helper) T cells in the meninges have been shown to contribute to learning and memory, providing key evidence that meningeal immunity can contribute to behaviour [12].

(6) **Immune cells or cytokines modulating vagal nerve activity** [13]. The vagus nerve has many roles, one of which is as a bidirectional immune–brain communication pathway, which can both sense and modulate peripheral immune activity. There is preliminary evidence for efficacy of vagal nerve stimulation as a treatment for psychiatric conditions including treatment-resistant depression [14]. Modulation of immune–brain communication is a potential mechanism for this effect [15].

6.4.3 Associations between Psychiatric Disorders and Immune Alterations

Alterations in the immune system have been observed in case–control studies of multiple psychiatric disorders, including depression, bipolar affective disorder, schizophrenia, autism, attention deficit hyperactivity disorder, post-traumatic stress disorder, obsessive–compulsive disorder (OCD) and other anxiety disorders. Some abnormalities appear to show at least some disorder specificity, for instance the association between NMDA receptor antibodies and psychosis, or the association between anti-striatal antibodies and OCD. However, some immune alterations are common to many

psychiatric disorders – among the most consistently reported findings across different conditions are:

- increased blood CRP
- increased blood pro-inflammatory cytokines, especially IL-6 and tumour necrosis factor (TNF)
- increased white blood cell counts in both myeloid and lymphoid lineages
- activation of the inflammasome, a cytosolic innate immune system sensor which responds to pathogen or host danger signals (including PAMPs, DAMPs and metabolic imbalance) to induce inflammation.

One challenge in immunopsychiatry is that it is difficult to interrogate the brain's immune system in patients, with very few circumstances in which a brain biopsy (the most scientifically informative sample) would be appropriate. Blood is easy to access and may contribute to (or reflect) immune activation in the brain, but, ideally, we want to know whether there is immunopathology in the central nervous system. Nonetheless, some small studies have provided evidence of brain immune activation in psychiatric disorders in post-mortem samples or by using neuroimaging techniques. For example, one positron emission tomography (PET) study using the translocator protein (TSPO) ligand as a proxy for microglial activation showed increased TSPO binding in multiple mood-relevant brain regions in depression compared to healthy controls [16]. It is not entirely clear what these and other TSPO PET results mean at the cellular level, or which cell types are contributing to this signal [17].

Notably, not all patients with psychiatric disorders show immune abnormalities, with increasing evidence that only a subset of patients have immune dysfunction. Importantly for clinical care, inflammation may relate to treatment resistance – for example, people with depression who have increased markers of inflammation are less likely to respond to conventional treatment with antidepressant medication [18]. This raises the prospect of stratified treatment – that we could improve outcomes by using some biomarker of immune dysfunction to detect those patients in whom the immune system contributes to symptoms, and then provide a different care pathway to those patients involving pharmacological or non-pharmacological immunomodulatory treatments. The barrier to this approach is that none of the immune markers assayed to date have yet to be shown to be satisfactory as clinical biomarkers. In particular,

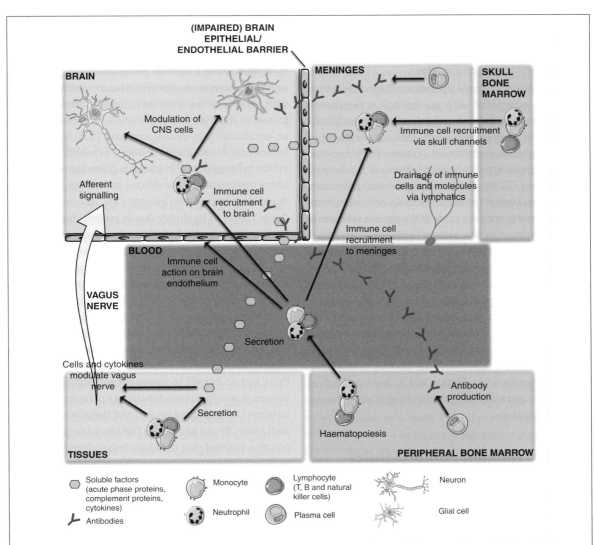

Figure 6.4.1 Pathways by which the immune system may act on the brain to induce behavioural change. A schematic of the principal anatomical structures involved in immune–brain communication (brain, meninges, lymphatics, skull bone marrow, peripheral tissues, peripheral bone marrow and vagus nerve). Arrows show how the movement of immune cells and inflammatory mediators between these compartments can contribute to the effects of the immune system on brain and behaviour. Cells, cytokines and antibodies can cross the blood–brain barrier to directly affect central nervous system (CNS) cells. Alternatively, cells and soluble components may act indirectly on the brain via effects on brain epithelium/endothelium; via the meningeal immune system; by the action of immune cells or cytokines on afferent vagal nerve signalling; or via the effects (not shown) of inflammation on neurotransmitter metabolism (see text for more details). Immune cells can be recruited to the central nervous system from the peripheral bone marrow, passing via the peripheral circulation, or be recruited directly from the skull bone marrow to the meninges, via channels in the skull. Parts of the figure were drawn by using pictures from Servier Medical Art, which is licensed under a Creative Commons Attribution 3.0 Unported License (https://creativecommons.org/licenses/by/3.0/).

high-sensitivity CRP assays are widely used in observational studies and have been used to stratify patients in clinical trials in psychiatry. However, increased CRP is not specific to psychiatric disorders, is affected by many environmental and biological factors unrelated to psychiatry, and varies substantially from day to day. For the case of psychosis, NMDA receptor antibodies may prove to be useful biomarkers (pending the results of clinical trials), but this assay captures only a small proportion of patients with immune dysfunction. To develop better biomarkers,

Another active avenue of investigation in immunopsychiatry is the gut–brain axis. Multiple psychiatric disorders have been associated with an altered microbiome and evidence of impaired gut barrier integrity, and inflammation in psychiatry may in part reflect increased bacterial translocation from the gut to the blood. Mice raised in germ-free environments, and mice treated with antibiotics and faecal microbiota transplants have been extensively used to investigate the effects of microbiota on behaviours relevant to psychiatry, demonstrating that microbiota are essential for appropriate stress responses and social behaviour, and can modulate anxiety/depressive behaviours [35]. The contribution of such alterations to symptoms in humans is yet to be demonstrated.

Conclusions and Outstanding Questions

In summary, results from human studies highlight the involvement of both the innate and adaptive immune system in psychiatric disorders. Experimental work in animals and in humans has demonstrated multiple mechanisms by which the immune system and the brain can interact to lead to symptoms, and there is growing evidence that the immune system makes a causal contribution to pathogenesis in psychiatry. Data suggest that there are likely both shared and distinct contributions of immunity to the pathogenesis of different psychiatric disorders. However, this is a field where there are far more questions than answers.

Outstanding Questions

- **What are the alterations in the immune system *doing*?** Many cells and molecules implicated in psychiatric conditions can have both pro- and anti-inflammatory functions in different contexts. For example, multiple psychiatric disorders are associated with increases in the cytokine IL-6 – is this causing damage, does this have a protective function or is it a pathologically unimportant by-product of some other more relevant process? It would be easier to understand the role of such immune mediators in psychiatry if we knew their cellular source (e.g. IL-6 can be produced by myeloid cells, lymphoid cells, adipose tissue, endothelial cells …), but these scientific questions remain outstanding.

- **_Where_ in the body is the important inflammation?** In psychiatric patient groups, it is much easier to assay the immune system in the periphery (by blood sampling) than in the brain, so most of our data on inflammation in psychiatry have been obtained using blood samples. But the activity of immune cells and molecules in the blood does not necessarily reflect what is going on in the brain or meninges (i.e. 'tissue immunity'). Moreover, it is unclear whether changes in the peripheral immune system make a causal contribution to psychiatric symptoms. This matters when designing new treatment strategies – for example, does a given blood biomarker reflect a mechanistically important process such that it can serve as a treatment target? Do we need our candidate immunomodulatory treatment to get into the brain or is it sufficient to block the cytokine or other factor in the periphery?

- **Which people are susceptible to the effects of inflammation and why?** Many people with psychiatric conditions have no evidence of immune abnormalities – it seems that only a subgroup of patients have immune dysfunction. Moreover, while psychiatric symptoms are more common in those with chronic illness, many people with immune abnormalities much more marked than those seen in idiopathic psychiatric conditions (e.g. the increased pro-inflammatory cytokines seen in patients with autoimmune diseases) do not develop psychiatric symptoms – why is this? We need to understand the variability in individuals' neural and psychological responses to inflammation, both for the benefit of psychiatric patient groups, and for the benefit of patients with psychological symptoms in the context of inflammatory 'medical' disorders including obesity, autoimmunity and infection.

- **How can we incorporate our emerging understanding of immunopsychiatric disease pathogenesis into clinical practice?** Many of the findings in immunopsychiatry (and indeed other areas of neuroscience) cut across traditional psychiatric diagnostic boundaries. Capitalising on this new understanding to improve patient care will require a wholescale revision of our approach to patient investigation and treatment.

REFERENCES

1. Dantzer R. Neuroimmune interactions: from the brain to the immune system and vice versa. *Physiol Rev* 2018; 98(1): 477–504.

2. Rua R, McGavern DB. Advances in meningeal immunity. *Trends Mol Med* 2018; 24(6): 542–559.

3. Louveau A, Smirnov I, Keyes TJ et al. Structural and functional features of central nervous system lymphatic vessels. *Nature* 2015; 523(7560): 337–341.

4. Aspelund A, Antila S, Proulx ST et al. A dural lymphatic vascular system that drains brain interstitial fluid and macromolecules. *J Exp Med* 2015; 212(7): 991–999.

5. Herisson F, Frodermann V, Courties G et al. Direct vascular channels connect skull bone marrow and the brain surface enabling myeloid cell migration. *Nat Neurosci* 2018; 21(9): 1209–1217.

6. Menard C, Pfau ML, Hodes GE et al. Social stress induces neurovascular pathology promoting depression. *Nat Neurosci* 2017; 20(12): 1752–1760.

7. Haroon E, Raison CL, Miller AH. Psychoneuroimmunology meets neuropsychopharmacology: translational implications of the impact of inflammation on behavior. *Neuropsychopharmacology* 2012; 37(1): 137–162.

8. Wohleb ES, Powell ND, Godbout JP, Sheridan JF. Stress-induced recruitment of bone marrow-derived monocytes to the brain promotes anxiety-like behavior. *J Neurosci* 2013; 33(34): 13820–13833.

9. Zandi MS, Irani SR, Lang B et al. Disease-relevant autoantibodies in first episode schizophrenia. *J Neurol* 2011; 258(4): 686–688.

10. Pollak TA, Lennox BR, Muller S et al. Autoimmune psychosis: an international consensus on an approach to the diagnosis and management of psychosis of suspected autoimmune origin. *Lancet Psychiatry* 2020; 7(1): 93–108.

11. Jezequel J, Johansson EM, Dupuis JP et al. Dynamic disorganization of synaptic NMDA receptors triggered by autoantibodies from psychotic patients. *Nat Commun* 2017; 8(1): 1791.

12. Derecki NC, Cardani AN, Yang CH et al. Regulation of learning and memory by meningeal immunity: a key role for IL-4. *J Exp Med* 2010; 207(5): 1067–1080.

13. Bluthe RM, Michaud B, Kelley KW, Dantzer R. Vagotomy attenuates behavioural effects of interleukin-1 injected peripherally but not centrally. *Neuroreport* 1996; 7(9): 1485–1488.

14. Bottomley JM, LeReun C, Diamantopoulos A, Mitchell S, Gaynes BN. Vagus nerve stimulation (VNS) therapy in patients with treatment resistant depression: a systematic review and meta-analysis. *Compr Psychiatry* 2019; 98: 152156.

15. Alen NV. The cholinergic anti-inflammatory pathway in humans: state-of-the-art review and future directions. *Neurosci Biobehav Rev* 2022; 136: 104622.

16. Setiawan E, Wilson AA, Mizrahi R et al. Role of translocator protein density, a marker of neuroinflammation, in the brain during major depressive episodes. *JAMA Psychiatry* 2015; 72(3): 268–275.

17. Perry VH. Microglia and major depression: not yet a clear picture. *Lancet Psychiatry* 2018; 5(4): 292–294.

18. Lanquillon S, Krieg JC, Bening-Abu-Shach U, Vedder H. Cytokine production and treatment response in major depressive disorder. *Neuropsychopharmacology* 2000; 22(4): 370–379.

19. Goebel A, Andersson D, Helyes Z, Clark JD, Dulake D, Svensson C. The autoimmune aetiology of unexplained chronic pain. *Autoimmun Rev* 2022; 21(3): 103015.

20. Goebel A, Krock E, Gentry C et al. Passive transfer of fibromyalgia symptoms from patients to mice. *J Clin Invest* 2021; 131(13): e144201.

21. Monje M, Iwasaki A. The neurobiology of long COVID. *Neuron* 2022; 110(21): 3484–3496.

22. Khandaker GM, Pearson RM, Zammit S, Lewis G, Jones PB. Association of serum interleukin 6 and C-reactive protein in childhood with depression and psychosis in young adult life: a population-based longitudinal study. *JAMA Psychiatry* 2014; 71(10): 1121–1128.

23. Harrison NA, Brydon L, Walker C, Gray MA, Steptoe A, Critchley HD. Inflammation causes mood changes through alterations in subgenual cingulate activity and mesolimbic connectivity. *Biol Psychiatry* 2009; 66(5): 407–414.

24. Wittenberg GM, Stylianou A, Zhang Y et al. Effects of immunomodulatory drugs on depressive symptoms: a mega-analysis of randomized, placebo-controlled clinical trials in inflammatory disorders. *Mol Psychiatry* 2020; 5(6): 1275–1285.

25. Raison CL, Rutherford RE, Woolwine BJ et al. A randomized controlled trial of the tumor necrosis factor antagonist infliximab for treatment-resistant depression: the role of baseline inflammatory biomarkers. *JAMA Psychiatry* 2013; 70(1): 31–41.

26. Perry BI, Upthegrove R, Kappelmann N et al. Associations of immunological proteins/traits with schizophrenia, major depression and bipolar disorder: a bi-directional two-sample Mendelian randomization study. *Brain Behav Immun* 2021; 97: 176–185.

27. Lynall ME, Soskic B, Hayhurst J et al. Genetic variants associated with psychiatric disorders are enriched at epigenetically active sites in lymphoid cells. *Nat Commun* 2022; 13(1): 6102.

28. Heidt T, Sager HB, Courties G et al. Chronic variable stress activates hematopoietic stem cells. *Nat Med* 2014; 20(7): 754–758.

29. Bellingrath S, Rohleder N, Kudielka BM. Effort–reward-imbalance in healthy teachers is associated with higher LPS-stimulated production and lower glucocorticoid sensitivity of interleukin-6 *in vitro*. *Biol Psychol* 2013; 92(2): 403–409.

30. Benros ME, Waltoft BL, Nordentoft M et al. Autoimmune diseases and severe infections as risk factors for mood disorders: a nationwide study. *JAMA Psychiatry* 2013; 70(8): 812–820.

31. Benros ME, Nielsen PR, Nordentoft M et al. Autoimmune diseases and severe infections as risk factors for schizophrenia: a 30-year population-based register study. *Am J Psychiatry* 2011; 168(12): 1303–1310.

32. Atladottir HO, Thorsen P, Schendel DE et al. Association of hospitalization for infection in childhood with diagnosis of autism spectrum disorders: a Danish cohort study. *Arch Pediatr Adolesc Med* 2010; 164(5): 470–477.

33. Lund-Sorensen H, Benros ME, Madsen T et al. A nationwide cohort study of the association between hospitalization with infection and risk of death by suicide. *JAMA Psychiatry* 2016; 73(9): 912–919.

34. Eisenberger NI, Berkman ET, Inagaki TK et al. Inflammation-induced anhedonia: endotoxin reduces ventral striatum responses to reward. *Biol Psychiatry* 2010; 68(8): 748–754.

35. Nagpal J, Cryan JF. Microbiota–brain interactions: moving toward mechanisms in model organisms. *Neuron* 2021; 109(24): 3930–3953.

National Neuroscience Curriculum Initiative online resources

Checking the Brain's Immune Privilege: Evolving Theories of Brain–Immune Interactions

Robert J. Fenstera and Jane L. Eisen

More Than a Gut Feeling: The Implications of the Gut Microbiota in Psychiatry
Pochu Ho and David A. Ross

This "stuff" is really cool: Christopher Bartley, *"Old Syndromes, New Eyes"* on brain-targeting antibodies and phage display

This "stuff" is really cool: Ryan Rampersaud, *"That's A Load of Crap!"* on mental health and the gut

7

Genetics

James Walters and Kimberley Kendall

James Walters and
Kimberley Kendall

7.1 Basic Genetic Principles and the History of Gene Identification

OVERVIEW

Sequencing of the human genome and the demonstration of a substantial heritability for many psychiatric conditions has enabled a new era of molecular psychiatric genetics research. Progress has been made towards goals of identifying 'risk genes' and associated biological pathways to establish new drug targets for psychiatric disorders, particularly in the last decade. In addition, genetic advances offer the prospect of informing more personalised treatments and improving diagnosis, classification and prediction. With the prospect of emerging genetic discoveries having real clinical impact comes the responsibility of establishing how best to communicate genetic findings to patients and their families. In the sections in this chapter, we provide an overview of basic genetics and review psychiatric genomic research advances over the last decade and beyond.

7.1.1 Structure of DNA

Deoxyribonucleic acid (DNA) is a molecule made up of nucleotides of different bases (guanine, adenine, cytosine and thymine), the order of which is called the DNA sequence. Segments of DNA form **genes**, which encode proteins and are comprised of (i) exons, which will be transcribed into messenger RNA (mRNA), (ii) introns – regions involved in functions such as regulation of gene expression and (iii) promoters, which control transcription and gene expression. DNA strands are organised into chromosomes, with 23 chromosomal pairs in each human non-reproductive cell: 22 pairs of autosomes (non-sex chromosomes) and one pair of sex chromosomes, typically XX (female) or XY (male).

The DNA sequence varies between humans at the level of single bases (e.g. a one-base change, called a single-nucleotide polymorphism (SNP) or a single nucleotide variant), as well as the number of copies of chromosomes or DNA regions. Human genetic research aims to discover how these genetic variations influence traits or clinical disorders. The individual genetic changes range from being common in the population (typically above 1%) to being much rarer (and can be **private** or unique to one individual).

7.1.2 Family-Based Studies

Family-based methods were the first genomic studies aimed at establishing the genetic contribution to the aetiology of psychiatric disorders. These include:

(i) **family studies** – families with multiple affected individuals are studied to establish the familial pattern and risk of the disorder in relatives

(ii) **twin studies** – twin pairs with one or both individuals affected are studied and compared to determine risk of the disorder in co-twins; conditions with genetic contributions exhibit higher disorder concordance rates in monozygotic twins (sharing 100% DNA sequence) compared to dizygotic twins (sharing ~50% DNA sequence)

(iii) **adoption studies** – adopted children and their biological and adoptive parents are studied, allowing assessment of the contribution of genetic and environmental (upbringing-related) risk factors.

These family studies formed the bedrock of psychiatric genetic epidemiology and allowed estimation of heritability (see Table 7.1.1), establishing genetic contribution to risk of a range of psychiatric disorders.

Table 7.1.1 Heritability estimates for psychiatric disorders calculated from family, twin and genetic association studies

Disorder	Heritability from family, twin and adoption studies	SNP-based heritability estimates
Autism	83% [2]	49–52% [3, 4]
Schizophrenia	79% [5]	41% [4]
Bipolar affective disorder	85% [6]	44% [4]
Attention deficit hyperactivity disorder	76% [7]	25% [4]
Major depressive disorder	37% [8]	18% [4]

Single-nucleotide polymorphism (SNP)-based heritability refers to common variation only.

7.1.3 Heritability

The aetiology of psychiatric disorders is multifactorial – liability to a disorder arises from both genetic and environmental factors. An individual's genetic make-up can convey a predisposition to develop a disorder. The genetic architecture of psychiatric disorders is complex – risk is increased by common genetic variants, each of which typically increases risk by a very small amount but collectively can account for a large proportion of genetic risk, and rare genetic variants, which typically increase risk by a much larger amount [1]. Under a proposed **liability threshold** model, multiple genetic and environmental factors jointly contribute to an individual's liability and once this crosses a particular threshold, the disorder is manifest. This model has been useful throughout psychiatric genetics research, not least in the calculation of heritability estimates for psychiatric disorders (Table 7.1.1). **Heritability** is the proportion of phenotypic variation in a disorder or trait that is explained by genetic factors. The estimation of heritability is specific to the population and environment studied at a particular time and thus can change across settings, although in general estimates of heritability for psychiatric disorders have been consistent across international study designs.

7.2 **Common Variation**

James Walters and
Kimberley Kendall

7.2.1 Genome-Wide Association Studies

Advances in the systematic mapping of human genetic variation and high throughput genotyping facilitated the development of genome-wide association studies (GWAS), which typically assess common genetic variants (those present at >1% frequency in the population). **Genotyping** can be performed either by sequencing to determine each individual's DNA sequence (see Subsection 7.3.2), or, much more cheaply and rapidly, using array-based technologies (DNA microarrays) to test genetic variation at specific predetermined locations across the genome. In GWAS, hundreds of thousands of single DNA base-pair changes (single-nucleotide polymorphisms (SNPs)) are genotyped throughout the genome using array-based technologies. These genotyped SNPs are typically selected as being representative of nearby SNPs that are in high linkage disequilibrium with them. **Linkage disequilibrium** refers to the non-random association of alleles at different positions (loci) in the genome. Blocks of alleles (haplotype blocks) are inherited together more often than expected by chance and thus are not independent. Hence, selected SNPs can capture commonly occurring genetic variation across the genome. In practice, the number of analysed SNPs can be increased to millions by **genotype imputation**, a statistical process that infers genotypes of non-genotyped SNPs using linkage disequilibrium derived from large population-based reference genetic data sets. The frequencies of genotyped and imputed SNPs are then compared between cases and controls, while controlling for population genetic differences, to identify SNPs associated with a disorder. What results is a list of SNPs, their effect sizes with confidence intervals and significance values for association with the disorder. An SNP is associated with a disorder if it achieves a *p* value at a genome-wide level of significance ($< 5 \times 10^{-8}$). This *p*-value threshold allows for the multiple testing (and possibilities for false discoveries or type-1 errors) inherent in variation across the genome and entailed in analysing millions of SNPs.

GWAS do not necessarily identify causal SNPs; rather, they identify a region around the associated SNP within which lies the causal association for a disorder. Thus, much of the work taking forward GWAS results concentrates on further characterising the origin of the causal association within this region. A simple method of estimating which genes are involved in the pathogenesis of a disorder is simply to look for those genes nearest to the risk variants identified by a GWAS. It seems the nearest-gene approach is often correct although variants can exert their effects via genes other than their closest gene. The identification of likely causal genes can be supplemented using additional methods such as **summary-based Mendelian randomisation**, which uses information from a GWAS of a phenotype (e.g. schizophrenia), along with information from GWAS of which genetic variants influence biological markers (e.g. variants that are associated with gene expression), to test whether the effect of a risk variant on a given phenotype is mediated by specific markers or genes.

GWAS have benefited tremendously from broader international collaboration, which has greatly increased sample sizes and thus statistical power. Most psychiatric genetic studies have been conducted in European and, to a lesser extent, East Asian populations. Researchers have recognised the need to represent the full diversity of human populations and this is imperative if genetics research is to be clinically translated.

Some examples of GWA studies conducted in psychiatric genetics are as follows:

- In major depressive disorder, a GWAS meta-analysis (maximum 246,363 cases, 561,190 controls) identified

102 variants associated with the disorder, 97 of which were also associated in a large replication sample. In combining SNP association statistics within genes, the authors undertook gene-based analyses to identify the particular genes that these SNPs indicated. They reported 269 individual genes as associated with depression along with gene sets corresponding to cellular components in the nervous system and biological pathways involved in synaptic function [9]. An earlier meta-analysis provided insights into the phenotypic heterogeneity (particularly relating to different diagnostic methods and common symptoms) and genetic overlaps between major depressive disorder and educational attainment, body mass and schizophrenia [10].

- A recent study in bipolar disorder (41,917 cases and 371,549 controls of European ancestry) identified 64 associated genomic regions and, using gene expression data, implicated 15 genes from these regions as potentially causal. The study also found that synaptic gene sets were important for bipolar disorder, and reported high genetic correlation between subtypes of bipolar disorder [11].

- In anxiety and stress-related disorders, a GWAS (12,655 cases, 19,225 controls) identified 68 variants. Across several analyses, associations with anxiety and stress-related disorders were found for the *PDE4B* (phosphodiesterase 4B) gene, which breaks down cyclic adenosine monophosphate, a second messenger, and so has a wide influence on brain development and function [12].

These GWAS have successfully identified SNPs, and hence regions of the genome, associated with disorders but, in order to gain biological insights, further downstream analyses are required. These techniques have advanced greatly in recent years.

7.2.2 GWAS and Post-GWAS Analysis of Schizophrenia: An Exemplar

In 2022, the Schizophrenia Working Group of the Psychiatric Genomics Consortium published the largest GWAS of schizophrenia to date. First, they did a primary GWAS and meta-analysed individual genotypes from people of European and East Asian ancestry (67,390 cases; 94,015 controls), with summary-level data from individuals of African-American and Latino ancestry (7,386 cases; 7,008 controls). They identified 313 independent SNPs, at 263 distinct loci, which were associated with schizophrenia at genome-wide levels of statistical significance. Second, they did a meta-analysis of their primary results for genome-wide significant SNPs with samples from deCODE Genetics Iceland (1,979 cases and 142,626 controls). They identified 342 SNPs at 287 loci associated with risk of schizophrenia [13]. To establish which variants and genes were most likely to explain the observed associations, and to aid their interpretation and follow-up, they then carried out a series of further (prioritisation) analyses:

- **Fine-mapping** – the group used a statistical fine-mapping procedure. This procedure helps to infer the most likely number of distinct causal variants responsible for the 287 associated loci – it prioritises which variants may be most important. Overall, *ATP2A2*, a gene previously implicated in risk of bipolar disorder, was identified, suggesting a role in schizophrenia, too. This analysis collectively generated a set of 434 protein-encoding genes containing at least one likely causal SNP. This collection of genes was commonly expressed in the brain, and was evolutionary constrained in that these genes cannot tolerate loss-of-function mutations. These fine-mapping procedures also prioritised genes having high-probability non-synonymous SNPs (SNPs that result in translation into altered proteins) or SNPs in untranslated regions. The value of such approaches is demonstrated by the high likelihood of causality assigned to a non-synonymous variant, rs13107325, within the *SLC39A8* gene. *SLC39A8* codes for a highly conserved (in evolutionary terms) metal ion (cation) transporter, now one of the most confidently implicated genes in schizophrenia.

- **Transcriptomic analysis and functional genomic annotation** – here, the authors used summary-based Mendelian randomisation (see Section 7.2.1) to implicate 101 genes in the pathogenesis of schizophrenia. Further analyses prioritised a group of 45 protein-encoding genes including the *ACE* (angiotensin converting enzyme) gene, which is the target of ACE inhibitor medications for hypertension, potentially highlighting a new treatment avenue in schizophrenia. Prioritised genes implicated synapse structure and function as being important in schizophrenia and gene-set analyses pointed to the involvement of neurotransmitter systems including gamma-aminobutyric acid and glutamate, as well as voltage-gated calcium and chloride channels [13].

Through these various state-of-the-art approaches this most recent GWAS has prioritised a list of high-confidence schizophrenia genes to be taken forward into wider experimental approaches to further characterise their role in aetiology. This study was the first to demonstrate a convergence of the genes and gene sets implicated by common variant (GWAS) research and by searches for rare coding variants in schizophrenia; genes involved in glutamatergic signalling (*GRIN2A* and *SP4*) were highlighted by both approaches.

7.2.3 Polygenic Risk Scoring

Individual SNPs increase disorder risk by a very small amount (typical odds ratios of 1.05–1.20) but, cumulatively, SNP effects can be appreciable. In 2009, the first attempt to evaluate the role of common variants *en masse* was published in a GWAS by the International Schizophrenia Consortium. The consortium used the results of their schizophrenia GWAS to derive a quantitative **polygenic risk score (PRS)** in non-overlapping independent case–control samples, based on summing the number of risk alleles of nominally associated SNPs weighted by their odds ratios [14]. The authors demonstrated that this PRS was significantly enriched amongst cases compared to controls in their independent target sample.

This method of polygenic scoring has been widely adopted and has provided insights into the genetic basis of psychiatric diagnoses and related traits. Polygenic scoring has now been extended to continuous traits such as height, body mass index and cognition. Further developments have also been made to refine how a PRS is derived [15–17] but the premise remains that an individual's PRS is generated by adding their number of risk alleles at each associated SNP weighted by their effect sizes [18].

Polygenic scores reflect an individual's common variation liability to develop an outcome of interest, whether a disorder or a trait. Within psychiatry, polygenic scores are not currently suitable for use in clinical practice given low sensitivities and specificities to predict affected status on an individual basis. However, this technique has provided insights into genetic overlaps between psychiatric disorders and across disorders and phenotypic traits.

7.2.4 Examination of Common Variation across Disorders

GWAS data have been successfully used to examine the genetic correlations (overlaps) between different psychiatric disorders as well as other traits. The two main approaches used here are **linkage-disequilibrium score regression (LDSC)** and PRS. LDSC examines relationships between the linkage disequilibrium of SNPs and their GWAS test statistics. This approach has become popular as it does not require individual-level genotype data and can be less computationally demanding than alternative approaches [19]. It does however require large, well-powered GWAS across the disorders or traits to be examined.

The Brainstorm Consortium examined genetic correlations between psychiatric and other phenotypes, using GWAS summary statistics from 265,218 patients and 784,643 controls. Using LDSC, they found significant genetic correlations between multiple psychiatric disorders, a phenomenon seen to a far lesser extent among neurological disorders. There were substantial genetic correlations between major depression and anxiety disorders, attention deficit hyperactivity disorder and post-traumatic stress disorder; between bipolar disorder and schizophrenia (the most strongly correlated conditions); and between anorexia nervosa and obsessive–compulsive disorder [20].

The availability of large discovery GWAS (training data sets) together with individual genotype data (target set) allows the use of polygenic scoring in examining genetic relationships between phenotypes and does not require the same large sample sizes as LDSC. This approach has proved productive in its application to the schizophrenia–bipolar disorder spectrum. In 2018, the Psychiatric Genomics Consortium used PRS analyses to examine relationships between disorder sub-phenotypes across this spectrum. They identified significant correlations between the schizophrenia PRS and the presence of psychotic features and the age at onset in bipolar disorder [21]. In parallel to this study, Allardyce and colleagues calculated the schizophrenia PRS in individuals with bipolar disorder, schizophrenia and controls. They reported significant associations between the PRS for schizophrenia and disorders across the schizophrenia–bipolar spectrum. The associations were stronger in disorders more phenotypically similar to schizophrenia – for instance,

7

the schizoaffective disorder–bipolar subtype showed a higher schizophrenia PRS than bipolar I disorder, which showed a higher schizophrenia PRS than bipolar II disorder. In addition, individuals with bipolar I disorder with a history of psychosis had a higher schizophrenia PRS than those with bipolar I disorder who had not experienced psychotic symptoms, providing further support to the concept of the schizophrenia–bipolar spectrum and helping to demonstrate a genetic contribution to the phenotypic overlaps between these disorders [22].

James Walters and
Kimberley Kendall

7.3 Rare Variation

In addition to the contribution from common variation, predisposition to many psychiatric disorders can also be increased by rare variants. A rare variant is one that occurs in the population at a rate of < 1% and rare variants identified to date have much larger effect sizes than individual common SNPs.

7.3.1 Structural Variation: Copy Number Variation

Structural variation refers to DNA variation involving at least 50 base pairs of genomic material. This variation may or may not result in a change in the amount of genetic material present: **unbalanced structural variation** includes insertions (gains of genetic material), deletions (losses) and duplications, while **balanced structural variation** (i.e. rearrangements) encompasses inversions (changes in the orientation of a DNA segment) and translocations (changes in the location of a DNA segment) [23, 24]. One important form of structural variation is **copy number variants (CNVs)** – structural variation involving deletions or duplications and affecting a region of more than 1,000 base pairs. CNVs may also be classified as macroscopic or microscopic depending on whether they are visible on microscopy. Examples of macroscopic CNVs include a change in the number of autosomes such as Down syndrome (trisomy 21) and number of sex chromosomes such as Klinefelter syndrome (XXY). For the remainder of this section, we will refer to unbalanced microscopic CNVs (deletions and duplications) given their relevance to psychiatry.

Most CNVs known to be associated with an increased risk of psychiatric disorders are recurrent – they occur at predictable genomic loci. Regions prone to CNV formation are those with highly repetitive sequences such as **low copy repeats**. During the chromosomal crossover that occurs during cell replication, these repetitive sequences can cause chromosomes to misalign, resulting in loss or gain of DNA sequence (non-allelic homologous recombination) [24]. The rates of rare CNVs detected in some neurodevelopmental and psychiatric disorders are shown in Table 7.3.1.

The recurrent, rare CNVs associated with developmental, neurological and psychiatric conditions are termed neuropsychiatric CNVs and are associated with wide-ranging impacts on diverse phenotypes and disorders across multiple body systems. The same neurodevelopmental CNVs can increase the risk of intellectual disability, autism, schizophrenia and depression [25, 29–32]. All neuropsychiatric CNVs seem to be associated with some degree of cognitive impairment, indeed the frequency of these CNVs is higher in disorders characterised by marked cognitive impairment. This increased CNV yield perhaps explains why the bulk of the UK's National Health Service (NHS) clinical testing for CNVs in psychiatric services is carried out in those with intellectual disabilities. Despite the wide-ranging effects of these CNVs in population studies many CNV carriers do not develop an overt psychiatric disorder or intellectual disability, although CNV carriers perform on average lower in cognitive tests compared to non-carriers [33–36]. Finally, these CNVs are also associated

Table 7.3.1 Rates of rare CNVs in some psychiatric disorders and controls

Disorder	CNV Rate (%)	Reference
Intellectual disability (ID)	16.8	[25]
Autism with ID	11.1	[25]
Autism without ID	10.2	[25]
Attention deficit hyperactivity disorder	12.2	[26]
Schizophrenia	2.5	[27]
Bipolar affective disorder	1.0	[28]
Controls	1.0	[27]

with physical phenotypes that can impact on an individual's quality of life and mortality risk, an aspect of potential clinical importance given the disparities of physical health in those with severe mental illness [37, 38].

7.3.2 Rare Single-Nucleotide Variants

Advances in genetic technologies and decreases in costs have begun to make feasible large-scale sequencing studies to identify the contribution of rare single-nucleotide variants to the risk of psychiatric disorders (typically <0.1% frequency in the population). In contrast to GWAS, sequencing studies genotype every base pair within the protein-coding parts of the genome

(**whole-exome sequencing (WES)**) or across the entire genome (**whole-genome sequencing (WGS)**). The relative expense of WGS has meant that most studies within neuropsychiatry to date have been based on WES. The field is in relative infancy as the sample sizes required to reliably detect rare variants and identify 'risk genes' are accrued. The fields of autism and developmental disorder research have led this endeavour thus far [39, 40] and it seems that these disorders demonstrate a greater burden of rare risk variants than schizophrenia and greater still compared to bipolar disorder. The largest autism study to date developed methods to incorporate WES rare variants from autism trios (variants present in an affected

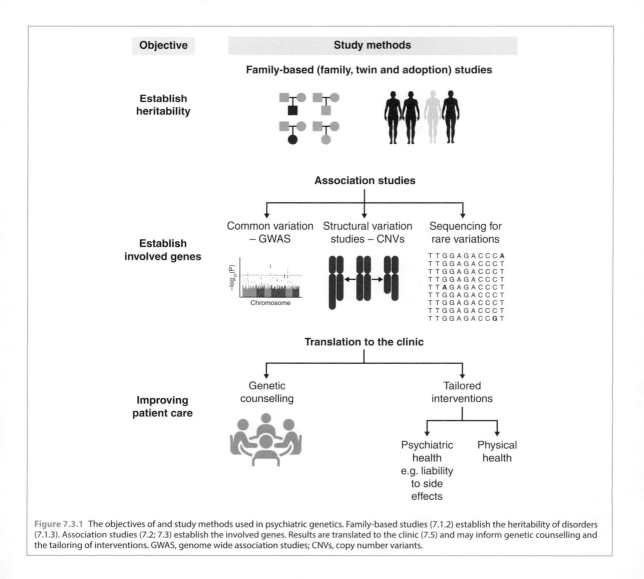

Figure 7.3.1 The objectives of and study methods used in psychiatric genetics. Family-based studies (7.1.2) establish the heritability of disorders (7.1.3). Association studies (7.2; 7.3) establish the involved genes. Results are translated to the clinic (7.5) and may inform genetic counselling and the tailoring of interventions. GWAS, genome wide association studies; CNVs, copy number variants.

family member (the proband) but not present in either of their unaffected parents) and case–control studies, identifying 102 associated genes with high probability. These genes showed enhanced expression in both excitatory and inhibitory neuronal cells, supporting the possibility that excitatory/inhibitory balance may play a part in autism. For the first time, the authors also found evidence suggestive of specificity of some risk genes acting independently in autism and in severe neurodevelopmental delay that does not include autism [40]. Within psychiatry the most meaningful studies to date have been in schizophrenia, showing enrichment of damaging rare variants within evolutionarily constrained, mutation-intolerant genes in schizophrenia cases compared with controls [41]. In addition, one gene, *SETD1A*, has been confidently implicated by rare loss-of-function variants in schizophrenia as well as in intellectual disability and severe developmental disorders [41]. Early indicators suggest that, as sample sizes get larger and analytic approaches evolve, rare variant studies within psychiatric disorders will reveal novel risk genes, which will provide clues to core functional mechanisms.

7.4 Epigenetics

James Walters and
Kimberley Kendall

Epigenetics is the umbrella term for processes by which gene expression can be altered without changes in DNA sequence, and represents a way in which genetics and environment can interact. The main epigenetic processes implicated in psychiatric disorders are DNA methylation and histone modification/chromatin structure.

- **DNA methylation** – methyl groups are added to cytosine bases that are followed by guanine bases, and these tend to cluster in gene expression regulatory regions (CpG islands), such as the promoter region that switches on transcription. DNA methylation in these regions usually results in the suppression of gene transcription, effectively switching the gene off [42].

- **Histone modification/chromatin structure** – chromatin is the DNA–histone protein complex present in cell nuclei that determines whether DNA molecules are available to transcription factors for transcription to occur. Modifications such as acetylation and methylation of histones control the switching of chromatin from tightly wound (heterochromatin – transcription will not occur) to more loosely wound (euchromatin – associated with transcription) and back again [42, 43].

Methylation changes in multiple genes have been reported in schizophrenia and related disorders, particularly in genetic pathways thought to be involved in brain development and psychiatric disorders [42, 43]. It is important to note that promoter methylation reported as disrupted in schizophrenia can be variable and influenced by treatment, genotype and environmental factors, opening up the possibility of examining links between genetics and environmental factors but also emphasising the need for methodological rigour in these studies [43].

7.5 | **The Clinical Application of Genetics in Psychiatry** | **James Walters and Kimberley Kendall**

7.5.1 Clinical Genetics Services and Psychiatry

In the UK, NHS medical genetics services are specialist tertiary services located in regional centres with clinical genetics and laboratory genetics services.

Clinical genetics is largely an outpatient specialty and is staffed by doctors, specialist nurses and genetic counsellors. These staff see patients and their families for clinical assessment, risk assessment, investigations (including genetic testing) and genetic counselling. The multidisciplinary team will often cover topics such as predictive testing, genetic risk and education around specific disorders, supported by onward referral when indicated. Clinicians within medical genetics often subspecialise in disease areas such as cancer genetics, and work alongside colleagues from other specialties.

Staff in laboratory genetics services carry out genetic testing using a range of techniques such as karyotyping and fluorescence *in situ* hybridisation ('FISH') to detect chromosomal abnormalities and array comparative genomic hybridisation to detect CNVs and, more recently, whole-exome and whole-genome screening.

A key part of any genetic service provision is specialist genetic counselling. According to the World Health Organization, genetic counselling is 'the process through which knowledge about the genetic aspects of illnesses is shared by trained professionals with those who are at an increased risk of either having a heritable disorder or of passing it on to their unborn offspring'. Genetic counselling encompasses the assessment and communication of risk, with discussions about the pros and cons of genetic testing, but is also supportive, providing education about inherited disorders and facilitating access to further support.

While psychiatry has not been an embedded specialty within clinical genetics to date, there are UK and wider examples of multidisciplinary teams and clinics being set up to begin to provide services for patients and their families. If communication and discussion of psychiatric genetic risk and testing is to prove informative for patients, families and clinicians, the design and delivery of psychiatric genetic services will be key. The involvement of multidisciplinary teams from genetics and psychiatry, alongside patients and their families, would seem to be a prerequisite if such services are to be delivered successfully.

Conclusions and Outstanding Questions

The field of psychiatric genetics has come a long way since the initial recognition that psychiatric disorders cluster in families and the birth of family, twin and adoption studies. Research findings are emerging rapidly due to advances in genetic technologies, the motivation of patients to take part in research and international collaboration. These elements have enabled the creation of large-scale data sets and research expertise, which have improved our understanding of the genetic architecture of psychiatric disorders and provided important insights into the underlying nature of mental illness.

Outstanding Questions

- How can we best move from genetic association results to the biological interpretation and mechanistic insights necessary for clinical translation?

- Can genotyping be used clinically to aid diagnosis, guide treatment or predict prognosis? The application of genetic findings in clinical psychiatry will need to include consideration of the ethical issues raised and patients, families and clinicians need to be central to these discussions.

REFERENCES FOR CHAPTER 7

1. Gratten J, Wray NR, Keller MC, Visscher PM. Large-scale genomics unveils the genetic architecture of psychiatric disorders. *Nat Neurosci* 2014; 17(6): 782–790.

2. Sandin S, Lichtenstein P, Kuja-Halkola R et al. The heritability of autism spectrum disorder. *JAMA* 2017; 318(12): 1182–1184.

3. Gaugler T, Klei L, Sanders SJ et al. Most genetic risk for autism resides with common variation. *Nat Genet* 2014; 46(8): 881–885.

4. Lee SH, Ripke S, Neale BM et al. Genetic relationship between five psychiatric disorders estimated from genome-wide SNPs. *Nat Genet* 2013; 45(9): 984–994.

5. Hilker R, Helenius D, Fagerlund B et al. Heritability of schizophrenia and schizophrenia spectrum based on the nationwide Danish twin register. *Biol Psychiatry* 2018; 83(6): 492–498.

6. McGuffin P, Rijsdijk F, Andrew M et al. The heritability of bipolar affective disorder and the genetic relationship to unipolar depression. *Arch Gen Psychiatry* 2003; 60(5): 497–502.

7. Faraone SV, Perlis RH, Doyle AE et al. Molecular genetics of attention-deficit/hyperactivity disorder. *Biol Psychiatry* 2005; 57(11): 1313–1323.

8. Sullivan P, Neale M, Kendler K. Genetic epidemiology of major depression: review and meta-analysis. *Am J Psychiatry* 2000; 157(10): 11.

9. Howard DM, Adams MJ, Clarke TK et al. Genome-wide meta-analysis of depression identifies 102 independent variants and highlights the importance of the prefrontal brain regions. *Nat Neurosci* 2019; 22(3): 343–352.

10. Wray NR, Ripke S, Mattheisen M et al. Genome-wide association analyses identify 44 risk variants and refine the genetic architecture of major depression. *Nat Genet* 2018; 50(5): 668–681.

11. Mullins N, Forstner AJ, O'Connell KS et al. Genome-wide association study of more than 40,000 bipolar disorder cases provides new insights into the underlying biology. *Nat Genet* 2021; 53(6): 817–829.

12. Meier SM, Trontti K, Purves KL et al. Genetic variants associated with anxiety and stress-related disorders: a genome-wide association study and mouse-model study. *JAMA Psychiatry* 2019; 76(9): 924–932.

13. Trubetskoy V, Pardiñas AF, Qi T et al. Mapping genomic loci implicates genes and synaptic biology in schizophrenia. *Nature* 2022; 604(7906): 502–508.

14. Common polygenic variation contributes to risk of schizophrenia that overlaps with bipolar disorder. *Nature* 2009; 460(7256): 748–752.

15. Choi SW, O'Reilly PF. PRSice-2: polygenic risk score software for biobank-scale data. *Gigascience* 2019; 8(7): giz082.

16. Chang CC, Chow CC, Tellier LC et al. Second-generation PLINK: rising to the challenge of larger and richer datasets. *Gigascience* 2015; 4: 7.

17. Vilhjálmsson BJ, Yang J, Finucane HK et al. Modeling linkage disequilibrium increases accuracy of polygenic risk scores. *Am J Hum Genet* 2015; 97(4): 576–592.

18. Lewis CM, Vassos E. Polygenic risk scores: from research tools to clinical instruments. *Genome Med* 2020; 12(1): 44.

19. Ni G, Moser G, Consortium SWG of TPG, Wray NR, Lee SH. Estimation of genetic correlation via linkage disequilibrium score regression and genomic restricted maximum likelihood. *Am J Hum Genet* 2018; 102(6): 1185.

20. The Brainstorm Consortium, Anttila V, Bulik-Sullivan B et al. Analysis of shared heritability in common disorders of the brain. *Science* 2018; 360(6395): eaap8757.

21. Ruderfer DM, Ripke S, McQuillin A et al. Genomic dissection of bipolar disorder and schizophrenia including 28 subphenotypes. *Cell* 2018;173(7): 1705–1715.e16.

22. Allardyce J, Leonenko G, Hamshere M et al. Association between schizophrenia-related polygenic liability and the occurrence and level of mood-incongruent psychotic symptoms in bipolar disorder. *JAMA Psychiatry* 2018; 75(1): 28–35.

23. Lee C, Scherer SW. The clinical context of copy number variation in the human genome. *Expert Rev Mol Med* 2010; 12: e8.

24. Kirov G, Rees E, Walters J. What a psychiatrist needs to know about copy number variants. *BJPsych Advances* 2015; 21(3): 157–163.

25. Girirajan S, Brkanac Z, Coe BP et al. Relative burden of large CNVs on a range of neurodevelopmental phenotypes. *PLoS Genet* 2011; 7(11): e1002334.

26. Williams NM, Franke B, Mick E et al. Genome-wide analysis of copy number variants in attention deficit hyperactivity disorder: the role of rare variants and duplications at 15q13.3. *Am J Psychiatry* 2012; 169(2): 195–204.

27. Rees E, Walters JT, Georgieva L et al. Analysis of copy number variations at 15 schizophrenia-associated loci. *Br J Psychiatry* 2014; 204(2): 108–114.

28. Green EK, Rees E, Walters JT et al. Copy number variation in bipolar disorder. *Mol Psychiatry* 2016; 21(1): 89–93.

29. Coe BP, Witherspoon K, Rosenfeld JA et al. Refining analyses of copy number variation identifies specific genes associated with developmental delay. *Nat Genet* 2014; 46(10): 1063–1071.

30. Cooper GM, Coe BP, Girirajan S et al. A copy number variation morbidity map of developmental delay. *Nat Genet* 2011; 43(9): 838–846.

31. Rees E, Kendall K, Pardiñas AFF et al. Analysis of intellectual disability copy number variants for association with schizophrenia. *JAMA Psychiatry* 2016; 73(9): 963–969.

32. Kendall KM, Rees E, Bracher-Smith M et al. Association of rare copy number variants with risk of depression. *JAMA Psychiatry* 2019; 76(8): 818–825.

33. Kendall KM, Rees E, Escott-Price V et al. Cognitive performance among carriers of pathogenic copy number variants: analysis of 152,000 UK Biobank subjects. *Biol Psychiatry* 2017; 82(2): 103–110.

34. Kendall KM, Bracher-Smith M, Fitzpatrick H et al. Cognitive performance and functional outcomes of carriers of pathogenic copy number variants: analysis of the UK Biobank. *Br J Psychiatry* 2019; 214(5): 297–304.

35. Stefansson H, Meyer-Lindenberg A, Steinberg S et al. CNVs conferring risk of autism or schizophrenia affect cognition in controls. *Nature* 2014; 505(7483): 361–366.

36. Männik K, Mägi R, Macé A et al. Copy number variations and cognitive phenotypes in unselected populations. *JAMA* 2015; 313(20): 2044–2054.

37. Crawford K, Bracher-Smith M, Kendall KM et al. Medical consequences of pathogenic CNVs in adults: analysis of the UK Biobank. *J Med Genet* 2019; 56(3): 131–138.

38. Owen D, Bracher-Smith M, Kendall K et al. Effects of pathogenic CNVs on physical traits in participants of the UK Biobank. *BMC Genomics* 2018; 867.

39. Kaplanis J, Samocha KE, Wiel L et al. Evidence for 28 genetic disorders discovered by combining healthcare and research data. *Nature* 2020; 586(7831): 757–762.

40. Satterstrom FK, Kosmicki JA, Wang J et al. Large-scale exome sequencing study implicates both developmental and functional changes in the neurobiology of autism. *Cell* 2020; 180(3): 568–584.e23.

41. Singh T, Kurki MI, Curtis D et al. Rare loss-of-function variants in *SETD1A* are associated with schizophrenia and developmental disorders. *Nat Neurosci* 2016; 19(4): 571–577.

42. Roth TL, Lubin FD, Sodhi M, Kleinman JE. Epigenetic mechanisms in schizophrenia. *Biochim Biophys Acta* 2009; 1790(9): 869–877.

43. Hannon E, Dempster EL, Mansell G et al. DNA methylation meta-analysis reveals cellular alterations in psychosis and markers of treatment-resistant schizophrenia. *elife* 2021; 10: e58430.

National Neuroscience Curriculum Initiative online resources

Polygenic Risk Scores: What Are They Good For?

Amanda B. Zheutlin and David A. Ross

Leaping Forward: The Surprising Role of Jumping Genes in Psychiatric Genetics

Maryem A. Hussein and David A. Ross

Psychiatric Pharmacogenomics: How Close Are We?

Matthew E. Hirschtritt, Aaron D. Besterman and David A. Ross

Leveraging the Power of Genetics to Bring Precision Medicine to Psychiatry: Too Little of a Good Thing?

Daniel Moreno-De-Luca, Michael E. Ross and David A. Ross

Small RNAs May Answer Big Questions in Mental Illness

Carrie Wright, David A. Ross and Daniel R. Weinberger

Genes Orchestrating Brain Function

Emily Olfson and David A. Ross"

This "stuff" Is really cool: Emily Olfson, *"Moving from Single Genes to Pathways"*

This "stuff" is really cool: Emily Olfson, *"Far from The Tree"* on de novo mutations *in psychiatry*

This "stuff" is really cool: Daniel Moreno De Luca, *"Genetic CBT"* on gene editing *in psychiatry*

8

Neurodevelopment and Neuroplasticity

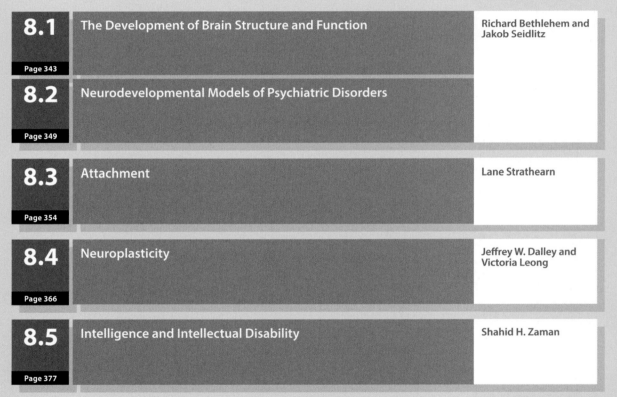

8.1

The Development of Brain Structure and Function

Richard Bethlehem and Jakob Seidlitz

OVERVIEW

Brain development is mediated by a series of coordinated and often genetically programmed events, simultaneously signalling the growth of the entire brain while harmoniously guiding the emergence of local structure, function and connections of numerous brain regions. This process of 'normative' or 'typical' brain development, from gestation through adolescence, creates a biological scaffold that gives rise to complex traits such as cognition, educational achievement and socio-affective functioning. In addition to the relevance of healthy brain development for these phenotypes (Paus et al., 2008; Gilmore et al., 2018), it is pivotally important for understanding neurodevelopmental disorders (e.g. autism, attention deficit hyperactivity disorder, anxiety disorders, depression, schizophrenia, etc.), which are conceptualised as arising from some form of deviation from typical brain maturation (see Section 8.2). Using non-invasive neuroimaging techniques, such as magnetic resonance imaging and diffusion tensor imaging, early studies have provided an intriguing first picture of brain growth trajectories and changes in structure, function and connectivity. Below, we highlight particularly critical periods of lifespan brain maturation and senescence, and describe the neurobiological phenomena at the microscale that are coincidental with these global and local effects queried at the macroscale.

8.1.1 Maturation of Brain Structure

The major biological axes of variation in the brain can be viewed in terms of composite metrics (i.e. 'building blocks') – classified into elements of size, scale, shape and composition (Jakob, 1899; Brodmann, 1909). The original histological investigations into these cerebral properties (specifically, cyto- and myeloarchitectonics) elucidated a highly diverse layer structure, which differentiates cortical areas with varying degrees of boundary specificity between parcellated brain regions. Intrinsic to this blueprint of cortical architecture is the notion of interconnectivity (microcircuitry). The six-layer neocortex is relatively consistent across the brain, with noticeable differences in the density, morphology (shape) and the positioning of neurons across the cortical layers (Jakob, 1899; Brodmann, 1909; Von Economo and Koskinas, 2008). During corticogenesis (see Figure 8.1.1A) *in utero*,

precursor cells (mainly radial glia) originating from the ventricular and inner/outer subventricular zones migrate radially to form the cortex inside to outside (from layer 6 near the white matter to layer 1 near the pial surface, respectively) and in the process forming the 'supragranular' layers 1–3, 'granular' layer 4, and 'infragranular' layers 5 and 6 (Rakic, 1974). These marked gradations in cortical microstructure emerge due to the varying profiles of pyramidal neuron density, and collectively form the basis of the cortical microcircuit (Gilbert and Wiesel, 1983; Rakic, 1988; Felleman and Van Essen, 1991), which grows and is simultaneously pruned throughout neonatal and postnatal development. See Section 8.4.1 for more on the development of neural circuits through synaptogenesis and pruning.

At a more global level, early brain formation during the prenatal stage largely takes place independent of

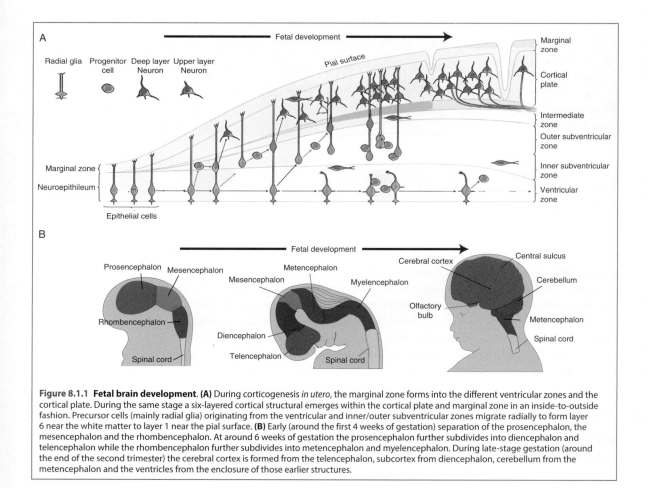

Figure 8.1.1 Fetal brain development. (A) During corticogenesis *in utero*, the marginal zone forms into the different ventricular zones and the cortical plate. During the same stage a six-layered cortical structural emerges within the cortical plate and marginal zone in an inside-to-outside fashion. Precursor cells (mainly radial glia) originating from the ventricular and inner/outer subventricular zones migrate radially to form layer 6 near the white matter to layer 1 near the pial surface. **(B)** Early (around the first 4 weeks of gestation) separation of the prosencephalon, the mesencephalon and the rhombencephalon. At around 6 weeks of gestation the prosencephalon further subdivides into diencephalon and telencephalon while the rhombencephalon further subdivides into metencephalon and myelencephalon. During late-stage gestation (around the end of the second trimester) the cerebral cortex is formed from the telencephalon, subcortex from diencephalon, cerebellum from the metencephalon and the ventricles from the enclosure of those earlier structures.

electrical activity and is strongly genetically driven. The basic subdivision from the aforementioned original layered single sheet of cells into prosencephalon, mesencephalon (which will later form the forward portion of the brainstem) and rhombencephalon (see Figure 8.1.1B) takes place during early gestation (~4 weeks old). The prosencephalon subsequently further divides into the telencephalon (which will later form the cerebral hemispheres) and the diencephalon (which will later form the collection of subcortical structures that make up the thalamic forebrain). See also Section 4.1.2 for more on the embryology of the nervous system. During the same gestational period the rhombencephalon will subdivide into the metencephalon (which will form the cerebellum), pontine flexure and myelencephalon (which will form the medulla oblongata). It should be noted that during this process of neurogenesis (i.e. the formation of new cells)

many more cells are formed than are sustained as there is a continuous process of apoptosis or programmed cell death. Overall, many more cells are formed than undergo apoptosis during early development, leading to overall rapid cortical expansion.

8.1.1.1 Grey Matter Maturation

At birth, although most structures are formed and organised in largely the same topology as adult brains, the total brain volume is estimated to be only about a third of the volume of an adult brain. Thus, formation of new tissue does not stop at birth. Furthermore, not all features that contribute to the total brain volume mature along the same trajectories (Figure 8.1.2). For example, in the first 2 years of life, grey matter volume, both cortical as well as subcortical, increases rapidly (estimated to increase by up to ~150% in the first year and a further increase of up to ~20% in the second year for cortical regions). Within those global volumetric changes, brain imaging studies also reveal similar rapid increases in morphological properties (Dahnke and Gaser, 2018) such as cortical thickness (the estimated distance between the grey/white matter boundary and the pial surface), surface area (in mm² of the pial surface of the cortex) and gyrification (formation and quantification of the characteristic folds of the cortex) (Figure 8.1.2A). The average cortical thickness is close to 100% that of the average adult brain by year 2 and slowly decreases over the course of the lifespan globally (Figure 8.1.2B). However, local microscale changes to these morphological properties also continue throughout development and there are likely regional variations in the precise developmental trajectories of each property. Brain surface area continues to expand after this initial rapid change in cortical thickness, peaking in early puberty in a similar fashion to global brain volume. Likewise, global cortical grey matter volume continues to expand and reaches its peak overall volume around the time of puberty onset after which there is a steady more linear decline. Interestingly, there are regional differences

during this stage of development whereby most regions follow an approximate cubic trajectory and mainly temporal and parietal regions exhibiting more quadratic or linear trajectories (Shaw et al., 2008) (Figure 8.1.2C). This decrease in grey matter volume continues till the end of life. Strong negative deviations from this decrease can be taken as signs of atrophy and are commonly associated with neurodegenerative disorders such as Alzheimer's disease and Parkinson's disease. It should be noted that most neurodegenerative conditions have strong regional specificity in terms of grey matter volume loss, and volumetric changes often precede the onset of symptoms (see Section 10.3).

8.1.1.2 White Matter Maturation

White matter volume, largely reflective of overall myelin content in the brain, follows a slightly different developmental trajectory (Figure 8.1.2B). Total white matter volume shows a mostly steady linear increase of around 10% annually in early development. However, there are also more fine-grained changes that indicate that the time of most rapid development takes place early on.

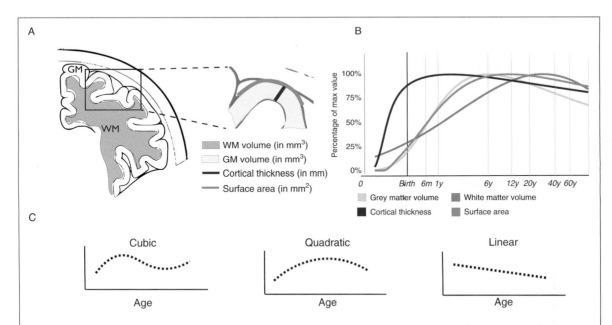

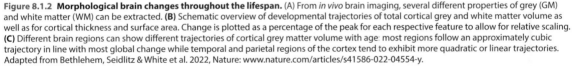

Figure 8.1.2 Morphological brain changes throughout the lifespan. (A) From *in vivo* brain imaging, several different properties of grey (GM) and white matter (WM) can be extracted. **(B)** Schematic overview of developmental trajectories of total cortical grey and white matter volume as well as for cortical thickness and surface area. Change is plotted as a percentage of the peak for each respective feature to allow for relative scaling. **(C)** Different brain regions can show different trajectories of cortical grey matter volume with age: most regions follow an approximately cubic trajectory in line with most global change while temporal and parietal regions of the cortex tend to exhibit more quadratic or linear trajectories. Adapted from Bethlehem, Seidlitz & White et al. 2022, Nature: www.nature.com/articles/s41586-022-04554-y.

The groundwork for axonal wiring, such as the major axonal tracts, as captured by white matter imaging, is largely laid out during preterm development. Pruning and fine-tuning of those connections rapidly takes off during the first 2 years of life. The pruning of unused connections and the further myelination of remaining fibres, whether genetically imprinted or as the result of neuronal activity, has a strong impact on the maturation of the brain's functional organisation. At a microstructural level, the previously mentioned basic layered nature of cyto- and myeloarchitecture in the cerebral cortex (Vogt, 1911; Von Economo and Koskinas, 2008) is also largely present at birth.

The pattern of white matter maturation diverges even more from grey matter development after this early period. While during childhood and adolescence overall white matter volume increases almost linearly, it generally peaks only well after 30 years, with a steeper decline of overall volume after 50 years (Figure 8.1.2B). Recent and classic histological studies emphasise that at a microstructural level this is likely not reflective of an indiscriminate increase in myelination, but rather an intricate reconfiguration dependent on the cortical layering, and varies across different brain regions (Paquola et al., 2019). The driving mechanisms of this reconfiguration can be both experience-dependent plasticity as well as genetic preprogramming. The interaction between these factors is an active field of research (de Faria et al., 2018).

8.1.2 Maturation and Localisation of Brain Function

Mapping functional changes during early development remains a challenge due to the fact that the neurovascular coupling system on which functional neuroimaging relies (i.e. how local perfusion responds to changes in neuronal activity) is also still maturing during early development. In addition, many factors that influence the accuracy of functional brain imaging are compounded when trying to assess this in early development. Head motion, differing levels of arousal caused by being in a loud and noisy machine as well as compliance and understanding of task instructions are more difficult in very early development. Early studies mapping the localisation and development of function have thus often relied on inferential approaches, such as linking structural development and behavioural development, or translational approaches across species. For example, visual attention in infants to some extent resembles behaviour seen in adult primates

and eye-tracking research shows that rapid eye movements are more strongly triggered by exogenous and not endogenous stimuli (Danka Mohammed et al., 2020). Exogenous stimuli draw attention to the stimulus itself (e.g. a light in peripheral vision catching our eye) and rely on subcortical structures while endogenous stimuli drive goal-directed attention (e.g. an arrow pointing toward a location that should be attended to) and rely on cortical executive function. Poor triggering of rapid eye movements by endogenous cues in infants indicates there is little top-down control of visual attention. During early development this pattern changes, which has led to the hypothesis that at birth a large part of the visual system is functionally driven by the evolutionary older subcortical system and, as both the visual cortex and frontal cortex (involved in executive function and top-down control) develop, this cortico-subcortical balance slowly shifts.

Despite difficulties in using conventional functional MRI in infants and neonates, studies have shown that the localisation of task-related activation specific to memory and response inhibition are largely present and stable by the time of adolescence while activation related to executive functioning still shows age-related changes from mid adolescence onwards (Paus et al., 2008). These changes are particularly apparent in the prefrontal and parietal cortices. In addition, studies have revealed ongoing functional activation changes during adolescent development in the brain's reward system (specifically regions in the ventral tegmental area and nucleus accumbens, which are heavily intertwined with the dopaminergic system). In recent years, the focus has shifted from studying the localisation of function in isolated brain systems to a network approach that assumes development of function in the brain takes shape in a systems-wide fashion involving an intricate process of inter-regional interactions. This notion of function in the brain as a distributed constellation of parallel circuits was also firmly established in early non-human primate studies (Goldman-Rakic, 1988). These early studies also confirm that the interaction and precise combination of distributed circuits giving rise to functional domains varies across development.

8.1.3 Maturation of Brain-Network Topology

While the assessment of regionally localised function is difficult, network analyses (see also Section 5.18) have revealed emerging organisational patterns during early brain development as well as continued changes to brain organisation later in life. Structural and diffusion-based neuroimaging shows that many of the building blocks of primary networks are already present at birth (Cao et al., 2016). For example, the network topology of the brain at birth already exhibits a modular structure, with certain areas serving as highly connected hubs that are also highly connected to each other (termed rich clubs). Further refinement of this configuration accelerates from birth when experience- and activity-dependent mechanisms start to exert their effects on development. In line with the protracted development of cognitive function at the behavioural level, functional neuroimaging shows, for example, that executive control networks develop later than networks associated with sensory and attention processing as well as compared to networks associated with self-awareness (e.g. the default mode network). In addition, between fetal and neonatal phases of development the cortico-subcortical organisation is further refined. In subsequent years, during teenage and adolescent development, further solidification of the basic network organisation takes place. Broadly, connections within networks increase or become stronger and connections between networks weaken or are pruned altogether. This process follows an asymptotic growth curve that peaks around 30 years, after which the pattern slowly reverses and a pattern of de-differentiation of the network architecture emerges.

Conclusions and Outstanding Questions

There are many different structural and functional properties that can be measured with non-invasive neuroimaging. Their varying but integrated trajectories of neurodevelopment are pivotal for brain health across the lifespan. Particularly early periods in the lifespan, especially the fetal and neonatal periods, see rapid changes in these properties, followed by a more gradual refinement and alteration over the rest of the lifespan.

Outstanding Questions

- What are the mechanisms driving early (fetal and neonatal) development of brain organisation?
- Are there specific genetic mechanisms that may put people at risk for atypical neurodevelopment?
- To what extent do factors impacting early-life brain development propagate throughout the lifespan and confer risk for atypical ageing and neurodegeneration?

8

REFERENCES

Bethlehem, R. A. I, J. Seidlitz, S. R. White et al. (2022). Brain charts for the human lifespan. *Nature* 604: 525–533.

Brodmann, K. (1909). *Vergleichende Lokalisationslehre der Grosshirnrinde in ihren Prinzipien dargestellt auf Grund des Zellenbaues von Dr. K. Brodmann*. J.A. Barth.

Cao, M., H. Huang, Y. Peng, Q. Dong, Y. He (2016). Toward developmental connectomics of the human brain. *Front Neuroanat* 10: 25.

Dahnke, R., C. Gaser (2018). Surface and shape analysis. In G. Spalletta, F. Piras, T. Gili (eds.), *Brain Morphometry*. Springer New York, pp. 51–73.

Danka Mohammed, C. Parvez, R. Khalil (2020). Postnatal development of visual cortical function in the mammalian brain. *Front Syst Neurosci* 14: 29.

de Faria, O., Jr, E. A. C. Pama, K. Evans et al. (2018). Neuroglial interactions underpinning myelin plasticity. *Dev Neurobiol* 78(2): 93–107.

Felleman, D. J., D. C. Van Essen (1991). Distributed hierarchical processing in the primate cerebral cortex. *Cereb Cortex* 1(1): 1–47.

Gilbert, C. D., T. N. Wiesel (1983). Clustered intrinsic connections in cat visual cortex. *J Neurosci* 3(5): 1116–1133.

Gilmore, J. H., R. C. Knickmeyer, W. Gao (2018). Imaging structural and functional brain development in early childhood. *Nat Rev Neurosci* 19(3): 123–137.

Goldman-Rakic, P. S. (1988). Topography of cognition: parallel distributed networks in primate association cortex. *Annu Rev Neurosci* 11: 137–156.

Jakob, C. (1899). Sobre el desarrollo de la corteza cerebral. *Rev Soc Méd Argent* 7: 397–403.

Paquola, C., R. A. I. Bethlehem, J. Seidlitz et al. (2019). Shifts in myeloarchitecture characterise adolescent development of cortical gradients. *eLife* 8: e50482.

Paus, Tomás, M. Keshavan, J. N. Giedd (2008). Why do many psychiatric disorders emerge during adolescence? *Nat Rev Neurosci* 9(12): 947–957.

Rakic, P. (1974). Neurons in rhesus monkey visual cortex: systematic relation between time of origin and eventual disposition. *Science* 183(4123): 425–427.

Rakic, P. (1988). Specification of cerebral cortical areas. *Science* 241(4862): 170–176.

Shaw, P., N. J. Kabani, J. P. Lerch et al. (2008). Neurodevelopmental trajectories of the human cerebral cortex. *J Neurosci* 28(14): 3586–3594.

Vogt, O. 1911. Die Myeloarchitektonik des Isocortex Parietalis. *J Psychol Neurol* 18: 379–390.

Von Economo, C., G. N. Koskinas (2008). *Atlas of Cytoarchitectonics of the Adult Human Cerebral Cortex* (transl. L. C. Triarhou). Karger.

National Neuroscience Curriculum Initiative online resources

The Architecture of Cortex – in Illness and in Health

Youngsun T. Cho, Julie L. Fudge and David A. Ross

Richard Bethlehem and Jakob Seidlitz

8.2 Neurodevelopmental Models of Psychiatric Disorders

OVERVIEW

The current era of diagnostics in psychiatry is nested within the axis between categorical labels which define distinct clusters of symptoms (e.g. the *Diagnostic and Statistical Manual of Mental Disorders*, 5th edition (DSM-5; American Psychiatric Association, 2013) and the *International Classification of Diseases*, 11th edition (ICD-11; World Health Organization, 2018)), and dimensional constructs which define continuous quantitative traits (e.g. the US National Institute of Mental Health Research Domain Criteria). Unlike neurological disorders such as Alzheimer's disease and Parkinson's disease, there is currently no conclusive evidence of a causal mapping of biological mechanisms to clinical symptomatology nor are there reliable neuropathophysiological correlates on which to base or confirm diagnoses. Thus, the quest for biomarkers in psychiatric disorders rests on the ability to untangle the convergent (shared) and divergent (distinct) effects in these conditions at multiple levels of biological scale – from molecular-scale genetics and transcriptomics, macroscale endophenotypes derived from neuroimaging, through to observable and quantifiable behavioural, cognitive and psychological phenomena.

In order to accurately ground psychiatry in biology, one major consideration is the added dimension of development, in the context of diagnosis, risk, onset and severity of a given disorder (Paus et al., 2008). Post conception, the genetic landscape in concert with the intrauterine environment determines the physical fate of the embryo through to birth. It is during this phase that critical morphological features of the brain are formed. Postnatally, childhood and adolescence are not only a period of physical growth, partly instantiated by puberty, but also in the development of complex behaviours and in personal expression and decision making. Because diagnosis of psychiatric disorders is determined based on aberrations in these constructs, this is the most common period of symptom onset and subsequent diagnosis. Given the rapid changes in brain development in these early years and the role of genetic and environmental risk factors, early development poses a particularly vulnerable period for the development of psychopathology (Figure 8.2.1). It is thus not

surprising that lifetime prevalence for most mental health conditions reaches 75% during or before adolescence (Jones, 2013), further underscoring the importance of ontogenesis in the emergence of psychiatric symptomatology. There are several conditions that are particularly marked by developmental atypicality and several approaches that emphasise the use of developmental models in studying psychiatric conditions, as discussed below.

8.2.1 Atypical Development in Psychiatric Disorders

8.2.1.1 Autism

Ever since autism was first described in the 1940s, researchers and clinicians have noticed that there is a considerable proportion of individuals with a larger than average head circumference (macrocephaly). More recent studies reveal that as many as 15% of boys with autism can be considered to have such macrocephaly (Sacco et al., 2015). Interestingly

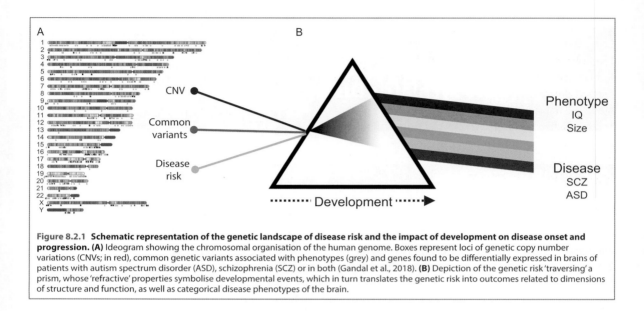

Figure 8.2.1 Schematic representation of the genetic landscape of disease risk and the impact of development on disease onset and progression. (A) Ideogram showing the chromosomal organisation of the human genome. Boxes represent loci of genetic copy number variations (CNVs; in red), common genetic variants associated with phenotypes (grey) and genes found to be differentially expressed in brains of patients with autism spectrum disorder (ASD), schizophrenia (SCZ) or in both (Gandal et al., 2018). **(B)** Depiction of the genetic risk 'traversing' a prism, whose 'refractive' properties symbolise developmental events, which in turn translates the genetic risk into outcomes related to dimensions of structure and function, as well as categorical disease phenotypes of the brain.

though, not all of these boys also have larger than average brains, underscoring the value of using MRI to study its neurobiology in more detail. Studies also reveal that this overgrowth mainly occurs in very early development, possibly *in utero*, and there is evidence that the average difference from a peer group diminishes during teenage development. Along similar lines, research also suggests there may be a significant subgroup of autistic individuals with microcephaly. Both these subgroups are hypothesised to result from atypical pruning of connections (e.g. reduced pruning of connections in macrocephaly and increased pruning in microcephaly). At a behavioural level, atypical pruning may be associated with broader differences in the way sensory input is processed and filtered, possibly associated with the sensory abnormalities often observed in autism. The potentially regionally specific pattern, morphological properties and implications for brain organisation that underlie these differences remain an active area of research. See Section 9.1.3 for more on the developmental biology of autism.

8.2.1.2 Schizophrenia

More often than not, patterns of atypical development are not obviously captured by abnormal maturational patterns of singular morphological properties (e.g. total grey or white matter volume). Schizophrenia, for example, exhibits a complex organised pattern of atypical

development (Alexander-Bloch et al., 2014). Specifically, there appears to be a network organisation in the atypicality whereby the areas that show atypical growth overlap with known modular organisation of the brain. This follows a longer-standing hypothesis of conceptualising schizophrenia as a developmental disorder (Jones et al., 1994) of altered brain connectivity, and complements genetic studies demonstrating that risk variants for schizophrenia affect genes linked to abnormal postnatal synaptic pruning (Sekar et al., 2016).

8.2.1.3 Neurodegenerative Disorders

Neurodegenerative disorders, somewhat like developmental disorders, also exhibit alterations in brain structure, function and organisation. For example, although there is a general slow decline in cortical grey and white matter volumes with old age, neurodegenerative diseases such as Alzheimer's disease and other forms of dementia often coincide with a more rapid decline compared to that observed in healthy ageing. In addition, the maturational connectivity pattern of decreasing within-network connectivity and increasing between-network connectivity seen in healthy ageing can also exhibit a more rapid profile in neurodegeneration. Specifically, in the case of Alzheimer's disease some of this network de-differentiation as well as the overall morphological pathology seems to specifically affect a network of memory-related brain regions.

8.2.2 Translational Models for Assessing Psychopathology

Throughout the history of basic ('bench') neuroscience, animal models (e.g. mammals such as rodents and non-human primates) have played a major role in determining the causal mechanisms and biological underpinnings of observable human phenomena and they can be specifically powerful in studying human brain development at the macroscale. However, in general, despite the widespread use of non-human animal models in the current era of psychiatric neuroscience and clinical trial research, there still remains the fundamental question about the translatability of findings in these models to humans.

8.2.2.1 Insights into Development from Genetic and Transcriptomic Studies

The increased accessibility of genotyping technologies has led to new bridges between human clinical research and the use of animal models. Genome-wide association studies (GWAS, see Section 7.2) studies are focused on determining associations between a particular trait or phenotype and single-nucleotide polymorphisms – specific alterations in the genome which are commonly present in the population and associated with the trait of interest (e.g. categorical: patients versus controls; or dimensional: height). Given that genetic predisposition and preprogramming are major factors in brain development these studies can potentially probe the causal mechanisms underlying psychopathology specifically and typical and atypical brain development more broadly.

A highly complementary approach to GWAS is whole-genome transcriptomic profiling through RNA sequencing. Whereas GWAS typically relies on DNA genotyping from blood samples and can identify alterations in the genetic code, RNA sequencing can estimate the level of gene expression. Gene expression can vary drastically across diverse tissue types and across development. Although accessing the human brain transcriptome is usually only possible through post-mortem tissue, there has been extensive work to identify specific genes that are differentially expressed in various brain regions between patients and controls. Studying how the expression of genes varies across development provides another window into the micro-level biological factors

underlying brain development and, in combination with neuroimaging, may shed light on the biology underlying atypical development specifically (Whitaker et al., 2016; Romero-Garcia et al., 2018; Seidlitz et al., 2020).

8.2.2.2 Modelling Development in vitro

Along with these whole-genome and transcriptome approaches to understanding the biology of mental illness, major advances in molecular biology and bioengineering have paved the way for mechanistic discovery in humans. Techniques such as induced pluripotent stem cell (iPSC) lines can be used to generate various neuronal and non-neuronal cell types that are present in human brain tissue, all from a saliva or blood sample from the participant (Dolmetsch and Geschwind, 2011). The ability to study these human-derived developing cell cultures in a dish holds immense potential to study fine-grained micro-level influences on cellular maturation. The fact that they can be derived from specific individuals, retaining their individual DNA profiles, allows the assessment of patient-specific atypicality. One underlying caveat with these methods is that there is some debate around how representative the resultant *in vitro* neurobiological properties are of *in vivo* brain structure and function. A step forward in expanding these two-dimensional *in vitro* protocols has been in the development of a three-dimensional version of these iPSC-derived cell cultures, mimicking brain tissue, also called 'organoids' (Lancaster et al., 2013). Commonly referred to as 'mini-brains', early proof-of-concept studies provided evidence on the neurobiological and biophysical feasibility of organoids as a model of early neurodevelopment and brain neurogenesis (Benito-Kwiecinski and Lancaster, 2020). One area of particular progress has been in the vascularisation (and consequent sustainability) of human cerebral organoids via successful transplant into a mouse model (Mansour et al., 2018). These combinatorial biological approaches to modelling the human brain in health and disease provide a seemingly clear bridge between basic neuroscience and clinical treatment.

8.2.2.3 Normative Models of Development

Finally, an overarching cross-domain methodological principle that can guide the field of psychiatry is normative modelling. This emerging statistical framework aims to capture individual differences through the establishment of normative variation of any given trait, psychological or cognitive construct, or biological metric. In practice, this is perhaps best conceptualised as being analogous to the growth charts used in a paediatrician's office. In the same fashion and given enough population data, one can construct a brain growth chart for brain development and estimate where on this trajectory each person falls at a given time during development. Subsequently, their developmental stage can be quantified and, if longitudinal data are available, it may be possible to make predictions on future estimates. The individually specific nature of this approach also better encapsulates the clinical reality of high heterogeneity within clinical cohorts. In other words, despite a common diagnostic label, no two patients with that label are generally exactly alike in their presentation of that diagnosis. Classical, so-called case–control studies often compare group means, which assumes a homogeneity within each group. Normative models do not rely on this assumption and may thus also be well equipped to study both categorical constructs as well as dimensional features while doing justice to individual variability, and have already proven specifically

useful in clinical populations (Marquand et al., 2019; Bethlehem et al., 2020; Lv et al., 2020).

Conclusions and Outstanding Questions

The quest for biomarkers in psychiatric disorders remains a central tenet of clinical neuroscience. Its success rests on the ability to untangle the convergent (shared) and divergent (distinct) effects at multiple levels of biological scale – from molecular-scale genetics and transcriptomics, macroscale endophenotypes derived from neuroimaging, through to observable and quantifiable behavioural, cognitive and psychological phenomena. To some extent, deviations from typical development may help elucidate these patterns at the level of the individual.

Outstanding Questions

- What are key biological markers in brain development that may put people at risk for a psychiatric condition?
- How can we efficiently parse clinical heterogeneity in the search for such biomarkers?

REFERENCES

Alexander-Bloch, A. F., P. T. Reiss, J. Rapoport et al. (2014). Abnormal cortical growth in schizophrenia targets normative modules of synchronized development. *Biol Psychiatry* 76 (6): 438–446.

American Psychiatric Association (2013). *Diagnostic and Statistical Manual of Mental Disorders*, 5th ed. (DSM-5). American Psychiatric Association,

Benito-Kwiecinski, S. , M. A. Lancaster (2020). Brain organoids: human neurodevelopment in a dish. *Cold Spring Harb Perspect Biol* 12(8): a035709.

Bethlehem, R. A. I., J. Seidlitz, R. (2020). A normative modelling approach reveals age-atypical cortical thickness in a subgroup of males with autism spectrum disorder. *Commun Biol* 3(1): 486.

Dolmetsch, R., D. H. Geschwind (2011). The human brain in a dish: the promise of iPSC-derived neurons. *Cell* 145(6): 831–834.

Gandal, M. J., P. Zhang, E. Hadjimichael et al. (2018). Transcriptome-wide isoform-level dysregulation in ASD, schizophrenia, and bipolar disorder. *Science* 362(6420): eaat8127.

Jones, P. B. (2013). Adult mental health disorders and their age at onset. *Br J Psychiatry Suppl* 54: S5–10.

Jones, P., R. Murray, P. Jones, B. Rodgers, M. Marmot (1994). Child developmental risk factors for adult schizophrenia in the British 1946 birth cohort. *Lancet* 344(8934): 1398–1402.

Lancaster, M. A., M. Renner, C.-A. Martin et al. 2013. Cerebral organoids model human brain development and microcephaly. *Nature* 501(7467): 373–379.

Lv, J., M. Di Biase, R. F. H. Cash et al. (2020). Individual deviations from normative models of brain structure in a large cross-sectional schizophrenia cohort. *Mol Psychiatry* 26(7): 3512–3523.

Mansour, A. A, J. T. Gonçalves, C. W. Bloyd et al. (2018). An *in vivo* model of functional and vascularized human brain organoids. *Nat Biotechnol* 36(5): 432–441.

Marquand, A. F., S. Mostafa Kia, M. Zabihi et al. (2019). Conceptualizing mental disorders as deviations from normative functioning. *Mol Psychiatry* 24: 1415–1424.

Paus, T., M. Keshavan, J. N. Giedd (2008). Why do many psychiatric disorders emerge during adolescence? *Nat Rev Neurosci* 9(12): 947–957.

Romero-Garcia, R., V. Warrier, E. T. Bullmore, S. Baron-Cohen, R. A. I. Bethlehem (2018). Synaptic and transcriptionally downregulated genes are associated with cortical thickness differences in autism. *Mol Psychiatry* 24: 1053–1064.

Sacco, R., S. Gabriele, A. M. Persico (2015). Head circumference and brain size in autism spectrum disorder: a systematic review and meta-analysis. *Psychiatry Res* 234(2): 239–51.

Seidlitz, J., A. Nadig, S. Liu et al. (2020). Transcriptomic and cellular decoding of regional brain vulnerability to neurogenetic disorders. *NatCommun* 11(1): 3358.

Sekar, A., A. R. Bialas, H. de Rivera et al. (2016). Schizophrenia risk from complex variation of complement component 4. *Nature* 530(7589): 177–183.

Whitaker, K. J., P. E. Vértes, R. Romero-Garcia et al. (2016). Adolescence is associated with genomically patterned consolidation of the hubs of the human brain connectome. *Proc Natl Acad Sci USA* 113(32): 9105–9110.

World Health Organization (2018). *International Classification of Diseases*, 11th ed. (ICD-11). World Health Organization.

8

<table>
<tr><td>**8.3**</td><td># Attachment</td><td>**Lane Strathearn**</td></tr>
</table>

OVERVIEW

Since articulated by John Bowlby in the late 1960s, attachment theory has become foundational for our understanding of how early experience may shape neurodevelopment and later psychopathology. Using well-validated instruments to measure attachment, such as the Strange Situation Procedure and the Adult Attachment Interview, variations in human attachment have been observed and linked to differences in brain, endocrine and behavioural responses. These observations closely parallel non-human animal models of caregiving and social behavior, which also provide more detailed data on neuroendocrine mechanisms. Understanding the neurobiology of attachment has also led to some novel approaches to therapeutic intervention.

8.3.1 Attachment Theory

8.3.1.1 John Bowlby: the Father of Attachment

Since John Bowlby first published his seminal works on the theory of attachment [1], the biological sciences have validated and expanded upon many of his hypotheses, linking early patterns of maternal caregiving with adult behaviour and risk for psychopathology [2]. Potential mechanisms include epigenetic changes affecting gene expression, the neuroendocrine regulation of stress, decision making and social behaviour. Bowlby's primary premise was that infants possess an innate biological need to form attachments with their caregivers in order to secure protection and nurturance essential for survival and reproductive success.

Parental behaviour is thought to be a crucial factor influencing infant neural development, with animal research identifying possible neuroendocrine mechanisms [2–4]. Since parental caregiving is provided by the mother in most mammalian species, animal research has primarily focused on maternal behaviour. Mechanisms include changes in hippocampal stress hormone receptor expression [2, 5, 6], cholinergic innervation [2] and DNA methylation affecting oxytocin and glucocorticoid

receptor gene expression [7]. See also Section 8.4.2 on the effects of stress on the developing brain. In animal models, maternal care has been linked with three infant developmental outcomes – cognition, parenting behaviour and stress reactivity – each of which may contribute to maternal caregiving and risk of psychopathology in the next generation [4].

8.3.1.2 Ainsworth's Strange Situation Procedure and Main's ABC+D Attachment Model

Following in Bowlby's footsteps, Mary Ainsworth operationalised his theory to test whether differences in early maternal sensitivity were linked to varying patterns of attachment behaviour in early childhood, developing the classic Strange Situation Procedure (SSP) to observe infant response to introductions, separations and reunions [3]. This involves exposing the child to episodes of mildly increasing stress, with repeated separations from the mother and introductions to a 'stranger'. Her work revealed that infants displayed patterns of behaviour which maximised the likelihood of caregiver proximity, and avoidance of potential danger. Three basic attachment strategies were identified: (i) type A, 'avoidant', which was characterised by avoidance of proximity or interaction with the caregiver during the reunion phase; (ii) type B, 'secure', characterised by the infant actively seeking proximity with the caregiver, resulting in diminished infant distress; and (iii) type C 'ambivalent/anxious', with the infant initiating contact with the caregiver, but also maintaining resistance and distress. A fourth type D 'disorganised' category was later added by Mary Main [4], to describe some infants with anomalous behaviour, characterised as a proposed *lack of* an organised response to frightening or frightened caregiver behaviour.

The so-called ABC+D attachment model ultimately led to the development of one of the most accepted and empirically validated measures of attachment in adulthood: the Adult Attachment Interview (AAI) [5], originally developed by Mary Main and colleagues. The AAI is a semi-structured interview used to identify differences in 'state of mind with regard to overall attachment history', an analysis of which characterises the subject's ability to describe attachment-related memories while simultaneously maintaining a coherent, cooperative discourse [6]. The coding schema was originally designed to match the four categories of Ainsworth's infant attachment, with relatively strong concordance observed at the level of secure (type B) versus insecure (type A or C) attachment [7].

8.3.1.3 Crittenden's Dynamic–Maturational Model of Attachment and Adaptation

Concurrent with this work, Patricia Crittenden developed the Dynamic–Maturational Model (DMM) of attachment and adaptation, which provided a strong theoretical foundation for later work on the neurobiology of attachment [8]. In this model, attachment patterns were formulated on the basis of specific memory systems in the brain (e.g. procedural, semantic, imaged, etc.) and the integration of cognitive and affective information processing, systems which become more complex with ongoing maturation and experience. Patterns of attachment were considered to be 'self-protective strategies', which varied dimensionally (i.e. along a spectrum rather than being either present or absent) in terms of the relative use of **cognitive**-contingent information or **affect**-arousing information to organise behaviour. Crittenden theorised that sensory stimulation was transformed into either temporally ordered 'cognitive' information (Type A), or intensity-based arousal or 'affective' information (Type

C). Type B organisation was thought to be a balanced integration of both sources of cognitive and affective information (Figure 8.3.1).

For example, Crittenden proposed that Type A individuals tended to dismiss their own feelings, intentions and perspectives, and rely more upon rules, procedural memory and learned temporal relations in predicting future outcomes. They behaved as if following the rule: 'Do the right thing – from the perspective of other people, without regard to your own feelings or desires'. She suggested that Type C individuals, in contrast, organised their behaviour around affective information such as fear, anger or desire for comfort. They tended to be preoccupied by their own feelings and perspectives, while omitting or distorting temporally ordered or cognitive information. They functioned as if under the dictum: 'Stay true to your feelings, and do not delay, negotiate or compromise'. Individuals with Type B or balanced patterns of attachment were able to integrate temporally ordered information regarding causal effect and more affect-based information such as emotional states of self and others and imaged memories, in order to form close relationships, make accurate decisions and predict future reward.

The AAI discourse also provided information on a modifying factor labelled 'unresolved trauma', defined not so much by recalled traumatic events, but on the impact of these events on current discourse and interpersonal functioning, indicative of past trauma that had not yet been adequately processed. One advantage of the AAI over self-report measures of attachment is its capacity to uncover distortions in information processing and perception, with the discourse revealing cognitive and/or affective discrepancies.

In contrast to the traditional coding method, Crittenden predicted that threatened children and adults would show highly **organised** (not 'disorganised') attachment strategies that reflected more complex Type A or C organisations than were seen in Ainsworth's A1–2, B and C1–2 patterns [8]. The new patterns, which acknowledged sexual development during adolescence and reflected the more advanced cognitive and affective capacities of adulthood, were numbered A3–8 and C3–8 and included organised A/C combinations (Figure 8.3.1). Higher-numbered categories were observed in individuals with more severe forms of psychopathology and in strategies

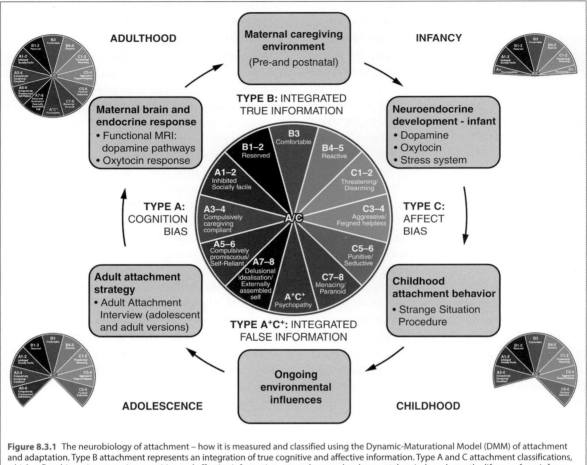

Figure 8.3.1 The neurobiology of attachment – how it is measured and classified using the Dynamic-Maturational Model (DMM) of attachment and adaptation. Type B attachment represents an integration of true cognitive and affective information. Type A and C attachment classifications, which reflect biases in processing cognitive and affective information, expand across developmental periods and over the lifespan, from infancy and childhood to adolescence and adulthood. The antithesis of Type B attachment is Type A+C+, which represents an integration of falsified or distorted cognitive and affective information. Adapted from [9].

with increasingly distorted or even falsified cognition and affect. Whereas secure Type B attachment was defined as the integration of **true** cognitive and affective information, its antithesis, labelled psychopathy, was defined as the integration of **falsified** or transformed cognitive and affective information.

For example, during one part of the AAI, interviewees are asked, 'Think of five words or phrases that describe your relationship with your mother [or other attachment figure], going as far back as you can remember.' Responses might include words such as 'warm', 'loving', 'affectionate', or perhaps, in some cases, 'stressful'. They are then asked to provide a specific memory that illustrates each descriptive word. Individuals with Type A3–4 attachment, in which negative affect is inhibited, may only use positive descriptive words or phrases to describe their attachment figure. However, when asked to provide a specific memory related to that word, they may be unable to do so. Typical responses are: 'I can't remember any specific times, but she was always just … warm and loving'. Later in the interview, when directly asked about episodes of trauma or neglect, these discrepancies become even more evident. Individuals who use a C3–4 strategy may use subtle forms of aggression, or feign helplessness, to elicit an affective response from the interviewer. Individuals with higher-numbered strategies may falsify or distort affect or cognition, such as smiling and laughing when describing traumatic life events (A7–8), or describing acts of cruelty or torture as helping a child to become more compassionate (C7–8).

8.3.2 Behavioural Studies of Attachment

As demonstrated in numerous studies, infants who are secure in their attachment relationships generally manifest with higher levels of self-esteem, self-reliance and self-regulation of impulses and emotions from preschool through to adolescence. They are also better able to form closer relationships, which evolves into an enhanced capacity for intimacy and self-disclosure in adolescence and adulthood [10]. In contrast, insecure attachment is associated with a higher risk for anxiety, eating and conduct disorders, post-traumatic stress disorder, borderline personality disorder and other forms of psychopathology [11]. For example, one study showed that women with borderline personality disorder had much higher rates of high-ordered A/C strategies in the DMM coding system, as well as extremely high rates of

unresolved loss or trauma [12]. Recognising patterns of adult attachment and unresolved childhood trauma may assist providers to formulate more effective treatment strategies for many psychiatric conditions.

8.3.3 Animal Models of Attachment

Research conducted primarily in rodents and non-human primates provides a framework for understanding the neurobiology of maternal caregiving and attachment (Figure 8.3.2). Variations in maternal behaviour, such as licking of rat pups, are associated with differences in pup neuroendocrine development, from the level of gene expression to behaviour. Animals that are exposed to different levels of maternal caregiving – either naturally occurring or experimentally induced – show differences in the epigenetic regulation of key genes involved in stress regulation and social behaviour, including the

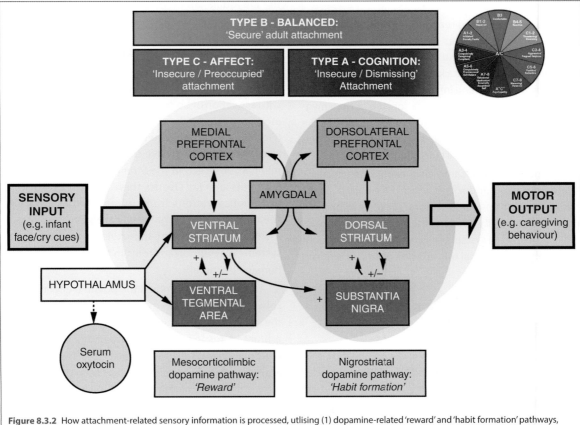

Figure 8.3.2 How attachment-related sensory information is processed, utlising (1) dopamine-related 'reward' and 'habit formation' pathways, and (2) oxytocin pathway connections. Different types of attachment are thought to utilise different brain pathways and regions. Adapted from J Neuroendocrinol (2011), 23(11), 1054–1065.

glucocorticoid [13] and oxytocin receptor genes, resulting in differences in gene expression, neuroendocrine feedback and response, and social and stress-related behaviours [14]. Offspring who are separated from their mothers, or experience low levels of licking and grooming, tend to display more anxious behaviour, and show lower levels of maternal caregiving toward their own offspring, which tends to perpetuate the cycle of stress and parental neglect.

Dopaminergic reward processing pathways are likewise affected by early-life experience and maternal care. Firing of dopamine neurons is stimulated by reward-related prediction errors (see Section 5.7), which enhances learning and reinforces patterns of behaviour, including maternal caregiving in response to infant cues. Infant behavioural cues elicit dopamine release in the ventral striatum of rodent dams and trigger responsive caregiving behaviours [15]. Animals with lower levels of maternal caregiving have a diminished dopamine response to infant cues.

Oxytocin release and receptor expression have also been linked to differences in caregiving behaviour in rodents as well as sheep and non-human primates. When the effect of oxytocin is blocked experimentally, maternal caregiving behaviour and infant responsiveness is diminished [16]. Oxytocin receptors are located in the amygdala, affecting stress and fear responses, as well as the ventral tegmental area and ventral striatum, influencing reward processing of social cues (Figure 8.3.2).

In summary, early caregiving experience appears to program neuroendocrine systems that are critically involved in learning and memory, social development and stress reactivity, namely, the dopamine, oxytocin, and glucocorticoid systems, which may partially account for the intergenerational transmission of attachment and psychopathology risk.

8.3.4 Studying the Neurobiology of Attachment in Humans

8.3.4.1 Maternal Attachment

Functional MRI (fMRI) has provided exciting opportunities to test models of attachment in human parents and children. The first neuroimaging study to examine neuroendocrine differences based on adult attachment classification examined the brain response of mothers when viewing their own infant's (compared with an unknown infant's) facial expressions [17]. Mothers with a Type B 'secure' pattern of attachment, based on the AAI (DMM model), showed greater brain activation of dopamine-associated reward pathways, including the ventral striatum and the medial prefrontal cortex, when viewing happy own-infant faces (Figure 8.3.3). Mothers with a Type A insecure/dismissing attachment pattern showed less reward activation and greater activation of the dorsolateral prefrontal cortex (DLPFC) when viewing sad own-infant faces; this area is associated with cognitive processing and habit formation, rather than affective reward response (Figure 8.3.2). Corresponding results were found using another measure of attachment, with decreased striatum (and ventral tegmental area) activation in those with a Type A attachment style, in response to smiling faces and positive feedback. In those with Type C attachment, increased activation of the amygdala, an emotion-processing region of the brain, was observed in response to angry faces and negative feedback [18].

Type B mothers also showed an enhanced peripheral oxytocin response when interacting with their infants, compared with Type A mothers, which was correlated with activation of both oxytocin- and dopamine-associated brain regions (hypothalamus and ventral striatum) (Figure 8.3.4). Mothers with secure attachment were also far more likely to have children with secure attachment, as observed in the Strange Situation Procedure 6-months later [7]. Overall, these results validate many of the observations from animal studies regarding the neurobiology of maternal caregiving and attachment and suggest that the oxytocin and dopamine systems play important roles in the establishment of human attachment.

Another study examined the possible effect of unresolved trauma on maternal brain responses. Based on the AAI, mothers with unresolved loss or trauma showed a blunted response in the amygdala when viewing their own infant's distressed face [19]. This diminished amygdala response was specifically seen when mothers viewed their own infant's sad faces, but not while viewing unknown-infant faces (Figure 8.3.5). Although symptoms of post-traumatic stress disorder were not measured,

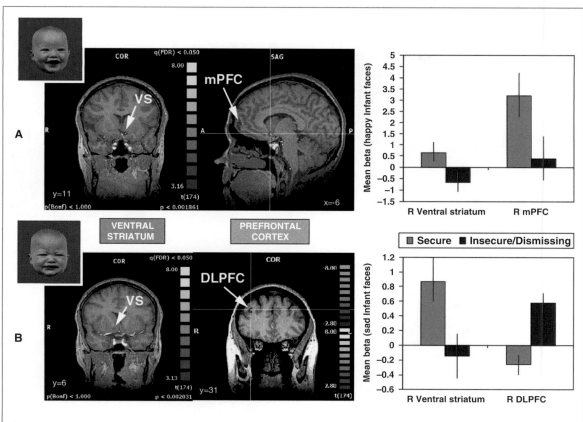

Figure 8.3.3 Brain responses to happy and sad own-infant faces, contrasting mothers with Type A (insecure/dismissing) and B (secure) attachment classifications (mean beta values ± the standard error of the mean). **(A)** Type B mothers show greater activation of the right ventral striatum (VS; $t = 3.1$, $p < 0.005$) and medial prefrontal cortex (mPFC; $t = 3.0$, $p < 0.01$) in response to own-happy infant faces. **(B)** Type B mothers show greater activation of the right ventral striatum ($t = 3.0$, $p < 0.01$) in response to own-sad infant faces. Type A mothers show greater activation of the dorsolateral prefrontal cortex (DLPFC). Adapted from [17].

these findings are consistent with well characterised symptoms of emotional numbing and disengagement when viewing emotionally salient stimuli.

One further example is of mothers with addiction problems, a vast majority of whom have evidence of unresolved trauma. These mothers showed deactivation of dopamine- and oxytocin-associated brain regions when viewing own- versus unknown-infant faces [20] (Figure 8.3.6). It is yet to be determined whether this abnormal brain response to infant cues is related to the drug use per se, or more proximal causes, such as early-life abuse, neglect or disturbed mother–infant attachment, which may affect the development of reward circuitry – and increase vulnerability to addiction.

8.3.4.2 Mothers, Fathers and Other Caregivers

With mothers most often acting as the primary caregiver, research studies have predominantly emphasised the mother–infant relationship. However, other recent studies have shown that fathers also play an important role in promoting the health, development and psychosocial well-being of their children. Both behavioural and neuroendocrine studies have indicated significant differences in how mothers and fathers typically interact with and respond to their children [21] (Figure 8.3.7). These differences may be associated with the changes that occur during pregnancy, parturition and lactation, which lead to neuroendocrine and behavioural adaptation [22].

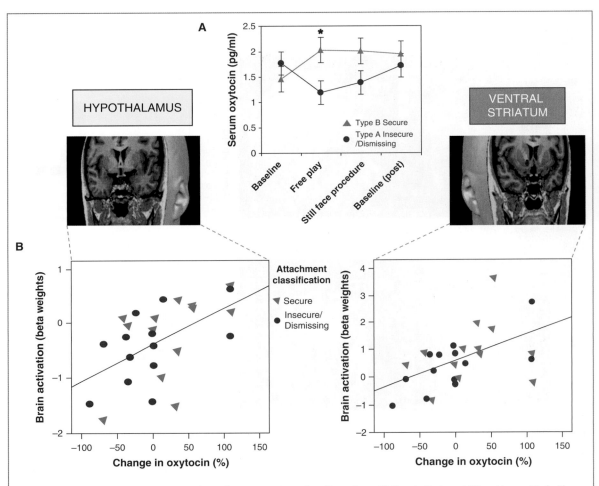

A

HYPOTHALAMUS

VENTRAL STRIATUM

B

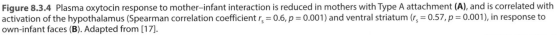

Figure 8.3.4 Plasma oxytocin response to mother–infant interaction is reduced in mothers with Type A attachment (**A**), and is correlated with activation of the hypothalamus (Spearman correlation coefficient $r_s = 0.6$, $p = 0.001$) and ventral striatum ($r_s = 0.57$, $p = 0.001$), in response to own-infant faces (**B**). Adapted from [17].

Although these adaptations are biologically restricted to the female parent, other neuroendocrine changes may also be associated with close interpersonal contact with the infant. For example, infant faces are socially salient stimuli that capture attention from fathers, mothers and non-parents alike. Studies suggest that parental exposure to infant cues, particularly those of one's own infant, are associated with changes in a parent's hormonal profile, and activation of brain regions associated with reward and attachment, which may facilitate parenting behaviours in both mothers and fathers [21, 23].

Several studies have looked at parental sex differences in response to viewing infant faces, as reviewed by Luo et al. [23]. Females, compared to males, tend to have a stronger attentional bias and preference for infant faces. Furthermore, neuroimaging studies have shown that primary caregiving mothers, compared to secondary caregiving fathers, have enhanced brain responses in limbic areas associated with reward and motivation when viewing infant video clips. However, primary caregiving fathers in same-sex relationships also show increased functional connectivity between both the limbic and socio-cognitive networks when viewing infant stimuli [24]. Thus, it may be that parental sex differences in responses to infant cues are shaped not only by underlying sex-specific biology, but also the type and amount of contact a parent

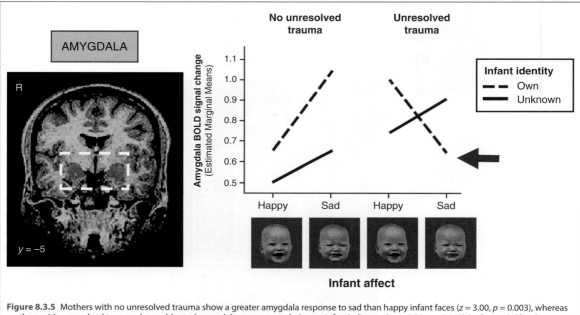

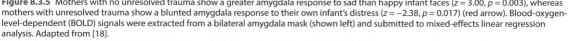

Figure 8.3.5 Mothers with no unresolved trauma show a greater amygdala response to sad than happy infant faces ($z = 3.00$, $p = 0.003$), whereas mothers with unresolved trauma show a blunted amygdala response to their own infant's distress ($z = -2.38$, $p = 0.017$) (red arrow). Blood-oxygen-level-dependent (BOLD) signals were extracted from a bilateral amygdala mask (shown left) and submitted to mixed-effects linear regression analysis. Adapted from [18].

has with his/her child during the early postpartum period. This has important implications for adoptive, foster and step parents, who do not undergo the biological changes associated with pregnancy, parturition and breastfeeding, but spend a large amount of time forming bonds with their infant during these formative early years.

8.3.5 From Neurobiology to New Therapies

With a substantial body of both animal and human research implicating endogenous oxytocin in the establishment and maintenance of attachment relationships, newer studies have explored the potential effects of intranasally administered oxytocin. While numerous placebo-controlled studies have demonstrated efficacy in specific narrowly defined outcomes, the results from clinical trials have been inconsistent, with meta-analyses in specific clinical populations generally revealing modest to no effect. However, others have suggested that moderating factors, such as sex, genetic variation and attachment experience [25], may obscure any effects. For example, several randomised controlled

trials of intranasal oxytocin have shown opposite effects depending on attachment security [26–29], with beneficial effects seen only in participants with low or anxious attachment styles.

Although much work is needed to understand how insecure attachment and unresolved trauma are best treated, preliminary evidence suggests that individuals with reorganising attachment strategies toward security (as measured by reflective and evaluative statements in the DMM–AAI) may be more likely to have children with secure attachment [30, 31]. If attachment strategies are adaptations to adverse experience, efforts to modify these strategies must focus on changing an individual's environment, in addition to the processing of cognitive and affective information. Symptom-based diagnoses, rather than attachment classifications, for conditions such as depression, eating disorders and borderline personality disorder, fail to identify the root causes of these conditions. Identifying the underlying attachment strategy, and its neurobiology, may help us to better direct treatment toward underlying mechanisms, rather than treating symptom manifestations alone.

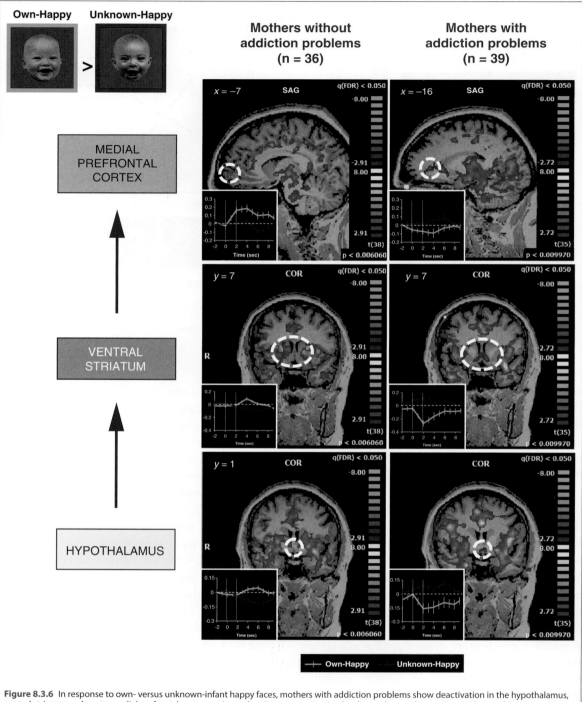

Figure 8.3.6 In response to own- versus unknown-infant happy faces, mothers with addiction problems show deactivation in the hypothalamus, ventral striatum and ventromedial prefrontal cortex, regions wherein strong activation has been observed in mothers without addiction problems (random effects analysis; FDR corrected $p < 0.05$). Insets show time courses extracted from the peak voxels in each (de)activated region, with the y-axis representing brain activation. Adapted from [20].

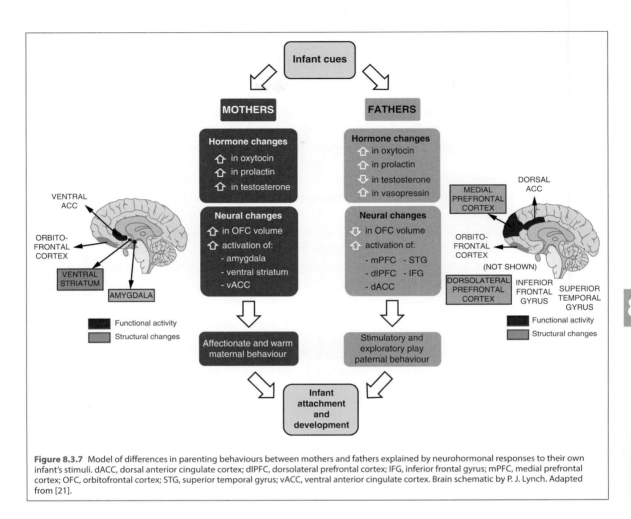

Figure 8.3.7 Model of differences in parenting behaviours between mothers and fathers explained by neurohormonal responses to their own infant's stimuli. dACC, dorsal anterior cingulate cortex; dlPFC, dorsolateral prefrontal cortex; IFG, inferior frontal gyrus; mPFC, medial prefrontal cortex; OFC, orbitofrontal cortex; STG, superior temporal gyrus; vACC, ventral anterior cingulate cortex. Brain schematic by P. J. Lynch. Adapted from [21].

Conclusions and Outstanding Questions

Research on the neurobiology of attachment helps psychiatrists and other mental health professionals look beyond current symptom profiles to neurodevelopmental pathways. Understanding biological mechanisms, such as epigenetic and neuroendocrine adaptation to stress and social experience, opens new opportunities for personalised patient care, to develop tailored intervention and prevention strategies for mental illness in childhood, adolescence and adulthood.

Outstanding Questions

- How does early-life experience affect epigenetic regulation of genes involved in reward processing, social development and stress regulation in humans?

- Do drugs such as intranasal oxytocin enhance brain reward responses in individuals with Type A attachment?

- Do psychotherapy and other forms of behavioural therapy affect brain responses to attachment-related cues?

- How can measures of attachment be better integrated into clinical assessments and treatment?

REFERENCES

1. J. Bowlby. *Attachment and Loss. Volume 1: Attachment.* Basic Books (1969/1982).

2. L. A. Sroufe. Attachment and development: a prospective, longitudinal study from birth to adulthood. *Attach Hum Dev* 7(4): 349–367 (2005).

3. M. D. Ainsworth, S. M. Bell. Attachment, exploration, and separation: illustrated by the behavior of one-year-olds in a strange situation. *Child Dev* 41(1): 49–67 (1970).

4. M. Main, J. Solomon. Procedures for identifying infants as disorganized/disoriented during the Ainsworth Strange Situation. In M. T. Greenberg, D. Cicchetti, E. M. Cummings (eds.), *Attachment in the Preschool Years: Theory, Research, and Intervention.* University of Chicago Press (1990), pp. 121–160.

5. C. George, N. Kaplan, M. Main. *Adult Attachment Interview*, 3rd ed. Department of Psychology, University of California, Berkley (1996).

6. M. Main. The organized categories of infant, child, and adult attachment: flexible vs. inflexible attention under attachment-related stress. *J Am Psychoanal Assoc* 48(4): 1055–1095 (1997).

7. P. E. Shah, P. Fonagy, L. Strathearn. Is attachment transmitted across generations? The plot thickens. *ClinChild Psychol Psychiatry* 15(3): 329–345 (2010).

8. P. Crittenden, A. Landini. *Assessing Adult Attachment.* W. W. Norton (2011).

9. L. Strathearn. Maternal neglect: oxytocin, dopamine and the neurobiology of attachment. *J Neuroendocrinol* 23(11): 1054–1065 (2011).

10. L. A. Sroufe. Infant–caregiver attachment and patterns of adaptation in preschool: the roots of maladaptation and competence. In M. Perlmutter (ed.), *Minnisota Symposium in Child Psychology.* Erlbaum Associates (1983), pp. 41-48.

11. L. A. Sroufe, B. Egeland, E. Carlson, W. A. Collin. *The Development of the Person: The Minnesota Study of Risk and Adaptation from Birth to Adulthood.* Guilford (2005).

12. P. M. Crittenden, L. Newman. Comparing models of borderline personality disorder: mothers' experience, self-protective strategies, and dispositional representations. *Clin Child Psychol Psychiatry* 15(3): 433–451 (2010).

13. I. C. G. Weaver, N. Cervoni, F. A. Champagne et al. Epigenetic programming by maternal behavior. *Nat Neurosci,* 7(8): 847–854 (2004).

14. M. J. Meaney. Epigenetics and the biological definition of gene x environment interactions. *Child Dev* 81(1): 41–79 (2010).

15. F. A. Champagne, P. Chretien, C. W. Stevenson et al. Variations in nucleus accumbens dopamine associated with individual differences in maternal behavior in the rat. *J Neurosci,* 24(17): 4113–4123 (2004).

16. E. B. Keverne, K. M. Kendrick. Oxytocin facilitation of maternal behavior in sheep. *Ann NY Acad Sci* 652: 83–101 (1992).

17. L. Strathearn, P. Fonagy, J. Amico, P. R. Montague. Adult attachment predicts maternal brain and oxytocin response to infant cues. *Neuropsychopharmacology* 34(13): 2655–2666 (2009).

18. P. Vrticka, F. Andersson, D. Grandjean, D. Sander, P. Vuilleumier. Individual attachment style modulates human amygdala and striatum activation during social appraisal. *PLoS One* 3(8): e2868 (2008).

19. S. Kim, P. Fonagy, J. Allen, L. Strathearn. Mothers' unresolved trauma blunts amygdala response to infant distress. *Soc Neurosci* 9(4): 352–63 (2014).

20. S. Kim, U. Iyengar, L. C. Mayes et al. Mothers with substance addictions show reduced reward responses when viewing their own infant's face. *Hum Brain Mapp* 38(11): 5421–5439 (2017).

21. P. Rajhans, R. P. Goin-Kochel, L. Strathearn, S. Kim. It takes two! Exploring sex differences in parenting neurobiology and behaviour. *J Neuroendocrinol* 31(9): e12721 (2019).

22. C. H. Kinsley, L. Madonia, G. W. Gifford et al. Motherhood improves learning and memory. *Nature* 402(6758): 137–138 (1999).

23. L. Luo, X. Ma, X. Zheng et al. Neural systems and hormones mediating attraction to infant and child faces. *Front Psychol* 6: 970 (2015).

24. E. Abraham, T. Hendler, I. Shapira-Lichter et al. Father's brain is sensitive to childcare experiences. *Proc Natl Acad Sci USA* 111(27): 9792–9797 (2014).

25. K. S. Macdonald. Sex, receptors and attachment: a review of individual factors influencing response to oxytocin. *Front Neurosci* 6: 194. (2013).

26. J. A. Bartz, J. Zaki, N. Bolger, K. N. Ochsner. Social effects of oxytocin in humans: context and person matter. *Trends Cogn Sci* 15(7): 301–9 (2011).

27. A. Venta, C. Ha, S. Vanwoerden et al. Paradoxical intranasal oxytocin effects on trust in inpatient and community adolescents. *J Clin Child Adolesc Psychol* 48(5): 706–715 (2017).

28. J. Bartz, D. Simeon, H. Hamilton et al. Oxytocin can hinder trust and cooperation in borderline personality disorder. *Soc Cogn Affect Neurosci* 6(5): 556–563 (2011).

29. J. A. Bartz, J. E. Lydon, A. Kolevzon et al. Differential effects of oxytocin on agency and communion for anxiously and avoidantly attached individuals. *Psychol Sci* 26(8): 1177–86 (2015).

30. U. Iyengar, S. Kim, S. Martinez, P. Fonagy, L. Strathearn. Unresolved trauma in mothers: intergenerational effects and the role of reorganization. *Front Psychol* 5(966), 1–9 (2014).

31. U. Iyengar, P. Rajhans, P. Fonagy, L. Strathearn, S. Kim. Unresolved trauma and reorganization in mothers: attachment and neuroscience perspectives. *Front Psychol* 10(110): 1–9 (2019).

8

<table>
<tr></tr>
</table>

8.4	**Neuroplasticity**	Jeffrey W. Dalley and Victoria Leong

OVERVIEW

Neurodevelopment begins *in utero* and continues throughout life. At each stage of development – from neurulation to adulthood – neural architecture is continuously and adaptively remodelled in response to experience. This experience-driven neural plasticity reaches its zenith during the early years of life, conferring an enormous potential for learning but also an innate vulnerability to the harmful effects of stress. In this section, we describe how brain development is shaped by sensory input, gonadal steroid hormones and experience over the lifespan. We cover concepts such as 'bloom' (synaptic overproliferation) and 'prune' (synaptic pruning), and present the evidence for critical periods of neuroplasticity for learning in humans. We specify critical periods for hormone-dependent organisational and activational effects from birth to adolescence, including sexually dimorphic neural plasticity. We also highlight specific examples of neuroplasticity during postnatal development and childhood such as language acquisition that may recruit activity-dependent plasticity mechanisms analogous to those that underlie the formation of ocular dominance columns in the primary visual cortex.

8.4.1 Neuroplasticity Mechanisms across the Lifespan

8.4.1.1 The Formation of Neural Circuits

The key stages of early brain development include neurogenesis, neuronal migration, cell death, differentiation, synaptogenesis, synaptic pruning and myelination. Remarkably, these stages do not occur in isolation, nor necessarily in a linear manner, as outlined in Figure 8.4.1.

During neurogenesis, neural stem cells make a transition from being proliferative and multipotent to being fully differentiated or specialised. When neurons are born, they migrate and disperse throughout the central nervous system, guided by glial cells and chemotactic cues. Although there is an early overabundance of neurons during brain development, programmed death of immature neurons, via apoptosis, subsequently serves to reduce the number of surplus neurons. Differentiation

involves the formation and outgrowth of axons and dendrites in order to form new synapses (synaptogenesis). The first synapses are observed around the 23rd prenatal week and rapid synaptic proliferation follows and continues until after birth. Synaptic proliferation is followed by pruning, which is the controlled and selective elimination of excess synapses. This process is **experience-dependent**, whereby only active synapses are conserved, and **non-uniform** across the brain. Thus, in visual and auditory cortices, adult synaptic levels are reached during childhood, while in the frontal lobe, adult levels are not reached until adolescence. Alterations in synaptic pruning may be implicated in the pathogenesis of neurodevelopmental disorders. For example, some evidence suggests that autism may be associated with deficits in dendritic spine pruning that lead to an excess of excitatory synapses during development (Tang et al., 2014). Myelination begins before birth and continues into

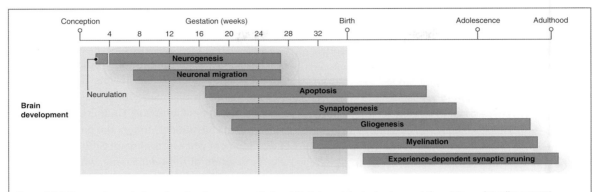

Figure 8.4.1 Temporal organisation of overlapping processes that contribute to early brain development (from Estes and McAllister, 2016).

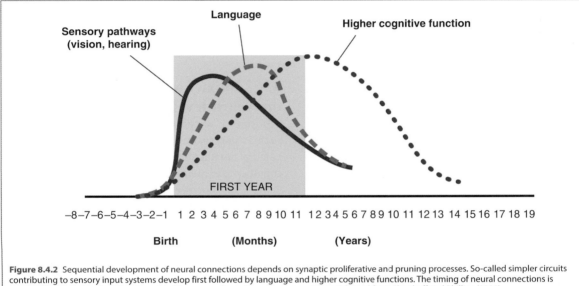

Figure 8.4.2 Sequential development of neural connections depends on synaptic proliferative and pruning processes. So-called simpler circuits contributing to sensory input systems develop first followed by language and higher cognitive functions. The timing of neural connections is genetically determined but the strength of the connections depends on experience. Adapted from Shonkoff and Phillips (2000).

adulthood, facilitating the speed and fidelity of cognitive processing. Neural systems develop sequentially; sensory circuits develop first, followed by early language skills and higher cognitive functions. Later, more complex brain circuits are established from earlier, simpler functional circuits, as illustrated in Figure 8.4.2.

8.4.1.2 The Role of Sex Hormones in Neurodevelopment

The developing brain is exquisitely sensitive to gonadal steroidal hormones, which fundamentally determine sexually dimorphic differences in the hard-wiring of male and female brains (McCarthy and Arnold, 2011);

see also Section 5.3 on sex and sex hormones. Much evidence points to a pivotal role of an initial testosterone spike in the perinatal phase, generated by the developing testes controlled by *SRY* gene expression on the Y chromosome, which **organises** neurogenesis, neuronal migration, synaptogenesis and apoptosis in the male brain. By contrast, ovarian steroid production is delayed until puberty whereupon oestrogen and other pubertal hormones further organise and **activate** sexually dimorphic brain circuits. The perinatal and pubertal periods thus represent critical periods for gonadal hormone-dependent differentiation of brain circuitry.

8.4.1.3 Plasticity and Sensitive Periods

While genes provide the basic blueprint for brain development, this is readily modifiable by experience-dependent plasticity. However, the impact of experience on brain plasticity is not continual throughout life. The capacity for plasticity is greater during early life than adulthood. Further, a developmental domain (such as vision or hearing) may display heightened plasticity within a relatively narrow window of time – or a so-called **sensitive period**. Before and after this period, neural systems are less responsive to restructuring by environmental influences (although in some cases, development may be rescued with early intervention). However, neuroplasticity is a double-edged sword, conferring both an advantage for learning and acquisition of cognitive abilities (e.g. language acquisition; see Case Study 8.4.1) but also as a window of vulnerability for the damaging effects of stress (see Section 8.4.2 below).

CASE STUDY 8.4.1 LANGUAGE DEVELOPMENT

Over the course of the first year of life, speech processing shifts from a universal mode to a native mode (Werker and Tees, 1984; Kuhl et al., 1992). Before 8–10 months of age, infants are able to discriminate the full range of phonetic contrasts that are used across the world's languages. By the end of their first year, infants lose their ability to discriminate between pairs of similar-sounding phonemes (called phoneme contrasts) that do not occur in their native language. Instead, infants demonstrate biased listening for phonemes that make up the sound inventory of their native language.

8.4.1.4 Neural Circuit Mechanisms of Sensitive Periods

Sensitive periods do not open or shut abruptly and may never close completely. Indeed, learning is possible throughout the lifespan. In general, however, the timing and opening of sensitive periods is controlled by the balance between excitatory and inhibitory neural circuits (Hensch, 2005). Molecular 'brakes' such as peri-neuronal nets, myelination and epigenetic mechanisms eventually consolidate the neural circuit to a stable state, closing the sensitive period. The excitatory–inhibitory balance is controlled by excitatory glutamatergic pyramidal cells and parvalbumin cells that utilise the inhibitory neurotransmitter gamma-aminobutyric acid (GABA). During development, the maturation of inhibitory parvalbumin-expressing neurons acts as a pivotal plasticity switch, itself modifiable by pharmacological intervention. Thus, agents that augment inhibitory GABAergic circuit function (e.g. benzodiazepines) trigger the precocious onset of development while disruption of GABAergic function (e.g. by deletion of the *Gad65* gene, which encodes a GABA-synthetic enzyme; Hensch et al., 1998) delays the opening of the sensitive neuroplasticity window (Hensch, 2005). Moreover, activation of the maternal immune system during pregnancy dramatically delays the postnatal excitatory-to-inhibitory GABA polarity shift in cortical microcircuits (Fernandez et al., 2019), reminiscent of animal models of autism (Ben-Ari, 2017).

8.4.2 Impact of Stress on Neurodevelopment

Exposure to uncontrollable stress during early life – such as maltreatment (abuse/neglect), poverty and parental mental disorder – can produce impairments in cognition and mental health that persist into adult life. Remarkably, however, not all children who experience early-life adversity suffer long-lasting ill effects, some children show resilience, or the ability to 'bounce back' after experiencing adverse life events, perhaps akin to the reported immunising effects of mild early-life stress on the hypothalamic pituitary axis function in adult rats (Levine et al., 1967).

The impact of stress differs depending on the stressor and the precise timing of the stress vis-à-vis the maturational time course of neural structures. This can be illustrated by case studies in humans – explicitly from an analysis of the effects of early institutionalisation and subsequent intervention (i.e. placement in foster care) on Romanian orphans in the 1980s (Nelson et al., 2007) – as well as experimental approaches where early social stressors in rodents and other experimental animals reveal sensitive periods of development for normal neurobehavioural maturation (Einon and Morgan, 1977). Ultimately, individual reactions to early stress depend on genetic and social factors that shape the balance of stress vulnerability and resilience mechanisms.

CASE STUDY 8.4.2 POVERTY

Poverty, or low socioeconomic status, is associated with a conglomerate of biological, environmental and psychosocial forms of 'toxic stress'. These include malnutrition, exposure to environmental toxins and physical danger, reduced sensory stimulation, lower-quality care and learning resources, parental distress and conflict. It is estimated that nearly 15 million children (20%) in the United States are currently living in poverty. A coherent body of neurocognitive research suggests that low socioeconomic status is associated with the largest disparities in childhood language development (explaining up to 30% of variance in language ability), and to a lesser extent with the development of memory and executive control (Farah et al., 2006; Noble et al., 2007). Although not as consistent as the link with cognitive function, low socioeconomic status is also known to have a significant impact on socio-emotional development, particularly in middle childhood and adolescence. Low socioeconomic status confers a higher risk for antisocial behaviour (e.g. aggressiveness and delinquency) and mental disorders (especially schizophrenia and personality disorders).

Neuroimaging studies have demonstrated a relationship between childhood poverty and reduced grey matter volume in the hippocampus and amygdala (e.g. Hanson et al., 2011; Luby et al., 2013). However, some of these studies failed to exclude participants on the basis of current or family psychiatric history (in fact, Luby et al., 2013 deliberately oversample preschoolers with depressive symptoms), thereby potentially confounding genetic effects. Hanson et al. (2013) also reported effects of low socioeconomic status on frontal and parietal brain development in a cohort of 77 infants and children, scanned longitudinally between 5 months and 4 years of age. Low socioeconomic status was found to be associated specifically with lower total grey matter, and lower frontal and parietal grey matter volume. Lower total grey matter was in turn associated with more problem behaviours at age 4, such as rule breaking, excessive aggression and hyperactivity. This study was notable because of the strict exclusion criteria used (e.g. maternal drug use during pregnancy, birth complications, child development disorders and family psychiatric history). These data suggest that frontal and parietal grey matter development are particularly impacted by low socioeconomic status, which would be expected to affect the development of executive functions such as planning and impulse control, as well as the development of attentional processes.

8.4.2.1 The Neural Effects of Adversity

There are many forms of early-life adversity, or 'toxic stress'. Children may experience abuse (emotional, physical or sexual), neglect (emotional or physical) or suffer the ill effects of household dysfunction (domestic violence, substance abuse or mental illness). Children who are exposed to stressors during early life have a higher risk of developing long-term impairments in cognition and mental health. Childhood maltreatment is a severe stressor, which, in addition to behavioural and cognitive problems, produces a cascade of physiological, neurochemical and hormonal changes, as well as enduring alterations in brain structure and function (Teicher et al., 2006). In rodents, the repeated separation of newborn pups from maternal contact leads to depressive behaviour in adulthood (Matthews et al., 1996) while isolating rats during adolescence causes increased aggression, anxiety

and abnormal reactions to reward-related stimuli (Burke et al., 2017). Negative social experiences during sensitive periods strengthen amygdala-dependent processes involved in fear and anxiety responses at the expense of hippocampal and prefrontal cortical substrates, subserving memory, learning and cognitive control (Radley et al., 2004; Bock et al., 2005). The hypothalamic–pituitary–adrenal (HPA) axis and its regulation by limbic cortical circuitry eventually becomes dysregulated by unmanaged stress and overproduces corticosteroids (e.g. cortisol). Hypercorticosteroidism in turn causes neuronal atrophy, especially within sensitive hippocampal subregions, and has been associated with increased risk for mental illnesses such as depression (de Kloet et al., 2005). Thus, toxic stress during early life often leads to poorly controlled stress responses that become overly reactive and slow to shut down when faced with threats throughout the lifespan

(Zhang et al., 2004). In humans, the impact of stress varies for different stressors (see Case Studies 8.4.2 and 8.4.3), and at different developmental timepoints depending on the maturation state of different brain regions.

To illustrate this point, uncontrollable stress during sensitive periods of development has deleterious effects on the developing foetus, caused in part by stress hormones (i.e. glucocorticoids) disrupting the normal programming events of the maturing brain (Gillies et al., 2014). Thus, whereas glucocorticoids may have adaptive developmental roles during late gestation, excessive glucocorticoid release during sensitive periods of development has negative outcomes for behavioural and emotional regulation that extend throughout adulthood. In this regard, the developing populations of dopamine neurons in the midbrain are exquisitely sensitive to the surrogate glucocorticoid stress agent, dexamethasone, when administered in the drinking water of rat dams during a critical embryonic stage (Virdee et al., 2014).

8.4.2.2 Resilience to Adversity

Not all children who experience early-life stress suffer poor developmental sequelae, some show positive adaptation or **resilience**. It is estimated that around 10–25% of maltreated children achieve resilient functioning (Walsh et al., 2010). Resilience is a dynamic developmental process with social (environmental) and biological component factors.

(1) **Social resilience factors**. At the individual level, positive self-esteem and ego-control (impulse control) positively predict adaptive functioning in maltreated children (Cicchetti et al., 1993). The family environment can also have a protective effect. Positive early caregiving and parental support can decrease the likelihood of adverse outcomes following early-life stress and moderate the impact of genetic vulnerability (Barr et al., 2004) and the effects of early-life stress. Associations between the degree to which parents offer love and affection, emotional commitment, reliability and consistency provide guidance and limit setting; and indices of adjustment are amongst the most extensive and reliable in developmental psychology. Finally, maltreated children who have a close reciprocal friendship or a network of friends are more likely to show resilience (Bolger and Patterson, 2003).

CASE STUDY 8.4.3 PARENTAL POSTNATAL DEPRESSION

Infants require warm and contingent social interaction with adult caregivers for healthy socio-emotional and cognitive development. The quality of a parent's interaction with their infant is profoundly affected by his or her own mental and physical health. Postpartum depression affects both mothers and fathers: it is estimated that 10–15% of new mothers experience postpartum depression, and around 10% of fathers become depressed in the perinatal period (Paulson and Bazemore, 2010). However, historically, maternal depression is more commonly studied. A depressed mother becomes anxious, irritated and fatigued; and may be withdrawn and insensitive (Murray, 2009). Depression particularly affects mother–infant responsiveness and quality of caregiving. A depressed mother tends to interact less with her infant and to be less tuned to her infant's social cues. Typical mothers speak to their infants using a prosodically enhanced register, infant-directed speech, that helps to engage the infant and regulate the infants' emotional state. Depressed mothers make less use of infant-directed speech, instead speaking with a flattened affect that is associated with the emotion of sadness.

This depressed pattern of interaction can profoundly affect infants' emotional development: babies vocalise less, display more negative emotion and show atypical neural processing of emotion (e.g. Dawson, 1992). Infants of mothers with postnatal depression are themselves at an increased risk for developing depression and other types of psychopathology (Murray, 2009), as well as later cognitive and language difficulties. However, much remains unknown about how early adverse social experiences become biologically embedded in the developing brain. According to one hypothesis, a depressed mother's lower maternal sensitivity elevates levels of stress in her infant. This chronically activates the infant's HPA axis, which overproduces stress hormones (glucocorticoids) that cause neuronal atrophy in key structures that subserve learning and emotional regulation, such as the hippocampus and amygdala.

(2) **Biological resilience factors**. In the last few decades, significant progress has been made in understanding the biological and genetic basis of psychological resilience. Variations in the expression of 'vulnerability genes' can modulate whether early stressors will lead to subsequent problems in stress hormone regulation and behavioural difficulties. A series of landmark studies by Caspi and colleagues (e.g. Caspi et al., 2003) highlighted several susceptibility genes that moderate an individual's vulnerability to developing antisocial behaviour (monoamine oxidase A, *MAO-A*), depression (serotonin transporter, *5-HTT*) and schizophrenia (catechol-O-methyltransferase, *COMT*) following adverse life events. However, mixed results have emerged following attempts to replicate some of these findings. A polymorphism of the brain-derived neurotrophic factor (*BDNF*) gene, Val66Met, is also associated with the development of depression in response to environmental adversity and stress (Gatt et al., 2009). Moreover, there may be epistatic interactions – where the effect of one gene on phenotype is dependent on another gene – that additionally regulate susceptibility genes (Pezawas et al., 2005).

8.4.3 Interventions to Rescue Stress-Induced Neuroplasticity

8.4.3.1 Exercise

In animal models, aerobic exercise seems to stimulate a cascade of neuroplastic mechanisms within the hippocampus that are associated with improved performance in tasks involving spatial or contextual memory. However, in humans, the evidence for the impact of exercise on cognition has been inconsistent – although several meta-analyses have found a tendency toward improvements in memory-based task performance, particularly in older age groups. Rodent studies have found that aerobic exercise increases the rate of hippocampal neurogenesis in the brain (e.g. van Praag et al., 2005). Exercise is also thought to enhance synaptic plasticity by stimulating long-term potentiation in young rodents and reversing age-related long-term potentiation decline in aged rodents (van Praag et al., 1999). Finally, neurotrophins such as BDNF are thought to play an important role mediating the effect of exercise on hippocampal neuroplasticity. In animal models, aerobic exercise is associated with an upregulation of hippocampal BDNF (Neeper et al., 1995), which is in turn correlated with improved memory performance. The therapeutic potential of aerobic exercise for treatment of psychiatric disorders has only recently begun to be explored and has mainly focused on the treatment of major depressive disorder or schizophrenia. Early results have been promising in terms of reducing affective symptomatology, although neural effects have been mixed. Some studies involving exercise interventions on patients with schizophrenia have reported increased hippocampal volume and improved memory performance (e.g. Pajonk et al., 2010), whereas other studies have found no impact (e.g. Rosenbaum et al., 2015). One possible direction for future research would be to investigate whether aerobic exercise may be included as a complementary treatment to the traditional pharmacological approach.

8.4.3.2 Mindfulness Meditation Training

Mindfulness describes a form of meditation that cultivates a non-judgemental awareness of the present moment. There has been increasing interest in the ways in which mindfulness might aid recovery from, or reduce susceptibility to illness, such as by reducing reactivity to stress. For example, Tang et al. (2007) reported that Chinese undergraduates who were randomly assigned to perform 5 days of an integrative body–mind training method (including aspects of mindfulness training) showed lower salivary cortisol and higher salivary immunoglobulin A concentrations in response to a stressful mental arithmetic challenge, compared with a control group who received relaxation training. Creswell et al. (2014) conducted a randomised control trial in which 66 adult participants were either given a brief 3-day mindfulness meditation training or a cognitive training control programme. Participants who received mindfulness training reported lower psychological stress reactivity to the Trier Social Stress Test, although their salivary cortisol reactivity was higher relative to the cognitive training control group. Recent brain-imaging studies have also found that mindfulness training is associated with lower amygdala activation in response to emotional stimuli and reduced functional connectivity between the right amygdala and subgenual anterior cingulate cortex in a community sample of stressed adults (e.g. Taren et al., 2015). There is also preliminary evidence that mindfulness meditation may interact with immune function. Davidson et al. (2003) found that adult employees who took part in a workplace mindfulness-based stress reduction programme showed increased left anterior EEG activation (a pattern associated with positive affect) as well as a more robust immune response to influenza vaccination compared to the control group. Further, the magnitude of participants' antibody titre rise was positively related to their change in neural activation. Greater increase in antibody titers to influenza vaccine and the magnitude of the EEG change predicted the magnitude of antibody response. Thus, mindfulness training may be effective in regulating the neural, endocrine and immune responses to psychosocial stress.

Conclusions and Outstanding Questions

The chapter highlights the extraordinary capacity for neuroplasticity in the developing central nervous system. Such neuroplasticity depends on a number of factors (e.g. sensory input, gonadal hormones, stress) and manifests across the lifespan in waves during so-called critical or sensitive periods, to dynamically regulate and constrain synaptic connections in primary sensory and association cortices. Genetic and environmental factors influence, respectively, the timing and strength of synaptic connections and underlie the phenotypic expression of cognitive abilities (e.g. language acquisition), vulnerability versus resilience to stress, and various neurodevelopmental disorders such as autism and schizophrenia.

Outstanding Questions

- How in precise terms do neuronal and molecular mechanisms determine the opening and closure of so-called sensitive periods of brain development?

- What scope exists for experimental interventions to reverse neuroplasticity associated with adverse environmental exposures in infants and young children (e.g. maltreatment, deprivation, maternal depression)?

- How is the balance between stress resilience and vulnerability moulded by neuroplasticity mechanisms?

REFERENCES

Barr CS, Newman TK, Shannon C et al. (2004). Rearing condition and rh5-HTTLPR interact to influence limbic hypothalamic–pituitary–adrenal axis response to stress in infant macaques. *Biological Psychiatry* 55: 733–738.

Ben-Ari Y (2017). NKCCl chloride importer antagonists attenuate many neurological and psychiatric disorders. *Trends in Neuroscience* 40, 536–554.

Bock J, Gruss M, Becker S, Braun K (2005). Experience-induced changes of dendritic spine densities in the prefrontal and sensory cortex: correlation with developmental time windows. *Cerebral Cortex* 15, 802–808.

Bolger KE, Patterson CJ (2003). Sequelae of child maltreatment: vulnerability and resilience. In Luthar SS (ed.), *Resilience and Vulnerability: Adaptation in the Context of Childhood Adversities.*Cambridge University Press, pp. 156–181.

Burke AR, McCormick CM, Pellis SM, Lukkes JL (2017). Impact of adolescent social experiences on behavior and neural circuits implicated in mental illness. *Neuroscience and Biobehavioural Reviews* 76: 280–300.

Caspi A, Sugden K, Moffitt TE et al. (2003). Influence of life stress on depression: moderation by a polymorphism in a *5-HTT* gene. *Science* 301: 386–389.

Cicchetti D, Rogosch F, Lynch M, Holt K (1993). Resilience in maltreated children: processes leading to adaptive outcome. *Development and Psychopathology* 5: 629–647.

Creswell JD, Pacilio LE, Lindsay EK, Brown KW (2014). Brief mindfulness meditation training alters psychological and neuroendocrine responses to social evaluative stress. *Psychoneuroendocrinology* 44: 1–12.

Davidson RJ, Kabat-Zinn J, Schumacher J et al. (2003). Alterations in brain and immune function produced by mindfulness meditation. *Psychosomatic Medicine* 65(4): 564–570.

Dawson G, Frey K, Panagitotides H et al. (1992). Infants of depressed mothers exhibit atypical frontal electrical brain activity during interactions with mother and with a familiar, non-depressed adult. *Child Development* 70(5): 1058–1066.

de Kloet ER, Joëls M, Holsboer F (2005). Stress and the brain: from adaptation to disease. *Nature Reviews Neuroscience* 6: 463–475.

Einon DF, Morgan MJ (1977). A critical period for social isolation in the rat. *Developmental Psychology* 10: 123–132.

Estes ML., McAllister AK (2016). Maternal immune activation: implications for neuropsychiatric disorders. *Science* 353: 772–777.

Farah MJ, Shera DM, Savage JH (2006). Childhood poverty: specific associations with neurocognitive development. *Brain Research* 1110: 166–174.

Fernandez A, Dumon C, Guimond D (2019). The GABA developmental shift is abolished by maternal immune activation already at birth. *Cerebral Cortex* 29: 3982–3992.

Gatt JM, Nemeroff CB, Dobson-Stone C (2009). Interactions between *BDNF* Val66Met polymorphism and early life stress predict brain and arousal pathways to syndromal depression and anxiety. *Molecular Psychiatry* 14: 681–695.

Gillies GE, Virdee K, McArthur S, Dalley JW (2014) Sex-dependent diversity in ventral tegmental dopaminergic neurons and developmental programming: a molecular, cellular and behavioral analysis. *Neuroscience* 12: 69–85.

Hanson JL, Chandra A, Wolfe BL, Pollak SD (2011). Association between income and the hippocampus. *PLoS One* 6: e18712.

Hanson JL, Hair N, Shen DG et al. (2013). Family poverty affects the rate of human infant brain growth. *PLoS One* 8(12): e80954.

Hensch TK (2005). Cortical period plasticity in local cortical circuits. *Nature Reviews Neuroscience* 6: 877–888.

8

Hensch TK, Fagiolini M, Mataga N et al. (1998). Local GABA circuit control of experience-dependent plasticity in developing visual cortex. *Science* 282(5393): 1504–1508.

Kuhl PK, Williams KA, Lacerda F, Stevens KN, Lindblom B (1992). Linguistic experience alters phonetic perception in infants by 6 months of age. *Science* 255: 606–608.

Levine S, Haltmeyer GC, Karas GC, Denenberg VH (1967). Physiological and behavioural effects of infantile stimulation. *Physiology and Behaviour* 2: 55–59.

Luby J, Belden A, Botteron K et al. (2013). The effects of poverty on childhood brain development: the mediating effect of caregiving and stressful life events. *JAMA Pediatrics* 167: 1135–1142.

Matthews K, Wilkinson LS, Robbins TW (1996). Repeated maternal separation of preweanling rats attenuates behavioural responses to primary and conditioned incentives in adulthood. *Physiology and Behaviour* 59: 99–107.

McCarthy MA, Arnold AP (2011). Reframing sexual differentiation of the brain. *Nature Neuroscience* 14: 677–683.

Murray L (2009). The development of children of postnatally depressed mothers: evidence from the Cambridge longitudinal study. *Psychoanalytic Psychotherapy* 23: 185–199.

Nelson CA, Zeanah CH, Fox NA et al. (2007). Cognitive recovery in socially deprived young children: the Bucharest early intervention project. *Science* 318(5858): 1937–1940.

Neeper SA, Gómez-Pinilla F, Choi J, Cotman C (1995). Exercise and brain neurotrophins. *Nature* 373: 109.

Noble KG, McCandliss BD, Farah MJ (2007). Socioeconomic gradients predict individual differences in neurocognitive abilities. *Developmental Science* 10: 464–480.

Pajonk F-G, Wobrock T, Gruber O et al. (2010). Hippocampal plasticity in response to exercise in schizophrenia. *Archives of General Psychiatry* 67: 133–143.

Paulson JF, Bazemore SD (2010). Prenatal and postpartum depression in fathers and its association with maternal depression: a meta-analysis. *JAMA* 303(19): 1961–1969.

Pezawas L, Meyer-Lindenberg A, Drabant EM (2005). *5-HTTLPR* polymorphism impacts human cingulate–amygdala interactions: a genetic susceptibility mechanism for depression. *Nature Neuroscience* 8: 828–834.

Radley JJ, Sisti HM, Hao J et al. (2004). Chronic behavioral stress induces apical dendritic reorganization in pyramidal neurons of the medial prefrontal cortex. *Neuroscience* 125: 1–6.

Rosenbaum S, Lagopoulos J, Curtis J et al. (2015). Aerobic exercise intervention in young people with schizophrenia spectrum disorders; improved fitness with no change in hippocampal volume. *Psychiatry Research: Neuroimaging* 232: 200–201.

Shonkoff J, Phillips D (eds) (2000). *From Neurons to Neighborhoods: The Science of Early Childhood Development*. National Academies Press.

Tang G, Gudsnuk K, Kuo SH et al. (2014). Loss of mTOR-dependent macroautophagy causes autistic-like synaptic pruning deficits. *Neuron* 83(5): 1131–1143.

Tang YY, Ma Y, Wang J et al. (2007). Short-term meditation training improves attention and self-regulation. *Proceedings of the National Academy of Sciences of the United States of America* 104(43): 17152–17156.

Taren AA, Gianaros PJ, Greco CM (2015). Mindfulness meditation training alters stress-related amygdala resting state functional connectivity: a randomized controlled trial. *Social Cognitive and Affective Neuroscience* 10(12): 1758–1768.

Teicher MH, Samson JA, Polcari A, McGreenery CE (2006). Sticks, stones, and hurtful words: relative effects of various forms of childhood maltreatment. *American Journal of Psychiatry* 163, 993–1000.

van Praag H, Christie BR, Sejnowski TJ, Gage FH (1999). Running enhances neurogenesis, learning, and long-term potentiation in mice. *Proceedings of the National Academy of Sciences of the United States of America* 96: 13427–13431.

van Praag H, Shubert T, Zhao C, Gage FH (2005). Exercise enhances learning and hippocampal neurogenesis in aged mice. *Journal of Neuroscience* 25: 8680–8685.

Virdee K, McArthur S, Brischoux F, Caprioli et al. (2014). Antenatal glucocorticoid treatment induces adaptations in adult midbrain dopamine neurons, which underpin sexually dimorphic behavioural resilience. *Neuropsychopharmacology* 39: 339–350.

Walsh WA, Dawson J, Mattingly MJ (2010). How are we measuring resilience following childhood maltreatment? Is the research adequate and consistent? What is the impact on research, practice, and policy? *Trauma, Violence, & Abuse* 11: 27–41.

Werker JF, Tees RC (1984). Cross-language speech perception: evidence for perceptual reorganization during the first year of life. *Infant Behavior & Development* 7: 49–63.

Zhang TY, Parent C, Weaver IAN, Meaney MJ (2004). Maternal programming of individual differences in defensive responses in the rat. *Annals of the New York Academy of Sciences* 1032: 85–103.

8

National Neuroscience Curriculum Initiative online resources

The Nature of Nurture: How Developmental Experiences Program Adult Stress Circuitry

Jennifer B. Dwyer and David A. Ross

Beyond Bootstraps: Pulling Children Up With Evidence-Based Interventions

Anya K. Bershad and David A. Ross

Poverty, Parenting, and Psychiatry

Kunmi Sobowale and David A. Ross

This "stuff" is really cool: Jenny Dwyer, *"Sad Synapses" on the synaptic effects of chronic stress*

Expert video: *Stacy Drury on Genetics, Neurodevelopment & Child Psychiatry*

Expert video: *Brian Dias on Intergenerational Trauma*

<table>
<tr><td>**8.5**</td><td>**Intelligence and Intellectual Disability**</td><td>Shahid H. Zaman</td></tr>
</table>

OVERVIEW

This chapter discusses the concept of intelligence from a neurodevelopmental and evolutionary perspective. I also discuss how measuring intelligence has helped us to refine the definition of intellectual disability, and how understanding intelligence has shed light on the nature of the mind and its relationship to cognition and behavioural disturbances as well as mental illness.

8.5.1 Defining Intelligence

There is some degree of controversy and debate about the definition of intelligence as definitions do vary. However, it can be defined as a '**general mental ability**'. The definition proposed by the American Psychological Association (see Neisser et al., 1996) is:

> Individuals differ from one another in their ability to understand complex ideas, to adapt effectively to the environment, to learn from experience, to engage in various forms of reasoning, to overcome obstacles by taking thought. Although these individual differences can be substantial, they are never entirely consistent: a given person's intellectual performance will vary on different occasions, in different domains, as judged by different criteria. Concepts of 'intelligence' are attempts to clarify and organize this complex set of phenomena.

Intelligence has enabled effective adaptation to the challenges presented by the environment and granted a huge survival advantage for our species. It is the ability to learn from experience and apply that learning to novel situations. Intelligence is not the ability to rote learn but to work out patterns to make sense of sensory information with little use of acquired knowledge or experience. For intelligence to understand ideas, learn, abstract, plan *and* solve problems, it needs to call on a number of cognitive processes, such as the ability to concentrate, reason, perceive, lay down memories and

Table 8.5.1 Types of adaptive behaviour

- **Practical skills** Activities of daily living (personal care); occupational skills; use of money; safety; health care; travel/transportation; schedules/routines; use of the telephone
- **Conceptual skills** Language; reading and writing; money, time and number concepts
- **Social skills** Interpersonal skills; social responsibility; self-esteem; gullibility; naïveté (i.e. wariness); follows rules/obeys laws; avoids being victimised; social problem solving

From Tassé et al. (2012).

to manipulate stored data, retrieve it and use it in the correct combination or order.

The expression of the degree of intelligence and the range of ability will be influenced by the person's developmental trajectory, that is determined by genetic inheritance, general physical health, the degree of adaptive skills (see Table 8.5.1) and on the psychological, social, educational and cultural environment experienced by the person (AAIDD, 2010).

8.5.2 Measures of Intelligence: The Invention and Discovery of IQ

The notion of measuring cognitive differences between individuals is a key approach of differential psychology, the aim of which is to quantify the phenotype, to understand its impact on individuals and to understand the underlying biological basis of the difference. The intellectual quotient (IQ) is often thought as the de facto measure of intelligence. It is the psychometric method for measuring intelligence which is a measure of *differences* between individuals; it reflects the range of ability in a population and is based on a statistical notion of correlation and covariance of tests of cognitive abilities (such as memory, attention, processing speed, reasoning, spatial perception, pattern recognition and vocabulary) between groups. Although evidence from brain lesion studies supports the relative independence of cognitive domains, differential psychology has shown that there is an overriding factor called '**general intelligence**' or '**g-factor**' (and IQ is one measure of it) that determines how well a person performs in all the subdomains of cognitive tests. So, the corollary of this is that if you score well say in a working memory task then your scores in other unrelated cognitive tests are also likely to be high and therefore your IQ score would also be high. However, tests of cognition in certain domains correlate much better with IQ than do others. Importantly, g is a well-established **psychometric construct** rather than a psychological one and assumes that if there is interrelatedness (as evaluated by a statistical method of factor analysis – see below) amongst results of tests then that is due to a latent variable (that is, an unobserved underlying explanatory variable, in this case 'g', that can be inferred from observed variables).

IQ tests were originally developed as a way of evaluating the academic abilities and needs of school children in France (**Alfred Binet** with **Théodore Simon**). Binet was tasked with developing tests that could be used to identify those children in primary education who were struggling academically. The tests evaluated included, for example, attention, memory and problem solving. The tests Binet devised allowed teachers to give the identified children further support, while also identifying those more able children who needed greater challenges. Binet was able to test enough children to develop a scale which produced normative scores from the statistical distribution of the test results, corrected for chronological age to produce a 'mental age' as the measure of IQ. The mental age was the expected test score when compared with the average score of a group of children aged the same age. So, if the child was able to answer well on questions normally expected of an older child, then that child's mental age would be higher than his or her peers. In Germany, **William Stern** simplified this to a ratio of mental age to chronological age and the intelligence

quotient was born. However, the concept of mental age is less reliable in adults, especially at the lower end of intellectual functioning.

The Binet test was further developed by **Lewis Terman** at Stanford so that it could be used in adults; it became the **Stanford–Binet Test** and it produced a number which became known as the IQ, which was Stern's ratio multiplied by 100. Importantly, a tested IQ score should be viewed as a likelihood score with a confidence interval and not as a single score number. This becomes especially important where interpretations of assessments of the degree of intellectual impairment based on tests determine which clinical or social services a person is eligible for.

Charles Spearman analysed the data from the Stanford–Binet test and discovered that individual cognitive tests were highly positively correlated with each other. For example, if you scored high in one modality, you were likely to score high in another one. Using factor analysis (a statistical measure of the degree of correlation between a set of parameters) he modelled cognition as having a g-factor and a **specific** or '**s-factor**'. He proposed a **hierarchical model of cognition** where the g-factor was a general cognitive ability or the driver or main determinant of the s-factor, and applicable to any cognitive task. Spearman's analysis has been replicated in many subsequent data sets supporting a hierarchical structure of cognitive ability, and he proposed that the g-factor is a mental function entity ('**mental energy**') with an underlying biological substrate. Much of the subsequent neurobiological research in intelligence has employed the g-factor (such as that measured by IQ tests) to provide evidence of biological links. There is less support for proponents of the theory that individual cognitive domains are essentially independent.

Alternative interpretations of the data have also been put forward. Instead of viewing the g-factor as mental energy, **Godfrey Thompson** proposed that there were multiple functional units in the brain, which when they cooperated with one another through 'bonds' also explained the correlations. This theory predicts that intelligence is a function of the efficiency or number of connections. Data available to date cannot distinguish between Spearman's and Thompson's models.

A proposal by **Thurston** interpreted the analysis of psychometric data supporting the case for individual '**primary mental abilities**' and not g-factor. These mental abilities were: verbal ability, perceptual speed, inductive reasoning, numerical ability, memory, deductive reasoning, word fluency and spatial visualisation.

Cattell and **Horn** developed the work of Spearman and Thurston and introduced the concept of '**fluid**' and '**crystallised**' **intelligence**, where the former corresponds with the g-factor and the latter with stored or acquired knowledge. With age and experience, and as the store of knowledge grows, crystallised intelligence increases and plateaus, but fluid intelligence weakens. **Carroll** further expanded the model and categorised fluid intelligence, crystallised intelligence, general memory/learning, visual perception, auditory perception, retrieval ability, cognitive speediness, processing and decision speed as belonging to **second-order cognition** or '**stratum II**', above which there is **stratum III** (which is g) or **third-order cognition**. **Stratum I** contains the individual cognitive tasks for which there are specific psychometric tests.

Similar to the Stanford–Binet test, **David Wechsler** developed the **Weschler Adult Intelligence Scale** (WAIS) test for adults and children. The WAIS and its successors are well validated, are the most consistent tests of IQ, and are widely used by clinical and other practitioner psychologists (see Figure 8.5.1). The WAIS test has subtests assessing: verbal ability (language), perceptual reasoning, working memory and processing speed, and from this the full-scale IQ is derived. The g-score is derived from a subset of the tests. The score achieved is **compared with** that expected (i.e. it is a measure of difference) in those of the same age, and it is assumed to have a Gaussian distribution with parameters set at a mean of 100 with a standard deviation of 15 and a range of 85 to 115 for 68% of the population. When IQ is measured in populations, it does indeed follow a normal distribution except at the lower IQ end where it is represented by conditions seen in people with intellectual disability. Measures of IQ tend to **remain stable** throughout a healthy life, but early in development IQ tests show a **greater variability** which could reflect the ongoing changing and evolving biological features of the brain and may be one reason why IQ tests are unreliable at the more severe end of intellectual impairment. A higher IQ during early life correlates with favourable socioeconomic and health outcomes.

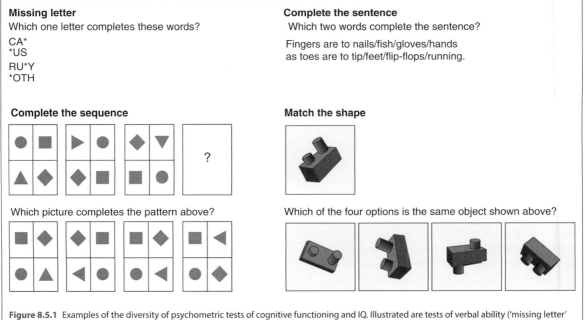

Figure 8.5.1 Examples of the diversity of psychometric tests of cognitive functioning and IQ. Illustrated are tests of verbal ability ('missing letter' and 'complete the sentence'), abstract non-verbal reasoning ('complete the sequence', a good measure of fluid intelligence) and visual spatial processing ('match the shape'). Adding a timing element to these tests provides a measure of processing speed (Reproduced from Plomin and von Stumm, 2018).

8.5.3 An Evolutionary Perspective on Intelligence

An evolutionary approach to understanding intelligence throws light on brain design and possible mechanisms (see O'Reilly and Carr, 2016 for a more detailed discussion). By studying the cognitive abilities of our common ancestors, we can begin to map the path, the genetic determinants and the design constraints that evolution imparted on cognitive structure, mechanism and function. From our ancestral precursors we learn of the **impact of bi-pedalism**, the **increase in the size of cranium**, the transformation from a life of hunting to agricultural tool making and usage, the necessity of social functioning, migration epochs and the development from a basic language to **symbolic representation**. Such changes suggest staged step-by-step elaborations in cognitive abilities where subsequent developments or features are influenced and restrained by previous ones. For example, the phase of evolution when there was an increase in the size of the cranium (but not in body size) and the emergence of right-handed dominance suggested brain structural development favouring **lateralisation of some functions**. About 2 million years ago, when the *Homo erectus* cranium underwent a further size increase, there is evidence that our ancestors began to engage in **prolonged periods of childhood nurturing**, suggesting a necessity for a prolonged period of postnatal development and child rearing, which made the impact of the child's environment very significant for brain development. *Homo neaderthalis* had larger craniums, they were advanced in hunting techniques, social behaviour and tool making, and they buried their dead, the significance of which is unknown. Importantly, the emergence of verbal language allowed concrete and abstract symbolic representations. So, there is a **selection pressure for technological, social and linguistic intelligence.** This helps explain the many cognitive abilities and behaviour recognised in *Homo sapiens*. There is genetic and other evidence of **cross breeding** with *Homo neaderthalis* and with other subspecies of archaic humans, such as the Denisovans after the migration from Africa, which had an impact on the evolved cognitive structures and behaviour in *Homo sapiens*. The elucidation of the genomes of our ancestors is helping us to establish the gene(s) involved in important aspects of cognitive evolutionary design on our species.

8.5.4 The Evolutionary Perspective and Models of Cognition

By scrutinising the behaviour of chimpanzees and other non-human primates and comparing the inferred cognitive abilities of our ancestors from archaeological and other evidence, models of intelligence and cognition have been proposed. For example, Donald (1993) suggests the evolution from ape to human required the trajectory of three phases or transitions, which have culminated in the emergence of our modern-day abilities, and that our species is best understood if we include **biological (anatomical) adaptations** as well as 'external' or **technological** ones. The biological ones include the emergence of 'mimetic' skills followed by language. Mimetic culture refers to the ability of hominids to use the whole body as a **communication and representational device**. It allowed the translation of event perceptions into action. Hominid body movements are voluntarily accessible for replay (such as playing a rhythm with a stick). Pre-dating the mimetic culture, Donald notes that modern apes and Australopithecines have an '**episodic culture**'. Modern ape culture is an episodic culture as apes live in the moment and the memory of the event is not elaborated beyond a happening in the episode. Their lives are a series of concrete events, **lacking semantic representation and so the ability to reflect on store of information or knowledge**. The emergence of language enriched representational ability and like mimesis is essentially a tool of the mind to model reality. From the use of language developed the **culture of storytelling, exchange of information and social interaction**. Donald puts forward a third transition, which is the 'technological transition', in which he proposes that the modern brain has learned to utilise **external stores of information**, representing a changing role of biological memory.

8.5.5 The Neurobiology of Intelligence: Genetics, Molecules, Cells and Networks

There have been many studies (using for example monozygotic and dizygotic twins) that show the influence of genes versus environment on intelligence to be 50% to 80%. Although general intelligence has been shown to be highly heritabile, it is polygenic, with numerous alleles having small effects, and environmental factors (such as socioeconomic status) play an important role in the expression or phenotypic manifestation of genes. Most of the genetic variance can be accounted for by the gene regulatory **non-coding intronic or intergenic regions of DNA**. These regions can control the expression of genes and are responsive to synaptic activity and plasticity and to the environment. The remaining 1.4% of associations are from exonic (protein-coding) regions: the 105 implicated genes tend to encode components of neurogenesis, neuronal differentiation, synaptic function, growth factors and bioenergetics. Therefore, the majority of variation in intelligence is not explained by alterations in protein sequence, structure or conformation. The majority of genes implicated are active during brain development (neuronal proliferation, neuronal migration, synaptogenesis, apoptosis and myelination) *in utero* and postnatally, and many of these continue to have roles in synaptic functioning and plasticity.

Macroscopic measures provided by structural MRI have been shown to correlate with intelligence. For example, **bigger brain volume**, **thicker cortex** (grey matter) especially in certain regions (frontal, parietal and temporal lobes) and the integrity of **associational white matter tracts** (axonal) positively correlate with higher intelligence. One study showed correlation of white matter integrity of the fibres between the frontal and temporal lobes in people with intellectual disabilities. By analysing the blood-oxygen-level-dependent signal of brain regions using functional MRI (fMRI), populations of active neurons are considered connected when other regions or 'nodes' are simultaneously active. This provides evidence for the existence of **interconnected brain areas forming networks** that are associated with particular cognitive functions. Measures of the efficiency derived from interconnectedness of fMRI networks and studies measuring brain glucose utilisation during a task (event-related) or at rest have provided support for the hypothesis of **'neuronal efficiency'** of intelligence. This hypothesis proposes that the brain works more efficiently in individuals that are more intelligent. For example, for a given cognitive task, an intelligent person's cortex would be activated less (by using less energy) than the cortex of one with a lower intelligence. Some but not all aspects of prefrontal cortical executive functions are necessary for intelligence (Duncan, 2005; Roca et al., 2010) as other regions of the brain are needed. The **parieto-frontal**

integration hypothesis (Jung and Haier, 2007) proposes that several specific brain regions interact with each other where they hold information (working memory), abstract and select responses for an output. When lesion-mapping studies were undertaken in adults, the following significant correlations were seen: left frontal cortex with verbal comprehension, parietal cortex with working memory and the right parietal cortex with perceptual organisation (Gläscher et al., 2009).

Although we know which brain regions are involved in intelligence, we also need to know which cell types are involved. Genome-wide association studies (GWAS) show that the same regions as those suggested by neuroimaging studies (e.g. the frontal cortex) are indeed involved in intelligence, and that astrocytes and oligodendrocytes are not, but that **pyramidal cells** (the most abundant neurons in the neocortex and hippocampus) and **medium spiny neurons** of the striatum are (Coleman et al., 2019). In 2018, Goriounova and colleagues (see Figure 8.5.2) showed in humans (from a sample who were undergoing surgery) that a higher IQ was associated with a thicker cortex, **larger dendrites** and faster action potentials, as measured in the temporal cortex, which may explain the faster processing speeds associated with intelligence. Larger dendritic compartments and longer neurites lead to the ability of these spaces to function relatively independently and so improve computational ability.

8.5.6 Defining Intellectual Disability: Its Uses and Limitations

When there is impaired cognition, it can lead to lower intellectual ability that can have an impact on the ability to function from day to day ('**adaptive functioning**'– see Table 8.5.1). If the time of the onset of the cognitive deficit occurs during the **early developmental period** *and* if it also impacts adaptive functioning, it can result in an intellectual disability (Table 8.5.2). Intellectual disability is not a unitary condition. People with intellectual disability are a **heterogeneous group** of people due to the very **large range of aetiologies** that can result in variable degrees of severity and ranges of impairment. The definition of intellectual disability is based on the World Health Organization notion of malfunctioning as a consequence of abnormal **underlying biology leading to disability**, which in turn can become a **handicap** if environmental or nurturing factors are unfavourable. Examples of causative

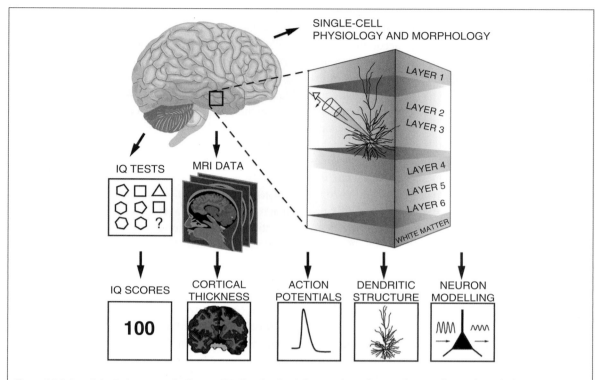

Figure 8.5.2 A study by Goriounova and colleagues (2018) undertaken in humans shows the area of temporal cortex from which tissue sample was obtained for *in vitro* brain-slice electrophysiological analysis of superficial layer pyramidal cells. The patients had undergone an IQ test using the WAIS test and cortical thickness was measured using MRI. By infusing biocytin dye using a glass microelectrode attached onto a single pyramidal cell, the morphology of dendrites and the rest of the neuronal processes were ascertained as well as electrophysiological parameters such as action potentials. Reproduced under a CC BY 4.0 licence.

Table 8.5.2 Clinical criteria of intellectual disabillity

- IQ below 70 (less than two standard deviations)
- Poor adaptive skills
- Cause of neurodevelopmental delay to have started during childhood (under age of 18 years)

From the British Psychological Society Division of Clinical Psychology (2015).

agents or adverse events include genetic, congenital, environmental, infectious, traumatic or exposure to toxins impacting the normal brain developmental trajectory during the earliest (and most sensitive) period of neurodevelopment (which is under 18 years, but especially *in utero* or during the early postnatal developmental period). The impact on brain functioning needs to have produced a tested IQ score of 70 or under (more than two standard deviations below the mean of the general population; mean = 100 and one standard deviation = 15). When there is an acute reduction in intelligence during adulthood (i.e.

when brain development is mostly complete), caused by an insult to the brain, for example from traumatic brain injury, this would not be termed intellectual disability. The treatment or the management of psychiatric disorders or mental illness related to intellectual disability needs to be specific to the cause of the disability (if known) or, if interventions designed to change behaviour psychologically or behaviourally (a functional approach) are being considered, adaptations need to be made such that the interventions take into account the specific mechanisms being hypothesised as 'causing' or explaining the behavioural phenotype. For example, the Prader–Willi syndrome behavioural phenotype includes the propensity to eat uncontrollably. However, this is unlike, say, an obsessive–compulsive disorder behaviour, or a behaviour due to sensory integration deficits that manifest in autism, affecting for example touch, olfaction or taste. All of these mechanisms may produce similar behaviour.

8.5.7 The Genetics, Syndromes, Behavioural Phenotypes and Behavioural Problems in Intellectual Disability

There are many (but individually rare) cases of genetically determined intellectual disability in the general population including those due to chromosomal abnormalities (aneuploidies), monogenic X-linked mutations, point mutations, copy number variants, and deletions and/or duplications of parts of the genome that have been identified as causing **intellectual disability syndromes**. Examples include Down syndrome, fragile X syndrome, phenylketonuria, Rett syndrome and Prader–Willi syndrome. The genes involved in these conditions overlap with those associated with intelligence and brain development.

Certain characteristic types of behaviour and cognitive profiles occur more commonly than expected in certain genetic syndromes associated with ID. These include autistic behaviours, anxiety traits, attention deficits and deficits in specific cognitive abilities or language function. Therefore, a person with a given syndrome may have greater strengths in some cognitive domains than in others. Studying such syndromes provides valuable insights for understanding of brain and behaviour and the mechanisms of gene action and the relationship to IQ. Much of the research has focused on the commoner syndromes such as Down syndrome, fragile X syndrome, Williams syndrome, Turner syndrome, velocardiofacial syndrome (22q11.2 deletion or DiGeorge syndrome) and Prader–Willi syndrome.

The prevalence of problem (or 'challenging') behaviour is much greater in people with intellectual disability than in the general population. There are several reasons hypothesised for this, including a poor understanding of expectations of social norms of behaviour, a poorly developed theory of mind, a less-well-developed executive functioning, greater difficulty in regulating emotions, poor self-image due to adverse early experiences, discrimination and fewer opportunities for development and learning. Mental illness is also more common for similar reasons and because of genetic and neurodevelopmental factors.

Conclusions and Outstanding Questions

Mental ability results in intelligence, which is a fundamental property of mind, and tested IQ is one useful but an incomplete measure of it. IQ measured early in life predicts a person's future outcomes, so a higher IQ correlates with favourable socioeconomic and health outcomes. The analysis of psychometric measures (tests of attention, speed of processing, memory, visual perception, etc.) has led to hierarchical models of the structure of intelligence. The neurobiology of intelligence is complex and the range of intellectual abilities can be explained by the variation in the efficiency with which nerve signals compute information and that depends on the efficiency of synapses, dendrites and axons (white matter) and the robustness of the networks formed from these elements. The emergence of intelligence has been a major advantage for our species, and understanding the evolutionary history gives clues about the design of our brains. The period during which brain development is the most sensitive is that in which insults result in impaired intellectual ability.

Outstanding Questions

- How is the brain able to learn from the specific, extracting abstractions or patterns and applying these to novel situations, that is, from the specific to the general?

- What components are needed to explain the biological nature of the g-factor at the molecular, cellular and network or systems levels?

- What can the study of intelligence learn from artificial intelligence and vice versa?

- How does intelligence emerge during development and what is its relation to the developing brain?

- Can we treat or ameliorate the effects of developmental intellectual impairment?

REFERENCES

American Association on Intellectual and Developmental Disabilities (AAIDD) (2010). *Intellectual Disability: Definition, Classification, and Systems of Supports*, 11th ed. AAIDD.

British Psychological Society Division of Clinical Psychology (2015). *Guidance on the Assessment and Diagnosis of Intellectual Disabilities in Adulthood*. The British Psychological Society.

Coleman JRI, Bryois J, Gaspar HA et al. (2019) Biological annotation of genetic loci associated with intelligence in a meta-analysis of 87,740 individuals. *Mol Psychiatry* 24(2): 182–197.

Donald, N (1993). Précis of origins of the modern mind: Three stages in the evolution of culture and cognition. *Behav Brain Sci* 16(4): 737–748.

Duncan J (2005). Frontal lobe function and general intelligence: why it matters. *Cortex* 41(2): 215–217.

Gläscher J, Tranel D, Paul LK et al. (2009) Lesion mapping of cognitive abilities linked to intelligence. *Neuron* 61(5): 681–691.

Goriounova NA, Heyer DB, Wilbers R et al. (2018). Large and fast human pyramidal neurons associate with intelligence. *elife*: e41714.

Jung RE, Haier RJ (2007). The parieto-frontal integration theory (P-FIT) of intelligence: converging neuroimaging evidence. *Behav Brain Sci* 30(2):135–154.

Neisser U, Boodoo G, Bouchard TJ, Jr et al. (1996) Intelligence: knowns and unknowns. *Am Psychol* 51: 77–101.

O'Reilly G, Carr A (2016). Intelligence. In Carr A, Linehan C, O'Reilly G, Noonan Walsh P, McEvoy J (eds.) *Handbook of Intellectual Disability and Clinical Psychology Practice*, 2nd ed. Routledge, pp. 81–106.

Plomin R, von Stumm S (2018). The new genetics of intelligence. *Nat Rev Genet* 19(3): 148–159.

Roca M, Parr A, Thompson R et al. (2010). Executive function and fluid intelligence after frontal lobe lesions. *Brain* 133(Pt 1): 234–247.

Tassé MJ, Schalock RL, Balboni G et al. (2012). The construct of adaptive behavior: its conceptualization, measurement, and use in the field of intellectual disability. *Am J Intellect Dev Disabil* 117(4): 291–303.

National Neuroscience Curriculum Initiative online resources

A Fragile Balance: Dendritic Spines, Learning, and Memory

Ruth F. Mccann and David A. Ross

9

Integrated Neurobiology of Specific Syndromes and Treatments

Meng-Chuan Lai and Simon Baron-Cohen

OVERVIEW

Autism is a heterogeneous, behaviourally defined, neurodevelopmental condition characterised by early-emerging atypical social communication and restricted, repetitive behaviours and interests. The underlying neurocognitive underpinnings may include difficulties
in social processing (particularly 'mentalising'), executive functioning, as well as strengths in
pattern recognition (attention to detail and rule-based reasoning or 'systemising'). Each of
these involves atypical brain connectivity. The underlying molecular neurobiology involves
developmentally sensitive and spatiotemporally specific genetic and gene–environmental
(e.g. neuroendocrine-immune) mechanisms, converging on neuronal synaptic functioning
and transcriptional regulation prenatally, and their cascade effects on brain development,
influenced by the autistic person's interaction with the environmental contexts from early
in life and across the lifespan. Future autism research needs to clarify the relations between
the genes and the environmental factors and their relations to neurocognitive architectures, to identify factors associated with plasticity in developmental trajectories and to
develop neurobiologically informed therapeutics and support strategies that are precisely
tailored to respect individual differences.

9.1.1 Autism: A Behaviourally Defined, Heterogeneous Neurodevelopmental Condition

Autism is a neurodevelopmental condition defined
behaviourally by early-emerging atypicalities in social
communication skills (including social–emotional reci-
procity, non-verbal communication and understanding,
developing and maintaining typical social relations),
alongside what is called restricted and repetitive behaviours and interests (including stereotyped and repetitive
behaviours, inflexible adherence to routines, sameness
or rituals, and fixated interests), which also includes
idiosyncratic sensory sensitivity. These atypical behaviours emerge in the early years, but the clinical diagnosis can be made at any time in life. Decades ago, autism
was regarded as a rare condition but, due to changing
diagnostic criteria, improved recognition and increased

awareness, autism is now relatively common. Today ~1%
of the global population has a formal diagnosis, with a
male:female (sex assigned at birth) ratio of 3–4:1.

The current definition of autism encompasses a
heterogeneous group of individuals sharing atypicalities
in social communication and restricted and repetitive
behaviours and interests, but who may differ in levels
of language, intellectual ability, co-occurring medical,
neurodevelopmental or psychiatric conditions, and
developmental trajectories. This umbrella label describes
a group of people at the high end of dimensions of autistic traits that are continuously distributed in the general
population. A clinical diagnosis is given when there is
significant functional impairment related to these high-
level traits, but the diagnosis encompasses a variety of
qualitatively different subgroups of individuals. Despite
the strong genetic aetiology (heritability estimates are

64–91%) [1], causal factors of autism are diverse. The vast heterogeneity across phenotype, neurobiology and aetiology is the rule rather than the exception in autism [2], especially considering the neurodevelopmental and psychiatric conditions with which it frequently co-occurs (e.g. attention deficit hyperactivity disorder (ADHD), anxiety disorders) [3]. Current intervention and support models are primarily behavioural and educational, focusing on maximising the autistic individual's potential in development and learning, minimising their barriers to adaptation and creating adequate environmental support to optimise the person–environment fit [4]. The autism and neurodevelopmental research field is leveraging the increasingly large and multi-level data and applying both hypothesis-driven and data-driven approaches to decompose this heterogeneity, to move towards the goals of precision in intervention and support [2].

9.1.2 The Neurocognitive Bases of Autism

In the past 50 years, several cognitive models have been empirically examined to understand how the autistic mind works differently, to explain how the behavioural profiles of autism unfold and to build a bridge between behaviour and biology [5]. The main models are summarised below but see [5] for a contemporary review of cognitive theories of autism. These cognitive models have also led to evidence-based intervention strategies such as naturalistic developmental behavioural interventions, social skills and theory of mind training [4]. Although current evidence finds no 'grand theory' for the cognitive basis of autism, each prevailing model explains part of the behavioural phenotype and its development in autism, and points to plausible underlying brain circuits or systems that explain a portion of the heterogeneity.

Historically, the 'deficit models' of theory of mind impairment, reduced social orientation and social motivation (in very early years) and executive dysfunction have been used to explain the unique early-onset social-communication difficulties in autism, with experimental supports from relatively small-sample studies. Accumulated evidence reveals a more complex picture.

First, the primary social cognitive difficulty experienced by autistic individuals lies in intuitive 'mentalising' (i.e. knowing what other people think or feel). This is further compounded by the natural complexity of social interactions, in which non-autistic people often show difficulties understanding autistic people (sometimes referred to as the 'double empathy problem').

Second, reduced orientation to social stimuli is not present at birth, but likely emerges in the first few months, reflecting a deviation from the typical infant's developmental transition from reflex-like social orientating to an experience-dependent, volitional social orienting [6]. Such deviation (and hence the later clinical autism phenotype) could be an alternative, adaptive developmental process with an unusual starting state of attention allocation (i.e. focal attention, repetition and withdrawal from social stimuli and contexts) underpinned by neurobiological differences (e.g. synaptic processing) [7].

Third, atypical motivation is neither specifically about social scenarios nor universally impaired in autistic individuals [8].

Finally, although executive dysfunction is common in autistic individuals, impedes adaptive function and explains parts of social and general cognitive features of autism, it does not link directly to the behavioural phenotypes of autism. Further, it does not seem to be autism-specific, but rather is present transdiagnostically with other neurodevelopmental conditions.

Another way of conceptualising the cognitive features of autism is viewing them as different or alternative (instead of impaired) ways of information processing [5]. These domain-general cognitive models posit that autistic people, from very early in life have:

(i) an attentional, sensory-perceptual and cognitive pattern biasing towards local details more than global contexts, which is not simply part of executive dysfunction but may reflect cognitive strengths alongside difficulties

(ii) challenges integrating multimodal and complex information and, perhaps in relation to this, have atypical allocation of attention ('monotropism', i.e. focusing attention on specific interests at any time and missing things outside of this attention tunnel)

(iii) an increased tendency to engage in rule-based, predictable and logical contexts, referred to as 'systemising'

(iv) reliance on greater weighting of sensory information in updating the probabilistic representations of the environment – an alternative, Bayesian view of autism.

The brain bases of these cognitive characteristics have been investigated primarily via neuroimaging methods. This literature is characterised by diverse findings and is mostly cross-sectional, with a relative paucity of longitudinal data from early in life to address causality, developmental mechanisms, plasticity and compensation. The findings (Figure 9.1.1) generally suggest that (i) individual variability is substantially higher in the autistic than the non-autistic population; (ii) brain correlates of autism tend to be widely distributed across cortical and subcortical regions; (iii) high heterogeneity of findings is critically associated with factors such as age, sex, gender, and co-occurring conditions; and (iv) hidden subgroups are likely to be the key to understanding the various neurobiological bases of autism.

At the whole-brain level, although an influential theoretical model of reduced global and increased local connectivity (corresponding to the information-processing cognitive models) has been proposed [9], findings have been variable. Studies on intrinsic brain functional organisation show mixed findings of hyper- and hypoconnectivity in autistic compared to non-autistic individuals, though trends of convergence have been shown regarding hypoconnectivity hubs in the sensorimotor regions and hyperconnectivity hubs in the prefrontal and parietal cortices [10], with various involvement of cortico-subcortical circuitries such as enhanced sensory cortex–subcortex connectivity. Neurophysiological studies using electro- or magnetoencephalography tend to show long-range underconnectivity in autism. Structurally, diffusion imaging studies tend to show altered white matter organisation (e.g. reduced fractional anisotropy) of long-range fibre tracts including the corpus callosum and various association fibres such as the superior longitudinal fasciculus, occipitofrontal fasciculus, inferior longitudinal fasciculus, uncinate fasciculus and cingulum.

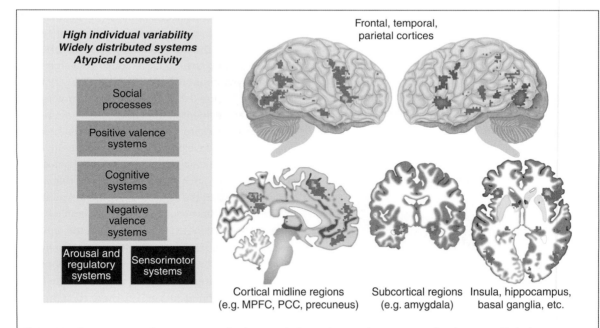

Figure 9.1.1 Neurocognitive architecture associated with autism. The brain substrates of autism are complex, characterised by high heterogeneity of findings, likely underpinned by substantial individual variability, involvement of widely distributed neural systems, and atypical structural and functional connectivity. Using the US National Institute of Mental Health Research Domain Criteria framework, the involvements of three systems (orange boxes) are most frequently reported, followed by emerging findings about other systems (yellow and blue boxes). The brain representations on the right illustrate regions mostly associated with autism, involving cortical and subcortical structures. These regions are identified based on a term-based automated meta-analysis conducted via Neurosynth.org on July 14, 2019 with the term 'autism', which involved 244 studies and 11,329 activations; 'hot' colour shows significant voxels in a uniformity test, indicating the degree to which the voxel is consistently activated in studies that use the term 'autism'. Abbreviations: MPFC, medial prefrontal cortex; PCC, posterior cingulate cortex.

Using the US National Institute of Mental Health Research Domain Criteria (RDoC) framework, neuroimaging findings suggest converging atypicality across all six systems but most atypicality centres around three of them (Figure 9.1.1). First, atypical social processes are commonly identified in autism, demonstrated by functional and anatomical differences in autistic compared to non-autistic people in the posterior superior temporal sulcus, temporoparietal junction, medial prefrontal cortex, fusiform face area, inferior frontal gyrus, amygdala, insula and cingulate cortex, many of these considered the 'social network' in the brain. Among these, an altered default-mode network and its developmental trajectory, which underlies atypical integration of information about self and other, is a prominent neurocognitive feature [11]. Second, findings regarding positive valence systems suggest atypical reward processing in autism, which encompasses not only decreased social but also decreased non-social reward processing, alongside increased reward processing associated with fixated interests [8]. Third, findings in cognitive systems are characterised by altered frontoparietal, dorsal attention and ventral attention networks [12], alongside altered neuromolecular composition (e.g. signalling via gamma-aminobutyric acid (GABA) neurotransmitters) in primary sensory cortices and their atypical responses across sensory modalities and during multimodal perception [13]. For the remaining RDoC systems, atypical negative valence systems in autism (e.g. amygdala, corticolimbic circuitry) may be highly related to the frequent co-occurrence of anxiety, emotion processing and regulation challenges [14]. There are fewer investigations so far into the arousal and regulatory systems and sensorimotor systems in autism, but atypicality has been reported.

9.1.3 The Molecular–Neurobiological Bases of Autism

One important development in the neurobiological understanding of autism is research into very early development, particularly the behavioural and brain development prior to the emergence of the clinical autism phenotype in infants who have older autistic siblings. These studies found a predictive feature of emerging autism, characterised by cortical surface-area hyper-expansion in the first year followed by brain-volume overgrowth in the second year [15]. This may be underpinned

by increased proliferation of neural progenitor cells that leads to surface-area hyper-expansion, which underpins atypical early sensorimotor and attentional experiences; this results in altered experience-dependent neuronal development, in particular reduced postnatal pruning, which further contributes to brain overgrowth, altered excitation–inhibition balance and atypical connectivity from the second year of life [15]. Such observations are in line with the idea that atypical early sensorimotor and attentional processes are primary in the emergence of autism, which results in downstream alterations in complex information processing and social communication [7, 13].

Further evidence supports the idea that the emergence of autism starts prenatally through a cascade of processes [16]. Genetic studies show that the aetiologies of autism are substantially contributed by large-effect, germline, heterozygous, rare, *de novo* coding genetic mutations [17]. In fact, structural variation and mutations to both coding and non-coding regions occur in more than 30% of individuals diagnosed with autism. Many of these genes are expressed prenatally in the brain, are biologically pleiotropic and have diverse functions across developmental timing and anatomical distribution. However, they do have spatiotemporal 'convergence' in encoding synaptic proteins and involving transcriptional regulation (Figure 9.1.2) [16, 17]. Such convergence is particularly evident in affecting cortical deep-layer glutamatergic excitatory projection (pyramidal) neurons during mid-fetal development and, less evidently, in the cerebellum and medial dorsal nucleus of thalamus early postnatally [17]. Such specific spatiotemporal alteration suggests that the neurodevelopmental processes towards autism start *in utero*, and hence highlights the impact of both genetics and prenatal gene–environment interactions [18]; for example, maternal polycystic ovary syndrome (marked by hyperandrogenic hormonal status) is associated with a 1.66 times increase in the likelihood of offspring autism [19]. These complex interactions may involve neuroendocrine–immune (e.g. the prenatal interaction between steroid hormones, microglia, neuronal gene expression and morphology) and microbiome–gut–brain processes, even into postnatal development [20].

The molecular bases of autism also involve common genetic variants, which additively add to the

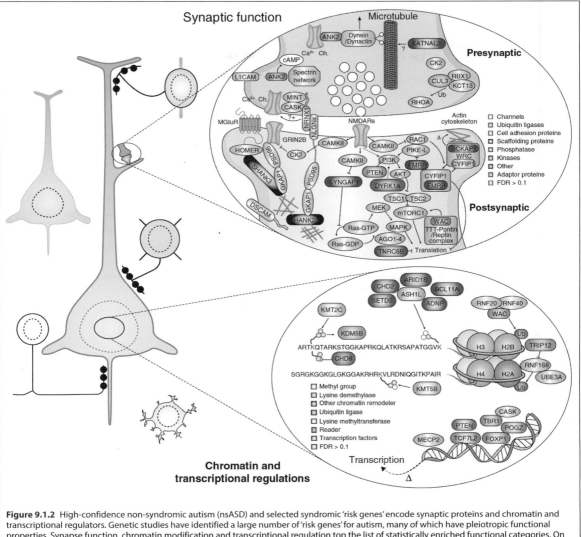

Figure 9.1.2 High-confidence non-syndromic autism (nsASD) and selected syndromic 'risk genes' encode synaptic proteins and chromatin and transcriptional regulators. Genetic studies have identified a large number of 'risk genes' for autism, many of which have pleiotropic functional properties. Synapse function, chromatin modification and transcriptional regulation top the list of statistically enriched functional categories. On the left, a simplified schematic of the major cellular components of neural circuits in the cerebral cortex is shown: pyramid-shaped glutamatergic excitatory projection neurons, GABAergic inhibitory interneurons and glial cells. On the right is shown the diverse intracellular distribution and pleiotropic roles of high-confidence (false discovery rate (FDR) < 0.1) nsASD 'risk genes' and selected syndromic 'risk genes'. Red outlined circles depict a view of the synapse with its many protein products of nsASD 'risk genes' (top) and the nsASD proteins in the nucleus (bottom). Proteins in synaptic signalling pathways encompass cell adhesion, scaffolding and signalling molecules. Nuclear protein products of nsASD 'risk genes' are mainly associated with chromatin modification and transcriptional control, suggesting that alterations in chromatin structure and gene expression may contribute to autism. Figure reproduced from [17].

aforementioned impact of rare variants [21]. Common variant effects are typically small and involve multiple genes; the largest study up to 2019 (involving 18,381 autistic individuals) shows that the polygenic architecture of autism is significantly shared with the risk of psychiatric disorders (i.e. schizophrenia, major depression), ADHD and higher educational attainment and intelligence [22]. Interestingly, the common-variant association with higher intelligence and educational attainment is only observed in individuals with a diagnosis of 'Asperger's syndrome' and those without intellectual disability, suggesting plausible subgroups of autism at the genetic level.

Conclusions and Outstanding Questions

Recent progress in genetics and molecular biology extends our understanding to the neurodevelopmental underpinnings of autism, both prenatally and postnatally. In light of the well-recognised multi-level heterogeneity of autism [2], challenges remain in (i) mapping out the relations between the genes and the environmental factors and their relations to neurocognitive architectures; (ii) identifying factors related to plasticity in developmental trajectories; (iii) developing neurobiologically informed therapeutics and support strategies that are tailored to precision medicine and appreciate individual differences. While the strongest evidence of early intervention focuses on enhancing caregiver–child synchrony and facilitating autistic children's joint attention and engagement with caregivers, rapidly emerging clinical trials are also evaluating agents modulating the neural excitation–inhibition balance (e.g. through glutamatergic or GABAergic systems) and neuropeptides (e.g. oxytocin, vasopressin and serotonin) [4]. Resolving the neuroscientific puzzles is key to answering the critical clinical question of 'what works for whom' in enhancing autistic individuals' adaptation and well-being.

Outstanding Questions

- What are the best ways to decompose the phenotypic, neurobiological, aetiological and developmental heterogeneity of autism?

- How will the progress in neuroscientific understanding of autism be translated into useful interventions and supports that improve autistic people's adaptation and well-being?

- To what extent and in what way can the neurocognitive and neurobiological underpinnings of autism be understood as reflecting aspects of neurodiversity?

REFERENCES

1. Tick B, Bolton P, Happé F, Rutter M, Rijsdijk F. Heritability of autism spectrum disorders: a meta-analysis of twin studies. *J Child Psychol Psychiatry* 2016; 57(5): 585–595.

2. Lombardo MV, Lai MC, Baron-Cohen S. Big data approaches to decomposing heterogeneity across the autism spectrum. *Mol Psychiatry* 2019; 24(10): 1435–1450.

3. Lai MC, Kassee C, Besney R et al. Prevalence of co-occurring mental health diagnoses in the autism population: a systematic review and meta-analysis. *Lancet Psychiatry* 2019; 6(10): 819–829.

4. Lai MC, Anagnostou E, Wiznitzer M, Allison C, Baron-Cohen S. Evidence-based support for autistic people across the lifespan: maximizing potential, minimizing barriers, and optimizing the person–environment fit. *Lancet Neurol* 2020; 19(5): 434–451.

5. Fletcher-Watson S, Happé F. *Autism: A New Introduction to Psychological Theory and Current Debate.* Routledge, 2019.

6. Shultz S, Klin A, Jones W. Neonatal transitions in social behavior and their implications for autism. *Trends Cogn Sci* 2018; 22(5): 452–469.

7. Johnson MH. Autism as an adaptive common variant pathway for human brain development. *Dev Cogn Neurosci* 2017; 25: 5–11.

8. Clements CC, Zoltowski AR, Yankowitz LD et al. Evaluation of the social motivation hypothesis of autism: a systematic review and meta-analysis. *JAMA Psychiatry* 2018; 75(8): 797–808.

9. Belmonte MK, Allen G, Beckel-Mitchener A et al. Autism and abnormal development of brain connectivity. *J Neurosci* 2004; 24(42): 9228–9231.

10. Holiga S, Hipp JF, Chatham CH et al. Patients with autism spectrum disorders display reproducible functional connectivity alterations. *Sci Transl Med* 2019; 11(481): eaat9223.

11. Padmanabhan A, Lynch CJ, Schaer M, Menon V. The default mode network in autism. *Biol Psychiatry Cogn Neurosci Neuroimaging* 2017; 2(6): 476–486.

12. Dichter GS. Functional magnetic resonance imaging of autism spectrum disorders. *Dialogues Clin Neurosci* 2012; 14(3): 319–351.

13. Robertson CE, Baron-Cohen S. Sensory perception in autism. *Nat Rev Neurosci* 2017; 18(11): 671–684.

14. McVey AJ. The neurobiological presentation of anxiety in autism spectrum disorder: a systematic review. *Autism Res* 2019; 12(3): 346–369.

15. Piven J, Elison JT, Zylka MJ. Toward a conceptual framework for early brain and behavior development in autism. *Mol Psychiatry* 2017; 22(10): 1385–1394.

16. Courchesne E, Pramparo T, Gazestani VH et al. The ASD living biology: from cell proliferation to clinical phenotype. *Mol Psychiatry* 2019; 24(1): 88–107.

17. Sestan N, State MW. Lost in translation: traversing the complex path from genomics to therapeutics in autism spectrum disorder. *Neuron* 2018; 100(2): 406–423.

18. Mandy W, Lai MC. Annual research review: the role of the environment in the developmental psychopathology of autism spectrum condition. *J Child Psychol Psychiatry* 2016; 57(3):271–292.

19. Katsigianni M, Karageorgiou V, Lambrinoudaki I, Siristatidis C. Maternal polycystic ovarian syndrome in autism spectrum disorder: a systematic review and meta-analysis. *Mol Psychiatry* 2019; 24(12): 1787–1797.

20. Gumusoglu SB, Stevens HE. Maternal inflammation and neurodevelopmental programming: a review of preclinical outcomes and implications for translational psychiatry. *Biol Psychiatry* 2019; 85(2): 107–121.

21. Weiner DJ, Wigdor EM, Ripke S et al. Polygenic transmission disequilibrium confirms that common and rare variation act additively to create risk for autism spectrum disorders. *Nat Genet* 2017; 49(7): 978–985.

22. Grove J, Ripke S, Als TD et al. Identification of common genetic risk variants for autism spectrum disorder. *Nat Genet* 2019; 51(3): 431–444.

National Neuroscience Curriculum Initiative online resources

Found in Translation: Autism Genetics and the Quest for Its Rosetta Stone

Jonathan Goldstein, David A. Ross and Daniel Moreno De Luca

This "stuff is really cool: Kartik Pattabiraman, *"Mystery of Autism"*

Attention Deficit Hyperactivity Disorder

Marina Mitjans and Bru Cormand

OVERVIEW

Attention deficit hyperactivity disorder (ADHD) is a childhood-onset disorder with a prevalence of 5%. It is clinically defined by symptoms of inattention, motor hyperactivity and impulsivity. In addition to the core symptoms, it has also been associated with impairment in cognitive domains. ADHD is highly heritable and multifactorial in origin; multiple genes and non-inherited factors contribute to the aetiology of the disorder. ADHD has been associated with slower maturation of long white matter tracts and decreased volume in brain regions relevant for executive function, sustained attention, impulse suppression and regulation of motor activity. In addition to structural brain changes, a range of brain networks and dysregulation of neurotransmitter signalling have also been associated with ADHD. However, no diagnostic neurobiological markers are currently available for clinical use.

9.2.1 What Is ADHD?

Attention deficit hyperactivity disorder (ADHD) is a neurodevelopmental disorder with an estimated worldwide prevalence of at least 5% in children and adolescents [1]. Its symptoms/functional impairment can persist into adulthood in as many as 65% of individuals with a childhood diagnosis. ADHD can present differently depending on the patient's sex: in children and adolescents, around 80% of ADHD cases are males, whereas in clinically diagnosed adults the proportion of males falls to 50% [1]. Comorbidity with other neurodevelopmental and psychiatric disorders is substantial.

According to the *Diagnostic and Statistical Manual of Mental Disorders*, 5th edition (DSM-5) and the *International Classification of Diseases*, 11th edition (ICD-11) [2, 3], childhood-onset ADHD begins before age 12 years and is defined by inattention, motor hyperactivity and impulsivity. In addition to the core symptoms, patients with ADHD also present impairment in other executive functions such as working memory or planning deficits. Alterations in other cognitive domains such as deficits in arousal and motivation have also been reported [1].

Among ADHD patients, the expression of all these symptoms and impairments is very heterogeneous.

9.2.2 Aetiology of ADHD

Family and twin studies suggest a strong genetic influence on ADHD with an estimated heritability between 70% and 80% [4]. Before the emergence of genome-wide association studies (GWAS) many candidate gene studies were performed. These studies have focused mainly on genes involved in the monoamine neurotransmitter systems, since monoamines had been implicated in ADHD pathophysiology by the mechanisms of action of drugs used in clinical management. There is meta-analytic support for associations between ADHD and variants in the genes encoding the D4 (*DRD4*) and D5 (*DRD5*) dopamine receptors, but due to methodological issues with candidate gene studies, these results must be interpreted with caution. Using high-throughput genotyping methodologies, the latest GWAS meta-analysis for ADHD used 38,691 ADHD cases and 186,843 controls and successfully identified risk single-nucleotide variants in 27 loci, implicating genes particularly involved in early brain development [5]. This study confirmed a polygenic architecture for ADHD and the proportion of heritability explained by these common variants is approximately 14%. Going beyond single-nucleotide polymorphisms, genetic studies have also shown enrichment of certain copy number variants [4] and increased load of rare protein-truncating variants in ADHD [5].

Numerous environmental exposures have also been associated with ADHD, including prenatal and perinatal factors such as early maternal deprivation, maternal smoking and alcohol use, low birth weight, premature birth and exposure to some environmental toxins [1]. However, rather than being specific to ADHD, these environmental factors are associated with several psychiatric disorders.

In summary, ADHD arises from several genetic and environmental risk factors, each having a small individual effect and acting together to increase susceptibility.

9.2.3 Brain Mechanisms of ADHD

ADHD has been associated with a range of brain alterations affecting different brain regions (Figure 9.2.1) and brain networks (Table 9.2.1), which can be related to different symptoms or cognitive domains that are affected in ADHD patients. We here describe the main findings at the neurotransmitter, structural and functional levels.

9.2.3.1 Neurotransmitter Alterations

Dysregulation in multiple neurotransmitter systems has been reported for most psychiatric disorders including ADHD, but results are often inconsistent across studies. The most studied neurotransmitter in ADHD has been dopamine since methylphenidate, the most prescribed and effective treatment for ADHD, acts as a dopamine reuptake inhibitor, increasing dopamine levels at the synaptic cleft. This fact, together with the dopamine-related candidate genes that have been associated with ADHD, and the role that dopamine plays in attention, has led to the dopamine hypothesis of ADHD. Using positron emission tomography, some studies have reported an increased number of dopamine transporters in the putamen and the caudate nucleus in adults and children with ADHD; however, these findings have not been replicated by other groups [6].

9.2.3.2 Structural Brain Alterations

Morphological structural imaging studies have shown total brain volumes 3–5% smaller in individuals with ADHD compared to unaffected controls, which could be attributed to a reduction of grey matter [7–9]. Meta-analyses have demonstrated reductions in the volume of multiple specific brain regions, most consistently the right globus pallidus, right putamen, caudate nucleus and cerebellum [10, 11].

Other morphological aspects, such as cortical thickness or cortical surface area, have also been explored in ADHD. A meta-analysis found a delay in cortical maturation in children with ADHD compared to children without, showing on average a 2–3-year delay in reaching peak thickness of much of the cerebrum, especially in the prefrontal cortex [12]. Interestingly, this study showed that ADHD patients who clinically remitted presented a normalisation of initial delays, while those with persistent ADHD showed either fixed non-progressive cortical deficits or a tendency to diverge from the trajectories observed in typically developing subjects [12]. Recently, the ENIGMA-ADHD group found that children with ADHD had lower total brain surface area compared to controls, with reductions in surface area in frontal cingulate, and temporal regions. Fusiform gyrus and temporal pole cortical thickness was also lower in children with ADHD. Neither surface area nor cortical thickness was found to be different in the adolescent or adult ADHD groups compared to control subjects [13].

Diffusion tensor imaging (DTI) studies have also been used to assess abnormalities in white matter structure in ADHD. A meta-analysis of DTI studies showed widespread alterations in white matter integrity, most pronounced in the right anterior corona radiata, right forceps minor, bilateral internal capsule and left cerebellum [14].

9.2.3.3 Brain Connectivity Alterations

Task-based functional MRI (fMRI) studies have focused on tasks related to cognitive domains affected in ADHD patients. A meta-analysis focusing only on inhibition tasks (including response inhibition and interference control) found lower activation in ADHD compared to healthy subjects in frontostriatal regions including the right inferior frontal cortex, supplementary motor area, anterior cingulate cortex and striatothalamic areas [15].

In reward processing paradigms, most studies report hypoactivation of the ventral striatum in anticipation of reward in patients with ADHD compared to controls. The ventral striatum is a central node within the reward

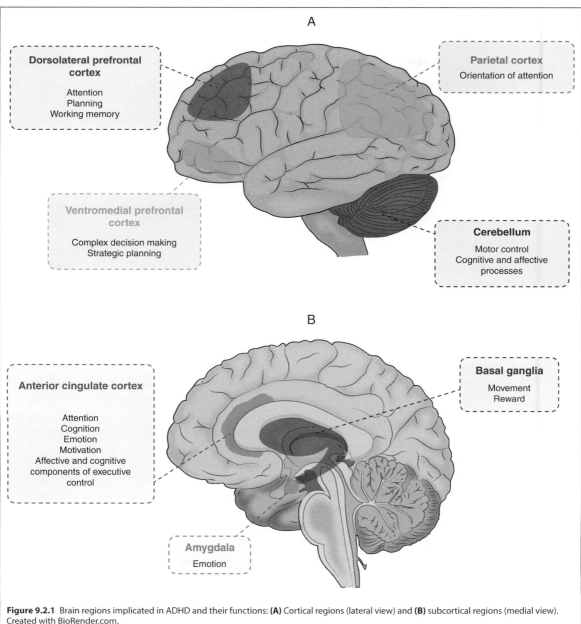

Figure 9.2.1 Brain regions implicated in ADHD and their functions: **(A)** Cortical regions (lateral view) and **(B)** subcortical regions (medial view). Created with BioRender.com.

network, and this hypoactivation possibly reflects a reduced desirability of delayed rewards in ADHD [16].

A meta-analysis combining different task-based fMRI studies (working memory, inhibition and attention tasks), which tried to find putative common alterations, found underactivation of the frontoparietal network (related to executive function) and the ventral attentional network (related to attention) [17]. The authors also found hyperactivation of somatomotor and visual networks, which could be the result of compensatory mechanisms in which children with ADHD may try to compensate for deficits in higher-order goal-directed executive functions using regions involved in sensory modalities [17].

Table 9.2.1 Brain networks involved in ADHD

Network	Brain regions involved	Function
Reward network	Ventromedial prefrontal cortex, orbitofrontal cortex, ventral striatum, thalamus, amygdala, cell bodies of dopaminergic neurons in the substantia nigra	Anticipation and receipt of reward
Ventral attentional network	Temporoparietal junction, ventral frontal cortex	Monitoring environment for emergence of salient stimuli and interrupting ongoing activity when necessary
Executive-control network	Frontal cortex, basal ganglia, dorsal anterior cingulate cortex, cerebellum	Planning, goal-directed behaviour, inhibition, working memory and flexible adaptation to context
Default-mode network	Medial prefrontal cortex, posterior cingulate cortex, medial temporal lobe, lateral parietal cortex	Involved in self-reflection, planning future activities, monitoring environment
Motor network	Motor cortices, supplementary motor area, putamen, thalamus, cerebellum	Involved in motor activity
Visual network	Occipital visual cortex and temporal structures	Maintenance of attention and suppression of attention to irrelevant stimuli

Resting-state fMRI studies in ADHD have shown reduced connectivity within the default-mode network and atypical interactions between the default-mode network and attentional networks, which might reflect a tendency toward distractibility, potentially due to impaired regulation of attentional resources in ADHD patients [18]. See Section 5.12.5 for more on the mechanisms of attentional deficits in ADHD.

Conclusions and Outstanding Questions

The biological mechanisms through which genetic and environmental factors act and interact in ADHD are not fully yet understood and, therefore, no diagnostic biomarkers are available. Although different neurobiological alterations have been identified in ADHD, no specific neurotransmitters, brain regions or circuits can accurately delineate the symptoms of the disorder and studies have yielded inconsistent findings. Some of these inconsistencies may reflect the clinical heterogeneity of ADHD, but other factors, such as the cross-sectional designs, small sample sizes and poor reproducibility of the studies, also play a role. Moreover, certain behavioural correlates are not unique to ADHD and there is evidence for substantial rates of comorbidity with other disorders,

which makes the understanding of the neurobiological basis of ADHD more complicated. Gaining insight into the neurobiology of ADHD would allow clinicians and researchers to:

(i) complement current diagnostic procedures, based on clinical interviews, with objective biological measures

(ii) develop new therapeutic strategies based on pathophysiology, including personalised treatment approaches

(iii) evaluate the effects of available treatments with objective tools.

Outstanding Questions

- Given the limitations of the current studies and the development of novel imaging techniques, what direction will the neuroimaging studies for ADHD follow?

- How can researchers improve on studies to find stronger, more robust associations between brain measures and ADHD?

- How can researchers deal with the heterogeneous nature of ADHD?

- Are the biological alterations observed in ADHD specific to ADHD or are they shared with other comorbid conditions?

REFERENCES

1. Faraone SV, Asherson P, Banaschewski T et al. Attention-deficit/hyperactivity disorder. *Nat Rev Dis Prim* 2015; 1: 15020.

2. American Psychiatric Association. *Diagnostic and Statistical Manual of Mental Disorders*, 5th ed. (DSM-5). American Psychiatric Association, 2013.

3. World Health Organization. *International Classification of Diseases*, 11th ed. (ICD-11). World Health Organization, 2018.

4. Faraone SV, Larsson H. Genetics of attention deficit hyperactivity disorder. *Mol Psychiatry* 2019; 24: 562–575.

5. Demontis D, Walters RK, Athanasiadis G et al. Genome-wide analyses of ADHD identify 27 risk loci, refine the genetic architecture and implicate several cognitive domains. *Nat Genet* 2023; 55: 198–208.

6. Gonon F. The dopaminergic hypothesis of attention-deficit/hyperactivity disorder needs re-examining. *Trends Neurosci* 2009; 32: 2–8.

7. Castellanos FX, Lee PP, Sharp W et al. Developmental trajectories of brain volume abnormalities in children and adolescents with attention-deficit/hyperactivity disorder. *JAMA* 2002; 288: 1740–1748.

8. Durston S, Hulshoff Pol HE, Schnack HG et al. Magnetic resonance imaging of boys with attention-deficit/hyperactivity disorder and their unaffected siblings. *J Am Acad Child Adolesc Psychiatry* 2004; 43: 332–340.

9. Greven CU, Bralten J, Mennes M et al. Developmentally stable whole-brain volume reductions and developmentally sensitive caudate and putamen volume alterations in those with attention-deficit/hyperactivity disorder and their unaffected siblings. *JAMA Psychiatry* 2015; 72: 490–499.

10. Stoodley CJ, Schmahmann JD. Functional topography in the human cerebellum: a meta-analysis of neuroimaging studies. *Neuroimage* 2009; 44: 489–501.

11. Frodl T, Skokauskas N. Meta-analysis of structural MRI studies in children and adults with attention deficit hyperactivity disorder indicates treatment effects. *Acta Psychiatr Scand* 2012; 125: 114–126.

12. Shaw P, Eckstrand K, Sharp W et al. Attention-deficit/hyperactivity disorder is characterized by a delay in cortical maturation. *Proc Natl Acad Sci USA* 2007; 104: 19649–19654.

13. Hoogman M, Muetzel R, Guimaraes JP et al. Brain imaging of the cortex in ADHD: a coordinated analysis of large-scale clinical and population-based samples. *Am J Psychiatry* 2019; 176: 531–542.

14. van Ewijk H, Heslenfeld DJ, Zwiers MP, Buitelaar JK, Oosterlaan J. Diffusion tensor imaging in attention deficit/hyperactivity disorder: a systematic review and meta-analysis. *Neurosci Biobehav Rev* 2012; 36: 1093–1106.

15. Hart H, Radua J, Nakao T, Mataix-Cols D, Rubia K. Meta-analysis of functional magnetic resonance imaging studies of inhibition and attention in attention-deficit/hyperactivity disorder: exploring task-specific, stimulant medication, and age effects. *JAMA Psychiatry* 2013; 70: 185–198.

16. Plichta MM, Scheres A. Ventral-striatal responsiveness during reward anticipation in ADHD and its relation to trait impulsivity in the healthy population: a meta-analytic review of the fMRI literature. *Neurosci Biobehav Rev* 2014; 38: 125–134.

17. Cortese S, Kelly C, Chabernaud C et al. Toward systems neuroscience of ADHD: a meta-analysis of 55 fMRI studies. *Am J Psychiatry* 2012; 169: 1038–1055.

18. Posner J, Park C, Wang Z. Connecting the dots: a review of resting connectivity MRI studies in attention-deficit/hyperactivity disorder. *Neuropsychol Rev* 2014; 24: 3–15.

9

National Neuroscience Curriculum Initiative online resources

Shifting Focus: From Group Patterns to Individual Neurobiological Differences in Attention-Deficit/Hyperactivity Disorder

Alison E. Lenet

Clinical neuroscience conversations: *From Circuit to Symptom: Understanding The Adhd Brain*

Alison E. Lenet, MD and Melissa R. Arbuckle

Expert video: *Philip Shaw on Childhood ADHD*

Alexandra Hayes and
Anne Lingford-Hughes

9.3	**Drug Use, Addiction, Tolerance, Withdrawal and Relapse**

OVERVIEW

Occasional or 'recreational' use of drugs of abuse may result in pleasurable effects such as euphoria and reduced anxiety. Regular use leads to dependence and addiction through a series of steps. Initial drug-seeking behaviour and positive reinforcement increase use and cause neural adaptations. Adaptations in key parts of the brain manifest as tolerance, where more drug is required to achieve the same effects, and to withdrawal in the absence of the drug. With repetitive use comes attribution of salience to the drug. Associated environmental items become conditioned stimuli that drive further, repetitive drug-seeking behaviour. These neuroadaptations play a critical role in perpetuating drug use that incurs social, mental and physical health harms (according to the *International Classification of Diseases*, 11th edition (ICD-11): abuse; or the *Diagnostic and Statistical Manual of Mental Disorders*, 5th edition (DSM-5): mild substance use disorder) as well as development of addiction for some (ICD-11: dependence; DSM-5: moderate to severe substance use disorder) [1, 2]. For all drugs of abuse, these neuroadaptations result in broadly similar changes in brain function, particularly in the mesolimbic system, despite the range of molecular targets (see Section 2.7). The wide range of molecular targets for different drugs of abuse, and the various underpinning neuroadaptations mean that the degree of tolerance and signs and symptoms of withdrawal differ between drugs, dependence on cocaine and alcohol being exemplar contrasts.

9.3.1 Initial Drug Use and the Mesocorticolimbic 'Reward' System

The dopaminergic mesocorticolimbic system is commonly referred to as the reward system and plays a key role in mediating the reinforcing properties of conventional rewards such as food and sex [3]. This system is also the target for drugs of abuse. Originating in the ventral tegmental area, the dopaminergic neurons project to key brain regions associated with reward processing including the nucleus accumbens, ventral striatum and prefrontal cortex [4]. The prefrontal cortex plays a critical role in top-down control of the striatal reward system such that its responses are moderated through their reciprocal connections (Figure 9.3.1). See Section 5.9.4 for more on reward circuitry. Regions within the prefrontal cortex have been shown to be involved with particular functions related to addiction:

- the orbitofrontal and anterior cingulate cortices are implicated in attributing salience to reward and driving goal-directed behaviour [6]

- the ventrolateral prefrontal cortex is implicated in impulse/inhibitory control and monitoring ongoing behaviour

- the dorsolateral prefrontal cortex is involved in working memory and is implicated in formation of memory that is biased toward drug-related stimuli.

Other brain areas that also receive dopaminergic projections and play important roles in the development of addiction include the amygdala and hippocampus, which encode memories related to rewarding stimuli.

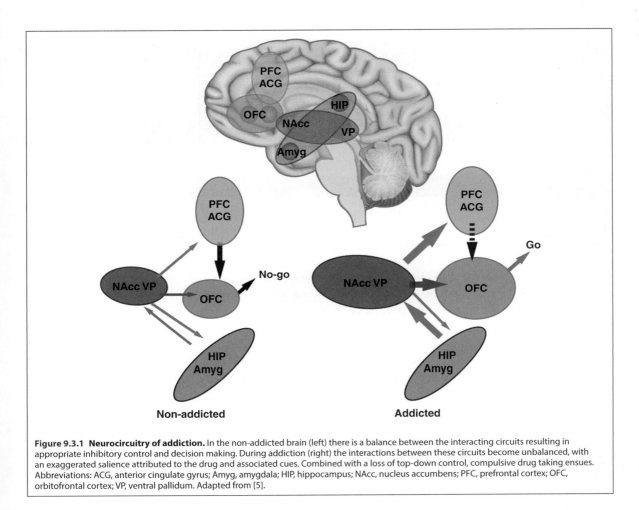

Figure 9.3.1 Neurocircuitry of addiction. In the non-addicted brain (left) there is a balance between the interacting circuits resulting in appropriate inhibitory control and decision making. During addiction (right) the interactions between these circuits become unbalanced, with an exaggerated salience attributed to the drug and associated cues. Combined with a loss of top-down control, compulsive drug taking ensues. Abbreviations: ACG, anterior cingulate gyrus; Amyg, amygdala; HIP, hippocampus; NAcc, nucleus accumbens; PFC, prefrontal cortex; OFC, orbitofrontal cortex; VP, ventral pallidum. Adapted from [5].

As drug use develops into regular use and dependence, these circuits become dysregulated. The motivational drive therefore to seek and consume the drug of abuse becomes more intense, memories associated with the drug are all-consuming and there is a loss of top-down control (see Figure 9.3.1, Table 9.3.1 and Section 2.7).

9.3.2 Interaction between Drugs of Abuse and the Mesocorticolimbic System

Stimulants such as cocaine and amphetamines directly target the dopaminergic system to increase extracellular dopamine in the nucleus accumbens in the absence of conventional rewards, creating feelings of pleasure, enjoyment and arousal. Both cocaine and amphetamines block the presynaptic dopamine transporter,

thus inhibiting reuptake of dopamine from the synapse. Amphetamines also increase the dopaminergic release rate from synaptic vesicles.

For all other drugs of abuse, increases in dopamine in the nucleus accumbens and ventral pallidum result from a change in firing of input dopaminergic neurons in the ventral tegmental area from tonic (background) to phasic burst firing. These dopaminergic neurons are modulated by inhibitory GABAergic interneurons, which act as a 'brake' on the dopamine system. A range of inhibitory receptors modulate GABAergic inhibition including mu-opioid, nicotinic and cannabinoid-1 receptors. Thus, drugs of abuse that activate these receptors indirectly increase the phasic firing of dopamine by inhibiting GABAergic inhibitory modulation of dopaminergic ventral tegmental area neurons and disinhibiting the pathway. Some drugs such as alcohol and stimulants

Table 9.3.1 The pharmacology of common drugs of abuse

Drug	Primary target	Acute effect	Key neuroadaptation with chronic consumption
Stimulants			
Cocaine	DAT	↑ dopamine	↓ dopaminergic activity
Amphetamine	DAT + MAO ↑ synaptic vesicle release	↑ dopamine	↓ dopaminergic activity
Nicotine	Nicotinic ACh receptor on dopaminergic VTA neurons	↑ dopamine	↓ dopaminergic activity
Sedatives/depressants			
Alcohol	GABA glutamate	↑ GABA-A function ↓ NMDA function	↓ GABA-A function ↑ NMDA function
Benzodiazepines	GABA	↑ GABA function	Unclear, likely reduced GABA-A function
Gamma-hydroxybutyric acid	GABA-B receptors, GHB receptors	↑ GABA function	Unclear
Cannabis	CB1 receptors	↑ dopamine via modulation of GABAergic input to dopaminergic neurons; modulates opioid systems	↓ CB1 receptor activity
Opiates: morphine, heroin, codeine, etc.	Mu-opioid receptors	Stimulate opioid receptors (mu is key), indirectly increase dopamine via modulation of GABAergic input to dopaminergic neurons	Reduced sensitivity of mu-opioid receptor, reduced noradrenergic activity

Abbreviations: ACh, acetylcholine; CB1, cannabinoid 1; DAT, dopamine transporter; GABA, gamma-aminobutyric acid; NMDA, N-methyl-D-aspartate; VTA, ventral tegmental area; ↑, increased; ↓, decreased.

promote the release of endogenous endorphins which contributes to their pleasurable effects via activation of the mu-opioid receptor. In humans, positron emission tomography studies have reported that stimulants robustly increase dopamine in the striatum, with some evidence to suggest alcohol has a similar effect. However, this has been less apparent following administration of other drugs of abuse including opiates and cannabis [7, 8]

While the role of the dopaminergic system in substance use and addiction has received much attention, the important contributions of a range of other mechanisms and neurotransmitter systems should not be forgotten. It is important to remember that addiction is a multi-neurotransmitter disorder and not just a dysregulation in the dopamine pathway, particularly when considering therapeutic targets (Figure 9.3.2).

9.3.3 Tolerance and Withdrawal

Tolerance is characterised clinically by an individual requiring a higher dose of a drug to achieve a response equivalent to that experienced following initial consumption. Neuroadaptive changes occur in order to maintain brain function homeostasis in the presence of an increasing amount of drug and its effects. Due to the wide range of pharmacological profiles of drugs of abuse, the mechanism underpinning tolerance will depend on the drug. Tolerance however generally involves adaptive changes such as downregulation and diminished sensitivity of receptors activated by the drug and changes in enzyme production and metabolism. While tolerance is an adaptive state observed with many drugs of abuse, it may not be evident in all cases. For example, behavioural tolerance to alcohol and opiates has been readily reported but is less common in stimulant use.

Once such neuroadaptive changes have occurred, abrupt cessation of the drug renders the brain unable to achieve homeostasis in the absence of adequate input. This in turn leads to withdrawal, generally accompanied by dysphoria, emotional stress and a decrease in cognitive ability as well as physical withdrawal symptoms such as headaches, nausea, muscle tension, tremors and aches [10]. However, the specific withdrawal symptoms experienced will depend on the extent of neuroadaptation that has occurred, the drug of abuse used and the individual. We will now focus on tolerance and withdrawal for two drugs – alcohol and opiates – given the important clinical implications of inappropriate management.

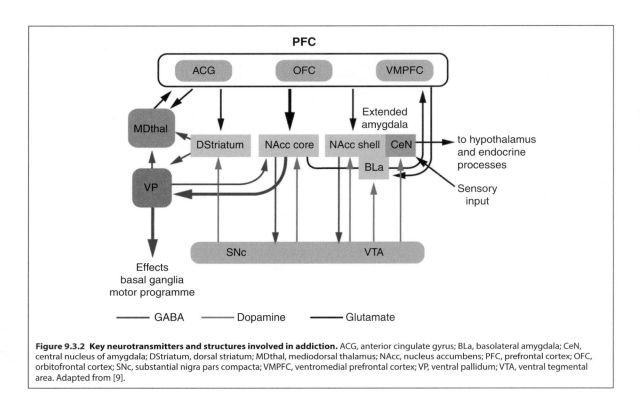

Figure 9.3.2 Key neurotransmitters and structures involved in addiction. ACG, anterior cingulate gyrus; BLa, basolateral amygdala; CeN, central nucleus of amygdala; DStriatum, dorsal striatum; MDthal, mediodorsal thalamus; NAcc, nucleus accumbens; PFC, prefrontal cortex; OFC, orbitofrontal cortex; SNc, substantial nigra pars compacta; VMPFC, ventromedial prefrontal cortex; VP, ventral pallidum; VTA, ventral tegmental area. Adapted from [9].

9.3.3.1 Alcohol

Tolerance to alcohol seen with regular, chronic consumption (not just a feature of dependence) is particularly associated with complementary neuroadaptations in the main inhibitory (GABA) and excitatory (glutamate) systems [11]. Acutely, alcohol boosts GABA-A (i.e. GABA–benzodiazepine) receptor function to enhance inhibitory activity, resulting in anxiolysis, sedation, etc. Chronic alcohol consumption results in reduced sensitivity of the GABA-A receptor to alcohol such that an individual may become less intoxicated or sedated and with very high consumption levels, as seen in alcohol dependence, where an individual may be over the drink–drive limit and not appear intoxicated. It is thought that the reduced sensitivity is due to a change in subunits in the GABA-A receptor [12]. Regarding the glutamate system, alcohol acts as an antagonist at the glutamate N-methyl-D-aspartate (NMDA) receptor which contributes to overall greater inhibition. To counter this antagonism, chronic alcohol consumption is therefore associated with upregulation of NMDA receptors. This is thought to underpin alcoholic 'blackouts' – alcohol-related memory loss during an episode of drinking.

In the continued presence of alcohol, the balance between GABAergic and glutamatergic function is maintained, but in its absence these neuroadaptations result in withdrawal. In particular, the hyper-glutamatergic state that results from lack of GABAergic inhibition is thought to be the main driver of the toxicity of alcohol withdrawal, underpinning withdrawal seizures and cell loss/atrophy [13]. Awareness of this neurobiology has led to use of medications that reduce glutamatergic hyperactivity in treating alcohol withdrawal. Clinically, alcohol withdrawal is generally treated by boosting GABAergic function with benzodiazepines or other drugs with anticonvulsant action, but medications that reduce glutamatergic hyperactivity (e.g. acamprosate) provide a complementary addition.

9.3.3.2 Opiates

Chronic opioid consumption is associated with reduced sensitivity of the mu-opioid receptor – the key receptor mediating analgesia, pleasurable rewarding effects and respiratory depression. It is important to note that tolerance to the various effects of opiates can develop at different rates. For example, tolerance to the euphoric effects of opiates occurs rapidly, thus underpinning further drug-seeking behaviour. However, tolerance to the respiratory depression effects of opioids happens more gradually and is incomplete. Tolerance of pupillary muscles is not clinically evident, so pupil size remains a good useful clinical indicator of opiate status. This desynchrony can be life-threatening as an individual will seek more of the drug to achieve the euphoric effect while putting themselves at risk of fatal respiratory depression. Furthermore, tolerance may differ between different opiate agonists since the reduction in sensitivity of the opiate receptor may occur through different mechanisms. This limited or lack of 'cross-tolerance', for instance between heroin and methadone, may contribute to overdose deaths. Given the life-threatening potential of these effects it is important we better understand the mechanisms underlying tolerance.

Opiate withdrawal ('cold turkey') manifests with a range of signs and symptoms associated with 'heightened arousal'. Mu-opiate receptors inhibit the production of noradrenaline in the locus coeruleus, which plays a key role in arousal and vigilance. To counter the low production of noradrenaline from chronic opiate exposure, activity of enzymes involved in noradrenaline synthesis is increased. While opiates are present, the overall noradrenergic activity is therefore maintained. However, in the absence of opiates, noradrenergic hyperactivity is revealed. This is the so-called 'noradrenergic storm' and is managed clinically by reducing noradrenergic activity with alpha-2-agonist medications such as lofexidine. Other signs and symptoms of withdrawal, such as nausea and diarrhoea, require alternative approaches to provide symptomatic relief.

9.3.4 Relapse

The risk of relapse and reinstatement of drug use remains high in individuals who successfully achieve abstinence. While the risk of relapse to dependent use never appears to disappear completely, it does reduce over time. As described, the neuroadaptations resulting from drug consumption begin to 'normalise' during withdrawal, a process that may take many weeks or longer. However, persisting altered neurobiology is clearly evident in addiction and likely underpins the risk of relapse. For instance, the dopaminergic mesolimbic system has been shown in many studies to be persistently dysregulated with hypofunction to 'normal' rewards but hyperactivity

to salient, that is, drug-related rewards. It should also be acknowledged that some of the differences seen between healthy controls and addiction in humans may be due to pre-existing vulnerabilities rather than purely secondary to drug consumption. However, this is unlikely to impact on clinical management of how to reduce the risk of relapse.

Relapse can be caused by a multitude of factors such as an attempt by the individual to reduce or overcome the withdrawal effects mentioned earlier. This is commonly the cause of relapse during acute withdrawal/early abstinence and the risk of this generally reduces over time in most. Relapse in response to environmental cues, low mood or stress, triggering the preoccupation/anticipation phase of addiction (craving), is also possible later in abstinence [10]. Environmental cues become associated with the pleasurable effect of the drug during the addiction process. When these are experienced during abstinence, this can induce an urge to use, which may lead to relapse. Relapse is often attributed to 'craving'; however, craving is difficult to measure clinically and does not always correlate well with relapse [14].

Conclusions and Outstanding Questions

Prolonged drug use and addiction lead to a range of neural adaptations. Such neural adaptations lead to dysregulation of our motivational drive, tolerance, withdrawal and relapse. In this section, we have discussed the neurotransmitter systems involved in these processes and outlined the divergent effects of different drugs of abuse. However, addiction is a multifaceted disorder so we must also consider how factors such as the environment and stress/mood may contribute to the initiation of drug use and the likelihood of relapse.

Outstanding Questions

- Tolerance to the behavioural and physiological effects of drugs may occur at different rates. In some cases, this can be life-threatening. In order to reduce this risk, we need to better understand the mechanisms underlying tolerance.
- Withdrawal is often implicated in perpetuating addiction, what neuroadaptations play a key role in this?
- The risk of relapse remains high in those who achieve abstinence. How can we investigate factors associated with relapse and identify those at higher risk?

REFERENCES

1. World Health Organization. *International Classification of Diseases*, 11th ed. (ICD-11). World Health Organization, 2018.

2. American Psychiatric Association. *Diagnostic and Statistical Manual of Mental Disorders*, 5th ed. (DSM-5). American Psychiatric Association, 2013.

3. Koob GF, Volkow ND. Neurobiology of addiction: a neurocircuitry analysis. *Lancet Psychiatry* 2016; 3(8): 760–73.

4. Adinoff B. Neurobiologic processes in drug reward and addiction. *Harv Rev Psychiatry* 2004; 12(6): 305–320.

5. Baler RD, Volkow ND. Drug addiction: the neurobiology of disrupted self-control. *Trends Mol Med* 2006; 12(12): 559–566.

6. Berridge KC, Kringelbach ML. Pleasure systems in the brain. *Neuron* 2015; 86(3): 646–664

7. Reid A, Lingford-Hughes A. Neuropharmacology of addiction. *Psychiatry* 2006; 5(12): 449–454.

8. Nutt DJ, Lingford-Hughes A, Eritzoe D, Stokes PR. The dopamine theory of addiction: 40 years of highs and lows. *Nat Rev Neurosci* 2015; 16(5): 305–312.

9. Turton S, Lingford-Hughes A. Neurobiology and principles of addiction and tolerance. *Alcohol Other Drug Disord* 2020; 48(12): 749–753.

10. Koob GF, Volkow ND. Neurocircuitry of addiction. *Neuropsychopharmacology* 2010; 35(1): 217–238.

11. Hoffman PL, Rabe CS, Grant KA et al. Ethanol and the NMDA receptor. *Alcohol* 1990; 7(3): 229–231.

12. Lingford-Hughes A, Watson B, Kalk N, Reid A. Neuropharmacology of addiction and how it informs treatment. *Br Med Bull* 2010; 96(1): 93–110.

13. Lobo IA, Harris RA. GABAA receptors and alcohol. *Pharmacol Biochem Behav* 2008; 90(1): 90–94.

14. Nutt DJ, Nestor LJ. *Addiction (Oxford Psychiatry Library)*. Oxford University Press, 2018.

National Neuroscience Curriculum Initiative online resources

Opioid Use Disorder: A Desperate Need for Novel Treatments

Brian S. Fuehrlein and David A. Ross

As Hopes Have Flown Before: Toward the Rational Design of Treatments for Alcohol Use Disorder

Noah A. Capurso and David A. Ross

Clinical Commentary: Perpetual Hunger: The Neurobiological Consequences of Long-Term Opioid Use

Tanner Bommersbach, David A. Ross and Joao P. De Aquino

What to say: *Perpetual Hunger: The Neurobiological Consequences of Long-Term Opioid Use*

Jane Eisen

Clinical neuroscience conversations: *Talking Pathways to Patients: Addiction*

Chris Karampahtsis, Michael Travis and Melissa Arbuckle

9

This "stuff" is really cool: Alex Moxam, *"Donut Pass Go" on habits and addiction*

9.4	Anxiety Disorders	Nathan Huneke, Bethan Impey and David Baldwin

OVERVIEW

Anxiety is a normal phenomenon that represents an 'alarm system', which allows preparation of physical and psychological responses to a perceived threat or danger (the 'fight-or-flight' response). Anxiety is usually appropriate, short-lived and controllable. When anxiety is present inappropriately, and its symptoms are abnormally severe, persistent and impair physical, social or occupational functioning, an 'anxiety disorder' can be diagnosed. In this section, we summarise what is known about the aetiology and neurobiology of the anxiety disorders included in the *International Classification of Diseases*, 11th edition (ICD-11) classification of mental disorders: generalised anxiety disorder, panic disorder with or without agoraphobia, specific phobia, social anxiety disorder and separation anxiety disorder [1]. As there is significant overlap in the neurobiology of these disorders, we discuss the anxiety disorders as a whole, highlighting specific aspects where relevant. Characteristic features of the anxiety disorders are shown in Table 9.4.1.

Table 9.4.1 Clinical features of anxiety disorders

Anxiety disorder	Characteristic features
Generalised anxiety disorder	Prolonged excessive worrying not restricted to particular circumstances – 'free floating' anxiety.
Panic disorder	Recurrent surges of severe anxiety ('panic attacks'), at least some of which are unexpected. Typically peak within 10 minutes and last 30–45 minutes. Patients often believe they are in imminent danger of death during the attack.
Agoraphobia	Fear and avoidance of situations from which escape is difficult (e.g. public spaces, crowds, public transportation).
Social anxiety disorder	Fear of being observed or appraised negatively by others in social or performance situations.
Specific phobia	Excessive fear of (and restricted to) single objects, animals, people or situations (e.g. bridges, spiders, heights, seeing blood) that are either avoided or endured with significant distress.
Separation anxiety disorder	Excessive fear of separation from those to whom an individual is attached. Commonly, there is persistent worry about potential harms to attachment figures or of unpleasant events leading to separation.

9.4.1 Anxiety and Fear Circuitry

Anxiety can be considered as the anticipation of threat, while fear can be considered as the avoidance of threat, or the immediate response to threat. These behaviours have slightly differing neurocircuitry, summarised in Figure 9.4.1.

The amygdala is central to anxiety processing in the brain. This complex structure comprising multiple subnuclei is part of the limbic system and is located in the anterior portion of the temporal lobe. The amygdala has two main functions in anxiety processing: identifying

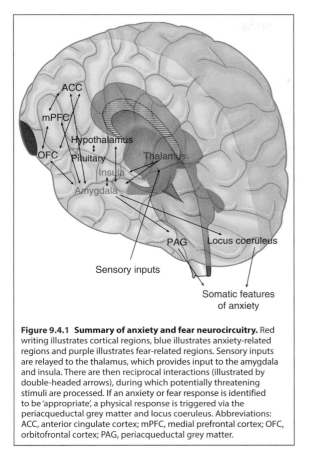

Figure 9.4.1 Summary of anxiety and fear neurocircuitry. Red writing illustrates cortical regions, blue illustrates anxiety-related regions and purple illustrates fear-related regions. Sensory inputs are relayed to the thalamus, which provides input to the amygdala and insula. There are then reciprocal interactions (illustrated by double-headed arrows), during which potentially threatening stimuli are processed. If an anxiety or fear response is identified to be 'appropriate', a physical response is triggered via the periacqueductal grey matter and locus coeruleus. Abbreviations: ACC, anterior cingulate cortex; mPFC, medial prefrontal cortex; OFC, orbitofrontal cortex; PAG, periacqueductal grey matter.

potential threats and coordinating an appropriate response [2]. Sensory afferents from the thalamus and sensory association cortices provide input into the basolateral complex of the amygdala. Reciprocal projections from here to cortical areas such as the anterior cingulate cortex and medial prefrontal cortex are involved in 'higher-order' processing of potentially threatening stimuli. The response to threat mediated by the amygdala is characterised by feelings associated with anxiety, such as apprehension, psychological symptoms such as worry, and endured distress. Therefore, this structure is likely to be important in anxiety-related disorders (e.g. generalised anxiety disorder). Consistent with this, functional neuroimaging studies show that patients with generalised anxiety disorder exhibit increased amygdala activity in response to threatening stimuli, with evidence of impaired control of amygdala responses by the anterior cingulate and medial prefrontal cortices [3].

The main output from the amygdala projects from its central nucleus to the hypothalamus and brainstem areas such as the periaqueductal grey matter. Activity in these regions is characterised by fear, a desire to escape and somatic responses to threatening stimuli, such as tachypnoea and increased blood pressure [4]. Accordingly, these structures are thought to be important in fear-related disorders (e.g. panic disorder and phobic disorders) [5]. However, this remains subject to debate, with neuroimaging studies showing inconsistent results regarding activation in the amygdala and subcortical regions when patients with panic disorder are exposed to non-specific and panic-specific threatening stimuli [6]. Better understanding of how the anxiety disorders relate to anxiety and fear circuitry might be important for improving clinical management.

9.4.2 Neurotransmitter Systems

Disturbed monoaminergic neurotransmission is probably common to all anxiety disorders. The serotonergic system is particularly important. Serotonin (5-hydroxytryptamine; 5-HT) inhibits **fight-or-flight** responses to threat mediated by the periaqueductal grey matter, but also facilitates anxiety responses mediated by the amygdala [7]. Treatment with selective serotonin reuptake inhibitors is therefore thought to reduce fear mediated by the periaqueductal grey matter in panic and phobic disorders, and improve symptoms in anxiety-related disorders by causing longer-lasting neuronal changes in the amygdala, possibly via the 5-HT2C receptor [7].

The noradrenergic system has been hypothesised to be 'hyperactive' in anxiety disorders as it is an important neurotransmitter in the autonomic nervous system. However, consistent evidence for such hyperactivity has only been found in panic disorder [8].

The gamma-aminobutyric acid (GABA) system is the most important inhibitory neurotransmitter system, and is strongly linked with the pathophysiology of anxiety disorders. Of the GABA receptor subtypes, GABA-A seems to be particularly linked with anxiety: the fast inhibitory action of GABA is mediated through this receptor; it includes the binding site of benzodiazepines, which enhance the actions of GABA; and negative GABA-A modulators produce anxiogenic-like effects [8]. Glutamate is the main excitatory neurotransmitter, and it is possible that a mismatch between glutamatergic and

GABAergic neurotransmission is important in the pathogenesis of anxiety disorders.

Endogenous opioids are also important in anxiety regulation. Evidence for altered opioidergic transmission has mainly been found in patients with panic disorder or specific phobia, suggesting a role in fear-related disorders. Endogenous opioid transmission appears to be important for the effectiveness of behavioural treatment in specific phobia [9]. It is thought that endogenous opioid activity might regulate panic states, but results from studies of the relationship between panic and endogenous opioid levels have been mixed [9]. Nevertheless, opioid peptides and receptors are located in brain areas involved in emotional regulation and in brainstem areas such as the periaqueductal grey matter. It is possible that opioidergic influence on anxiety is mediated through interactions with other neurotransmitter systems: opioid pathways have reciprocal connections with GABAergic interneurons, and endogenous opioid release is controlled by serotonin activation [9]. As with depression, opioid agonists and partial agonists might be investigated as potential medications for anxiety disorders in future.

There is accumulating research implicating neuropeptides in anxiety disorders. These include orexin and oxytocin [8]. Orexin is a hypothalamic peptide and orexin neurons innervate limbic structures; they are activated in response to emotionally salient stimuli and lead to excitation of noradrenergic neurons and so modulate emotional response [10]. There is evidence that orexin-1 receptor antagonist may be a potential treatment for panic disorder. Oxytocin might attenuate anxiety in social anxiety disorder and separation anxiety disorder [8].

9.4.3 Genetic Predispositions to Anxiety Disorders

9.4.3.1 Common Genetic Variants
Cross-sectional and longitudinal studies show much 'comorbidity' between anxiety disorders, and there may be common genetic predispositions. In a meta-analysis of European GWAS studies, the rs1709393 allele on the intron of non-coding RNA locus *LOC152225* on chromosome 3q12.3 was found to be associated with lifetime diagnosis of generalised anxiety disorder, social anxiety disorder, panic disorder, agoraphobia and specific phobias [11]. Polymorphisms in the serotonergic and catecholaminergic systems have been linked to generalised anxiety disorder [12].

9.4.3.2 Neurotic Personality Subtype
'Neuroticism' is a personality dimension that characterises trait propensity to negative thoughts and emotion. A high genetic correlation has been found between generalised anxiety disorder and neuroticism, estimated at 0.80 across genders [13]. The neurobiology of neuroticism is increasingly understood. Functional imaging has shown decreased functional connectivity in the amygdala and cingulate cortex and altered connectivity in the default-mode network (involved in episodic memory and semantic processing) [14]. Therefore, there is an overlap between the areas of the brain involved in neuroticism and anxiety. Enhanced understanding of neuroticism might contribute to knowledge of an individual's likelihood of developing an anxiety disorder, and therefore its prevention.

9.4.4 Anxiety Disorders across the Lifespan
The prevalence of different anxiety disorder subtypes changes over the life course. Phobias predominate in childhood. Panic disorder is most common in adolescence and early adulthood as autonomic responses change with age. Although separation anxiety disorder was initially thought to be an exclusively childhood disorder, it is increasingly understood to affect adults as well. Generalised anxiety disorder is most common in older age and this may be linked to neurodegeneration causing reduced connectivity within the brain [15].

9.4.5 Inflammation
The majority of anxiety research (at the cellular-neuroscience level) has focused upon neurons and neurotransmitters. However, research into depression and psychosis provides increasing evidence for a potential role for inflammation in the disease pathology (see Section 6.4). There is a small amount of evidence that inflammation may also play a role in anxiety. Generalised anxiety disorder has been associated with raised levels of

C-reactive protein and panic disorder may be associated with raised peripheral inflammation. Although research so far has focused on peripheral inflammation, it is likely that the immune system within the brain (involving astrocytes and microglia) is also involved. Thus far, anti-inflammatory medication has shown limited efficacy; improved understanding of a role for inflammation in anxiety could allow novel drug treatments to be developed [16].

Conclusions and Outstanding Questions

Neurobiological treatments for anxiety disorders are presently not optimal, as many patients do not respond to first-line therapies or experience unwanted side effects. Development of novel therapies and interventions requires a good understanding of the underlying neurobiology of these disorders. However, the neurobiology driving anxiety disorders is complex and remains poorly understood, as we have discussed in this section. Future work aimed at further characterising the aetiopathophysiology of these disorders is vital.

Outstanding Questions

- Can we further delineate the genetic and epigenetic factors that predispose to developing anxiety disorders? Will these factors indicate novel neurobiological mechanisms underpinning anxiety disorders?

- How do neurotransmitters such as serotonin and neuropeptides such as orexin or endogenous opioids interact in anxiety disorders? Could these neuropeptides be therapeutic targets?

- How does the neurobiology of anxiety disorders change across the lifespan? Could there be different treatment targets in different age groups?

9

REFERENCES

1. World Health Organization. *International Classification of Diseases*, 11th ed. (ICD-11). World Health Organization, 2018,

2. Fox AS, Oler JA, Tromp do PM et al. Extending the amygdala in theories of threat processing. *Trends Neurosci* 2015; 38: 319–329.

3. Mochcovitch MD, da Rocha Freire RC, Garcia RF et al. A systematic review of fMRI studies in generalized anxiety disorder: evaluating its neural and cognitive basis. *J Affect Disord* 2014; 167: 336–342.

4. Davis M. The role of the amygdala in fear and anxiety. *Annu Rev Neurosci* 1992; 15: 353–375.

5. Corchs F, Nutt DJ, Hince DA et al. Evidence for serotonin function as a neurochemical difference between fear and anxiety disorders in humans? *J Psychopharmacol* 2015; 29: 1061–1069.

6. Bandelow B, Baldwin D, Abelli M et al. Biological markers for anxiety disorders, OCD and PTSD – a consensus statement. Part I: neuroimaging and genetics. *World J Biol Psychiatry* 2016; 17: 321–365.

7. Deakin J. The origins of '5-HT and mechanisms of defence' by Deakin and Graeff: a personal perspective. *J Psychopharmacol* 2013; 27: 1084–1089.

8. Bandelow B, Baldwin D, Abelli M et al. Biological markers for anxiety disorders, OCD and PTSD: a consensus statement. Part II: neurochemistry, neurophysiology and neurocognition. *World J Biol Psychiatry* 2017; 18: 162–214.

9. Colasanti A, Rabiner E, Lingford-Hughes A et al. Opioids and anxiety. *J Psychopharmacol* 2011; 25: 1415–1433.

10. Soya S, Sakurai T. Orexin as a modulator of fear-related behavior: hypothalamic control of noradrenaline circuit. *Brain Res* 2020; 1731: 146037.

11. Otowa T, Hek K, Lee M et al. Meta-analysis of genome-wide association studies of anxiety disorders. *Mol Psychiatry* 2016; 21: 1391.

12. Gottschalk MG, Domschke K. Genetics of generalized anxiety disorder and related traits. *Dialogues Clin Neurosci* 2017; 19: 159.

13. Hettema JM, Prescott CA, Kendler KS. Genetic and environmental sources of covariation between generalized anxiety disorder and neuroticism. *Am J Psychiatry* 2004; 161: 1581–1587.

14. Gentili C, Cristea IA, Ricciardi E et al. Not in one metric: neuroticism modulates different resting state metrics within distinctive brain regions. *Behav Brain Res* 2017; 327: 34–43.

15. Lenze EJ, Wetherell JL. A lifespan view of anxiety disorders. *Dialogues Clin Neurosci* 2011; 13: 381.

16. Baldwin DS, Hou R, Gordon R et al. Pharmacotherapy in generalized anxiety disorder: novel experimental medicine models and emerging drug targets. *CNS Drugs* 2017; 31: 307–317.

National Neuroscience Curriculum Initiative online resources

The Parable of Panic: Suffocation, Social Attachment, and the Critical Role of an Integrative, Biopsychosocial Formulation

Andrew M. Novick and David A. Ross

What to say: The Parable of Panic: *Suffocation, Social Attachment, and The Critical Role of an Integrative, Biopsychosocial Formulation*

9

<table>
<tr><td>**9.5**</td><td>**Post-Traumatic Stress Disorder**</td><td>Eric Vermetten</td></tr>
</table>

OVERVIEW

Psychological trauma is different from ordinary stressors, and has been defined as 'experiencing, witnessing, or being confronted with an event or events that involved actual or threatened death or serious injury, or a threat to the physical integrity of self or others' (American Psychiatric Association, 2013). These events can leave the individual with intense terror, fear and paralysing helplessness. They can also disrupt the integrity of a person, and the sense that the world is predictable and safe. In a majority of exposures there is a gradual return to daily life with no residual symptoms. If symptoms persist or start to manifest and are related to the so called 'index trauma', the diagnosis of post-traumatic stress disorder (PTSD) can be made. Over time, the events qualifying for traumatic stress have been extensively debated. Prior and cumulative effects of trauma exposure are a particularly important determinant of risk for PTSD.

The fact that PTSD was not officially recognised as a diagnosis earlier than 1980 probably contributes to the persistent deficit in drugs targeting PTSD-specific symptoms. It was first included in the DSM-III, 40 years ago (American Psychiatric Association, 1980), but only recently have large-scale trajectory analyses yielded information on risk markers defined at multiple phenotypic levels. PTSD affects multiple biological systems such as brain circuitry and neurochemistry, and cellular, immune, endocrine and metabolic function. There is a need for algorithms that predict individual trajectories in responses to traumatic stress by incorporating genetic factors, sex-specific profiles, brain developmental processes, cumulative biological and psychological effects of early childhood (e.g. 'vulnerable' phenotype) and other lifetime stressful events, as well as social factors that promote resilience (Kim and Uddin, 2020; Vermetten and McFarlane, 2020; Burback et al., 2023).

9.5.1 Epidemiology

9.5.1.1 Prevalence
A 'potential traumatic experience or event' in the phenomenological pure sense of the word is: a direct threat to one's own life or that of a loved one, accompanied by horror, helplessness and intense fear. On average, one-third of those who are exposed develop complaints of stress after the trauma, and a minority (ranging from 5% to 15%) develop PTSD. Yet, even if only a minority of trauma-exposed individuals develops PTSD, it is one of the most prevalent psychiatric diseases worldwide (Kessler et al., 2017). There is no fixed incubation period between exposure and the occurrence of complaints. This can vary from a few weeks to many years.

9.5.1.2 Predictors and Risk Factors
An important predictor for the occurrence of PTSD is the relationship of the potential traumatic experience to personal distance, with a dose–response relationship dependent on the extent of the threat to one's own physical integrity; the predictive value of being raped for developing PTSD is about four times greater than that of witnessing a rape. Other predictors include genetic vulnerability, early childhood trauma, female gender, previous hospitalisation, involvement of children, the perceived (duration of the) threat, the duration of

peritraumatic dissociation and absence of social support or aftercare (Brewin et al., 2000).

Recently reported genetic association studies indicate that the effects contributing to the disorder may be mediated, in part, by gene–environment interactions involving polymorphisms within two key genes, *CRHR1* (corticotropin-releasing hormone receptor 1) and *FKBP5*, which regulates responsiveness of steroid hormone receptors that play a role in stress. Data suggest that these genes regulate hypothalamic–pituitary–adrenal (HPA) axis function in conjunction with exposure to child maltreatment or abuse (Mehta and Binder, 2012). In addition, a large and growing body of preclinical research (i.e. research in animals) suggests that increased activity of the amygdala–HPA axis induced by experimental manipulation of the amygdala mimics several of the physiological and behavioural symptoms of stress-related psychiatric illness in humans. Notably, interactions between the developing amygdala and HPA axis underlie critical periods for emotional learning, which are modulated by developmental support and maternal care. These translational findings support an integrated hypothesis: high levels of early-life trauma lead to disease through the developmental interaction of genetic variants with neural circuits that regulate emotion, together mediating risk and resilience in adults (Ressler, 2020).

9.5.2 Clinical Features of PTSD

PTSD can be diagnosed, given an index trauma, after 4 weeks of a combination of rather heterogeneous symptoms, which include: involuntary intrusions, often in the form of nightmares or flashbacks during the day; persistent attempts to avoid stimuli associated with the trauma; a blunting of general, normal human reactions; avoidance of feelings and memories; the impossibility of remembering aspects of the trauma; a reduced interest in important activities; feelings of detachment or alienation; the limited ability to express affect; the experience of a limited future; changes in cognition and mood that are related to the traumatic event, and that have since worsened; increased irritability (difficulty falling asleep, accompanied by irritability); feelings of helplessness, fear and horror; excessive vigilance; memory and concentration problems; and excessive shock reactions (American Psychiatric Association, 2013). These symptoms have focused scientific interest in this area

on stress regulation, memory processing, emotional regulation and maintenance of consciousness.

PTSD shows considerable comorbidity with other psychiatric disorders, most commonly depressive disorder and substance dependence (mainly in men). PTSD also increases the risk of cardiovascular and metabolic problems. Stress-axis disruption in the presence of increased sympathetic and decreased parasympathetic tone can also contribute to inflammation and to effects on brain areas that are crucial for the regulation of anxiety (such as the prefrontal cortex, insula, amygdala and hippocampus).

The specific diagnostic symptom clusters included in DSM-5 include intrusion symptoms, avoidance symptoms, symptoms of negative cognition or mood, and altered arousal. The DSM-5 diagnostic criteria for PTSD include acute, chronic and delayed onset forms of the disorder (American Psychiatric Association, 2013). However, the diagnostic pattern of symptoms is the same for each type of PTSD despite emerging evidence from network analyses that the internal structure and linkage or clustering of symptoms change with the passage of time. This limitation of phenomenological definitions of psychiatric disorders in general has been raised as a significant deficiency as it does not address the fluidity of the phenomenology of a disorder across time, particularly as it changes in the earlier stages of the disorder. It also takes no account of the secondary phenomena, which represent adaptations or consequences of the primary symptoms.

9.5.3 Neurobiological and Psychobiological Mechanisms

The pathophysiology of PTSD can be linked to not one but several neurobiological mechanisms related to traumatic stress. Preclinical studies that investigated the effects of stress on neural processes such as learning and memory retention were initially used to model PTSD as humans experience it. These studies suggested that an altered fear response mechanism, behavioural sensitisation and failure of the extinction of fear play an important role in the pathophysiology of PTSD (Charney et al., 1993; Yehuda et al., 2015). A fourth process identified as impaired in PTSD and proposed in the recent Research Domain Criteria description of PTSD is maintenance of consciousness, which can be seen in trauma-related and altered states of consciousness and dissociation (Schmidt and Vermetten, 2018). These neuro- or psychobiological mechanisms are briefly described below.

9.5.3.1 Behavioural Sensitisation (Enhanced Stress Sensitivity)

Insomnia, poor concentration, hypervigilance and exaggerated startle response are traits related to the increased susceptibility to stress (sensitisation) seen in patients with PTSD. 'Sensitisation' may be defined as an increase in a certain response due to the presentation of a specific stimulus. In military veterans with PTSD, for example, a traumatic event, or series of events they witnessed, is thought to cause the onset of PTSD (Stam, 2007). Patients become more aroused and hypervigilant, among other characteristics, than do healthy individuals when presented with trauma-related stimuli. It is the experience or recurrent experience of trauma that facilitates or sensitises this process. It is therefore possible to state that PTSD is a certain type of behavioural sensitisation, in which trauma exposure causes the onset of increased stress sensitivity. Although few human subject studies have investigated these symptoms on a neurobiological level, more advances have been made in preclinical settings.

The neural circuitry underlying the increased sensitivity to stress cannot be localised to a specific anatomical or functional neurological component. In patients with PTSD, the (over)sensitisation is most apparent in the structures and mechanisms involved in the stress response. For example, in PTSD, cells in the pituitary and hypothalamus are thought to be sensitised to glucocorticoid receptor signalling (Yehuda et al., 2015), making them more susceptible to the effects of stress. In peripheral blood white cells (used as they are easily accessible), methods for assessing HPA axis function include measuring the expression of the glucocorticoid receptor and testing the extent to which dexamethasone can inhibit the cellular proliferation of T cells *in vitro* (such inhibition is a normal physiological function of glucocorticoids). Interestingly, trauma exposure alone, without PTSD, is sufficient to induce at least some changes in glucocorticoid function. For example, in a study comparing veterans with PTSD, traumatised veterans without PTSD and healthy controls, trauma exposure alone was found to alter peripheral blood cell glucocorticoid receptor binding characteristics, whereas resistance of T-cell proliferation

to dexamethasone only occurred in PTSD (de Kloet et al., 2007). See Sections 6.2 and 6.3 for more background on stress and glucocorticoids.

9.5.3.2 Fear Conditioning

One of the most characteristic features of PTSD is that 'anxiogenic' memories (e.g. of the traumatic experience) can remain, seemingly indelible for years or decades without causing problems, and then can be reawakened by various sorts of stimuli and stressors (see Liberzon and Sripada, 2007). The strength of traumatic memories relates, in part, to the degree to which certain neuromodulatory systems, particularly catecholamines and glucocorticoids, are activated by the traumatic experience at the time of the trauma. Release of these stress hormones promotes the encoding of memories of the stressful event. Long-term alterations in these catecholaminergic and glucocorticoid systems may also be responsible for symptoms of fragmentation of memories, but also for hyperamnesia (enhancement of memory), amnesia, deficits in declarative memory, delayed recall and other aspects of the wide range of memory distortions in anxiety and traumatic stress-related disorders. Experimental and clinical investigations provide evidence that memory processes remain susceptible to modulating influences after information has been acquired. The brain mechanisms by which sensory representations (such as colors, objects or individuals) are selected for episodic encoding are not fully understood. It is thought that, with long-term storage, memories are shifted from the hippocampus to the neocortical areas, as the neocortex gradually comes to support stable long-term storage (see Section 5.14 for more on memory). The shift in memory storage to the cortex may represent a shift from conscious representational memory to unconscious memory processes that indirectly affect behaviour. 'Traumatic cues' such as a particular sight or sound reminiscent of the original traumatic event will trigger a cascade of anxiety and fear-related symptoms, often without conscious recall of the original traumatic event. In patients with PTSD, however, the traumatic stimulus is always potentially identifiable. In contrast, in panic or phobic disorder patients, symptoms of anxiety may be related to fear responses to a traumatic cue (in individuals who are vulnerable to increased fear responsiveness), even where there is no possibility that the original fear-inducing stimulus will ever be identified.

Thus, patients with PTSD have symptoms that reflect a more or less continuous perception of threat with unconsciously processed fear responses (see Vermetten et al., 2007). The animal model of contextual fear conditioning represents a good model for these symptoms. In this paradigm, an animal is introduced to a new environment (the conditioned stimulus), then after a few minutes given an electric foot shock (the unconditioned stimulus), such that on later returning to that environment it will show the characteristic fear behaviour of freezing. Preclinical data suggest that the hippocampus (as well as the bed nucleus of the stria terminalis (BNST) and periaquaeductal grey) plays an important role in contextual fear, and that increased responding to conditioned stimuli is due to hippocampal dysfunction. Hippocampal atrophy in PTSD therefore provides a possible neuroanatomical substrate for abnormal contextual fear conditioning and chronic symptoms of feelings of threat and anxiety. Interestingly, in light of studies showing abnormal noradrenergic function in PTSD, the BNST has some of the densest noradrenergic innervation of any area in the brain.

The startle reflex has been used to study fear conditioning in PTSD in humans. Startle is a useful method for examining fear responding in both animals and humans and is mediated by the amygdala and connected structures. Damage to the amygdala does not prevent patients from learning the relationship between the conditioned and the unconditioned stimuli, but it abolishes conditioned autonomic responses. In contrast, damage to the hippocampus does not affect conditioned autonomic responses, but does prevent learning of the conditioned stimulus–unconditioned stimulus association.

9.5.3.3 Failure of Extinction

The process of fear extinction is closely linked to the conditioning of fear. When a person is exposed to a normally dangerous situation from which no aversive events result, this situation elicits a smaller fear response than before – as the process is repeated, this leads to smaller and smaller responses. This is called extinction. Unconscious emotional processes affect this process – for example patients with anxiety disorders show greater resistance to extinction of conditioned responses to angry facial expressions, but not to neutral facial expressions, compared with controls. In patients with PTSD, extinction does not occur efficiently, and fear of certain situations fails to be extinguished. In

military veterans this may be identified by persistent, fearful responses to large, noisy crowds, fireworks and doors slamming, among other forms of traumatic recall (Milad et al., 2009). Therefore, some permanence in fear conditioning in patients is due to a dysfunction in the extinction of fear. Ultimately, this can be the cause of the persistence of the traumatic memories. The neural mechanisms involved in the extinction of fear greatly overlap with those involved in fear acquisition, as just described. It is hypothesised that in delayed onset cases of PTSD topics of guilt and shame may be dominant drivers of the symptomatology, with less of an amygdalocentric focus (Lanius et al., 2010a)

The main structures involved in the extinction of fear are the medial prefrontal cortex and the amygdala (Quirk et al., 2006). N-methyl-D-aspartate (NMDA) receptors and voltage-gated calcium channels are essential to extinction processes (Charney, 2004). Other systems include the neurotransmitters GABA, noradrenaline and dopamine. During a fearful response of the amygdala, the medial prefrontal cortex is activated and attempts to regulate the initial response to the threat so that fear is contained and managed appropriately. If this prefrontal activation is absent, or occurs to a lesser extent, the amygdala does not receive sufficient inhibitory feedback, resulting in higher autonomic arousal and exaggerated responses. The amygdala–medial prefrontal cortex connection (feedback process) is thought to be mediated by GABA interneurons, which may be malfunctioning in PTSD, as evidenced by a reduction in GABA-A receptor binding in the medial prefrontal cortex (Geuze et al., 2008).

Numerous studies have also examined the psychophysiology and neuroendocrine status of patients with chronic PTSD. Psychophysiological studies demonstrated autonomic reactivity manifested by increased heart rate and skin conductance in response to trauma-related cues, and exaggerated startle responses. These findings recapitulated symptoms of general hyperarousal and distress following traumatic reminders in PTSD.

9.5.3.4 Trauma-Related Dissociation and Altered States of Consciousness

Neuroimaging studies have implicated decreased activity of prefrontal regions and increased activity of limbic structures in the pathophysiology of PTSD (Francati et al., 2007; Sartory et al., 2013). Interestingly, however, studies have shown that psychobiological responses to recalling

9

traumatic experiences can differ significantly among individuals with PTSD and that not all PTSD patients show the same brain activation patterns in response to traumatic script-driven imagery. Lanius and colleagues (2002) found that approximately 70% of PTSD patients reported reliving their traumatic experience in response to traumatic scripts, also showing an increase in heart rate. The other 30% of PTSD subjects reported experiences of derealisation, depersonalisation and a feeling of emotional detachment and did not show a significant increase in heart rate when exposed to a traumatic script. Thus, similarly to the epidemiological studies discussed above, neurobiological studies have identified a dissociative subtype of PTSD that can be distinguished from non-dissociative PTSD. Moreover, these non-dissociative and dissociative response types have been associated with opposite patterns of activity in brain regions involved in arousal and emotion regulation. Patients who relived their traumatic experiences upon exposure to traumatic scripts showed less activation of the medial prefrontal cortex, anterior cingulate and thalamus during script-driven recall of traumatic events (Lanius et al., 2010b). This is consistent with the decreased prefrontal activation that most PTSD neuroimaging studies to date have reported. However, PTSD patients in a dissociative state showed more activation in the medial prefrontal cortex, anterior cingulate, medial frontal gyrus, inferior frontal gyrus, superior and middle temporal gyri, occipital lobe and parietal lobe during symptom provocation compared to control subjects (Lanius et al., 2002). Thus, although patients with re-experiencing/hyperaroused PTSD exhibit lower activation of prefrontal regions that are implicated in arousal modulation and emotion regulation, dissociative PTSD patients show higher activation of these prefrontal regions. The corticolimbic model of dissociation postulates that, once a threshold of anxiety is reached, the medial prefrontal cortex inhibits emotional processing in limbic structures, resulting in dissociative symptoms. Furthermore, there are indications that dissociation is associated with activity in the temporal lobes and insular cortex and an increase in prefrontal cortex volume. It has been proposed that dissociation is a regulatory strategy to restrain extreme arousal in PTSD through hyperinhibition of limbic regions.

Repeated and prolonged exposure to potential traumatic experiences can lead to a pattern of emotional disruption on a range of dimensions, as opposed to a single trauma (so-called type I trauma) in which fear typically is the more central problem. Chronic traumatisation (so-called type II trauma) is more often associated with attachment problems, a disturbed affect, and dissociation as an important coping strategy. The main issues here are disturbances in affect regulation, alterations in consciousness, changes in self-perception, changes in the perception of the other/perpetrator, changes in relationships with others and changes in meaning. These patients often describe not feeling, not remembering, not knowing oneself and as if 'it concerned someone else'. These so-called dissociative responses can be seen in part as an inevitable coping style, but possibly also as a serious consequence of chronic overloading of various neuronal systems. Traumatic stress and traumatic dissociation are known to be associated with a range of symptoms and conditions in PTSD, but also in depression, somatisation, substance abuse and eating disorders. It is proposed that peritraumatic dissociation results in insufficient encoding of the trauma memory and that persistent dissociation prevents memory elaboration, resulting in memory fragmentation and PTSD (Lanius et al., 2012).

In summary, two distinct response types in PTSD subjects exist: a re-experiencing/hyperaroused subtype and a dissociative subtype. These response types are characterised by different psychophysiological and neural responses to the recall of traumatic memories (see Table 9.5.1 and Figure 9.5.1).

A more comprehensive model of PTSD neurocircuitry acknowledges the interaction of three other systems beyond the frontolimbic circuits in PTSD: the default-mode network, salience network and central executive network. The default-mode network plays a key role in self-related processes, emotion regulation, social cognition, autobiographical memory and future oriented thinking. The salience network is involved in the detection of personally salient internal and external stimuli in order to direct behaviour with the goal of maintaining homeostasis. The central executive network is critical to working memory and cognitive control of thought, emotion and behaviour. Fluctuations in the activity of these circuits may explain how people with PTSD shift into dramatically different states in an attempt to regulate their extreme emotional responses to cues or trains of thought (see Yehuda et al., 2015; Shalev et al., 2017).

Table 9.5.1 Overview of features that distinguish dissociative PTSD form non-dissociative PTSD

	Dissociative PTSD	**Non-dissociative PTSD**
Epidemiology	More severe PTSD symptoms, complex, chronic	More often associated with trauma in adult life
	Associated with early-life trauma/repetitive trauma	Less cumulative trauma
	Higher level of comorbid psychiatric disorders	
Reaction after exposure to traumatic stimuli	Dissociation, numbing	Fear/anxiety-driven
	Suppression of autonomic response	Increased autonomic arousal
	No increase in heart rate	Increased heart rate
	No increase in skin conductance	Increased skin conductance
Phenomenology	Dissociation	Re-experiencing
Imaging	Anterior cingulate cortex ↑	Anterior cingulate cortex ↓
	Medial prefrontal cortex ↑	Medial prefrontal cortex ↓
	Amygdala ↓	Amygdala ↑
	Right anterior insula ↓	Right anterior insula ↑
Concept	Emotional overmodulation	Emotional undermodulation

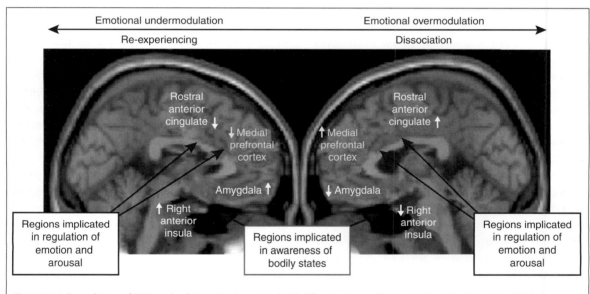

Figure 9.5.1 Two subtypes of PTSD can be distinguished, associated with different patterns of brain activation. Non-dissociative PTSD is associated with re-experiencing of trauma and emotional undermodulation; dissociative PTSD is associated with emotional overmodulation.

9.5.4 Neuroscience-Based Treatment Strategies

Trauma-focused psychotherapy and pharmacotherapy are first-line treatment options, but often must be combined with management of comorbid medical problems, such as chronic pain or sleep disturbance. PTSD treatment guidelines have unequivocally designated psychotherapy as a first-line treatment. There is an urgent need to discover novel compounds and new treatment strategies for PTSD. Despite demonstrations of numerous neurobiological alterations in PTSD, there are few medications with demonstrated efficacy for this disorder.

9.5.4.1 Psychological Treatments

Exposure-based or trauma-focused treatment is still advised as 'gold standard' (Rauch et al., 2012). Exposure means exposure to traumatic memories and the accompanying feelings and thoughts. The neuroscientific concepts rely on fear extinction, stimulus desensitisation as well as reconsolidation of new learning. This is not an easy or simple procedure and is often associated with cognitive avoidance or therapeutic resistance. Typically, this is done over time courses of several sessions of one specific therapeutic modality, over several months, and contains phases of **psychoeducation**, **emotional stabilisation**, **working through** and **closure**. Other potentially effective therapies include imagery rehearsal, brief psychodynamic therapy and hypnosis. Psychoeducation and supportive interventions are also important components of therapy.

The specific methods used, which have much in common, include: eye movement desensitisation and reprocessing (EMDR), cognitive behavioural therapy, prolonged exposure, narrative exposure therapy (NET) and brief eclectic psychotherapy for PTSD (BEPP) (Schnyder et al., 2015; Watkins et al., 2018). With EMDR the aim is to uncouple the traumatic event(s) and the associated emotions, so that the memory of the event(s) and the associated context are experienced as less emotionally stressful. EMDR is especially useful in single trauma and in the situation when the trauma is treated shortly after exposure. Exposure in combination with an explicit external focus of attention leads to larger PTSD symptom reduction than exposure alone. Eye movements have no advantage compared to visually fixating on a non-moving hand. Novel forms of psychotherapy, such as motion-assisted multi-modular memory desensitisation and reconsolidation, are used where motion is introduced as a way to bypass cognitive avoidance and increase openness (Nijdam and Vermetten, 2018). Third-wave cognitive behavioural therapies are increasingly used, with mindfulness therapies and acceptance and commitment therapies. New developments in immersion and virtual reality exposure therapy are also gradually starting to be used (Deng et al., 2019; Emmelkamp and Meyerbroker, 2021). Rituals can be very important; mourning rituals, writing letters, literally burying memories or commemorating through annual festivals. Particular attention is paid to this at BEPP, but also at NET. Rituals can channel an unprocessed emotion, give meaning and thereby promote social coherence. So-called non-verbal therapies (psychomotor therapy, yoga and other body-focused therapies) are also increasingly popular, but these have still not been adequately studied in scientific research.

However, exposure treatments should be used with caution in patients with significant emotional overmodulation, such as dissociative and numbing symptoms. Such symptoms can prevent emotional engagement with trauma-related information and thereby reduce treatment effectiveness. Grouping all PTSD patients into the same diagnostic category may hinder proper understanding of post-traumatic psychopathology.

9.5.4.2 Pharmacotherapies

Medication is typically used to support the psychological approaches to treatment outlined above. Evidence for neurobiological dysfunction in PTSD, such as dysregulation of both main arms of the stress response system, the HPA axis and the locus coeruleus–noradrenaline system, as well as dysfunctional responses of other neurotransmitter systems, including serotonin, gamma-aminobutyric acid (GABA) and glutamate, suggest a role for pharmacotherapeutic interventions in the treatment of PTSD; however, data obtained from randomised controlled trials still suggest limited efficacy (Stein et al., 2006; Williams et al., 2022).

Of the approved pharmacotherapeutic options for PTSD, selective serotonin reuptake inhibitors (SSRIs), tricyclic antidepressant medication and monoamine oxidase inhibitors have been evaluated in placebo-controlled trials. Although all of these are effective as antidepressant medication, and also show some anxiolytic and antipanic effects, it is important to realise that their effectiveness in PTSD is not simply mediated through improvement in anxiety and depression, that is, PTSD symptoms respond independently from the anxiolytic or antidepressant effect. Tricyclic antidepressant medication has modestly beneficial effects on hyperarousal and re-experiencing, but not on avoidance and numbing symptoms. Monoamine oxidase inhibitors appear somewhat more effective than tricyclics, and affect mainly intrusion/re-experiencing and sometimes avoidance symptoms.

Both categories are associated with broad side-effect profiles, and drop-out rates are consequently high. SSRIs have a more favourable side-effect profile, also have some anxiolytic properties and are more effective in reducing all three PTSD symptom clusters. They therefore currently form the first-line psychopharmacological treatment option for PTSD.

Classic anxiolytic medications have not been as extensively tested in PTSD. Benzodiazepines have not proved to be very effective, and are also problematic because of the development of dependence and subsequent withdrawal symptoms, which may actually exacerbate PTSD symptoms (Guina et al., 2015).

Antiadrenergic drugs (such as alpha-2 agonists or beta blockers) have received very little attention in clinical trials, despite evidence for adrenergic dysregulation in PTSD. The alpha-adrenergic blocker prazosin has been shown to alleviate sleep disturbance caused by nightmares in several studies (see Raskind et al., 2018; Hendrickson et al., 2021). Some authors recommended starting pharmacotherapy in new PTSD patients with an antiadrenergic agent such as clonidine or propranolol early after exposure. Also, clonidine can be effective in this respect, where the reduced adrenergic activity is often accompanied by a reduction in dissociative symptoms (Philipsen et al., 2004; Friedman, 2016).

9.5.4.3 Medication-Assisted Psychotherapies

New developments include agents such as ketamine, oxytocin, propanolol and D-cycloserine. These have as yet only anecdotal support, and some are used in low doses or as adjunct to psychotherapy, but more research is required. The compound methylenedioxymethamphetamine (MDMA) is seen as very promising as a catalyst within the context of psychotherapy (Mitchell et al., 2021). MDMA may serve as a serotonergic (5-HT2A) receptor enhancer that modulates mesolimbic dopamine activity, mediating oxytocin release, stimulated by 5-HT1A receptors (Thompson et al., 2007). How its mechanism of action affects fear extinction, mood enhancement or other pro-social processes still needs to be better understood. One hypothesis is that MDMA may interfere with storage (or reconsolidation) of traumatic memories that are reactivated during therapeutic sessions (van Elk and Yaden, 2022; Godes et al., 2023).

Conclusions and Outstanding Questions

Despite various guidelines and evidence-based interventions, approximately two-thirds of all patients do not respond adequately to an evidence-based intervention and do not achieve symptomatic recovery in the longer term (Kitchine et al., 2019). New interventions are therefore very much needed (see Burback et al., 2023).

There is a need for precision psychiatry driven by clinical neurosciences. Simple reductionist models do not fit well with the clinical reality, nor do they adequately address 'illness' – the patient's experience of the problem, which implies subjective suffering. Moreover, in a heterogeneous condition such as PTSD it is important to account for an array of individual differences. Since there are 65,000 ways of diagnosing PTSD, there may be an equal number of ways to deliver therapies (Galatzer-Levy et al., 2013). As rigorous as scientific approaches need to be, it is impossible to fit all patients into one model.

Outstanding Questions

- There is convincing evidence on PTSD symptom trajectories that several phenotypes of the disorder can be distinguished, supporting a staging typology of PTSD (i.e. multiple illness stages, as seen elsewhere in medicine). How can knowledge of these stages facilitate the selection of interventions that are proportionate to patients' current needs and risk of illness progression, facilitate interpretation of biomarker data and guide service delivery (McFarlane et al., 2017; Nijdam et al., 2023)?

- What is the relation between moral injurious distress and the role of guilt and shame as drivers for chronicity of PTSD (Vermetten and Jetly, 2018; Vermetten et al., 2023)? Accumulating evidence suggests a link between transgression of moral values and symptoms of guilt and shame, anger, suicidal ideation and PTSD in military servicemen and veterans (Koenig et al., 2019), as well as in healthcare workers (Griffin et al., 2019).

- Prediction of responses to traumatic stress is a holy grail since this may help secondary prevention and contribute to fostering resilience (Vermetten and McFarlane, 2020). Can neuroscience improve algorithms of phenotypic response patterns to help predict individual trajectories following traumatic stress?

9

REFERENCES

American Psychiatric Association (1980). *Diagnostic and Statistical Manual of Mental Disorders*, 3rd ed. (DSM-3). American Psychiatric Association

American Psychiatric Association (2013). *Diagnostic and Statistical Manual of Mental Disorders*, 5th ed. (DSM-5). American Psychiatric Association,

Brewin, C. R., Andrews, B., Valentine, J. D. (2000). Meta-analysis of risk factors for posttraumatic stress disorder in trauma-exposed adults. *Journal of Consulting and Clinical Psychology* 68(5): 748.

Burback, L., Brémault-Phillips, S., Nijdam, M. J., McFarlane, A., Vermetten, E. (2023). Treatment of posttraumatic stress disorder: a state-of-the-art review. *Current Neuropharmacology*: doi 10.2174/1570159X21666230428091433.

Charney, D. S. (2004). Psychobiological mechanisms of resilience and vulnerability: implications for successful adaptation to extreme stress. *American Journal of Psychiatry*, 161(2), 195–216.

Charney, D. S., Deutch, A. Y., Krystal, J. H., Southwick, S. M., Davis, M. (1993). Psychobiologic mechanisms of post-traumatic stress disorder. *Archives of General Psychiatry* 50(4): 294–305.

Deng, W., Hu, D., Xu, S. et al. (2019). The efficacy of virtual reality exposure therapy for PTSD symptoms: a systematic review and meta-analysis. *Journal of Affective Disorders* 257: 698–709.

Emmelkamp, P. M., Meyerbröker, K. (2021). Virtual reality therapy in mental health. *Annual Review of Clinical Psychology* 17: 495–519.

Francati, V., Vermetten, E., Bremner, J. D. (2007). Functional neuroimaging studies in posttraumatic stress disorder: review of current methods and findings. *Depression and Anxiety* 24(3): 202–218.

Friedman, M. J. (2016). Adrenergic mediation of dissociative symptoms in posttraumatic stress disorder. *Journal of Clinical Psychiatry* 77(4): 548–549.

Galatzer-Levy, I. R., Bryant, R. A. (2013). 636,120 ways to have posttraumatic stress disorder. *Perspectives on Psychological Science* 8(6), 651–662.

Geuze, E., Van Berckel, B. N. M., Lammertsma, A. A. et al. (2008). Reduced GABA A benzodiazepine receptor binding in veterans with post-traumatic stress disorder. *Molecular Psychiatry* 13(1): 74–83.

Godes, M., Lucas, J., Vermetten, E. (2023). Perceived key change phenomena of MDMA-assisted psychotherapy for the treatment of severe PTSD: an interpretative phenomenological analysis of clinical integration sessions. *Frontiers in Psychiatry* 14.

Griffin, B. J., Purcell, N., Burkman, K. et al. (2019). Moral injury: an integrative review. *Journal of Traumatic Stress* 32(3): 350–362.

Guina, J., Rossetter, S. R., DeRhodes, B. J., Nahhas, R. W., Welton, R. S. (2015). Benzodiazepines for PTSD: a systematic review and meta-analysis. *Journal of Psychiatric Practice* 21(4): 281–303.

Hendrickson, R. C., Millard, S. P., Pagulayan, K. F., Peskind, E. R., Raskind, M. A. (2021). The relative effects of prazosin on individual PTSD symptoms: evidence for pathophysiologically-related clustering. *Chronic Stress* 5: 2470547020979780.

Kessler, R. C., Aguilar-Gaxiola, S., Alonso, J. et al. (2017). Trauma and PTSD in the WHO world mental health surveys. *European Journal of Psychotraumatology* 8(suppl. 5): 1353383.

Kim, G. S., Uddin, M. (2020). Sex-specific and shared expression profiles of vulnerability and resilience to trauma in brain and blood. *Biology of Sex Differences* 11: 1–19.

Kitchiner, N. J., Lewis, C., Roberts, N. P., Bisson, J. I. (2019). Active duty and ex-serving military personnel with post-traumatic stress disorder treated with psychological therapies: systematic review and meta-analysis. *European Journal of Psychotraumatology* 10(1): 1684226.

de Kloet, C. S., Vermetten, E., Bikker, A. et al. (2007). Leukocyte glucocorticoid receptor expression and immunoregulation in veterans with and without post-traumatic stress disorder. *Molecular Psychiatry* 12(5): 443–453.

Koenig, H. G., Youssef, N. A., Pearce, M. (2019). Assessment of moral injury in veterans and active duty military personnel with PTSD: a review. *Frontiers in Psychiatry* 10: 443.

Lanius, R. A., Williamson, P. C., Boksman, K. et al. (2002). Brain activation during script-driven imagery induced dissociative responses in PTSD: a functional magnetic resonance imaging investigation. *Biological Psychiatry* 52(4): 305–311.

Lanius, R. A., Vermetten, E., Loewenstein, R. J. et al. (2010a). Emotion modulation in PTSD: clinical and neurobiological evidence for a dissociative subtype. *American Journal of Psychiatry* 167(6): 640–647.

Lanius, R., Frewen, P., Vermetten, E., Yehuda, R. (2010b). Fear conditioning and early life vulnerabilities: two distinct pathways of emotional dysregulation and brain dysfunction in PTSD. *European Journal of Psychotraumatology* 1(1): 5467.

Lanius, R. A., Brand, B., Vermetten, E., Frewen, P. A., Spiegel, D. (2012). The dissociative subtype of posttraumatic stress disorder: rationale, clinical and neurobiological evidence, and implications. *Depression and Anxiety* 29(8): 701–708.

Liberzon, I., Sripada, C. S. (2007). The functional neuroanatomy of PTSD: a critical review. *Progress in Brain Research* 167: 151–169.

McFarlane, A. C., Lawrence-Wood, E., Van Hooff, M., Malhi, G. S., Yehuda, R. (2017). The need to take a staging approach to the biological mechanisms of PTSD and its treatment. *Current Psychiatry Reports* 19(2): 10.

Mehta, D., Binder, E. B. (2012). Gene × environment vulnerability factors for PTSD: the HPA-axis. *Neuropharmacology* 62(2): 654–662.

Milad, M. R., Pitman, R. K., Ellis, C. B. et al. (2009). Neurobiological basis of failure to recall extinction memory in posttraumatic stress disorder. *Biological Psychiatry* 66(12): 1075–1082.

Mitchell, J. M., Bogenschutz, M., Lilienstein, A. et al. (2021). MDMA-assisted therapy for severe PTSD: a randomized, double-blind, placebo-controlled phase 3 study. *Nature Medicine* 27(6): 1025–1033.

Nijdam, M. J., Vermetten, E. (2018). Moving forward in treatment of posttraumatic stress disorder: Innovations to exposure-based therapy. *European Journal of Psychotraumatology* 9(1), 1458568.

Nijdam, M. J., Vermetten, E., McFarlane, A. C. (2023). Toward staging differentiation for posttraumatic stress disorder treatment. *Acta Psychiatrica Scandinavica* 147(1): 65–80.

Philipsen, A., Richter, H., Schmahl, C. et al. (2004). Clonidine in acute aversive inner tension and self-injurious behavior in female patients with borderline personality disorder. *Journal of Clinical Psychiatry* 65(10): 1414–1419.

Quirk, G. J., Garcia, R., González-Lima, F. (2006). Prefrontal mechanisms in extinction of conditioned fear. *Biological Psychiatry* 60(4): 337–343.

Raskind, M. A., Peskind, E. R., Chow, B. et al. (2018). Trial of prazosin for post-traumatic stress disorder in military veterans. *New England Journal of Medicine* 378(6): 507–517.

Rauch, S. A., Eftekhari, A., Ruzek, J. I. (2012). Review of exposure therapy: a gold standard for PTSD treatment. *Journal of Rehabilitation Research and Development* 49(5): 679–688.

Ressler, K. J. (2020). Translating across circuits and genetics toward progress in fear-and anxiety-related disorders. *American Journal of Psychiatry* 177(3): 214–222.

Sartory, G., Cwik, J., Knuppertz, H. et al. (2013). In search of the trauma memory: a meta-analysis of functional neuroimaging studies of symptom provocation in posttraumatic stress disorder (PTSD). *PloS One* 8(3): e58150.

9

Schmidt, U., Vermetten, E. (2018). Integrating NIMH research domain criteria (RDoC) into PTSD research. *Current Topics in Behavioral Neurosciences* 38; 68–91.

Schnyder, U., Ehlers, A., Elbert, T. et al. (2015). Psychotherapies for PTSD: what do they have in common? *European Journal of Psychotraumatology* 6(1): 28186.

Shalev, A., Liberzon, I., Marmar, C. (2017). Post-traumatic stress disorder. *New England Journal of Medicine* 376(25): 2459–2469.

Stam, R. (2007). PTSD and stress sensitisation: a tale of brain and body. Part 1: human studies. *Neuroscience & Biobehavioral Reviews* 31(4): 530–557.

Stein, D. J., Ipser, J. C., Seedat, S., Sager, C., Amos, T. (2006). Pharmacotherapy for post traumatic stress disorder (PTSD). *Cochrane Database of Systematic Reviews* 1: CD002795.

Thompson, M. R., Callaghan, P. D., Hunt, G. E., Cornish, J. L., McGregor, I. S. (2007). A role for oxytocin and 5-HT1A receptors in the prosocial effects of 3, 4 methylenedioxymethamphetamine ("ecstasy"). *Neuroscience* 146(2): 509–514.

van Elk, M., Yaden, D. B. (2022). Pharmacological, neural, and psychological mechanisms underlying psychedelics: a critical review. *Neuroscience & Biobehavioral Reviews* 140: 104793.

Vermetten, E., Jetly, R. (2018). A critical outlook on combat-related PTSD: review and case reports of guilt and shame as drivers for moral injury. *Military Behavioral Health* 6(2): 156–164.

Vermetten, E., McFarlane, A. C. (2020). Predicting future risk of PTSD. *Nature Medicine* 26(7): 1012–1013.

Vermetten, E., Dorahy, M. J., Spiegel, D. (2007). *Traumatic Dissociation: Neurobiology and Treatment*. American Psychiatric Publishing, Inc.

Vermetten, E., Jetly, R., Smith-MacDonald, L., Jones, C., Bremault-Phillip, S. (2023). Moral injury in a military context. In Warner, C. H. Castro, C. A. (eds.), *Veteran and Military Mental Health: A Clinical Manual*. Springer International Publishing, pp. 231–261.

Watkins, L. E., Sprang, K. R., Rothbaum, B. O. (2018). Treating PTSD: a review of evidence-based psychotherapy interventions. *Frontiers in Behavioral Neuroscience* 12: 258.

Williams, T., Phillips, N. J., Stein, D. J., Ipser, J. C. (2022). Pharmacotherapy for post traumatic stress disorder (PTSD). *Cochrane Database of Systematic Reviews* 3: CD002795.

Yehuda, R., Hoge, C. W., McFarlane, A. C. et al. (2015). Post-traumatic stress disorder. *Nature Reviews Disease Primers* 1: 15057.

National Neuroscience Curriculum Initiative online resources

Predicting Posttraumatic Stress Disorder: From Circuits to Communities

Alfred P. Kaye and David A. Ross

From Generation to Generation: Rethinking "Soul Wounds" and Historical Trauma

Stefanie L. Gillson and David A. Ross

An Integrated Neuroscience Perspective on Formulation and Treatment Planning for Posttraumatic Stress Disorder An Educational Review

David A. Ross, Melissa R. Arbuckle, Michael J. Travis, Jennifer B. Dwyer, Gerrit I. Van Schalkwyk and Kerry J. Ressler

Witnessing Modern America: Violence and Racial Trauma

J. Corey Williams, Terrell D. Holloway and David A. Ross

9

What to say: Predicting Posttraumatic Stress Disorder: From Circuits to Communities

Andrew Novick and Ashley Walker

Clinical neuroscience conversations: PTSD

Donna Sudak

This "stuff" is really cool: Nicole Zabik, *"1224 HOURS" on avoidance and PTSD*

This "stuff" is really cool: Remmelt Shur, *"Hidden Scars" on epigenetic changes in trauma and PTSD*

This "stuff" is really cool: Georgina Burcher, *"Developing A Picture of PTSD" on the neurobiology of post-intensive care PTSD*

Expert video: *Kerry Ressler on Fear & PTSD*

9.6

Obsessive–Compulsive and Related Disorders

Eileen M. Joyce and Naomi A. Fineberg

OVERVIEW

Of the obsessive-compulsive and related disorders (OCRDs), obsessive–compulsive disorder (OCD) remains the most well studied. In this section we review the integrated neurobiology of the OCRDs, focusing on OCD as the exemplar, touching upon phenotypes, cognitive endophenotypes and neural circuitry. Converging evidence from the neurosciences identifies core deficits in behavioural inhibition, cognitive flexibility, habit learning, fear extinction and safety signalling, underpinned by specific abnormalities in corticostriatal–thalamic circuits. Treatments found to be effective include serotonin reuptake inhibitor drugs, cognitive behavioural forms of psychotherapy, invasive or non-invasive neuromodulation or ablation of specific nodes or tracts within the corticostriatal–thalamic circuits. We conclude with a synthesis of the theoretical neural mechanisms leading to successful therapeutic intervention.

OCD is the archetypal and most studied disorder in the *International Classification of Diseases*, 11th edition (ICD-11) category of OCRDs [1]. In ICD-11 and DSM-5 [2], OCRDs were grouped together because they share a common phenotype and aetiology, principally involving the performance of compulsions. Alongside OCD, disorders also characterised by prominent obsessions comprise: body dysmorphic disorder, hypochondriasis and olfactory reference disorders. Anxiety is commonly experienced alongside core symptoms of OCRDs and comorbidity with anxiety disorder is high. However, increasing evidence from the neurosciences implicating the involvement of brain-based mechanisms and neural circuitry different from the core mechanisms underpinning anxiety disorders led to the establishment of OCRDs as separate from anxiety disorders, first by the DSM-5 and subsequently the ICD-11. See Table 9.6.1.

9.6.1 Cognitive Mediators

Patients with obsessive–compulsive disorder (OCD) show impairments on a range of cognitive functions when tested formally. These can explain symptom formation and enable investigation of neural mechanisms.

9.6.1.1 Impaired Inhibition and Cognitive Flexibility

Patients with OCD are impaired on tests of inhibition and cognitive flexibility. For example, they show difficulty inhibiting habitual or automatic behavioural responses when signalled to do so. They also show inflexibility in the use of environmental cues to change behaviour in an adaptive manner. This is apparent when testing the ability to form an attentional set, that is, a bias to respond to the relevant features of complex stimuli. Patients with OCD can form an attentional set during experimental testing but have difficulty in shifting their attention when circumstances change and other features of the stimuli become more relevant. In clinical terms, this may manifest as an inability to shift attention away from a pointless ritual. Deficits in inhibition and cognitive flexibility can also be seen in other obsessive compulsive or related disorders (OCRDs) such as trichotillomania, body dysmorphic disorder, hoarding disorder, as well as unrelated disorders such as schizophrenia. However, these deficits are also found in the healthy first-degree relatives of patients with OCD, showing that they are not merely epiphenomena (secondary effects) of illness but markers, or endophenotypes, of the neurobiological abnormality [3, 4].

Table 9.6.1 Obsessive–compulsive and related disorders (OCRDs): Adapted from the ICD-11/DSM-5 definitions

Obsessive–compulsive disorder	This represents the archetype. Core symptoms comprise obsessions and compulsions. Obsessions are unwanted, distressing, recurrent or persistent intrusive thoughts, images or urges. Obsessions follow themes often relating to harm, but also to things needing to feel right or other unrelated themes. Compulsions are repetitive unwanted behaviours or mental acts aimed at neutralising obsessional thoughts and reducing distress or performed according to rigid rules. Although compulsions are purposeful, they are either excessive or not logically related to the outcome they aim to achieve. Distress reduction is usually brief, leading to a cycle of thoughts and behaviour that is preoccupying, thereby limiting function.
Body dysmorphic disorder	Characterised by the persistent preoccupation with perceived defects in appearance that are in reality either minor or not noticeable. Individuals are excessively self-conscious and show compulsive behaviours such as checking or disguising their appearance. Distress is significant and interferes with everyday functioning.
Olfactory reference disorder/ olfactory reference syndrome	Characterised by the persistent preoccupation with the unwarranted belief that an offensive smell is being emitted from the body. Individuals are excessively self-conscious and show compulsive behaviours such as checking their body for odour and seeking reassurance. Distress is significant and interferes with everyday functioning.
Hypochondriasis[a]	Characterised by the persistent preoccupation about having a serious or progressive disease and compulsive searching for medical reassurance. Individuals may show a catastrophic misinterpretation of bodily symptoms that are often normal sensations. The preoccupation persists or reoccurs after reassurance by a normal medical assessment. Distress is significant and interferes with everyday functioning.
Hoarding disorder	Characterised by the accumulation of objects, regardless of value, secondary to compulsive acquisition of or difficulty in discarding possessions.
Trichotillomania	Characterised by recurrent hair pulling, leading to significant hair loss from any region of the body, occurring either in brief episodes or sustained periods.
Excoriation disorder	Characterised by recurrent skin picking causing lesions anywhere on the body, occurring either in brief episodes or more sustained periods.

[a] Note in DSM-5 this is not classified as an OCRD and is termed Illness Anxiety Disorder and is classified in the Somatic Symptom And Related Disorders section.

9.6.1.2 Excessive Habit Formation

Compulsions can be thought of as excessive, maladaptive habits [5]. The development of habits reflects the interaction of two distinct learning processes [6]. One mediates learning about the relevance of events and the shaping of actions to obtain a valued outcome, that is, goal-directed behaviour. The other mediates habit formation. This occurs when actions are repeated to the extent that they become independent of either the value of the outcome or the relationship between the response and the outcome, and are triggered by events alone. Thus, with repetition, the same behaviour can shift from being goal-directed to a habit [6]. Patients with chronic OCD are often unable to give a cogent reason for performing some of their compulsions, such as checking, counting or repeating rituals, and volunteer that they have become 'bad habits'. One hypothesis proposes that habit learning is abnormally excessive in OCD, resulting in compulsions [5]. A variant of this suggests that under normal circumstances goal-directed and habit learning are balanced, serving to enable flexible switching between the two; however, in OCD, goal-directed learning is impaired so that habit learning dominates [4]. This was tested in a study where actions were learned to avoid an

electric shock to the right or left hand; a specific stimulus signalled which hand would be shocked. After repetition learning, the participants were told they would no longer receive a shock to one hand. OCD patients continued to respond to the stimulus no longer predicting shock more than healthy controls and when questioned described a strong urge to keep responding [7]. Other studies of OCD employing different designs have similarly found dysfunctional goal-directed behaviour, resulting in a bias towards excessive habit formation [8, 9]. See Section 5.8 for more on habits and OCD.

9.6.1.3 Impaired Fear Extinction and Safety Signalling

Impaired inhibition and cognitive flexibility resulting in dysfunctional goal-directed learning and excessive habit formation may explain the development of compulsions in OCD. Although not tested experimentally, this formulation may also be applicable to obsessions; that is, patients with OCD experience abnormal and highly salient thoughts which, like behaviours, cannot be inhibited and through repetition become habitual. This explanation does not take into account the role of anxiety, however, which often serves to maintain compulsions in OCD. This has been tested with fear-conditioning paradigms in which a neutral event (a conditioned stimulus) is repeatedly paired with an electric shock (an unconditioned stimulus) so that an automatic fear response (the galvanic skin response, namely the change in skin conductance due to sweating) is elicited by the conditioned stimulus alone. Patients with OCD showed normal conditioned stimulus–unconditioned stimulus association learning but in extinction, when the conditioned stimulus no longer signalled an impending shock, they continued to display the fear response more than normal. Impaired fear extinction indicates that OCD patients have difficulty modulating their emotional response when a previously threatening event becomes non-threatening, a concept known as safety signalling [10, 11]. In OCD, impaired safety signalling and persistent fear responses may interact with abnormal goal-directed learning to promote excessive habit formation and thereby generate compulsive symptoms [8].

9.6.2 Neural Mechanisms

OCD has long been thought to reflect abnormalities of corticostriatal–thalamic circuits [5, 12]. Corticostriatal–thalamic circuits emanate from different areas of the frontal cortex, which project to the striatum in a topographical manner. Parallel circuits are formed by ongoing striatal projections to the pallidum, thence to the thalamus and finally back to the original cortical area. Individual corticostriatal–thalamic circuits process information concerning emotion/motivation, cognition or movement (Figure 9.6.1). These circuits are not fully segregated as some projections interconnect within the striatum. Thus, information can flow both within and across circuits so that motor responses can be influenced by emotional, motivational and cognitive states [13].

Early neuroimaging studies of OCD found hyperactivity of the orbitofrontal cortex, dorsal anterior cingulate cortex and their striatal targets [12]. Converging evidence suggests that an essential function of the orbitofrontal cortex is to encode the reward/punishment value of environmental stimuli and initiate appropriate responses when changes in value are detected [14]; see Section 5.15 for more on frontal lobe function. Within this remit the functions of the lateral and medial orbitofrontal cortex differ, with both having relevance for the psychopathology of OCRDs. The medial orbitofrontal cortex, with ventromedial prefrontal cortex, has a central role in

rapidly updating the value of stimuli, for example when they change from threatening to non-threatening. The lateral orbitofrontal cortex mediates inhibition of previously rewarded behaviour and switching of responses to new stimuli of importance.

In OCD, abnormal medial orbitofrontal cortex/ventromedial prefrontal cortex activity has been found in relation to impaired fear extinction, safety signalling and shock-avoidance learning [10, 11], whereas reduced behavioural flexibility has been associated with abnormal functional connectivity of outputs from the lateral orbitofrontal cortex to the striatum [4]. Whether these circuits are abnormally hyperactive or hypoactive depends on the particular cognitive function under investigation. In addition, the precise relationship between these abnormalities and clinical symptoms has yet to be elucidated. Existing evidence points to disrupted lateral orbitofrontal cortical and medial orbitofrontal/ventromedial prefrontal cortical circuitry, which normally work together to update the value of environmental events and initiate behaviour change.

Whereas the orbitofrontal cortex encodes the value of stimuli, the dorsal anterior cingulate cortex encodes the value of actions, known as error or conflict monitoring. In addition, dorsal anterior cingulate cortical activity has been shown to correlate with the galvanic skin response during fear conditioning [15]. In OCD, abnormal dorsal anterior cingulate cortex circuit function may contribute to the development of compulsive responses and excessive fear expression [15].

Most neuroimaging studies are conducted in adults with OCD yet the majority develop OCD during adolescence [16]. Studies have shown abnormalities of corticostriatal–thalamic circuits in young people, which are similar to those of adults, but there are also differences. As yet there are few longitudinal studies to shed light on when brain changes emerge and mature during development and how they can be embedded in a bio-psychosocial model of OCD [17].

9.6.3 The Neurobiological Basis of Current Treatments

Although the discovery of pharmacological and physical treatments for OCD was serendipitous, understanding the neural effects of successful interventions will inform cognitive neuroscience and the tailoring of new treatments.

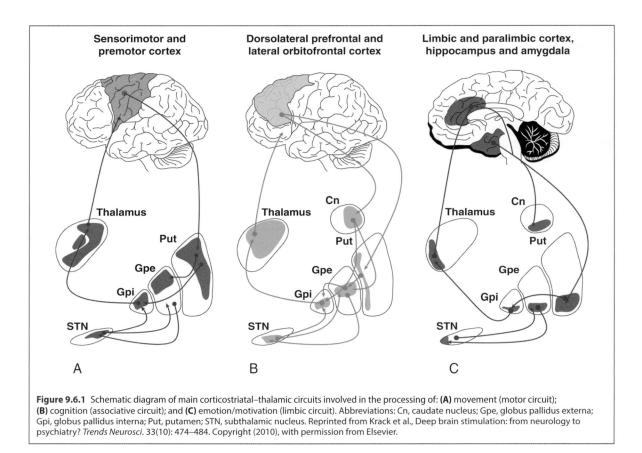

Figure 9.6.1 Schematic diagram of main corticostriatal–thalamic circuits involved in the processing of: **(A)** movement (motor circuit); **(B)** cognition (associative circuit); and **(C)** emotion/motivation (limbic circuit). Abbreviations: Cn, caudate nucleus; Gpe, globus pallidus externa; Gpi, globus pallidus interna; Put, putamen; STN, subthalamic nucleus. Reprinted from Krack et al., Deep brain stimulation: from neurology to psychiatry? *Trends Neurosci.* 33(10): 474–484. Copyright (2010), with permission from Elsevier.

9.6.3.1 Pharmacotherapy

Medications with the strongest evidence for efficacy are selective serotonin reuptake inhibitors (SSRIs; Table 9.6.2). Effective psychological therapies include variants of cognitive behaviour therapy (CBT) [20]. There have been few randomised controlled trials (RCTs) directly comparing different pharmacological and psychological treatments. To circumvent this, a network meta-analysis compared the effects of placebo drug with different OCD treatments using direct and indirect data from 54 different RCTs and 6,652 patients [21]. Using a change in the Y–BOCS as the outcome measure, the SSRIs fluoxetine, fluvoxamine, paroxetine, sertraline, citalopram and escitalopram were equally and significantly effective (group effect size [ES]: 3.62), clomipramine was not significantly more effective than SSRIs (ES: 4.66) and psychological therapies (CBT, BT, CT) were equally and significantly effective (ES: 7.98–10.41). However, the study found that most of the psychological therapy studies included patients who

had already been stabilised on antidepressant medication and so were in reality testing combination treatment. Given the equivalent efficacy of SSRIs, individual choice is based on adverse effects such as weight gain, sexual problems and ECG changes.

Early neuroimaging studies showing hyperactivity in the orbitofrontal cortex, dorsal anterior cingulate cortex and striatum found that activity was normalised following successful treatment with CBT or an SSRI [11]. The effect of SSRIs suggests that reduced serotoninergic modulation of corticostriatal–thalamic circuits may be one cause of OCD symptoms. Support comes from findings that tryptophan-induced serotonin depletion in humans and manipulation of serotonin (5-hydroxytryptamine; 5-HT) receptors in rodents produce OCD-like behaviour [4].

Despite optimum treatment with medication and psychological therapy, 40% do not have an adequate response. A successful strategy is to increase the use of SSRIs above recommended limits with careful monitoring [22].

Table 9.6.2 Evidence-based treatment strategies for OCRDs[a]

Disorder	Pharmacotherapy[b]	Psychotherapy[c]	Other	Assessment instrument
OCD	SSRI Clomipramine Adjunctive-dopamine antagonist	**CBT, ERP, CBT with ERP**	Cingulotomy Capsulotomy **Deep brain stimulation** **Repetitive transcranial magnetic stimulation**	Y-BOCS
Body dysmorphic disorder	SSRI Clomipramine	**CBT with ERP**		BDD Y-BOCS
Hypochondriasis	SSRI	CBT ERP		H-Y-BOCS HAI/SHAI Whiteley Index
Hoarding disorder	SSRI (in comorbid OCD) Venlafaxine	CBT for hoarding		Savings Inventory Revised
Trichotillomania	Clomipramine *N*-Acetylcysteine Olanzapine	HRT ACT DBT		NIMH-TSSS Mass Gen H-HPS Y-BOCS-TM
Excoriation disorder	SSRI *N*-Acetylcysteine Naltrexone	HRT ACT–BT		NE-YBOCS

[a] Abbreviations: BDD Y-BOCS, body-dysmorphic disorder Yale–Brown Obsessive Compulsive Scale; HAI/SHAI, Health Anxiety Inventory/Short Health Anxiety Inventory; H-Y-BOCS, hypochondriasis Yale–Brown Obsessive Compulsive Scale; NE-YBOCS (Yale–Brown Obsessive Compulsive Scale – modified for neurotic excoriation); NIMH-TSSS, National Institute for Mental Health trichotillomania symptom severity scale; SSRI, selective serotonin reuptake inhibitor; Y-BOCS, Yale–Brown Obsessive Compulsive Scale; Y-BOCS-TM, Yale–Brown Obsessive Compulsive Scale – trichotillomania. The Yale–Brown Obsessive Compulsive Scale for OCD [18] is the standard assessment instrument measuring OCD severity and has been adapted into different versions for assessing other OCRDs. Treatments in bold text represent those found to be efficacious in one or more head-to-head randomised controlled trials of fair comparison.

[b] OCD is by far the most robustly investigated disorder in terms of treatment trials. The pharmacotherapies with randomised controlled trial (RCT) evidence of efficacy as monotherapies, including long-term efficacy and relapse prevention, comprise the serotonergic agents clomipramine and SSRIs. Adjunctive dopamine antagonists, including first- and second-generation agents, also appear efficacious in SSRI-resistant OCD, at least in the short term. Higher doses of SSRIs, within recommended limits, are usually required for efficacy in OCD compared to standard doses used to treat depression and anxiety. Clomipramine is less well tolerated than SSRIs and is usually reserved as a second-line treatment after SSRIs [19].

[c] The psychological therapies with RCT evidence of efficacy are: behaviour therapy, that is, exposure and response prevention (ERP); cognitive therapy (CT); and cognitive–behavioural therapy (CBT). ERP involves exposure to the feared object together with prevention of the compulsive response. CT aims to change obsessional thoughts and CBT combines CT with behavioural experiments aimed at challenging obsessional beliefs. The form of CBT usually recommended in treatment guidelines for OCD and body dysmorphic disorder includes ERP (www.NICE.org.uk).

Another is to add a dopamine receptor antagonist; RCT evidence supports the use of haloperidol, risperidone, quetiapine, olanzapine and aripiprazole [19] (Table 9.6.2). There is evidence that striatal dopamine release is increased in OCD [22]. Dopamine projections from midbrain nuclei interact with corticostriatal–thalamic circuits in the striatum and, along with reciprocal projections back to the midbrain, form a 'spiral' of connections enabling information flow across the corticostriatal–thalamic circuits [13]. Thus, in OCD, dopamine receptor antagonists may act by disrupting abnormal information processing within and across orbitofrontal, ventromedial prefrontal and dorsal anterior cingulate cortical circuitry.

9.6.3.2 Neurosurgery

Notwithstanding optimal treatment, 10% of patients with OCD remain severely symptomatic. Dorsal anterior cingulotomy and ventral anterior capsulotomy are neurosurgical options where the respective brain areas are lesioned under stereotactic guidance. These are reserved for the most extremely disabled patients and rarely performed (Figure 9.6.2). Studies have shown that 41% and 54% of patients respectively have a meaningful response to these procedures [23]. Cingulotomy is likely to be effective because it targets the dorsal anterior cingulate cortical region, previously shown in neuroimaging studies to be active during fear conditioning and hyperactive in OCD with subsequent normalisation after successful SSRI therapy [15]. The most effective site for capsulotomy is the ventral aspect of the anterior limb of the internal capsule. Lesions here transect axons from the orbitofrontal, ventromedial prefrontal and dorsal anterior cingulate cortices, travelling to the thalamus and brainstem, thereby influencing the function not only of

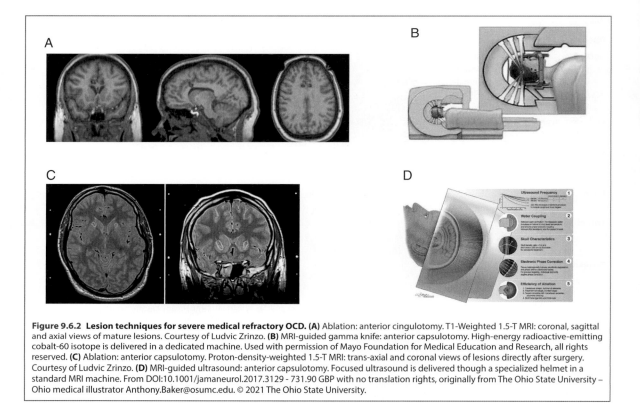

Figure 9.6.2 Lesion techniques for severe medical refractory OCD. (A) Ablation: anterior cingulotomy. T1-Weighted 1.5-T MRI: coronal, sagittal and axial views of mature lesions. Courtesy of Ludvic Zrinzo. **(B)** MRI-guided gamma knife: anterior capsulotomy. High-energy radioactive-emitting cobalt-60 isotope is delivered in a dedicated machine. Used with permission of Mayo Foundation for Medical Education and Research, all rights reserved. **(C)** Ablation: anterior capsulotomy. Proton-density-weighted 1.5-T MRI: trans-axial and coronal views of lesions directly after surgery. Courtesy of Ludvic Zrinzo. **(D)** MRI-guided ultrasound: anterior capsulotomy. Focused ultrasound is delivered though a specialized helmet in a standard MRI machine. From DOI:10.1001/jamaneurol.2017.3129 - 731.90 GBP with no translation rights, originally from The Ohio State University – Ohio medical illustrator Anthony.Baker@osumc.edu. © 2021 The Ohio State University.

the corticostriatal–thalamic circuits but also brainstem dopamine, noradrenaline and serotonin nuclei known to modulate mood.

9.6.3.3 Neuromodulation

Deep brain stimulation (DBS) is emerging as a promising procedure for severe SSRI- and CBT-resistant OCD (Figure 9.6.3), with particular emphasis on two brain targets: the anterior limb of the internal capsule (ALIC) and the anteromedial subthalamic nucleus; 50–65% of patients with treatment-resistant OCD who are eligible for DBS have a meaningful response with similar response rates for ALIC and anteromedial subthalamic nucleus targets. ALIC DBS affects the same white matter tracts as capsulotomy. It may seem paradoxical that both severing and stimulating the same fibres leads to similar clinical outcomes. However, ALIC DBS has been shown to decrease pathological hyperactivity in ventral prefrontal cortex. For example, DBS normalised excessive corticostriatal connectivity and decreased the cortical EEG changes elicited by symptom provocation [24]. This suggests that

ALIC DBS has a net inhibitory action on corticostriatal–thalamic circuitry. The subthalamic nucleus receives uninterrupted projections from frontal cortex forming the hyperdirect pathway. The subthalamic nucleus is also part of the basal ganglia (Figure 9.6.1) and input from the hyperdirect pathway provides a 'stop' mechanism so that behaviours already being programmed can be inhibited. Anteromedial subthalamic nucleus DBS may regulate abnormal information processing in the hyperdirect pathway from the dorsal anterior cingulate and orbitofrontal cortices and enable patients to interrupt their compulsive cycle of repetitive acts and thoughts.

Non-invasive external modulation of abnormal areas of the cerebral cortex using repetitive transcranial magnetic stimulation (TMS) or, more recently, transcranial direct current stimulation, is being studied in OCD. A significant problem for repetitive TMS is of magnetisation not reaching inaccessible cortical areas such as dorsal anterior cingulate and orbitofrontal cortices (see Section 9.20 on brain stimulation). New head-coil designs have recently addressed this problem with deep TMS of

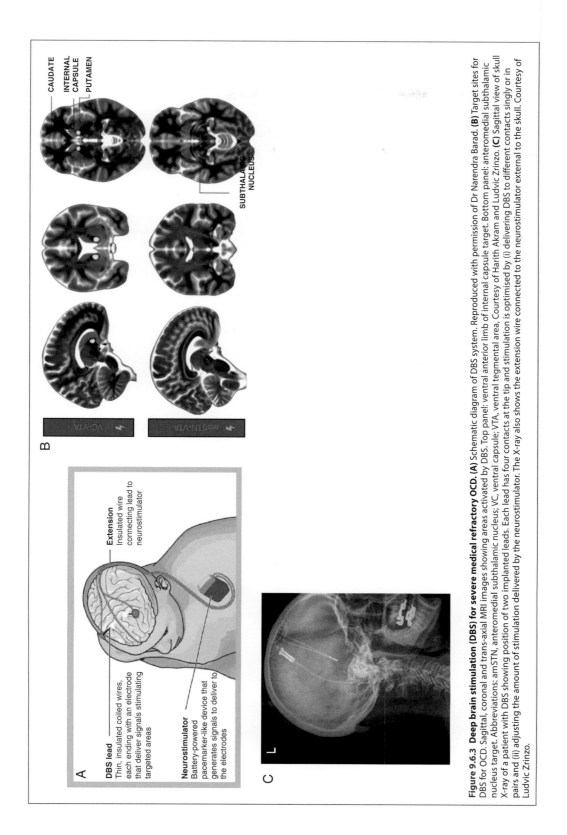

Figure 9.6.3 Deep brain stimulation (DBS) for severe medical refractory OCD. (A) Schematic diagram of DBS system. Reproduced with permission of Dr Narendra Barad. **(B)** Target sites for DBS for OCD. Sagittal, coronal and trans-axial MRI images showing areas activated by DBS. Top panel: ventral anterior limb of internal capsule target. Bottom panel: anteromedial subthalamic nucleus target. Abbreviations: amSTN, anteromedial subthalamic nucleus; VC, ventral capsule; VTA, ventral tegmental area. Courtesy of Harith Akram and Ludvic Zrinzo. **(C)** Sagittal view of skull X-ray of a patient with DBS showing position of two implanted leads. Each lead has four contacts at the tip and stimulation is optimised by (i) delivering DBS to different contacts singly or in pairs and (ii) adjusting the amount of stimulation delivered by the neurostimulator external to the skull. The X-ray also shows the extension wire connected to the neurostimulator external to the skull. Courtesy of Ludvic Zrinzo.

the dorsal anterior cingulate cortex showing particular promise for OCD [25].

Conclusions and Outstanding Questions

Advances in cognitive neuroscience have led to a sea change in the understanding of OCRDs. They are considered disorders of neural networks that mediate learning about the significance of environmental events and initiate adaptive flexible behaviour. Evidence suggests that dysfunctional imbalanced circuits, emanating from medial and lateral orbitofrontal and dorsal anterior cingulate cortices, result in excessive habitual thoughts and/or

actions. There are effective treatments for OCRDs but a significant number of patients do not have an adequate response and there remain major challenges for the development of better interventions.

Outstanding Questions

- How does OCD develop? Can we use behavioural endophenotypes to predict those at risk and intervene early?
- For those who do not respond to medication and CBT, can effective external brain modulation techniques be developed that are available for the many and even for home use?

REFERENCES

1. World Health Organization. *International Classification of Diseases*, 11th ed. (ICD-11). World Health Organization, 2018,

2. American Psychiatric Association. *Diagnostic and Statistical Manual of Mental Disorders*, 5th ed. (DSM-5). American Psychiatric Association, 2013.

3. Fineberg NA, Apergis-Schoute AM, Vaghi MM et al. Mapping compulsivity in the DSM-5 obsessive compulsive and related disorders: cognitive domains, neural circuitry, and treatment. *Int J Neuropsychopharmacol* 2018; 21(1): 42–58.

4. Robbins TW, Vaghi MM, Banca P. Obsessive–compulsive disorder: puzzles and prospects. *Neuron* 2019; 102(1): 27–47.

5. Graybiel AM, Rauch SL. Toward a neurobiology of obsessive–compulsive disorder. *Neuron* 2000; 28(2): 343–347.

6. Dickinson A. Actions and habits: the development of behavioral autonomy. *Philos Trans R Soc London B* 1985; 308(1135): 67–78.

7. Gillan CM, Morein-Zamir S, Urcelay GP et al. Enhanced avoidance habits in obsessive–compulsive disorder. *Biol Psychiatry* 2014; 75(8): 631–638.

8. Gillan CM, Robbins TW. Goal-directed learning and obsessive–compulsive disorder. *Philos Trans R Soc London B* 2014; 369(1655): 20130475.

9. Voon V, Derbyshire K, Ruck C et al. Disorders of compulsivity: a common bias towards learning habits. *Mol Psychiatry* 2015; 20(3): 345–352.

10. Apergis-Schoute AM, Gillan CM, Fineberg NA et al. Neural basis of impaired safety signaling in obsessive compulsive disorder. *Proc Natl Acad Sci USA* 2017; 114(12): 3216–3221.

11. Milad MR, Furtak SC, Greenberg JL et al. Deficits in conditioned fear extinction in obsessive–compulsive disorder and neurobiological changes in the fear circuit. *JAMA Psychiatry* 2013; 70(6): 608–518.

12. Saxena S, Brody AL, Schwartz JM, Baxter LR. Neuroimaging and frontal-subcortical circuitry in obsessive–compulsive disorder. *Br J Psychiatry Suppl* 1998; 35: 26–37.

13. Haber SN. Corticostriatal circuitry. *Dialogues Clin Neurosci* 2016; 18(1): 7–21.

14. Rolls ET. The functions of the orbitofrontal cortex. *Brain Cogn* 2004; 55(1): 11–29.

15. Milad MR, Rauch SL. Obsessive–compulsive disorder: beyond segregated cortico-striatal pathways. *Trends Cogn Sci* 2012; 16(1): 43–51.

16. Fineberg NA, Hengartner MP, Bergbaum CE et al. A prospective population-based cohort study of the prevalence, incidence and impact of obsessive–compulsive symptomatology. *Int J Psychiatry Clin Pract* 2013; 17: 170–178.

17. Hauser TU. On the development of OCD. *Curr Top Behav Neurosci* 2021; 49: 17–30.

18. Goodman WK, Price LH, Rasmussen SA, Mazure C et al. The Yale–Brown Obsessive Compulsive Scale. I. Development, use, and reliability. *Arch Gen Psychiatry* 1989; 46: 1006–1011.

19. Grancini B, Craig KJ, Cinosi E et al. Pharmacotherapy for OCD. In Simon NM, Hollander E, Rothbaum BO, Stein DJ (eds.), *The American Psychiatric Association Publishing Textbook of Anxiety, Trauma, and OCD-Related Disorders*, 3rd ed. American Psychiatric Publishing, 2019, pp. 321–352.

20. Reid JE, Laws KR, Drummond L et al. Cognitive behavioural therapy with exposure and response prevention in the treatment of obsessive–compulsive disorder: a systematic review and meta-analysis of randomised controlled trials. *Compr Psychiatry* 2021; 106: 152223.

9

21. Skapinakis P, Caldwell DM, Hollingworth W et al. Pharmacological and psychotherapeutic interventions for management of obsessive–compulsive disorder in adults: a systematic review and network meta-analysis. *Lancet Psychiatry* 2016; 3: 730–739.

22. Fineberg NA, Reghunandanan S, Simpson HB et al. Obsessive–compulsive disorder (OCD): practical strategies for pharmacological and somatic treatment in adults. *Psychiatry Res* 2015; 227: 114–125

23. Brown LT, Mikell CB, Youngerman BE et al. Dorsal anterior cingulotomy and anterior capsulotomy for severe, refractory obsessive–compulsive disorder: a systematic review of observational studies. *J Neurosurg* 2016; 124(1): 77–89.

24. Figee M, Luigjes J, Smolders R et al. Deep brain stimulation restores frontostriatal network activity in obsessive–compulsive disorder. *Nat Neurosci* 2013; 16(4): 386–387.

25. Carmi L, Tendler A, Bystritsky A et al. Efficacy and safety of deep transcranial magnetic stimulation for obsessive–compulsive disorder: a prospective multicenter randomized double-blind placebo-controlled trial. *Am J Psychiatry* 2019; 176(11): 931–938.

9.7 **Major Depressive Disorder**

Alexander Kaltenboeck and
Catherine Harmer

OVERVIEW

Major depression is a debilitating mental health condition that affects many people and causes a great deal of suffering worldwide. Yet, our understanding of its etiology and pathophysiology is still poor. Neuroscientists have studied depressive disorders from different perspectives and have reported a range of abnormalities on different levels of neurobiological description. Based on these findings, various, mutually not necessarily exclusive, theories have been put forward to explain the development and maintenance of depressive symptoms. The clinical relevance of these theories and how they relate to each other will have to be the subject of future neuroscientific research on depression.

9.7.1 What Constitutes Major Depression?

Depressive disorders are diagnosed using standard criteria outlined in agreed classification systems, such as the *Diagnostic and Statistical Manual of Mental Disorders* (currently DSM-5, published by the American Psychiatric Association [1]) or the *International Classification of Diseases* (currently ICD-10, published by the World Health Organization). A major depressive episode is typically characterised by the prolonged presence of low mood or anhedonia, accompanied by a number of other symptoms such as decreased energy, weight loss, sleeping difficulties or cognitive problems. Furthermore, it is important that symptoms have caused significant distress or impairment in functioning and cannot be attributed to another medical condition or taken substance. Major depression is relatively common, with estimates of lifetime risk in the general community going as high as about 20%. Combined with the difficulty in fully treating all its symptoms, this has led to the condition being identified as one of the leading causes of disability across the world.

Given the complexity of the central nervous system, neuroscientific research tries to understand the brain by studying it from different perspectives and on different spatial and temporal scales, ranging from molecules and cells, to neural circuits and macroscopic brain regions, to individual behaviour and subjective experience. In the case of major depression, this has led to the discovery of a wide range of abnormalities that are associated with the condition. This in turn has stimulated a number of – mutually not necessarily exclusive – neuroscientific theories that explain the development of depression on different levels of neuroscientific description (see Figure 9.7.1).

9.7.2 Neurochemical Perspective

For a long time, the clinical neuroscience of depression has focused heavily on neurotransmitter systems (the 'neurochemical perspective') to explain the development of depressive symptoms and the effects of antidepressant interventions. This was guided by observations that efficacious antidepressant drugs (e.g. tricyclics, selective serotonin reuptake inhibitors (SSRIs), serotonin and noradrenaline reuptake inhibitors (SNRIs)) potentiate serotonin and/or noradrenaline signalling and has culminated in the classic theory that depression results from insufficient or impaired monoamine (serotonin, noradrenaline and dopamine) neurotransmission. Early reports of monoaminergic dysfunction in patients with depression were often based on relatively limited

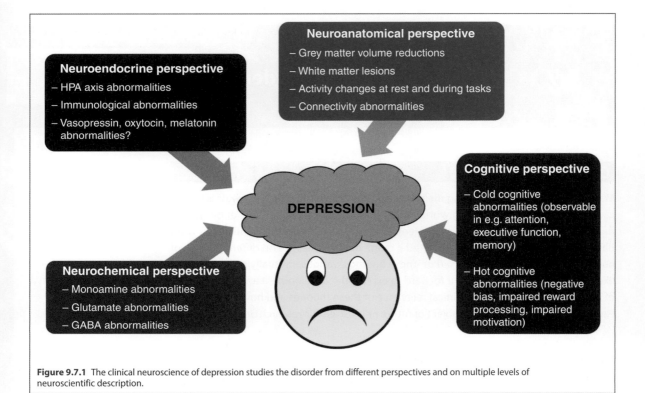

Figure 9.7.1 The clinical neuroscience of depression studies the disorder from different perspectives and on multiple levels of neuroscientific description.

methodologies (e.g. measurements of neurotransmitters, precursors or metabolites in plasma, cerebrospinal fluid or post-mortem brain tissue, or neuroendocrine challenge tests) but have more recently found further support from studies using improved techniques such as brain imaging with radiolabelled receptor ligands. Taken together, these observations generally suggest that major depression is associated with some sort of abnormality in monoaminergic neurotransmission, but the exact nature of the abnormality remains unclear.

In addition, it has also become increasingly clear that at least some monoamine abnormalities can be observed in patients in remission as well. This has given rise to the idea that some monoamine dysfunctions could also represent a general neurobiological vulnerability to develop depression in the first place or, alternatively, lasting neurobiological damage ('scars') resulting from previous depressive episodes and/or their treatment.

Interestingly, when monoaminergic pathway activity is manipulated experimentally (which can be done, for example, by artificially decreasing the availability of the serotonin precursor tryptophan), only those who had previously suffered from depression tend to experience depression-like symptoms. In contrast, healthy people without significant risk factors generally do not show symptoms of depression following these manipulations, which indicates that impaired monoaminergic neurotransmission alone is probably not sufficient for the development of depression.

While historically the monoaminergic system has received most attention in the clinical neurosciences of depression, accumulating evidence now suggests that the condition might also be associated with alterations in the gamma-aminobutyric acid (GABA) system and the glutamate system. In the plasma and cerebrospinal fluid of depressed patients, for example, GABA levels have been described to be lowered and the density of specific GABAergic interneurons in cortical regions also seems to be decreased. Furthermore, studies using magnetic resonance spectroscopy have documented a decrease of GABA in occipital cortex and anterior cingulate cortex in patients with major depression.

Paralleling these findings, abnormalities in the glutamatergic system have also been observed in plasma, serum, cerebrospinal fluid and brain tissue of depressed patients and magnetic resonance spectroscopy studies hint at decreased levels of glutamate especially in anterior brain regions. In addition, the glutamatergic N-methyl-D-aspartate (NMDA) receptor antagonist ketamine can exert rapid (but unfortunately only transient) antidepressant effects.

For more detailed discussions of the neurochemical perspectives on depression, please see [2–7].

9.7.3 Neuroendocrine and Neuroimmunological Perspective

In patients with major depression, a number of abnormalities in the hypothalamic–pituitary–adrenal (HPA) axis have been observed, most importantly subtle signs of cortisol hypersecretion. These include increased 24-hour urinary cortisol levels as well as elevated plasma and cerebrospinal fluid concentrations of cortisol, blunted suppression of cortisol secretion after dexamethasone administration, elevated waking salivary cortisol, increased adrenal gland volumes and decreased numbers of central and peripheral glucocorticoid receptors. Furthermore, patients with hypercortisolism due to Cushing's disease often develop depressive symptoms and patients with depression often suffer from comorbidities and long-term consequences (such as, for example, cardiovascular disease, diabetes mellitus or hippocampal volume reduction) that are consistent with hypercortisolism. This has led to the suggestion that excessive HPA axis activity might represent an important pathophysiological factor in the development of depressive symptoms and could conceivably be linked to increased stress. Animal and human research furthermore indicates that early-life stress could potentially set the HPA axis to a hyperactive or hypersensitive state that can persist into adulthood, thereby potentially providing a mechanism for how early-life adversity, which is a common risk factor for depression, could translate into later mental health problems.

Similar to neurochemical abnormalities associated with depression, some abnormalities in the HPA axis (e.g. increased waking salivary cortisol) can also be observed in non-depressed individuals who are at risk for the disorder, potentially representing a trait-like vulnerability marker.

More recently, other hormones, such as vasopressin, oxytocin or melatonin, have also been discussed in the context of depression but their pathophysiological relevance is unclear to date.

Depressive disorders have also been associated with abnormalities in the immune system, which can be found in a subgroup of patients. One example of this are elevated levels of inflammatory biomarkers such as C-reactive protein, tumour necrosis factor alpha or interleukin 6. In addition, treatment with certain immune-modulating drugs (e.g. interferon alpha) as well as systemic inflammation can induce depression-like symptoms ('sickness behaviour'). In contrast, clinical trials using anti-inflammatory treatments for depression have yielded some promising results. To date, it is unclear how exactly inflammatory processes could translate into depressive symptomatology. Some authors have suggested that cytokines could induce the expression of a tryptophan-metabolising enzyme (called indoleamine 2,3-dioxygenase), which could subsequently decrease the availability of the serotonin precursor tryptophan and increase the concentration of neurotoxins such as quinolinic acid. See Section 6.4 for more discussion of the role of inflammation in depression.

For a more comprehensive summary and discussion of neuroendocrine and neuroimmunological processes potentially related to depression and for further reading, please see [2, 3, 8–12].

9.7.4 Neuroanatomical Perspective

Neuroanatomical investigations in patients with major depression have revealed both structural and functional abnormalities in the limbic–corticostriatal–pallidothalamic pathway, which encompasses the orbitofrontal cortex, anterior cingulate cortex, basal ganglia, hippocampus, parahippocampus and amygdala.

In patients with depression, structural abnormalities have been found both in the grey matter as well as in the white matter. Examples of grey matter abnormalities that have been described include volume decreases of the hippocampus, frontal cortex, orbitofrontal cortex, cingulate cortex and basal ganglia. What exactly causes these volume changes is unclear to date but increased neuronal and glial cell death as well as diminished adult neurogenesis have been suggested as potential mechanisms (and could be plausibly related to prolonged exposure to elevated cortisol levels).

Especially in late-life depression, white matter lesions are also commonly observed. They are thought to result from ischaemic damage and might lead to depression by disrupting mood-regulating connections between limbic areas and the frontal cortex. Since higher levels of white matter lesions have been associated with poorer clinical outcome, a prominent symptom profile featuring apathy and psychomotor retardation, and greater clinical severity, some researchers have proposed that depression attributed to white matter abnormalities might represent a causally distinct subtype of major depressive disorder.

Functional neuroimaging studies in patients with depression have investigated potential abnormalities in brain activity at rest as well as when patients were engaged in cognitive tasks. These have yielded various abnormalities in blood flow and/or metabolism in different regions (e.g. the orbitofrontal, dorsolateral and dorsomedial cortices, anterior cingulate cortex and amygdala). When functional connectivity was assessed in patients with depression, evidence has emerged for focal and global connectivity abnormalities, suggesting that proper communication between different areas might be disturbed. In the limbic–corticostriatal–pallidothalamic circuit, several functional networks can be distinguished, including the cognitive control network, default-mode network, affective network and salience network. Interestingly, connectivity abnormalities have been reported both within these networks as well as between them.

For a more comprehensive discussion of structural and functional neuroanatomical abnormalities that have been linked to depression, and for further reading, see [2, 13–16].

9.7.5 Cognitive Perspective

Major depressive disorder has been associated with a range of abnormalities in how the brain processes information from the internal and external environment. Psychotherapeutic theories (such as those developed in the context of cognitive therapies) have long postulated that abstract high-level constructs such as 'dysfunctional attitudes' may play a causal role in the development of depression and have identified them as an important target for therapeutic interventions. Paralleling these ideas, dysfunctions in information processing associated with depression can also be observed in more basic cognitive domains such as perception, attention or memory, and can be captured using objective neuropsychological tests.

Cognitive impairments associated with major depression have been categorised into 'cold' (= emotion-independent) and 'hot' (= emotion-dependent) abnormalities. Cold cognitive impairments associated with depression are independent of the emotional valence of a processed stimulus and include altered attention, executive function and memory. Some cold cognitive abnormalities (e.g. memory impairments) have also been described in first-degree relatives of patients with depression. Furthermore, cold cognitive impairments seem to be more severe in patients with chronic or recurrent depression and might be predictive of poor treatment response regardless of symptom severity. This has led some authors to propose that at least a subgroup of patients with depression might benefit from cognition-enhancing interventions to improve their treatment outcome.

Hot cognitive abnormalities manifest as mood-congruent negative biases in the processing of emotional stimuli and abnormal processing of rewarding and punishing experiences. Negative biases can be captured using behavioural tasks that include positive as well as negative emotional stimuli. Healthy people generally exhibit a tendency to prioritise the processing of positive stimuli in these tasks, while in non-medicated depressed patients such positive biases are either less pronounced or completely reversed towards a prioritisation of negative input. Negative biases associated with depression have been described in different cognitive domains, including perception, attention, working memory and memory.

Importantly, different drugs (e.g. citalopram, reboxetine, mirtazapine, bupropion) have been shown to acutely induce a state of more positively biased emotional information processing – and this effect is observable in both healthy volunteers as well as patients with depression. These observations have led to the development of a cognitive neuropsychological model of antidepressant treatment action. According to this model, negative biases in hot cognition are not a mere epiphenomenon of depressed mood, but rather play a crucial causal role in its development. The drugs used for treating depression, according to the model, might thus exert their

HOW DO ANTIDEPRESSANT DRUGS USED TO TREAT DEPRESSION WORK?

Most of the currently available drugs used to treat depression target monoamine neurotransmitter function by, for example, inhibiting the reuptake of serotonin, noradrenaline or dopamine. This has led to theories that depression is caused by a deficit in monoamine function, which is remediated by treatment. However, a purely neurotransmitter-based explanation for drug action is challenged by the observation that, while monoamine levels are affected early in treatment, the effects on symptoms of depression take weeks to appear. This has led to two broad theoretical explanations for what happens during this delayed clinical onset.

The first, the **neurotrophic theory**, suggests that drug treatment triggers cellular processes involved in plasticity (such as proliferation of neuronal progenitor cells and expression of brain-derived neurotrophic factor (BDNF)). These effects could reverse potentially stress-induced and cortisol-mediated decreases in plasticity and cell function in depression.

The second, the **cognitive neuropsychological model of antidepressant treatment action**, highlights early effects of the drugs on the processing of positive versus negative information. These early effects can reverse negatively biased emotional information processing in depression and are believed to gradually reduce symptoms as the more positively biased processing influences mood, thoughts and behaviour over time (see Figure 9.7.2).

There is evidence for both of these theories and – as for the pathophysiology of depression – they may relate to different levels of description rather than opposing viewpoints. Future studies are needed to understand their relationship and how we can capitalise on these effects to improve the treatment of depression. For a more detailed discussion, see [23].

clinical effects by attenuating negative biases due to their shared ability to push emotional information processing towards positivity.

Some authors have extended this model to also incorporate a neuroscientific account of how psychological interventions (e.g. cognitive therapy) could work. Very briefly, the idea is that the prolonged presence of negative biases could feed the development and maintenance of negative beliefs (e.g. 'dysfunctional attitudes') about the world. These beliefs in turn could then exert top-down influence on hot cognition and further perpetuate and solidify the negative biases that gave rise to them in the first place. Drugs used to treat depression, in this model, are thought to tackle the low-level negative biases while psychotherapy is hypothesised to target the high-level negative beliefs. In principle, intervening on either level could break the vicious circle and thus lead to an improvement in mood. However, some patients may need treatment on both levels to develop a satisfactory response. See also Figure 9.7.2.

Other hot cognitive abnormalities that have been associated with depression are abnormal reward and punishment processing and abnormal motivation-related processes. For example, patients with depression have been shown to exhibit hypersensitivity to negative and hyposensitivity to positive feedback during reinforcement learning and decreased motivation in effort-based tasks. Future studies into these abnormalities might be especially helpful to improve our understanding of the clinically often difficult-to-treat symptom that is anhedonia (see Section 5.13).

For a more comprehensive summary and discussion of cognitive perspectives on depression, see [17–24].

9.7.6 Linking Individual Symptoms to Neurobiology

One long-standing question in the clinical neurosciences of major depression has been whether it is possible to map individual symptoms of depression to distinct neural processes (for example, to allow the development of more precise symptom-guided treatments).

Some authors have suggested that specific signs and symptoms of depression could indeed be traced to abnormal structure and/or function of specific circumscribed brain regions or, more plausibly, networks of brain regions. For example, the inability of depressed patients

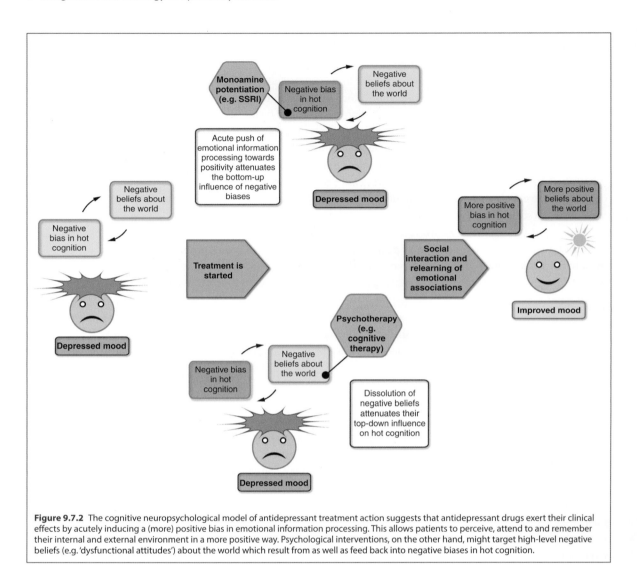

Figure 9.7.2 The cognitive neuropsychological model of antidepressant treatment action suggests that antidepressant drugs exert their clinical effects by acutely inducing a (more) positive bias in emotional information processing. This allows patients to perceive, attend to and remember their internal and external environment in a more positive way. Psychological interventions, on the other hand, might target high-level negative beliefs (e.g. 'dysfunctional attitudes') about the world which result from as well as feed back into negative biases in hot cognition.

to feel joy or pleasure may relate to dysfunctions within the reward circuitry of the brain involving the nucleus accumbens and the ventral striatum. Diminished ability to think or concentrate, on the other hand, could be related to impaired dorsolateral and dorsomedial prefrontal activity. Finally, impaired emotional processing might be linked to dysfunctions in limbic structures including the amygdala and the anterior cingulate cortex.

It has also been argued that depressive symptoms can be separated into those representing a lack of positive affect (anhedonia, lack of energy, etc.) and those relating to increased negative affect (low mood, guilt, irritability,

etc.). According to this theory, symptoms pertaining to decreased positive affect can be linked to impaired dopamine and noradrenaline pathway activity and thus patients who suffer from such symptoms might benefit particularly from drugs that target these systems (e.g. bupropion). On the other hand, symptoms linked to increased negative affect have been suggested to relate to impaired serotonergic and (again) noradrenergic activity. They might thus be more sensitive to drugs targeting these systems (e.g. SSRIs, SNRIs).

The simplicity and elegance of these theories notwithstanding, their predictions have not been properly evaluated to date. Furthermore, recent network approaches to psychopathology picture depression as the result of a dynamic interplay of symptoms that can be causally and reciprocally linked, that is, experiencing one symptom can cause other symptoms, some of which in turn might contribute to the maintenance of the first symptom. This, of course, raises further questions about whether symptoms could and should be conceptualised as independent neurobiological dysfunctions. Thus, more work will be needed to understand if it is possible to parse separable neural processes to individual symptoms or symptom clusters. For a more comprehensive discussion and further reading, please refer to [2, 25, 26].

Conclusions and Outstanding Questions

Major depressive disorder can be studied from different perspectives and on multiple levels of neuroscientific description. Neurochemical, neuroanatomical, neuroendocrine and cognitive perspectives on the pathophysiology of depression have revealed various abnormalities associated with the condition and suggested different – mutually not necessarily competing – theories of how depressive symptoms might develop. Future research will have to elucidate the causal relevance of different abnormalities, clarify how different levels of description could be linked mechanistically, establish whether and how individual symptoms of the disorder can be traced on each level of description and explore whether including other levels of description could offer additional insights.

Outstanding Questions

- What is the causal relevance of the various abnormalities that have been associated with depression on different levels of neuroscientific description? Which ones contribute to symptom development and which ones are mere epiphenomena (secondary effects)?
- What are the mechanisms that link abnormalities on different levels of description with each other?
- Could there be other important levels of description that have not been appreciated sufficiently to date (e.g. changes in the microbiome)?
- How can we explain the effects of antidepressant interventions on different levels of neuroscientific description?
- Could there be shared neurobiological mechanisms through which drugs and psychotherapy exert their clinical effects?

REFERENCES

1. American Psychiatric Association. *Diagnostic and Statistical Manual of Mental Disorders*, 5th ed. (DSM-5). American Psychiatric Association, 2013.

2. Harrison P, Cowen P, Burns T, Fazel M. Depression. In *Shorter Oxford Textbook of Psychiatry*, 7th ed. Oxford University Press, 2018, pp. 193–232.

3. Cowen P. Neuroendocrine and neurochemical processes in depression. In DeRubeis RJ, Strunk DR, eds., *The Oxford Handbook of Mood Disorders*. Oxford University Press, 2017, pp. 190–200.

4. Ruhé HG, Mason NS, Schene AH. Mood is indirectly related to serotonin, norepinephrine and dopamine levels in humans: a meta-analysis of monoamine depletion studies. *Mol Psychiatry* 2007; 12(4): 331–359.

5. Cowen P. Serotonin and depression: pathophysiological mechanism or marketing myth? *Trends Pharmacol Sci* 2008; 29(9): 433–436.

6. Sanacora G, Zarate CA, Krystal JH, Manji HK. Targeting the glutamatergic system to develop novel, improved therapeutics for mood disorders. *Nat Rev Drug Discov* 2008; 7(5): 426–437.

7. Sanacora G. Cortical inhibition, gamma-aminobutyric acid, and major depression: there is plenty of smoke but is there fire? *Biol Psychiatry* 2010; 67(5): 397–398.

8. Pariante CM, Lightman SL. The HPA axis in major depression: classical theories and new developments. *Trends Neurosci* 2008; 31(9): 464–468.

9. Pariante CM. The glucocorticoid receptor: part of the solution or part of the problem? *J Psychopharmacol* 2006; 20: 79–84.

10. Dantzer R, O'Connor JC, Freund GG, Johnson RW, Kelley KW. From inflammation to sickness and depression: when the immune system subjugates the brain. *Nat Rev Neurosci* 2008; 9(1): 46–56.

11. Krishnadas R, Cavanagh J. Depression: an inflammatory illness? *J Neurol Neurosurg Psychiatry* 2012; 83(5): 495–502.

12. Capuron L, Miller AH. Immune system to brain signaling: neuropsychopharmacological implications. *Pharmacol Ther* 2011; 130(2): 226–238.

13. Disabato B, Bauer IE, Soares JC, Sheline Y. Neural structure and organization of mood pathology. In DeRubeis RJ, Strunk DR eds., *The Oxford Handbook of Mood Disorders*. Oxford University Press, 2017, pp. 214–224.

14. Arnone D, McIntosh AM, Ebmeier KP, Munafò MR, Anderson IM. Magnetic resonance imaging studies in unipolar depression: Systematic review and meta-regression analyses. *Eur Neuropsychopharmacol* 2012; 22(1): 1–16.

15. Herrmann LL, Masurier ML, Ebmeier KP. White matter hyperintensities in late life depression: a systematic review. *J Neurol Neurosurg Psychiatry* 2008; 79(6): 619–624.

16. Price JL, Drevets WC. Neurocircuitry of mood disorders. *Neuropsychopharmacology* 2010; 35(1): 192–216.

17. Roiser J, Sahakian BJ. Information processing in mood disorders. In DeRubeis RJ, Strunk DR eds., *The Oxford Handbook of Mood Disorders*. Oxford University Press, 2017, pp. 179–189.

18. Roiser JP, Sahakian BJ. Hot and cold cognition in depression. *CNS Spectr* 2013; 18(3): 139–149.

19. Harmer C, Pringle A. Neuropsychological mechanisms of depression and treatment. In DeRubeis RJ, Strunk DR eds., *The Oxford Handbook of Mood Disorders*. Oxford University Press, 2017, pp. 201–213.

20. Harmer CJ, Goodwin GM, Cowen PJ. Why do antidepressants take so long to work? A cognitive neuropsychological model of antidepressant drug action. *Br J Psychiatry* 2009; 195(2): 102–108.

21. Roiser JP, Elliott R, Sahakian BJ. Cognitive mechanisms of treatment in depression. *Neuropsychopharmacology* 2012; 37: 117–136.

22. Eshel N, Roiser JP. Reward and punishment processing in depression. *Biol Psychiatry* 2010; 68(2): 118–124.

23. Harmer CJ, Duman RS, Cowen PJ. How do antidepressants work? New perspectives for refining future treatment approaches. *Lancet Psychiatry* 2017; 4(5): 409–418.

24. MacKenzie LE, Uher R, Pavlova B. Cognitive performance in first-degree relatives of individuals with vs without major depressive disorder: a meta-analysis. *JAMA Psychiatry* 2019; 76(3): 297.

25. Stahl SM. Mood disorders. In *Stahl's Essential Psychopharmacology: Neuroscientific Basis and Practical Applications*. 4th ed. Cambridge University Press, 2013, pp. 237–283.

26. Guloksuz S, Pries L-K, van Os J. Application of network methods for understanding mental disorders: pitfalls and promise. *Psychol Med* 2017; 47(16): 2743–2752.

National Neuroscience Curriculum Initiative online resources

Reshaping the Depressed Brain: A Focus on Synaptic Health

Danielle M. Gerhard and David A. Ross

The Habenula: Darkness, Disappointment, and Depression

Alfred Kaye and David A. Ross

Changing the Way We Think About (and With) Antidepressants

Andrew M. Novick and David A. Ross

What to say: Reshaping The Depressed Brain: A Focus on Synaptic Health

Robert Fenster

What to say: Changing The Way We Think About (and with) Antidepressants

Andrew Novick

This "stuff" is really cool: Dani Wentzel, *"Simple Logic", on BDNF, antidepressants and exercise*

This "stuff" is really cool: Allison Waters, *"The Ins and Outs of Brain-Based Treatment" on using neuroimaging to predict treatment response*

Expert video: *Paul Holtzheimer on Neuroscience & Depression*

Expert video: *Etienne Sibille on The Cellular & Molecular Basis of Depression*

9.8 Bipolar Affective Disorder

Nefize Yalin and Allan H. Young

OVERVIEW

Bipolar affective disorder is characterised by episodes of (hypo)mania and depression, and well-being states called euthymia [1]. The neurobiology of bipolar affective disorder is highly complex with several biological pathways putatively involved [1]. Despite the large amount of research on the pathophysiology of bipolar affective disorder, diagnosis still depends solely on symptomatology, and validated biological markers for diagnostic accuracy and treatment decisions remain to be determined [1]. This section summarises present findings on the biological mechanisms of bipolar affective disorder and highlights future research priorities.

9.8.1 Genetics of Bipolar Affective Disorder

Genetic factors in bipolar affective disorder were first highlighted by family and twin studies, which showed concordance rates of 8% to 10% in first-degree relatives and 40% to 70% in monozygotic twins [2]. These findings paved the way for molecular genetic studies in bipolar affective disorder and initial research centred on linkage studies showed that no loci of large effect are involved in the aetiology [2]. The linkage studies were followed by association studies and the research on candidate genes failed to provide any consistent findings. Nevertheless, genome-wide association studies (GWAS) revealed that variants in *TRANK1*, *ANK3*, *ODZ4*, *CACNA1* and *NCAN* genes are associated with susceptibility to bipolar affective disorder, supporting a polygenic aetiology for bipolar affective disorder, with risk being distributed across a large number of loci [2]. Recently, copy number variation studies have found that 1q21.1 duplication, 3q29 deletion and 16p11.2 duplication are associated with bipolar affective disorder [2]. Currently, genetic research on bipolar affective disorder focuses on whole-genome and exome sequencing as well as epigenetic modifications (DNA methylation, DNA hydroxymethylation and histone modifications), which are thought originate from

environmental influences including early-life adversities and treatments used in bipolar affective disorder [3]. Potentially, these approaches may enhance our understanding of the role of genetics in this disorder.

9.8.2 Neurotransmitters and Signal Transduction Systems in Bipolar Affective Disorder

Despite the large number of studies that have investigated the role of different neurotransmitter systems in bipolar affective disorder, evidence is still insufficient to allow definitive conclusions. For serotonin and noradrenaline, the most consistent findings are reduced serotonergic activity in the depressive phase and increased noradrenergic function in the manic phase [4]. With regard to dopamine, increases in dopamine 2 and 3 receptor availability were found in mania, whereas elevations in dopamine transporter levels were reported in euthymia and depression [5]. In terms of cholinergic systems, studies showed catecholaminergic–cholinergic imbalance in bipolar affective disorder, suggesting that the depressive phase might be associated with increases in cholinergic compared to catecholaminergic function while the reverse might be true of the manic phase [4]. Finally, glutamate levels are possibly increased in bipolar affective disorder, with abnormalities in expression of glutamate receptors in brain areas associated with the disease [6]. Studies combining molecular neuroimaging with genetic and other biological markers are needed to improve our knowledge on the role of neurotransmitters in bipolar affective disorder neurobiology.

The importance of signal transduction systems in bipolar affective disorder was initially indicated by lithium's ability to inhibit protein kinase C, a key enzyme in the phosphoinositide system [7]. Although later research on this cascade gave inconclusive results for protein kinase C levels in bipolar affective disorder, decreased levels of phosphoinositol and inositol monophosphatase and increased levels of phosphatidylinositol-4,5-bisphophate and calcium have repeatedly been demonstrated in bipolar affective disorder patients [7] (Figure 9.8.1). Another highly studied pathway is the adenylate cyclase cascade, which was found to be overactive in bipolar affective disorder with increased levels of stimulatory G-protein, adenylyl cyclase and protein kinase A [7] (Figure 9.8.2). One other signal transduction system that needs to be mentioned is the Wnt pathway. Dysregulation of this cascade in bipolar affective disorder manifests with increased glycogen synthase kinase 3 beta activation, beta-catenin phosphorylation and lysosomal destruction [7] (Figure 9.8.3). Regarding future directions,

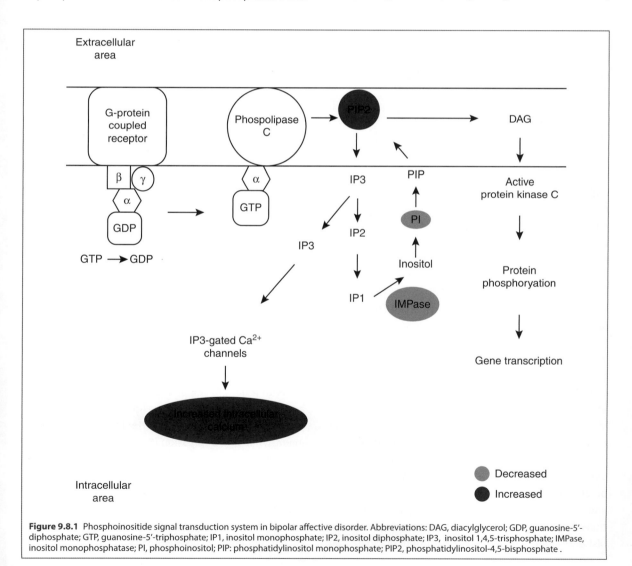

Figure 9.8.1 Phosphoinositide signal transduction system in bipolar affective disorder. Abbreviations: DAG, diacylglycerol; GDP, guanosine-5'-diphosphate; GTP, guanosine-5'-triphosphate; IP1, inositol monophosphate; IP2, inositol diphosphate; IP3, inositol 1,4,5-trisphosphate; IMPase, inositol monophosphatase; PI, phosphoinositol; PIP: phosphatidylinositol monophosphate; PIP2, phosphatidylinositol-4,5-bisphosphate .

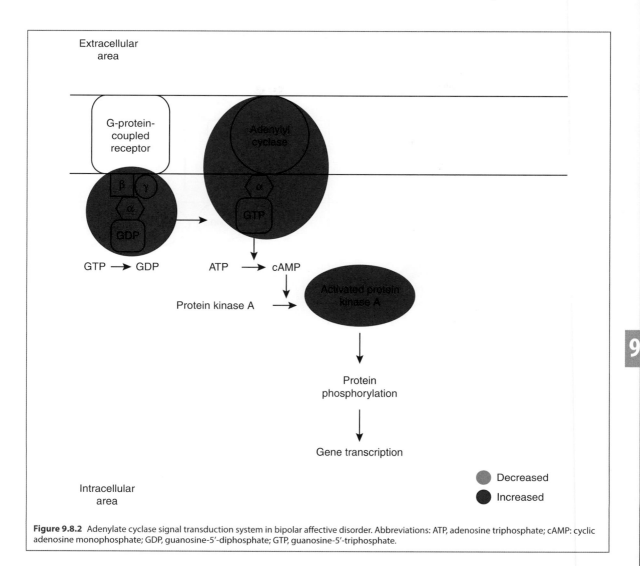

Figure 9.8.2 Adenylate cyclase signal transduction system in bipolar affective disorder. Abbreviations: ATP, adenosine triphosphate; cAMP: cyclic adenosine monophosphate; GDP, guanosine-5′-diphosphate; GTP, guanosine-5′-triphosphate.

human studies with bigger samples directly examining signal transduction abnormalities in the bipolar affective disorder brain are needed. Furthermore, more research is warranted on the role of extracellular signal-regulated kinases/mitogen-activated protein kinases and anti- and pro-apoptotic cascades in bipolar affective disorder.

9.8.3 Insights from neuroimaging in Bipolar Affective Disorder

There is now a 20-year history of neuroimaging studies of bipolar affective disorder, with the majority of studies conducted using structural MRI (sMRI), functional MRI (fMRI), diffusion tensor imaging (DTI) and magnetic resonance spectroscopy (MRS). So far, meta and mega analyses on sMRI have revealed grey matter volume reductions in the right insula, left anterior cingulate cortex, left inferior frontal cortex, bilateral hippocampus and thalamus, decreased cortical thickness in the left inferior frontal cortex, fusiform and rostral middle frontal cortex, decreased white matter volume in the posterior corpus callosum extending to the posterior cingulate cortex and enlarged lateral ventricles in bipolar affective disorder patients compared to healthy controls [8–11] (Figure 9.8.4). Although these sMRI alterations seem

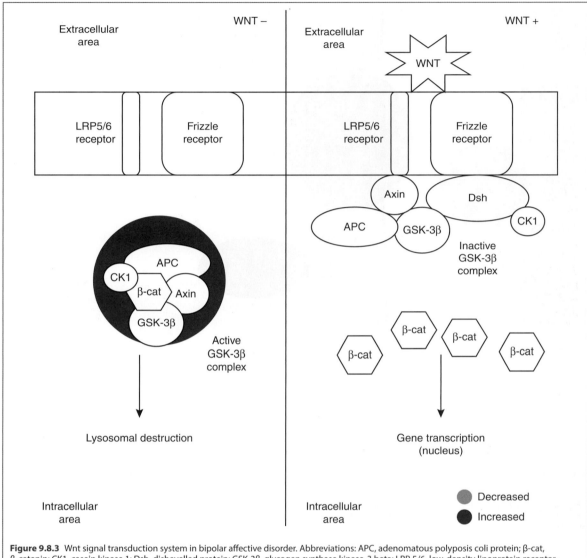

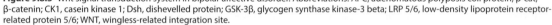

Figure 9.8.3 Wnt signal transduction system in bipolar affective disorder. Abbreviations: APC, adenomatous polyposis coli protein; β-cat, β-catenin; CK1, casein kinase 1; Dsh, dishevelled protein; GSK-3β, glycogen synthase kinase-3 beta; LRP 5/6, low-density lipoprotein receptor-related protein 5/6; WNT, wingless-related integration site.

to be independent from age, gender, age of onset and bipolar affective disorder subtypes across studies, they appear to be modulated by duration of illness, mood states and medications used in the bipolar affective disorder treatment including lithium and those with antiepileptic and antipsychotic action [8–11]. With regard to DTI studies, decreased fractional anisotropy in whole corpus callosum, bilateral cingulum, right posterior temporoparietal and left anterior and posterior cingulate cortices in bipolar affective disorder patients were shown compared to healthy controls [12, 13]. Considering MRS studies, in bipolar affective disorder patients compared to healthy controls there is evidence of decreased levels of N-acetylaspartate in the basal ganglia, lower N-acetylaspartate/creatinine ratio in the hippocampus and increased levels of glutamate and glutamine in frontal lobe and whole brain [6, 14]. Finally, meta-analysis of fMRI studies revealed underactivation in the inferior

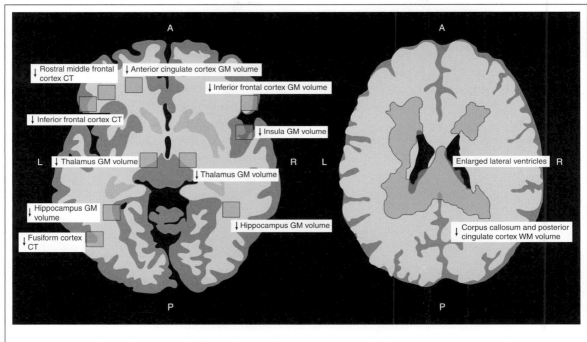

Figure 9.8.4 Structural MRI changes in bipolar affective disorder. Abbreviations: CT, cortical thickness; GM, grey matter; WM, white matter.

frontal cortex, lingual cortex and putamen during both cognitive and emotional tasks and overactivation in the putamen, pallidum and medial temporal lobe structures during emotional tasks in bipolar affective disorder patients in comparison to healthy controls [15] (Figure 9.8.5). Although the neuroimaging research to date has enhanced our understanding of bipolar affective disorder pathophysiology, it has also emphasised the need to incorporate multimodal biological measures into neuroimaging studies with prospective designs in order to find more clinically related biomarkers [16]. Future studies in this area should focus on implementing novel big data techniques into neuroimaging, conducting large-scale transdiagnostic studies, utilising new neuroimaging techniques such as functional MRS and quantitative MRI, as well as machine learning and multimodal imaging in order to better understand the bipolar affective disorder brain.

9.8.4 Peripheral Biological Markers in Bipolar Affective Disorder

Candidate peripheral biological markers (PBM) in bipolar affective disorder include markers of hypothalamic–pituitary–adrenal (HPA) axis function, inflammation, oxidative stress and brain-derived neurotrophic factor (BDNF). The HPA axis was the first peripheral biological marker investigated and a recent meta-analysis revealed that bipolar affective disorder patients have increased blood levels of cortisol (basal and post-dexamethasone) and adrenocorticotrophic hormone compared to healthy controls and while the rise in cortisol is positively associated with the manic phase it is negatively associated with antipsychotic use [17]. In terms of inflammatory markers, the manic and euthymic states were associated with increased C-reactive protein, interleukin (IL)-6, soluble IL-2 receptor and soluble IL-6 receptor; manic and depressive states were associated with increased tumour necrosis factor alpha (TNFα); and manic states were associated with increased soluble TNFα receptor 1 and IL-1 receptor antagonist [18]. Regarding BDNF and oxidative stress, BDNF levels were decreased in manic and depressive states while lipid peroxidation, deoxyribonucleic acid/ribonucleic acid damage and nitric oxide were significantly increased in bipolar affective disorder [1]. Larger prospective studies combining these peripheral markers with other biological parameters

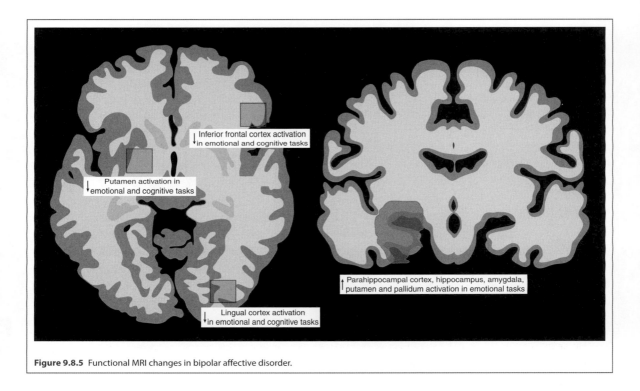

Figure 9.8.5 Functional MRI changes in bipolar affective disorder.

such as genetics, neurochemistry and neuroimaging are needed to enhance our understanding of their relationship with risk, course of disease, disease progression and treatment response.

Conclusions and Outstanding Questions

Bipolar affective disorder is a highly heritable disease with a clear polygenic component to the aetiology. The exact role of neurotransmitter systems is still uncertain, whereas imbalance in signal transduction systems may hold promise with future work. Neuroimaging studies highlight decreased grey and white matter, disturbance in brain networks during emotional and cognitive tasks and imbalanced metabolites in several brain cortices. Increased inflammation and oxidative stress as well as decreased BDNF levels are also likely to be a key part of bipolar affective disorder pathophysiology. Future studies should focus on integrating multimodal neuroimaging,

genetics, neurotransmitters, signal transduction systems and peripheral biological markers in order to understand the relevance of these with risk to disease, course of disease, disease progression and treatment response.

Outstanding Questions

- How do different types of neurobiological markers relate to each other in bipolar affective disorder pathopysiology?

- What is the exact relevance of the proposed neurobiological markers with disease risk, course of disease, disease progression and treatment response in bipolar affective disorder?

- Could clinical phenotyping increase precision in neurobiological studies?

- What could be the best study design and modality choice to model neurotransmitters and signal transduction systems pathways in bipolar affective disorder?

REFERENCES

1. Teixeira AL, Salem H, Frey BN, Barbosa IG, Machado-Vieira R. Update on bipolar disorder biomarker candidates. *Expert Rev Mol Diagn* 2016; 16(11): 1209–1220.

2. Goes FS. Genetics of bipolar disorder: recent update and future directions. *Psychiatr Clin North Am* 2016; 39(1): 139–155.

3. Legrand A, Iftimovici A, Khayachi A, Chaumette B. Epigenetics in bipolar disorder: a critical review of the literature. *Psychiatr Genet* 2021; 31(1): 1–12.

4. Manji HK, Quiroz JA, Payne JL et al. The underlying neurobiology of bipolar disorder. *World Psychiatry* 2003; 2(3): 136–146.

5. Ashok AH, Marques TR, Jauhar S et al. The dopamine hypothesis of bipolar affective disorder: the state of the art and implications for treatment. *Mol Psychiatry* 2017; 22(5): 666–679.

6. Gigante AD, Bond DJ, Lafer B et al. Brain glutamate levels measured by magnetic resonance spectroscopy in patients with bipolar disorder: a meta-analysis. *Bipolar Disord* 2012; 14(5): 478–487.

7. Niciu MJ, Ionescu DF, Mathews DC, Richards EM, Zarate CA, Jr. Second messenger/signal transduction pathways in major mood disorders: moving from membrane to mechanism of action, part II: bipolar disorder. *CNS Spectr* 2013; 18(5): 242–251.

8. Bora E, Fornito A, Yucel M, Pantelis C. Voxelwise meta-analysis of gray matter abnormalities in bipolar disorder. *Biol Psychiatry* 2010; 67(11): 1097–1105.

9. Hibar DP, Westlye LT, Doan NT et al. Cortical abnormalities in bipolar disorder: an MRI analysis of 6503 individuals from the ENIGMA Bipolar Disorder Working Group. *Mol Psychiatry* 2018; 23(4): 932–942.

10. Pezzoli S, Emsell L, Yip SW et al. Meta-analysis of regional white matter volume in bipolar disorder with replication in an independent sample using coordinates, T-maps, and individual MRI data. *Neurosci Biobehav Rev* 2018; 84: 162–170.

11. Hibar DP, Westlye LT, van Erp TG et al. Subcortical volumetric abnormalities in bipolar disorder. *Mol Psychiatry* 2016; 21(12): 1710–1716.

12. Favre P, Pauling M, Stout J et al. Widespread white matter microstructural abnormalities in bipolar disorder: evidence from mega- and meta-analyses across 3033 individuals. *Neuropsychopharmacology* 2019; 44(13): 2285–2293.

13. Nortje G, Stein DJ, Radua J, Mataix-Cols D, Horn N. Systematic review and voxel-based meta-analysis of diffusion tensor imaging studies in bipolar disorder. *J Affect Disord* 2013; 150(2): 192–200.

14. Kraguljac NV, Reid M, White D et al. Neurometabolites in schizophrenia and bipolar disorder: a systematic review and meta-analysis. *Psychiatry Res* 2012; 203(2–3): 111–125.

15. Chen CH, Suckling J, Lennox BR, Ooi C, Bullmore ET. A quantitative meta-analysis of fMRI studies in bipolar disorder. *Bipolar Disord* 2011; 13(1): 1–15.

16. Ching CRK, Hibar DP, Gurholt TP et al. What we learn about bipolar disorder from large-scale neuroimaging: findings and future directions from the ENIGMA Bipolar Disorder Working Group. *Hum Brain Mapp* 2022; 43(1): 56–82.

17. Belvederi Murri M, Prestia D, Mondelli V et al. The HPA axis in bipolar disorder: systematic review and meta-analysis. *Psychoneuroendocrinology* 2016; 63: 327–342.

18. Rowland T, Perry BI, Upthegrove R et al. Neurotrophins, cytokines, oxidative stress mediators and mood state in bipolar disorder: systematic review and meta-analyses. *Br J Psychiatry* 2018; 213(3): 514–525.

9

<table>
<tr><td>

9.9   **Psychosis**

</td><td>

Paul C. Fletcher

</td></tr>
</table>

OVERVIEW

Psychosis refers to the state of having a set of experiences and beliefs that do not accord with accepted reality and that seem to arise and persist in ways that do not reflect the evidence available. It is important to remember that the term is descriptive and is not in itself a diagnosis. Indeed, it emerges across a wide range of psychiatric, neurological and other physical disorders as well, in various forms, as a consequence of stress, trauma, drug use and other perturbations to the nervous system. Moreover, attention has more recently focused on the existence of attenuated psychosis-like thinking distributed within the healthy population: a phenomenon that has long been recognised (Taine, 1871) and that become a focus for systematic study more recently (e.g. van Os et al., 2009).

This chapter considers psychosis as a broad descriptive entity. It rejects, as arid and misguided, polarised debates over whether psychosis is a brain disorder or is primarily caused by external factors such as trauma since (i) any coherent view of brain function should acknowledge the profound influence of external factors on neural processes; (ii) conversely, a model that rejects the importance of neurobiology in understanding how the experiences of psychosis can be caused by events such as trauma is blinkered.

The concern here is with how the brain participates in a dynamic, adaptive interaction with its world and how this interaction may become disturbed. The discussion does not offer definitive statements about core pathophysiology in psychosis since this is likely to vary markedly across the different circumstances in which it occurs. What follows proposes that a deeper understanding of the general mechanisms by which psychosis may arise will prove very helpful in understanding these many circumstances and, ultimately, will be applicable to individual people and their treatment. Following consideration of the core features of psychosis, subsequent sections highlight the challenges in understanding it before exploring attempts to develop an adequate explanatory model,

one that applies at different levels of description, from the neurobiological to the social.

9.9.1 Hallucinations and Delusions: The Core Features of Psychosis

Psychosis has been defined and described in a number of different ways (Liddle, 2001). Though certain features (e.g. disorganised thought and behaviour, abnormal speech) are considered by some to be a core part of the psychotic state, for present purposes, a narrower view is taken: psychosis refers to a loss of contact with reality. It comprises abnormal beliefs (delusions) and perceptions (hallucinations). Therefore, an important prelude to understanding psychosis is likely to comprise a consideration of the ways in which a person constructs and experiences their perceptions and beliefs as well as how the content and expression of those phenomena shapes a person's model of reality, a principle that recurs.

A **delusion** is a firmly held belief that is out of keeping with a person's educational and cultural background. It persists even when there is strong evidence contradicting it. Delusions tend to be described in terms of their content (persecutory, grandiose, somatic, etc.) but there is much to be learned from focusing too on how they emerge, how a person experiences them and how they fluctuate across time and context. A **hallucination** is a percept without a corresponding explanatory stimulus. Hallucinations tend to be defined according to their sensory modality (and, indeed, can occur in any of the sensory modalities), their form (e.g. a voice) and by their content (e.g. third-person commentary with a persecutory content). See Sims (2008) for an overview and examples of these phenomena.

9.9.1.1 Are Hallucinations and Delusions Fundamentally Different Phenomena?

Hallucinations are perceptions and delusions are beliefs. While the latter assertion has been challenged on a number of grounds, the arguments over whether delusions can be called beliefs will not be considered here. It is fruitful to ask whether hallucinations are truly distinct phenomena since this has important implications for the perturbations that may underlie them. There are several reasons for questioning the dichotomy:

- Hallucinations often entail a belief about the reality of the perception, one that is intimately related to its experience.
- Delusional beliefs often seem to comprise a perceptual component. For example, delusions of control often present not just as a belief that one is under the control of another agent but also as a feeling or physical perception.
- A deeper, computational neuroscientific understanding of the nature of perception, and something that has profound implications for our models of psychosis, emphasises the fact that a delusion is an inference based on sensory evidence integrated with prior expectation.

On these grounds, perceptions and beliefs, and therefore delusions and hallucinations, share important features when viewed at a deeper level. This presents a potential conflict between perspectives that consider psychosis at different levels, and points to the importance of seeking precision in the language and concepts that we use.

9.9.1.2 Additional Perceptual Changes

Hallucinations are generally distinguished from **illusions**, which are misperceptions of a stimulus. However, there are many instances where the distinction is not clear-cut and there are notable changes in perceptual processing during the early stages of psychosis (Chapman, 1966) that do not fit easily into either definition. Indeed, the distinction is blurred even further when one realises that hallucinations and illusions are not far-removed from normal perceptual process. As observed in a remarkably comprehensive early treatment of psychosis: 'illusions are merely the sprinkling of fragments of genuine hallucination on a background of true perception' (Gurney et al., 1886).

9.9.2 The Neuroscience of Psychosis: Ambiguities and Challenges

Psychosis presents a major challenge to any attempt at a neuroscience-based explanation. Its complexity and variability of presentation, together with its tendency to emerge in many different contexts, makes identification of a core pathology elusive. But more profoundly challenging is the fact that psychosis is defined and described in terms of the highest levels of our experiences of, and beliefs about, reality. In order to represent psychosis in neuroscientific terms, therefore, we would need a comprehensive knowledge of how the brain represents and experiences the world. Since such knowledge is a long way off, we should be humble in making any brain-based assertions and we should, furthermore, beware of the widely prevalent assumptions that identifying something in the brain correlated with psychotic experience constitutes an explanation or an understanding. While such correlative observations are interesting and may, ultimately, contribute to a deeper understanding of how, why and where psychosis may arise, alone, they are inherently ambiguous since one cannot determine whether they reflect a cause or consequence of, or a compensation for, the clinical phenomena (Lewis, 2000).

A further profound challenge emerges when we recognise that observations at the neurobiological level do not link in a straightforward way to higher-level – psychological, clinical, subjective – phenomena. Observing that activity in brain area X correlates with the presence, absence or profundity of a symptom, may tell us that activity in X is associated with that symptom (albeit with the caveats alluded to above). If we knew precisely what computations are carried out in area X, we might conclude that such computations are related to the clinical phenomenon but, in general, we do not have such an understanding of regional brain function so we are left simply with an interesting but, in explanatory terms, very limited observation.

In brief, if we knew the cognitive or computational underpinnings of a clinical experience, say, a hallucination, we could map this experience onto brain observations and thereby learn more about the brain. Or if we knew what a brain region did and then observed that it was reliably active in association with a hallucination, we would have learned something important about the nature of hallucinations. But, if we have neither a full understanding of hallucinations nor of the functional role of the brain region, clearly our correlative observation must be interpreted very carefully if we are to avoid the risk of what Jaspers referred to as 'pseudo-insight through terminology' (Jaspers, 2013). This is a profound limitation of functional neuroimaging applications generally but is not unique to them. This is not to say that neurobiological observations may not prove useful and important in distinguishing patients from controls, or in identifying subtypes of psychosis, or in predicting clinical trajectories, outcomes and treatment effects. But they have far to go before they may be considered as plausible mechanistic explanations for psychosis.

9.9.3 Models of Psychosis

Part of our drive towards neuroscientific understanding must lie in the development, testing and refining of mechanistic models that have the potential to link multiple explanatory levels (so-called consilience). Currently, many see the models that hold greatest promise in this regard are those offering computational accounts of brain, behaviour and experience (Montague et al., 2011). They can be framed in terms of brain processes as well as cognition and offer inputs for social and cultural insights, though they face a number of difficulties (Teufel and Fletcher, 2016). Critically, they can be experimentally informed and tested. The following two subsections consider several influential models of psychosis and how they have shaped our understanding.

An array of models and explanations have been proposed to account for the features of psychosis (often in the context of schizophrenia). However, approaches that show validity and experimental support in accounting for hallucinations (most notably, so called **monitoring hypotheses**) are often less compelling when applied as explanations for delusions. Conversely, explanations for delusional thinking (for example, **information-processing bias accounts** and the **aberrant salience hypothesis**) are not convincingly applicable to hallucinations. This apparent selectivity of explanatory models might not necessarily concern us: if hallucinations and delusions are truly separate phenomena, it might make sense that their underlying causes, and hence the explanations that we must propose, can be distinct and need not refer to each other. In this respect, an important and influential perspective is that the psychotic state requires two dissociable impairments: one that accounts for the altered perceptual experiences, and one that accounts for altered beliefs, that is, for the fact that these new experiences are incorporated into an altered, and apparently bizarre and improbable, model of reality. This **two-factor theory** (see below) can be contrasted with the perspective that the disturbances in perception and belief that characterise psychosis may be accounted for by the same factor, though the differences may not be irreconcilable.

The following subsections briefly describe influential models of hallucinations and delusions before going on to more comprehensive accounts that seek to account for both the delusions and hallucinations simultaneously, either appealing to two factors or else rejecting the distinction and seeking a comprehensive account based on one factor.

9.9.4 Models of Hallucinations: Altered Self-Monitoring

One of the striking features of hallucinations is that internally generated experiences are interpreted as arising from an external source. An auditory hallucination, for example, has been accounted for as arising from a tendency to attribute inner speech to an outside agent. This idea is fully and elegantly outlined by Frith (1992), who lays out the hypothesis that core symptoms of schizophrenia arise when internally generated actions are misinterpreted as being external in origin. It is an important characteristic of this model that it draws on principles of neurology, psychology and neurophysiology and thus, unlike a number of predecessors, generates testable experimental predictions within these domains. In appealing, for example, to the notions of corollary discharge and inter-regional relationships in the brain (Ford and Mathalon, 2004, 2005), the model has allowed the fruitful and informative application of neuroimaging to understanding hallucination and delusion (Figure 9.9.1).

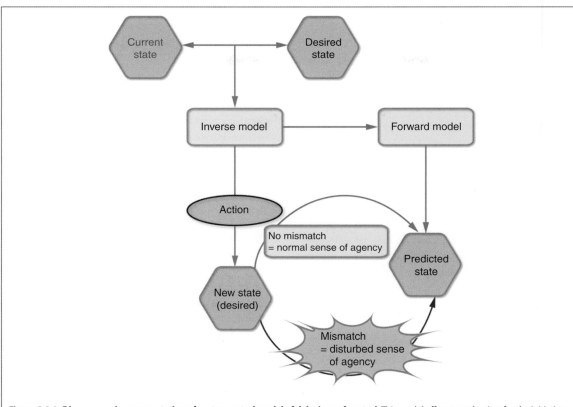

Figure 9.9.1 Diagrammatic representation of motor control model of delusions of control. This model offers a mechanism for the initiation and control of goal-directed actions (Wolpert and Kawato, 1998; see also Frith, 2005). If a person's desired state differs from their current state, an 'inverse model' forms the basis for calculating the sequence of motor commands that would attain the goal state. In parallel, a 'forward model' generates a prediction of the state that would be attained if the actions proposed by the inverse model were carried out. If necessary, this could be used to modify the inverse model. Otherwise, actions can be carried out to achieve the desired state, bringing the person into a new state that has been predicted using the forward model. It has been suggested that a satisfactory accordance between the new state and the prediction of that state is a key component of the 'sense of agency', that is, the sense that one has willed and achieved an action. Conversely, a mismatch at this point, in the form of a prediction error, could provide a sense that one was not the agent of an action (and hence, perhaps, that one is under the control of an external agent). It has been suggested that this erroneous mismatch signal, perhaps arising from a faulty forward model, is the basis for delusions of control and other symptoms of psychosis in which an internally generated event is falsely attributed to an external source.

As well as successfully accounting for auditory hallucinations in terms of misattributed inner speech, this model provides a compelling explanation for how delusions of control may arise when the sensory consequences of an internally-generated movement are not anticipated, leading to the powerful experience that the movement was not intended and, hence, must have been initiated by an external agent (Frith 1992). As with auditory hallucinations, the model has inspired formal experimental testing: for example, it has been shown that the phenomenon of anticipatory force-cancellation in schizophrenia is altered (Shergill et al., 2005).

9.9.5 Models of Delusions

While altered self-monitoring has been related to delusions, its applicability is less convincing when considering altered beliefs, for which there is no clear understanding of what might constitute predictions or, indeed, sensory consequences. Rather, influential models of delusions have tended to appeal to altered inference processes, that is, to an alteration in how conclusions are drawn on the basis of existing evidence. Some models assert that delusions are associated with an alteration in the experiences that constitute the evidence while others suggest that experience/evidence is unchanged but that the nature of inference process is altered. Examples of each are briefly described below.

9.9.5.1 Aberrant Salience: Altered Experience Giving Rise to Altered Beliefs

Maher (1974) put forward eloquent accounts of how delusional beliefs may arise as a consequence of, or more precisely, as explanations for, changes in perceptual experiences. This idea has been at the core of a number of ensuing accounts that framed the emergence of delusions as a learning or inference process (Miller, 1976; Hemsley, 2005). In particular, the account proposed by Kapur (2003) – the so-called **aberrant salience hypothesis** – has been highly influential. This draws together three ideas and, in doing so, provides not just a credible account for how delusions might arise but also a means of relating delusions to neurobiological underpinnings, including dopamine dysregulations (see Section 4.6.3 for background on dopaminergic pathways in the brain). The ideas are:

(1) Dopaminergic firing is dysregulated in schizophrenia.

(2) Dopamine firing forms the basis for attribution of attention to events and objects and it is critical in allocating them motivational salience – that is, this firing is the basis for attending to and acting upon events and stimuli.

(3) If there is aberrant dopamine firing (for example, inappropriately high firing to an irrelevant event), it results in disruption of 'the normal process of contextually driven salience attribution and leads to aberrant assignment of salience to external objects and internal representations'.

(4) Therefore, delusions, according to this framework, are top-down explanations that the individual uses in the attempt to make sense of experience. As Kapur states: 'Since delusions are constructed by the individual, they are imbued with the psychodynamic themes relevant to the individual'. Once the person arrives at an explanation, they are relieved by this insight and then continue to look for confirmatory evidence.

In addition, Kapur's account provides a framework for understanding how dopamine blockade may treat delusions. He suggests that the action of the drugs used for treating psychosis may be to 'dampen' this increase in motivational salience: 'Anti-psychotics do not excise

symptoms, rather they attenuate the salience of the distressing ideas and percepts, allowing patients to reach their own private resolution of these matters' (Kapur, 2003).

9.9.5.2 Altered Inference: Jumping to Conclusions

The key feature of another set of explanations is that delusional thinking is underpinned by inferential biases, rather than by normal inference acting on abnormal experiences. One noteworthy feature of these models is that they frame the emergence of a delusion in terms of biases that are frequently found in healthy people. In doing so, they help to develop the idea of psychosis as a continuum of normal experience. They have also provided a powerful framework within which to consider cognitive–behavioural treatment approaches in delusional states.

Several inferential alterations have been proposed. I shall mention one: that psychosis – and particularly delusions – arise from a tendency to 'jump to conclusions' or, more precisely, to develop a strong inference on the basis of less information sampling. There have been further suggestions that there is inflexibility once the inference has been made – a so-called **bias against disconfirmatory evidence**). It has been consistently shown that people with, or prone to, delusions, sample less evidence before making a decision, a finding that accords well with the idea that delusional reasoning is based on altered processing of available evidence. While this has compelling face validity, the emergent picture is a complex one, with a recent study (Dudley et al., 2016) demonstrating that, while schizophrenia is associated with reduced information sampling, delusions are actually associated with more.

9.9.6 Explaining Abnormal Experiences and Abnormal Beliefs: Two-Factor Theory

Based on observations of delusional thinking in the context of brain injury, and drawing on the principles of neuropsychology, a compelling case (e.g. Coltheart, 2007; Langdon, 2011) has been made that single-factor theories (abnormal experience or abnormal inference), such as those described above, are insufficient to account for psychosis. Rather, two factors must be invoked: (1) an abnormal perception which accounts for the **content** of the belief and (2) an abnormal inference which accounts for the **failure to reject** the belief.

The two-factor theory provides a very valuable perspective as it points to important omissions in the ideas above. Indeed, it seems undeniable that, if we are to elucidate fully the mechanisms by which psychosis arises, it is inevitable that we must consider both changed perceptions and changed beliefs. And, if perceptions and beliefs are different, if they have different properties and arise and persist through different mechanisms, embracing two-factor theory seems to be not just advisable but inevitable. In the next subsection, however, the possibility is raised that, though perception and belief are descriptively distinct, at a deeper level, they share important properties, raising the possibility that perceptions and beliefs – and hence hallucinations and delusions – can be considered together and can arise as a consequence of a single mechanistic disturbance.

9.9.7 A Single Underlying Disturbance in Psychosis: Predictive Processing and Related Theories

The most recent developments in theoretical models of psychosis have roots spread across a number of eras, and disciplines, including, among others, cybernetics, information theory, reinforcement learning, artificial intelligence and visual neuroscience. Core to them is a recognition that the profound problem faced by a brain trying to make sense of a world is the need to derive a model of the causes of its sensory input. These causes are essentially ambiguous. That is, any given pattern of sensory impressions could have an infinite number of causes and the challenge is to identify the most probable. That we can do this by relying on prior knowledge is an idea that goes back to von Helmholtz who stated: 'Objects are always imagined in the field of vision as would have to be there in order to create the same impression on the nervous mechanism' (von Helmholtz, 1867). In short, perception is a constructive (imaginative) act in which the percept accords with what is most probable.

This idea of perception as inference to the most likely cause has important connotations for how we may understand psychosis. It is central to so-called **predictive coding** (Rao and Ballard, 1999), the idea of the brain as an organ of prediction, and to the view that our experiences of the world are generated by an integration of sensory input and past experience (Friston, 2012). It introduces a framework for understanding information processing as a hierarchical system of message-passing in which higher areas generate predictions about upcoming signals and thereafter process the prediction error – the deviation of the upcoming signals from the top-down expectations.

This view, that our model of reality arises from a complex and fine balance between feedforward signals and feedback predictions, offers a comprehensive framework for considering the computational and neurobiological instantiation of perceptions and beliefs and also offers us new and testable ways of thinking about psychosis (Fletcher and Frith, 2009; Adams et al., 2013). Notably, it considers psychosis as a sub-optimal model of the world, with delusions and hallucinations emerging from a shift in the feedforward–feedback balance. For example, excessive top-down expectation could generate percepts that do not accord with reality (hallucinations) while excessive weighting of feedforward signals could lead to a powerful, though erroneous, drive to update the world model, to develop new and delusional beliefs. That is, delusions and hallucinations can be considered in the setting of a single alteration or disturbance.

Moreover, within this framework, two other useful features emerge: first, the nature of the balance and how it is maintained can be highly different across different people, as can the ways in which it can become perturbed. Second, the contents of delusions and hallucinations cannot be seen as separate from the prior experiences (and, hence, predictions) of the person in question. This is illustrated in a simple example shown in Figure 9.9.2. Past trauma or adversity may change prior expectations and generate an explanatory framework for sensory inputs. This is important, it counsels strongly against neglecting the individual's past experiences and their consequent repertoire of explanations and predictions since these will profoundly shape how they experience and respond to any perturbation of the balance. Furthermore, and related to this, while the framework is potentially useful for understanding how psychotic experiences might ultimately emerge, it also entertains a wide range of underlying causal possibilities. One can imagine many ways in which the priors may be shifted (e.g. by traumatic past experience), the inputs may be perturbed (e.g. by sensory

9

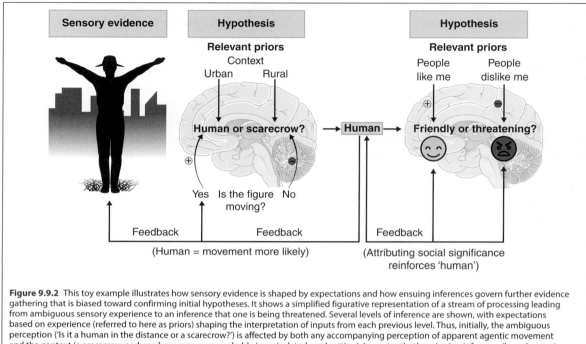

Figure 9.9.2 This toy example illustrates how sensory evidence is shaped by expectations and how ensuing inferences govern further evidence gathering that is biased toward confirming initial hypotheses. It shows a simplified figurative representation of a stream of processing leading from ambiguous sensory experience to an inference that one is being threatened. Several levels of inference are shown, with expectations based on experience (referred to here as priors) shaping the interpretation of inputs from each previous level. Thus, initially, the ambiguous perception ('Is it a human in the distance or a scarecrow?') is affected by both any accompanying perception of apparent agentic movement and the context (a scarecrow perhaps becomes more probable in an isolated rural setting). Importantly, the winning inference (here, human) both becomes the substrate for the next level of inference ('Is there a meaningful social gesture?') and generates the modified expectations for ensuing input (for example, movement may be more readily perceived and attended to when the overarching hypothesis is 'human'). Put simply, the inference 'human' means that further inputs are processed in a way that confirms it as the correct hypothesis. At a higher level, the percept may be attributed a social significance ('Threatening?', 'Friendly?') depending on the person's prior expectations (which of course, may be highly complex and intricate). Importantly, as well as leading to a further updating of ever higher-level inferences, the interpretation at this level provides further confirmatory evidence that the lower inferences ('movement' and 'human') are correct and meaningful. After all, if the percept has social significance, it confirms that the figure is human, and if it is human, movement is highly probable.

damage or deprivation) or the integration of signals may be changed to produce altered inferences (e.g. by drugs). In short, this is truly a biopsychosocial model.

9.9.8 Linking to Neurochemical Underpinnings

One of the attractions of computational modelling of mental symptoms is in the potential to provide a link between higher-level subjective experiences, cognitive processes and the underlying neurobiology, including neurochemistry. (It should be noted, though, that this is not without challenges and limitations; see Teufel and Fletcher, 2016). Sophisticated attempts have been made to explicate predictive processing and related models in terms of the existing understanding of neurotransmitter systems in the brain (e.g. Friston, 2010) and thereby to embed the ideas more deeply in cerebral cortex microcircuitry (Shipp, 2016). A general suggestion is that the content of both top-down predictions and the

upcoming prediction-error signals is mediated by 'driving' neurotransmission (predominantly glutamatergic) while modulatory neurotransmitters, notably dopamine and acetylcholine, underpin 'precision' by changing the gain on driving neurotransmitters (e.g. Kanai et al., 2015). In essence, this would mean that, say, a putative dopaminergic disturbance in psychosis might exert its effect through changing the gain on glutamatergically mediated prediction-error signals (for a comprehensive description of applying the model to psychosis, see Adams et al., 2013).

It is important to recognise that this work embedding predictive processing in underlying neurochemistry is largely theoretical and remains at a speculative stage, though there is empirical support for links between aspects of glutamatergic transmission and the top-down/bottom-up signalling processes that are key to the predictive processing ideas outlined above (Self et al., 2012). Crucially, however, computational approaches, exemplified by predictive processing, offer a framework for generating testable hypotheses about how perturbations, both pharmacological and non-pharmacological (Corlett et al., 2009), may underpin complex mental symptoms, thereby linking different levels of description and generating a real potential for much-needed consilience in psychiatry (Kapur, 2003).

9.9.9 Psychosis Models: Competing or Complementary?

It is easy to see these and other explanatory models for psychosis as being in competition, with the task of the researcher to weigh up the validity of each and select the one that, for the moment, performs best. This is not necessarily so. Models provide different explanations at different levels and are constructed with a variety of aims in mind (see Teufel and Fletcher (2017) for fuller discussion). Importantly they do not necessarily compete with each other: for example, it may be that the family of predictive processing models easily encompass reality monitoring models, the latter providing specific instances of more general and extensive principles that are made explicit in the latter (Griffin and Fletcher, 2017). Even seemingly discordant ideas, such as one-factor versus two-factor theories, may be reconciled when we recognise that they are pitched at different levels of explanation. Thus, while examining the state of psychosis at one level of description, it makes sense to consider both alterations in experience and in belief. But, recognising that, at a deeper (computational and neurobiological) level, perception is a form of inference, and thus overlaps with belief, it remains possible that one underlying perturbation may encompass changes that, at the higher level, tend to be described using two different terminologies. Such considerations should precede all attempts to adjudicate between apparently competing models.

Conclusions and Outstanding Questions

The term psychosis provides a description for an altered model of reality that may arise across a range of circumstances and with a large set of possible underlying causes.

I have argued here that it will be valuable to develop a mechanistic understanding of how the features of psychosis arise and persist and have offered some sketches of how existing models, functioning at different levels of explanation, and with different explanatory aims and scope, may offer useful frameworks for scrutinising psychosis and for identifying causal pathways by which it arises. The increasingly sophisticated approaches to non-invasive human neuroscience will demand such frameworks if they are to fulfil their potential since, alone, they provide only partial and ambiguous insights. Attempts to embed high-level descriptions of the experience, characteristics and circumstances of psychosis in fundamental principles emerging from neuroscience will be immensely challenging and, without suitable models, likely impossible.

Outstanding Questions

- Computational psychiatry approaches to clinical syndromes inevitably involve simplified models that, perforce, do not account for the complete phenomenology of psychotic experiences. Can we extend these models to provide a more comprehensive account of why, for example, delusional beliefs are so fixed and seemingly impervious to evidence, or why they tend to involve recurring themes, such as persecution?

- While computational accounts of symptoms offer the prospect of linking complex experiences to neurobiology, the reality is that we have only a rudimentary understanding of the brain basis for predictive processing. Can we extend and enhance this by harnessing advances in neuroscientific understanding of the functional architecture of predictive processing hierarchies?

- What are the implications for therapeutic interventions of developing this model of mechanisms underlying psychotic experiences?

- Can we employ this framework for understanding psychosis to improve stratification of clinical groups, thereby making research questions more precise and treatments more targeted?

9

REFERENCES

Adams RA, Stephan KE, Brown HR, Frith CD, Friston KJ (2013). The computational anatomy of psychosis. *Front Psychiatry* 30(4):47.

Chapman J (1966). The early symptoms of schizophrenia. *Br J Psychiatry* 112(484): 225–251.

Coltheart M (2007). Cognitive neuropsychiatry and delusional belief. *Q J Exp Psychol (Hove)* 60(8): 1041–1062.

Corlett PR, Frith CD, Fletcher PC (2009). From drugs to deprivation: a Bayesian framework for understanding models of psychosis. *Psychopharmacology* 206(4): 515–530.

Dudley R, Taylor P, Wickham S, Hutton P (2016). Psychosis, delusions and the "jumping to conclusions" reasoning bias: a systematic review and meta-analysis. *Schizophr Bull* 42(3): 652–665.

Fletcher PC, Frith CD (2009). Perceiving is believing: a Bayesian approach to explaining the positive symptoms of schizophrenia. *Nat Rev Neurosci* 10(1): 48–58.

Ford JM, Mathalon DH (2004). Electrophysiological evidence of corollary discharge dysfunction in schizophrenia during talking and thinking. *J Psychiatr Res* 38(1): 37–46.

Ford JM, Mathalon DH (2005). Corollary discharge dysfunction in schizophrenia: can it explain auditory hallucinations? *Int J Psychophysiol* 58(2–3): 179–189.

Friston, K (2010). The free-energy principle: a unified brain theory? *Nat Rev Neurosci* 11, 127–138.

Friston K (2012). Prediction, perception and agency. *Int J Psychophysiol* 83(2): 248–252.

Frith CD (1992). *The Cognitive Neuropsychology of Schizophrenia*. Lawrence Erlbaum Associates.

Frith, CD (2005). The self in action: lessons from delusions of control. *Consciousness Cogn* 14: 752–770.

Griffin JD, Fletcher PC (2017). Predictive processing, source monitoring, and psychosis. *Annu Rev Clin Psychol* 8(13): 265–289.

Gurney E, Myers FWH, Podmore F (1886). *Phantasms of the Living*. Trubner & Co.

Hemsley DR (2005). The development of a cognitive model of schizophrenia: placing it in context. *Neurosci Biobehav Rev* 29(6): 977–988.

Jaspers, K (2013). *Allgemeine Psychopathologie*. Springer-Verlag.

Kanai R, Komura Y, Shipp S, Friston K (2015). Cerebral hierarchies: predictive processing, precision and the pulvinar. *Philos Trans R Soc London B* 370(1668): 20140169.

Kapur S (2003). Psychosis as a state of aberrant salience: a framework linking biology, phenomenology, and pharmacology in schizophrenia. *Am J Psychiatry* 160(1): 13–23.

Langdon R (2011). The cognitive neuropsychiatry of delusional belief. *Wiley Interdiscip Rev Cogn Sci* 2(5): 449–460.

Lewis DA (2000). Distributed disturbances in brain structure and function in schizophrenia. *Am J Psychiatry* 157: 1–2.

Liddle PF (2001). *Disordered Mind and Brain: The Neural Basis of Mental Symptoms*. Gaskell.

Maher BA (1974). Delusional thinking and perceptual disorder. *J Individ Psychol* 30(1): 98–113.

Miller R (1976). Schizophrenic psychology, associative learning and the role of forebrain dopamine. *Med Hypotheses* 2(5): 203–211.

Montague PR, Dolan RJ, Friston KJ, Dayan P (2012). Computational psychiatry. *Trends Cogn Sci* 16(1): 72–80. Erratum in *Trends Cogn Sci* 2012; 16(5): 306.

Rao RP, Ballard DH (1999). Predictive coding in the visual cortex: a functional interpretation of some extra-classical receptive-field effects. *Nat Neurosci* 2(1): 79–87.

Self MW, Kooijmans RN, Supèr H, Lamme VA, Roelfsema PR (2012). Different glutamate receptors convey feedforward and recurrent processing in macaque V1. *Proc Natl Acad Sci USA* 109(27): 11031–11036.

Shergill SS, Samson G, Bays PM, Frith CD, Wolpert DM (2005). Evidence for sensory prediction deficits in schizophrenia. *Am J Psychiatry* 162(12): 2384–2386.

Shipp S (2016). Neural elements for predictive coding. *Front Psychol* 7: 1792.

Sims A (2008). *Sims' Symptoms in the Mind: An Introduction to Descriptive Psychopathology*. Saunders Elsevier.

Taine H (1871). *On Intelligence*. L. Reeve and Co.

Teufel C, Fletcher PC (2016). The promises and pitfalls of applying computational models to neurological and psychiatric disorders. *Brain* 139(Pt 10): 2600–2608.

van Os J, Linscott RJ, Myin-Germeys I, Delespaul P, Krabbendam L (2009). A systematic review and meta-analysis of the psychosis continuum: evidence for a psychosis proneness–persistence–impairment model of psychotic disorder. *Psychol Med* 39(2): 179–195.

von Helmholtz H (1867). *Handbook of Physiological Optics*. Verlag von Leopold Voss.

Wolpert DM, Kawato M (1998). Multiple paired forward and inverse models for motor control. *Neural Networks* 11: 1317–1329.

National Neuroscience Curriculum Initiative online resources

Guided by Voices: Hallucinations and the Psychosis Spectrum

Albert R. Powers, Philip R. Corlett and David A. Ross

Clinical neuroscience conversations: Auditory-Verbal Hallucinations

Demian Rose

This "stuff" is really cool: Kunmi Sobowale, *"In Case of a Fire"* on integrating prior beliefs with context

9

Expert video: *Demian Rose on Hallucinations*

Expert video: *Oliver Howes on First Episode Psychosis*

**Emilio Fernandez-Egea and
Peter B. Jones**

OVERVIEW

Described over a century ago, schizophrenia still presents personal, clinical and scientific challenges, and is increasingly considered a concept rather than a single disorder. It has become a paradigmatic psychiatric disorder while remaining something of an enigma. Defined by a syndrome of psychotic phenomena (positive phenomena such as delusions, hallucinations or disordered thought structure) and negative features resulting from motivation and emotional dysfunction, schizophrenia is defined by symptoms lasting at least 4 weeks and impairment for 6 months or more [1, 2]. Where the illness is short-lived, the clinical syndrome is defined as a schizophrenia-related diagnosis [1]. The clinical presentation usually encompasses features prominent in other psychiatric conditions such as cognitive dysfunction, motor abnormalities, obsessional phenomena or depression. These additional features not included in the definition of schizophrenia underscore its pervasive neural dysfunction; they influence management and often shape the clinical outcome. The seeds of schizophrenia may be sown in early life with aberrant childhood development in multiple domains [2], but the clinical syndrome typically presents in early adulthood (Figure 9.10.1); abnormal neural connectivity may underlie these seemingly remote phenomena. About a quarter of patients will have a single episode, half will suffer relapsing episodes and another quarter will experience persistent psychotic illness.

Being such an extensive concept, much neuroscience relevant to schizophrenia is covered elsewhere in this textbook including limitations of animal models (Section 3.3) and sex differences (Section 5.3). Here, we describe key anatomical, electrophysiological, biochemical and brain-circuitry findings, with special emphasis on dopamine function. We go on to detail the neurobiology of core symptom domains of schizophrenia: psychotic, negative, cognitive, motor and affective. We also consider proposals for unifying neurobiological mechanisms such as dysconnectivity, abnormal neurodevelopment or pleiotropy with immunological dysfunction.

9.10.1 Anatomy: Macro- and Microscopic

Seminal CT studies showed that schizophrenia is associated with enlargement of the lateral and third ventricles and of the subarachnoid area, between the meninges and the brain [5], suggesting a reduction in temporal and frontal cortical volumes. Higher-resolution imaging modalities (e.g. MRI and voxel-based morphometry, Chapter 3) consistently show decreased whole-brain volume in schizophrenia, especially in the temporal lobe, hippocampus, amygdala, thalamus, anterior cingulate cortex and basal ganglia [6], accounting for the early CT findings. Over the course of the illness, progressive volume loss may occur in frontal and temporal grey matter areas [7].

White matter abnormalities are also widespread in schizophrenia. Diffusion tensor imaging studies (DTI, see Chapter 3) show decreased white matter integrity (measured with fractional anisotropy or mean diffusivity) across association tracts (intrahemispheric), commissural tracts (interhemispheric) and projection tracts (ascending

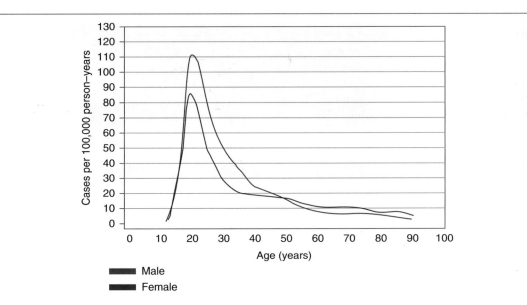

Figure 9.10.1 Schizophrenia as a neurodevelopmental disorder. The age-at-onset function is one of the most replicable characteristics of schizophrenia and is prime facie evidence that schizophrenia is a developmental syndrome, as seen in the composite figure drawn on the basis of published evidence (e.g. Solmi et al. [3]). In contrast to neurodevelopmental disorders presenting during early childhood, its onset is bound to the subsequent epoch of dramatic brain development between puberty and the late twenties (see Section 8.2), although onset is often presaged by earlier developmental manifestations in a wide variety of domains: motor, social, cognitive and language. The neuroscientific basis of these early developmental phenomena may be recapitulated following puberty, with abnormal neural connectivity being a potential unifying mechanism for these and the psychosis syndrome (see text). Causes of schizophrenia are best seen in this developmental or life-course framework: genetic and early-life environmental (physical, psychological or social) events disrupt normal brain development, making it vulnerable to later-life stressors (cannabis, psychosocial trauma including racism, and other factors), which act as triggers of a hyperdopaminergic state in the striatum, leading to the core psychosis syndrome. In addition to epidemiological data [4], supporting evidence for a developmental view of schizophrenia comes from minor physical anomalies, structural brain abnormalities seen before the onset (see Subsection 9.10.1) and the excess of abnormal cognitive and neurodevelopmental findings in schizophrenia patients. Early intervention services have been created worldwide to provide fast-track access to care; these are predicated on these life-course, developmental models but do not yet support or refute them experimentally. The figure also shows that around 17 people per 1,000 experience schizophrenia during their lifetime, double that for related psychoses and marginally more common in men.

and descending fibres), mainly at the inferior longitudinal fasciculus, inferior fronto-occipital fasciculus, corpus callosum and cingulum bundle (see Section 4.5 for the neuroanatomy of these tracts).

Modern histopathological post-mortem studies have shown cytostructural abnormalities in schizophrenia. These abnormalities are mostly found in prefrontal, hippocampal and thalamic areas, involving pyramidal neurons, interneurons and glia [8]. The decreased grey matter volumes seen on neuroimaging could reflect either fewer cells or smaller cells (or a combination): histological studies of pyramidal neurons in the prefrontal cortex indicate that, rather than fewer neurons, increases in cell packing are due to a reduction in neuron density, reduced soma (cell body) size, reduced dendritic field (the extent of dendritic branching) and reduced spine density. Fewer oligodendrocytes have been reported in various

brain areas in schizophrenia [9]. Molecular changes in prefrontal cortical interneurons include decreased expression of glutamate decarboxylase, reelin, parvalbumin, somatostatin and cholecystokinin.

Overall, these findings suggest subtle but widespread abnormalities in both grey and white matter: in particular, reduced connectivity between neurons both locally and globally.

9.10.2 Event-Related Potentials, Pre-Pulse Inhibition and Latent Inhibition

Electrophysiological studies have shown abnormal information filtering and processing in schizophrenia. Abnormalities in EEG theta and gamma bands have been described but the major abnormalities were found using event-related potentials. This technique measures a characteristic series of EEG waves after a specific event (e.g. noise), measured as positive (P) or negative (N) deflections in the EEG and time elapsed (in milliseconds). Schizophrenia is consistently associated with deficits in the P50 (a positive response 50 msec after the stimulus), N100 and P300 amplitudes in auditory stimuli, and the N400 response to semantic priming. This suggests abnormal sensory gating [10], a process by which irrelevant stimuli are separated from meaningful ones, while mismatch negativity studies indicate decreased ability to detect auditory change (e.g. a change in the noise pattern).

Other electrophysiological studies have focused on startle reflexes, that is, reflexes intended to prepare a person to deal with a sudden change. Two phenomena are particularly important: pre-pulse inhibition occurs when a low-intensity pre-stimulus reduces the reaction to a more intense stimulus which follows it; startle habituation refers to the phenomenon where repeated presentation of a stimulus leads to a smaller response to that stimulus. A related phenomenon is called latent inhibition, in which pre-exposure to a stimulus on its own delays subsequent association of that stimulus to an outcome. Interestingly, all these effects are abnormal in people with schizophrenia and are biomarkers underpinning several animal models of schizophrenia [11].

Overall, in schizophrenia there may be a reduced ability to predict future events based on past experience: responses to familiar events are abnormally large, and responses to surprising events are abnormally small. The resulting excess of unpredictable information may lead to errors in the attribution of relevance (salience), poor executive function and abnormal goal-directed behaviour (motivation).

9.10.3 Functional Connectivity in Schizophrenia

Bar the neurodegenerative dementias, the evidence implicating abnormal connectivity as a mechanism for psychiatric illness is strongest for schizophrenia: symptoms may emerge from disturbances in synchronisation of communication between brain areas, rather than a localised lesion [12].

The combination of diffuse white matter and diffuse EEG changes implicates particular brain networks, that is, groups of regions that show synchronous activity during functional neuroimaging. As reviewed in Section 5.18, the study of the connectome (the brain as a set of networks) using graph theory (and other methods) has demonstrated network abnormalities in schizophrenia. The default-mode network – active during waking and at rest – is key: people with schizophrenia show abnormalities both during the resting state and when they are asked to shift attention. An influential meta-analysis using DTI information has shown that abnormal hubs in schizophrenia were mostly concentrated in frontal and temporal cortical regions [13].

9.10.4 Genetics

The genetics of schizophrenia has been extensively covered elsewhere (Section 2.6 and Chapter 7). Although it is highly heritable, the environment is also key, and there is no 'schizophrenia gene'; rather, many (at least hundreds of) alleles confer a slightly increased risk, pointing to dopamine and glutamate pathways (see below) but also to genes not directly associated with classical neurotransmitter pathways, such as the immune system, synaptic plasticity and neurodevelopment. There is considerable overlap between the genes implicated in different mental disorders.

9.10.5 Neurochemistry of Schizophrenia

Abnormal synaptic function is the hallmark of schizophrenia. Dopamine is at the core of our mechanistic and therapeutic understanding but is not the only neurotransmitter implicated (see Section 2.3 for more on dopaminergic transmission).

9.10.5.1 Dopamine

Dopamine neurotransmission is key to the motivation–reward system (the process of ascertaining what is relevant or pleasurable, Section 5.9) and to motor control (see Section 5.6). It has recently also been implicated in processes relevant to the positive symptoms of schizophrenia, namely associative learning [14] and hallucinations [15]. Its importance in schizophrenia symptoms is well established (Figure 9.10.2). For instance, the antipsychotic efficacy of different dopamine-blocking drugs is directly associated with their affinity to the D2 receptor [16]. The use of dopamine agonists in Parkinson's disease

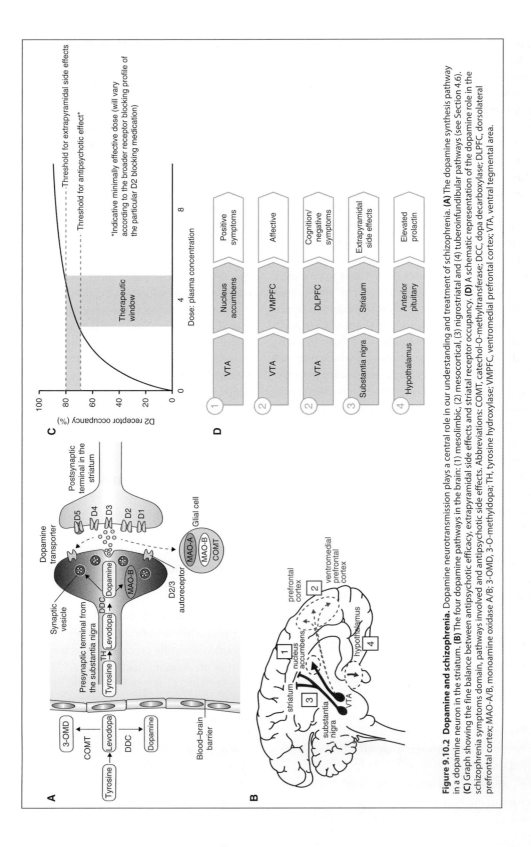

Figure 9.10.2 Dopamine and schizophrenia. Dopamine neurotransmission plays a central role in our understanding and treatment of schizophrenia. **(A)** The dopamine synthesis pathway in a dopamine neuron in the striatum. **(B)** The four dopamine pathways in the brain: (1) mesolimbic, (2) mesocortical, (3) nigrostriatal and (4) tuberoinfundibular pathways (see Section 4.6). **(C)** Graph showing the fine balance between antipsychotic efficacy, extrapyramidal side effects and striatal receptor occupancy. **(D)** A schematic representation of the dopamine role in the schizophrenia symptoms domain, pathways involved and antipsychotic side effects. Abbreviations: COMT, catechol-O-methyltransferase; DCC, dopa decarboxylase; DLPFC, dorsolateral prefrontal cortex; MAO-A/B, monoamine oxidase A/B; 3-OMD, 3-O-methyldopa; TH, tyrosine hydroxylase; VMPFC, ventromedial prefrontal cortex; VTA, ventral tegmental area.

treatment is associated with psychotic symptoms in a dose-dependent manner.

Several mechanisms are thought to elevate presynaptic dopamine release in schizophrenia including dysfunction of the *N*-methyl-D-aspartate (NMDA) receptor (glutamatergic pathway) and GABAergic interneurons, sensitisation by stress and by psychostimulants, and cannabis use. Single-photon emission computed tomography (SPECT) and positron emission tomography (PET) techniques (Section 3.1.5) can distinguish dopamine synthesis from dopamine release or postsynaptic dopamine receptor density *in vivo*. Imaging during the prodromal phase of schizophrenia shows excess neural dopamine synthesis capacity, linked with subclinical psychotic symptoms [17]. In people with established schizophrenia, both excess synthesis and excess release of dopamine are observed. Postsynaptic D2 receptor supersensitivity has also been observed in PET and SPECT studies. However, these results are confounded by the effects of long-term D2 blockade by drugs with antipsychotic action, which results in increased homeostatic postsynaptic synthesis of the D2 G-protein receptor (see below). Note, this phenomenon is also important in the pathogenesis of treatment-related tardive dyskinesia where reduction in the drug dose may be related to a transient worsening of the movement disorder until this system re-equilibrates.

All currently used drugs for psychosis exert their main action through postsynaptic receptor antagonism. In the G-protein-receptor tribe, there are two main dopamine receptors: the D2 family (with D2, D3 and D4 subtypes) and the D1 family (D1 and D5 subtypes). Clinically, a 50% striatal blockade of D2/D3 is required to achieve antipsychotic action, whereas blockade above 80% has no greater efficacy but leads to side effects: a rule that guides titration of dose in clinical practice. See also [18] .

9.10.5.2 Other Neurotransmitters

A number of other neurotransmitters have been implicated in schizophrenia, either by their role in increasing the release of dopamine (e.g. in part by the glutamate pathway and NMDA receptors) or as a primary/independent dysfunction, suggesting potential novel therapeutic opportunities.

Most (~70%) patients with first-episode psychotic disorder respond to dopamine-blocking drugs [19] . For the remainder, defined as having treatment-resistant schizophrenia if they do not respond to at least two drugs, evidence suggests there is no excess presynaptic dopamine synthesis. This highlights the heterogeneity of the syndrome: magnetic resonance spectroscopy shows increased glutamate metabolites in the frontal cortex [20] and might, when alternative treatment approaches are available, help clinicians identify who may be resistant to conventional D2 blocking antipsychotic therapy and so reduce the delay in accessing the right therapies. As it stands, such an approach might hasten the use of clozapine.

The endocannabinoid (cannabinoid) system is also implicated in schizophrenia: tetrahydrocannabinol in cannabis (marijuana) can lead to psychotic phenomena, while cannabidiol is under investigation as a therapeutic agent. The alpha-7-nicotinic receptor also has a potential role in enhancing cognition in schizophrenia. Similarly, the serotonin (5-hydroxytryptamine; 5-HT) pathway may play a role: agonism of 5-HT2A might also cause psychotic symptoms, underpinning the efficacy of second-generation (atypical) drugs with antipsychotic action (D2/5-HT2A antagonists).

9.10.6 The Immunology of Schizophrenia

Recent paradigm shifts mean the brain is no longer considered an immune-privileged organ. A fast-growing research field is starting to address central and peripheral immune function in schizophrenia and other mental disorders. See Section 6.4 for further details.

9.10.7 The Neuroscience of Specific Schizophrenia Symptoms

9.10.7.1 Psychosis

Psychotic symptoms are the core criteria for schizophrenia. Also called positive (as a *de novo* emergence of psychic phenomena) or reality-distortion symptoms, they are vivid experiences for patients, impacting their behaviour and mood and impairing their social and working life. Hallucinations refer to sensory perceptions without a stimulus (e.g. hearing voices); delusions are strongly held abnormal beliefs based on insufficient evidence (and maintained in the face of contradictory evidence) that are unusual for the person's cultural and education background.

The emergence of psychotic symptoms could be hypothesised using the anatomical, electrophysiological and biochemical abnormalities mentioned above. Social adversities (e.g. trauma) might prime brain attention which, combined with the excess of unpredictable information in the brain, poor communication between key brain areas and attribution of relevance to innocuous factors, can lead to the onset of psychotic symptoms [21]. Cognitive and computational neuroscience attempts to explain the mechanisms by which abnormal dopamine function might lead to the emerge of psychotic symptoms. Fletcher in this volume (Section 9.9) reviews theories leading to abnormal perception and delusion using a cognitive neuroscience framework and the central role of dopamine in salience, reward and learning. See also [22].

Thought disorganisation (formal thought disorder) betrayed in written or spoken language is often included as part of schizophrenia. Typical examples are 'loose association' of ideas or words (clanging or word salad). These symptoms have been linked with abnormal event-related potentials and abnormal synchrony between brain areas.

9.10.7.2 Cognitive Symptoms

Neurocognitive deficits are key in schizophrenia. They are present before the onset of psychosis, during acute exacerbations and during periods of remission. They are important because they are key predictors of functional outcome and are poorly treated (or even exacerbated) by drugs for psychosis. Attention (Section 5.12), memory (Section 5.14) and executive functions (Section 5.15) are particularly affected, with performance about 1.5 standard deviations below healthy controls [23]. Executive dysfunction implicates the prefrontal cortex, including the dorsolateral prefrontal, anterior cingulate and orbitofrontal cortices, with extensive, dopamine-dependent communication with other brain subcortical areas such as the amygdala, hippocampus and basal ganglia.

9.10.7.3 Negative Symptoms

There are five domains of a negative symptom complex or 'deficit syndrome', significantly impairing normal function:

(1) anhedonia: lack of sense of pleasure during activity or the anticipated pleasure from a future activity

(2) asociality: reduced social activity accompanied by decreased interest in forming close relationships with others

(3) avolition: a reduction in the initiation of and persistence in activity

(4) alogia, a quantitative reduction of words spoken

(5) blunted affect, a decrease in the outward expression of emotion (facial or vocal expression or reduction in expressive gestures).

Factor analytic studies indicate that domains 1, 2 and 3 co-occur as a motivation and pleasure (MAP) complex, independently of 4 and 5 as an emotional expression dimension [24]. There is an overlap between cognitive and negative symptoms: motivation and pleasure are associated with impaired executive and goal-directed function, whereas expression is associated with global impairment in cognition. Furthermore, there are trans-diagnostic commonalities. For instance, avolition in schizophrenia can be studied using the same prism of apathy as in depression or neurodegenerative disorder (Section 5.13). Dopamine dysfunction has been the main (but not the only) focus of study in the context of reduced reward sensitivity, pleasure experience and emotion regulation. See Section 5.9 for more on the role of dopamine in reward and pleasure. Clinically, this means that depression, extrapyramidal drug side effects (see below) and even positive psychotic symptoms need exclusion (and treatment) when assessing negative symptoms.

9.10.7.4 Motor Symptoms

Abnormal movements, such as spontaneous dyskinesia and parkinsonism, are present developmentally (and transiently) in children who will develop schizophrenia as adults and are common in treatment-naïve patients [25]. Indeed, Kraepelin's conceptualisation of schizophrenia merged Kahlbaum's catatonia with two other entities (paranoia and hebephrenia); interest in motor symptoms intrinsic to schizophrenia faded with the advent of medication with antipsychotic action and the attendant drug-induced motor symptoms [25]. They are of great interest due to commonalities in the reward-learning and prediction-error systems that may have evolved to support motor behaviour and are implicated in psychosis.

Dyskinesias are present in about 12% of cases: abnormal involuntary movements of the orofacial, limb, trunk and respiratory musculature. Parkinsonism symptoms are seen in 20%, mostly as rigidity or tremor associated with dopamine dysfunction [26]. That these symptoms can also be caused by the antipsychotic-induced dopamine antagonism in the basal ganglia (mesostriatal dopamine pathway) complicates their assessment in clinical practice.

Catatonia [27] is potentially life-threatening. Characterised by periods of psychomotor immobility (stupor catatonia) with limited episodes of non-goal-directed hyperactivity (excited catatonia), sometimes evolving to malignant catatonia (motor symptoms plus autonomic dysregulation), patients might present spectacular symptoms such a catalepsy, waxy flexibility, echolalia, echopraxia, grimacing, stereotypy or mutism. Interestingly, catatonia has been linked to GABAergic dysfunction in the basal ganglia (see Section 5.6), hence the therapeutic efficacy of benzodiazepines, or the risk of triggering a catatonic stuporous state during the withdrawal of agents with potent gamma-aminobutyric acid (GABA) action (e.g. clozapine, benzodiazepines or alcohol). Finally, catatonia is starting to be considered (again) transdiagnostically as it can occur not only in schizophrenia and related disorders but also in major affective disorder (depression and bipolar), associated to autism or even as an independent entity.

9.10.7.5 Affective Symptoms

Depressive and manic symptoms are common in people with schizophrenia, and clinical depression is experienced by at least half of patients during their illness. There are different approaches to the depression in schizophrenia patients, including considering it as intrinsic to the illness, a side effect of medication, an expression of negative symptoms or a psychological response to the psychotic illness and its consequences. It is likely that a combination of these factors is responsible for affective symptoms, and the underlying mechanisms are shared with those detailed for major depressive disorder (Section 9.7) and bipolar affective disorder (Section 9.8).

9.10.7.6 Other Phenomena

We have limited this chapter to the symptoms most closely related to the disorder. Nevertheless, patients with schizophrenia experience high comorbidity with other symptoms/disorders [28]. Reviewing the neurobiology of these might be also useful for a more comprehensive understanding. Comorbid problems often include post-traumatic stress disorder (Section 9.5), anxiety disorder (Section 9.4), obsessive–compulsive disorder (Section 9.6 and Section 5.8 on habit formation), metabolic complications (Section 5.1), substance misuse (Section 9.3) and autism (Section 9.1).

Conclusions and Outstanding Questions

We are far from fully understanding the neuroscience underlying schizophrenia and it remains unclear whether the schizophrenia syndrome is a collection of discrete aetiopathological disorders with similar manifestations, or a single entity with diverse clinical expression.

Outstanding Questions

- Will study of neurotransmitter systems beyond dopamine yield new therapeutics?
- Does immune dysfunction illuminate the obscure but unequivocal link between schizophrenia and physical health, perhaps offering new therapeutic approaches?
- Is schizophrenia preventable?
- Key for patients, families and clinicians and related to the therapeutic obstinacy of negative and cognitive symptoms: how can life functioning be improved when psychotic symptoms are controlled?

REFERENCES

1. American Psychiatric Association. *Diagnostic and Statistical Manual of Mental Disorders*, 5th ed. (DSM-5). American Psychiatric Association, 2013.

2. Jones P, Murray R, Rodgers B, Marmot M. Child developmental risk factors for adult schizophrenia in the British 1946 birth cohort. *Lancet* 1994; 344(8934): 1398–1402.

3. Solmi M, Radua J, Olivola M et al. Age at onset of mental disorders worldwide: large-scale meta-analysis of 192 epidemiological studies. *Mol Psychiatry* 2022; 27(1): 281–295.

4. Radua J, Ramella-Cravaro V, Ioannidis JPA et al. What causes psychosis? An umbrella review of risk and protective factors. *World Psychiatry* 2018; 17(1): 49–66.

5. Johnstone EC, Frith CD, Crow TJ, Husband J, Kreel L. Cerebral ventricular size and cognitive impairment in chronic schizophrenia. *Lancet* 1976; 2(7992): 924–926.

6. Ellison-Wright I, Bullmore E. Anatomy of bipolar disorder and schizophrenia: a meta-analysis. *Schizophrenia Research* 2010; 117(1): 1–12.

7. Ho B-C, Andreasen NC, Nopoulos P et al. Progressive structural brain abnormalities and their relationship to clinical outcome. *Archives of General Psychiatry* 2003; 60(6): 585–594.

8. Jaaro-Peled H, Ayhan Y, Pletnikov MV, Sawa A. Review of pathological hallmarks of schizophrenia: comparison of genetic models with patients and nongenetic models. *Schizophrenia Bulletin* 2010; 36(2): 301–313.

9. Glantz LA, Lewis DA. Decreased dendritic spine density on prefrontal cortical pyramidal neurons in schizophrenia. *Archives of General Psychiatry* 2000; 57(1): 65.

10. Amann LC, Gandal MJ, Halene TB et al. Mouse behavioral endophenotypes for schizophrenia. *Brain Research Bulletin* 2010; 83(3-4): 147–161.

11. Thaker GK. Neurophysiological endophenotypes across bipolar and schizophrenia psychosis. *Schizophrenia Bulletin* 2008; 34: 760–773.

12. Fornito A, Bullmore ET. Reconciling abnormalities of brain network structure and function in schizophrenia. *Current Opinion in Neurobiology* 2015; 30: 44–50.

13. Crossley NA, Mechelli A, Scott J et al. The hubs of the human connectome are generally implicated in the anatomy of brain disorders. *Brain* 2014; 137(8): 2382–2395.

14. Lee JY, Jun H, Soma S et al. Dopamine facilitates associative memory encoding in the entorhinal cortex. *Nature* 2021; 598(7880): 321–326.

15. Schmack K, Bosc M, Ott T, Sturgill JF, Kepecs A. Striatal dopamine mediates hallucination-like perception in mice. *Science* 2021; 372(6537): eabf4740.

16. Seeman P, Lee T, Chau-Wong M, Wong K. Antipsychotic drug doses and neuroleptic/dopamine receptors. *Nature* 1976; 261(5562): 717–719.

17. McCutcheon RA, Merritt K, Howes OD. Dopamine and glutamate in individuals at high risk for psychosis: a meta-analysis of *in vivo* imaging findings and their variability compared to controls. *World Psychiatry* 2021; 20(3): 405–416.

18. Stahl SM. *Stahl's Essential Psychopharmacology*. Cambridge University Press, 2013.

19. Kahn RS, Wolfgang Fleischhacker W, Boter H et al. Effectiveness of antipsychotic drugs in first-episode schizophrenia and schizophreniform disorder: an open randomised clinical trial. *Lancet* 2008; 371: 1085–1097.

20. Jauhar S, Veronese M, Nour MM et al. Determinants of treatment response in first-episode psychosis: an ^{18}F-DOPA PET study. *Molecular Psychiatry* 2019; 24(10): 1502–1512.

21. Howes OD, Murray RM. Schizophrenia: an integrated sociodevelopmental–cognitive model. *Lancet* 2014; 383(9929): 1677–1687.

22. McKenna P. *Delusions: Understanding the Un-Understandable*. Cambridge University Press, 2017.

23. Marder SR. The NIMH-MATRICS project for developing cognition-enhancing agents for schizophrenia. *Dialogues in Clinical Neuroscience* 2006; 8(1): 109–113.

24. Ahmed AO, Kirkpatrick B, Galderisi S et al. Cross-cultural validation of the 5-factor structure of negative symptoms in schizophrenia. *Schizophrenia Bulletin* 2019; 45(2): 305–314.

25. Pappa S, Dazzan P. Spontaneous movement disorders in antipsychotic-I patients with first-episode psychoses: a systematic review. *Psychological Medicine* 2009; 39: 1065–1076.

26. Mateos JJ, Lomeña F, Parellada E et al. Decreased striatal dopamine transporter binding assessed with [123I] FP-CIT in first-episode schizophrenic patients with and without short-term antipsychotic-induced parkinsonism. *Psychopharmacology* 2005; 181(2): 401–406.

27. Fink M, Taylor MA. *Catatonia: A Clinician's Guide to Diagnosis and Treatment*. Cambridge University Press, 2006.

28. Plana-Ripoll O, Pedersen CB, Holtz Y et al. Exploring comorbidity within mental disorders among a Danish national population. *JAMA Psychiatry* 2019; 76(3): 259–270.

National Neuroscience Curriculum Initiative online resources

Addressing Cognitive Deficits in Schizophrenia: Toward a Neurobiologically Informed Approach

Ashley E. Walker, Jerrod D. Spring and Michael J. Travis

Kraepelin's Crumbling Twin Pillars: Using Biology to Reconstruct Psychiatric Nosology From the Bottom Up

Joao P. De Aquino and David A. Ross

What to say: Kraepelin's Crumbling Twin Pillars: Using Biology to Reconstruct Psychiatric Nosology from The Bottom Up

Robert Boland

Clinical neuroscience conversations: *Endophenotypes and Psychosis*

This "stuff" is really cool: Melanie Grubisha, *"Franklin's Future" on bridging genetics and neuropathology in schizophrenia*

9.11 **Borderline Personality Disorder**

Patrick Luyten, Peter Fonagy and Chloe Campbell

OVERVIEW

This chapter considers the neuroscience of borderline personality disorder, also known as emotionally unstable personality disorder, focusing on three domains: neuroendocrinological, structural and functional findings. Research in these areas is related to clinical understanding of borderline personality disorder as characterised by (1) emotional dysregulation, (2) impulsivity and (3) social dysfunction. In patients with borderline personality disorder, the hypothalamic–pituitary–adrenal (HPA) axis tends to show elevated continuous cortisol output and blunted cortisol following psychosocial challenges. The amygdala and hippocampus differ from healthy controls in terms of both reduced volume and measurable activity, and the dorsolateral prefrontal cortex tends to be less active. The neurobiology of borderline personality disorder can be characterised as a proneness to flooding by cortisol, with the amygdala working to heighten the affective meaning of stressful stimuli, and the prefrontal cortex underperforming in the task of downregulating emotional experience. The chapter also considers genetic findings in relation to borderline personality disorder.

9.11.1 Neuroscientific Approaches to Borderline Personality Disorder

Borderline personality disorder is perhaps paradigmatic of the complex and inter-reacting nature of neurobiology, genes and environment in mental health disorder. Our understanding of the neurobiology of borderline personality disorder has developed rapidly in recent years, and evidence is increasingly accruing that implicates the basic stress response and structural and functional differences in brain areas concerned with emotion and cognition. Here, we provide a brief overview of these findings and situate these within a multilevel perspective on the aetiology of borderline personality disorder.

The *Diagnostic and Statistical Manual of Mental Disorders*, 5th edition (DSM-5) [1] uses the following nine criteria for borderline personality disorder, of which a minimum of five must be apparent for a diagnosis: (1) a pattern of unstable intense relationships, (2) inappropriate, intense anger, (3) frantic efforts to avoid abandonment, (4) affective instability, (5) impulsive actions, (6) recurrent self-harm and suicidality, (7) chronic feelings of emptiness or boredom (dysphoria), (8) transient, stress-related paranoid thoughts and (9) identity disturbance and severe dissociative symptoms. The range of these criteria means that borderline personality disorder is a heterogeneous diagnosis. The high rates of comorbidity associated with the disorder add to the heterogeneity, and have complicated research on its neurobiology. However, there is increasing consensus that the overarching characteristics of borderline personality disorder are **emotional dysregulation**, **impulsivity** and **social dysfunction**. Neurobiological systems underpinning these areas of functioning have been identified. We discuss these findings in a developmental model that takes in **genetic and environmental stressors** and **forms of response to stress** that shape social–cognitive function.

An integrated neurobiological perspective on borderline personality disorder tends to point towards an approach that considers the range of biological systems associated with this disorder as generating a low threshold for the activation of an **interpersonal emergency functioning system**: the stimulation of the attachment system; the loss of the capacity for reflective, controlled mentalising (the ability to understand actions by both other people and oneself in terms of thoughts, feelings, wishes and desires, an essential social–cognitive process for affect regulation and effective social functioning); and the consequent resort to impulsive unregulated responses to fend off the emergency. Following Ruocco and Corcone's systematic review [2], we categorise findings on the neurobiology of borderline personality disorder into three main areas: **neuroendocrinological**, **structural neuroimaging** and **functional neuroimaging**.

9.11.2 Neuroendocrinology of Borderline Personality Disorder

One recent meta-analysis of basal cortisol levels in individuals with borderline personality disorder versus non-psychiatric controls found a significant pooled effect size showing reduced mean cortisol levels in those with the disorder, with a reported effect size (standardised mean difference) of 0.32 [3]. The authors suggest that impaired functioning of the hypothalamic–pituitary–adrenal (HPA) axis may be a maladaptation to stressors (see Figure 9.11.1). A more comprehensive recent meta-analysis of HPA axis functioning found that individuals with borderline personality disorder showed no significant difference from healthy controls in singular cortisol assessment, with substantial levels of heterogeneity between studies [5]. Restricting the review to five studies that compared continuous cortisol output (by measuring either salivary cortisol during the day or urinary cortisol overnight or across 24 hours [5]) in patients with borderline personality disorder versus healthy controls indicated the existence of increased cortisol levels in the former group (Hedges' $g = 0.52$). Borderline personality disorder patients' cortisol response to psychosocial challenges was blunted relative to controls and individuals with other personality disorders [5]. It is possible that the patients with the disorder have increased adrenal responsiveness to endogenous adrenocorticotropic hormone. The most likely model uses the allostatic load hypothesis to interpret blunted cortisol response as a compensatory downregulation of the negative feedback mechanism regulating

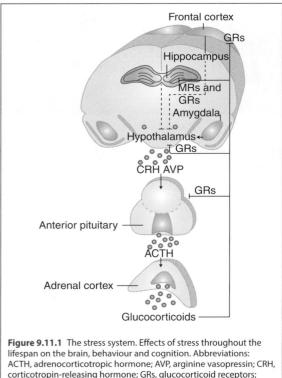

Figure 9.11.1 The stress system. Effects of stress throughout the lifespan on the brain, behaviour and cognition. Abbreviations: ACTH, adrenocorticotropic hormone; AVP, arginine vasopressin; CRH, corticotropin-releasing hormone; GRs, glucocorticoid receptors; MRs, mineralocorticoid receptors. Redrawn from Lupien et al. [4].

the HPA axis [6]. It is currently unknown at which level of the HPA axis these disruptions are situated for individuals with borderline personality disorder. Increased cortisol secretion throughout the day would account for the experience of constant tension and hypervigilance to negative experience that is characteristic of this disorder. See Section 6.2 and Section 6.3 for more on the HPA axis in stress and psychiatric disorders.

Herpertz and Bertsch [7] have made a case for how the oxytocin system may be implicated in the biological foundations of borderline personality disorder. They review evidence of the role of oxytocin in the modulation of the following biobehavioural mechanisms: (1) the brain salience network, favouring adaptive social approach behaviour; (2) the affect regulation circuit, normalising top-down processes; (3) the mesolimbic circuit (see Figure 9.11.2), improving social reward experiences; and (4) the modulation of brain regions involved in cognitive and emotional empathy [7]. Accumulating evidence implies that oxytocin facilitates social learning. This

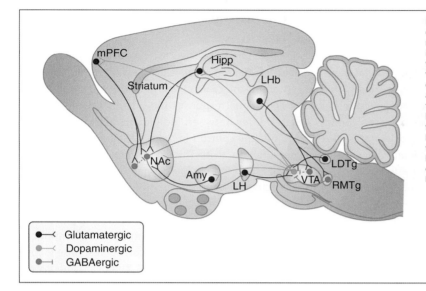

Figure 9.11.2 The mesocorticolimbic dopaminergic reward circuit in the rodent brain. The pathway of interest includes the ventral tegmental area (VTA), which projects directly and indirectly via the amygdala (Amy)/bed nucleus of the stria terminalis to the nucleus accumbens (NAc). Thalamic projections to the prefrontal and cingulate cortex are believed to activate cells that ultimately feed back to the VTA. Other abbreviations: Hipp, hippocampus; LDTg, laterodorsal tegmentum; LH, lateral hypothalamus; LHb, lateral habenula; mPFC, medial prefrontal cortex; RMTg, rostromedial tegmentum. Redrawn from Russo and Nestler [9].

applies to negative instances (mistrust) as well as positive instances (trust). In other words, we learn not only when to trust someone but also when to mistrust them, which may explain many of the anomalous findings in relation to borderline personality disorder [8]. These mechanisms 'may not be specific for borderline personality disorder but rather may be common to a host of psychiatric disorders in which disturbed parent–infant attachment is a major etiological factor' [7, p. 840].

9.11.3 Brain Structure in Borderline Personality Disorder

Volume reductions in the hippocampus and amygdala have been consistently found in individuals with borderline personality disorder compared with non-psychiatric controls. A meta-analysis found that these structures are reduced by up to 14% in patients with the disorder, and the reductions do not seem to be related to state-of-illness factors or comorbidity with other psychiatric disorders [10]. Similar findings were reported by Nunes et al. [11]. Hence, volumetric reductions in the hippocampus and amygdala, areas of the brain concerned with the regulation of behaviour and emotions, might be 'promising candidate endophenotypes for BPD [borderline personality disorder]' [10, p. 251].

9.11.4 Functional Neuroimaging in Borderline Personality Disorder

Two recent meta-analyses of functional MRI in borderline personality disorder found slightly inconsistent results. The first meta-analysis revealed heightened activation during processing of negative emotional stimuli in the left amygdala, left hippocampus and posterior cingulate cortex, as well as diminished activation in the prefrontal regions, including the dorsolateral prefrontal cortex [12]. In contrast, the second meta-analysis showed heightened activity in the insula and less activation in the subgenual anterior cingulate cortex in individuals with the disorder, but did not find amygdala hyperactivity [10]. These discrepant findings might reflect the fact that individuals with borderline personality disorder may be more stimulated by ambiguous or neutral facial expressions than controls, and that the salience of such faces may fluctuate in different contexts, confounding the results of different studies [2]. The differing functional activity of these areas that are concerned with executive function and affect regulation (in addition to the volumetric changes described above) is congruent with the heightened emotional reactivity and reduced downregulatory activity of executive function that are associated with borderline personality disorder.

9.11.5 Genetics of Borderline Personality Disorder

A review of 39 prospective studies found that exposure to different types of trauma, including emotional abuse, neglect and physical and sexual abuse, was associated with increased risk for borderline personality disorder [13]. This review provides support for more recent formulations emphasising the broader socioecological context in the aetiology of the disorder, as it found that patients typically are exposed to a broader adverse context characterised by parental psychopathology, lower socioeconomic status and/or violence. However, although the prevalence of (complex) trauma in borderline personality disorder is often up to 90%, and patients with the disorder typically report higher levels of trauma than individuals with other personality disorders, genetic factors, including gene–environment correlations and interactions, play an important role in the aetiology of borderline personality disorder. It has an estimated heritability of 40–50% [14]. A study of over 5,000 twins and almost 1,300 siblings found that the unique environmental variance explaining features of the disorder increased linearly with the number of traumatic life events to which an individual had been exposed (from 54% with no events to 64% with six events) [15]. This suggests that traumatic events increase borderline psychopathology even when genetic influences have been taken into account. In a nationally representative birth cohort of over 1,100 families with twins in the UK, maltreatment was highly associated with borderline personality disorder, but only in those with a family history of psychopathology as an index of genetic vulnerability [16]. In families without a history of psychopathology, maltreatment was reported by only 7% of individuals with the disorder, compared with almost 50% of those with a history of psychopathology. Hence, consistent with our more recent theoretical formulations, vulnerability to borderline personality disorder is best considered within a multifactorial socioecological framework. The literature still lacks information in relation to genome-wide association studies (GWAS) with borderline personality disorder and currently no reliable GWAS risk score exists to our knowledge.

Conclusions and Outstanding Questions

Understanding of the neuroscience of borderline personality disorder has grown steadily in recent decades. The regions of the brain concerned with affect regulation and emotional response – the amygdala and hippocampus – differ between individuals with this disorder and healthy controls in terms of reduced volume and measurable activity. The dorsolateral prefrontal cortex, which assists in the regulation of emotion, tends to be less active. In addition, the HPA axis, which produces and regulates cortisol in response to stress, has been shown to function differently in borderline personality disorder, with patients showing elevated continuous cortisol output and a blunted cortisol response following psychosocial challenges [5]. The overall neurobiological picture is of a brain that is prone to being flooded by cortisol, with the amygdala working to heighten the affective meaning of stressful stimuli, and the prefrontal cortex underperforming in the task of downregulating emotional experience.

A note of caution is needed with this account. Many characteristics of this neurobiological picture are associated with other disorders. Neurobiological models that draw upon a singular model of mental disorder most commonly invoke dysfunction of the prefrontal cortex [17]. There is evidence from meta-analytic studies of reduced grey matter volume in the prefrontal cortex and limbic regions of individuals with mental disorder in general [18]. Similarly, HPA axis dysregulation has been associated with depression, post-traumatic stress disorder (PTSD) and psychosis. While there is clearly a component of heritability in the aetiology of borderline personality disorder, genetic research has struggled to identify biomarkers unique to particular disorders. In other words, the neurobiology of borderline personality disorder accounts for the characteristic difficulties in emotion regulation and executive function, but these difficulties are also features of other disorders, and similar neurobiological differences are accordingly found in these other disorders – PTSD presenting perhaps the most consistently similar picture. The World Health

Organization's *International Classification of Diseases*, 11th edition (ICD-11) has recently reconceptualised personality disorders according to three levels of severity, with the diagnostic option of one or more trait domains (negative affectivity, detachment, disinhibition, dissociality and rigid perfectionism) [19]. In addition, across these dimensions, there is a qualifier: the borderline pattern qualifier. Such an approach indicates that the difficulties in executive function and emotion regulation that are so consistently implicated in borderline personality disorder may be understood as a general factor that drives psychiatric symptom severity more generally [20].

Outstanding Questions

- It is not clear whether neurobiological findings in borderline personality disorder are specifically associated with the disorder or whether they are best related to trauma or other transdiagnostic vulnerability factors such as attachment insecurity.

- As a result of the heterogeneity of borderline personality disorder in terms of presenting symptoms and etiology, many neurobiological findings have not been replicated in meta-analyses.

- Many neurobiological alterations in borderline personality disorder might be the consequence of the disorder and associated features. Further longitudinal research is needed in this area.

9

REFERENCES

1. American Psychiatric Association. *Diagnostic and Statistical Manual of Mental Disorders*, 5th ed. (DSM-5). American Psychiatric Association, 2013.

2. Ruocco, A. C., D. Carcone. A neurobiological model of borderline personality disorder: Systematic and integrative review. *Harvard Review of Psychiatry* 2016; 24(5): 311–329.

3. Thomas, N., C. Gurvich, A.-R. Hudaib, E. Gavrilidis, J. Kulkarni. Systematic review and meta-analysis of basal cortisol levels in borderline personality disorder compared to non-psychiatric controls. *Psychoneuroendocrinology* 2019; 102: 149–157.

4. Lupien, S., B. McEwen, M. Gunnar, C. Heim. Effects of stress throughout the lifespan on the brain, behaviour and cognition. *Nature Reviews Neuroscience* 10; 2009: 434–445.

5. Drews, E., E. A. Fertuck, J. Koenig, M. Kaess, A. Arntz. Hypothalamic–pituitary–adrenal axis functioning in borderline personality disorder: a meta-analysis. *Neuroscience and Biobehavioral Reviews* 2019; 96: 316–334.

6. McEwen, B. S. Allostasis and allostatic load: implications for neuropsychopharmacology. *Neuropsychopharmacology* 2000; 22(2): 108–124.

7. Herpertz, S. C., K. Bertsch. A new perspective on the pathophysiology of borderline personality disorder: a model of the role of oxytocin. *American Journal of Psychiatry* 2015; 172(9): 840–851.

8. Xu, L., B. Becker, K. M. Kendrick. Oxytocin facilitates social learning by promoting conformity to trusted individuals. *Frontiers in Neuroscience* 2019; 13: 56.

9. Russo, S., E. Nestler. Brain reward circuitry in mood disorders. *Nature Reviews Neuroscience* 2013; 14:609–625.

10. Ruocco, A. C., S. Amirthavasagam, K. K. Zakzanis. Amygdala and hippocampal volume reductions as candidate endophenotypes for borderline personality disorder: a meta-analysis of magnetic resonance imaging studies. *Psychiatry Research: Neuroimaging* 2012; 201(3): 245–252.

11. Nunes, P. M., A. Wenzel, K. Tavares Borges et al. Volumes of the hippocampus and amygdala in patients with borderline personality disorder: a meta-analysis. *Journal of Personality Disorders* 2009; 23(4): 333–345.

12. Schulze, L., C. Schmahl, I. Niedtfeld. Neural correlates of disturbed emotion processing in borderline personality disorder: a multimodal meta-analysis. *Biological Psychiatry* 2016; 79(2): 97–106.

13. Stepp, S. D., S. A. Lazarus, A. L. Byrd. A systematic review of risk factors prospectively associated with borderline personality disorder: taking stock and moving forward. *Personality Disorders: Theory, Research, and Treatment* 2016; 7(4): 316–323.

14. Distel, M. A., T. J. Trull, C. A. Derom et al. Heritability of borderline personality disorder features is similar across three countries. *Psychological Medicine* 2008; 38(9): 1219–1229.

15. Distel, M. A., C. M. Middeldorp, T. J. Trull et al. Life events and borderline personality features: the influence of gene–environment interaction and gene–environment correlation. *Psychological Medicine* 2011; 41(4): 849–860.

16. Belsky, J. The development of human reproductive strategies: progress and prospects. *Current Directions in Psychological Science* 2012; 21(5): 310–316.

17. Macdonald, A. N., K. B Goines, D. M. Novacek, E. F. Walker. Prefrontal mechanisms of comorbidity from a transdiagnostic and ontogenic perspective. *Development and Psychopathology* 2016; 28(4): 1147–1175.

18. Wise, T., J. Radua, E. Via et al. Common and distinct patterns of grey-matter volume alteration in major depression and bipolar disorder: evidence from voxel-based meta-analysis. *Molecular Psychiatry* 2016; 22(10): 1455–1463.

19. World Health Organization. *International Classification of Diseases*, 11th ed. (ICD-11). World Health Organization, 2018.

20. McClure, G., D. J. Hawes, M. R. Dadds. Borderline personality disorder and neuropsychological measures of executive function: a systematic review. *Personality and Mental Health* 2016; 10(1): 43–57.

National Neuroscience Curriculum Initiative online resources

Clinical neuroscience conversations: *Talking Pathways to Patients: Borderline Personality Disorder*

Michael Jibson

Clinical neuroscience conversations: *Epigenetics & Trauma*

9

| 9.12 | **Self-Harm and Suicidality** | Paul O. Wilkinson and Anne-Laura van Harmelen |

OVERVIEW

Self-harm is common; with a prevalence in adolescents of 17–26% it is an issue of enormous public health importance. In absolute terms, few people with suicidal thoughts go on to attempt suicide, but self-harm is strongly associated with completed suicide [1]. It is important to understand the differences between those with suicidal thoughts only and those who go on to complete suicidal actions – this will help us to identify higher-risk individuals and to design effective interventions to reduce suicide attempts. Some clinical (e.g. cannabis use) and environmental (e.g. exposure to self-harm in others) variables have been shown to be associated with transition from suicidal thoughts to attempts [2] but predictive power is low. It is possible that biological markers will have stronger predictive power so it is important to understand the biological basis of self-harm so we can know which putative prognostic markers to test. Understanding the biology of suicidal thoughts will help us to design treatments that reduce these.

Self-harm and suicidality are complex phenomena involving an interplay between emotions, social environment, cognitive processes (including rumination, memory biases and impulsivity) and capability [3]. No medications have been approved for use in self-harm. Some psychological therapies are effective against self-harm; however, courses of treatment are long and expensive, hence acceptability is limited and they are not widely available [4]. Understanding the biological profile of people with self-harm may help us to select and test candidate pharmacological agents – drugs which are known to influence the biological pathways implicated in self-harm may themselves reduce self-harm.

There is some controversy as to whether self-harm should be categorised as suicidal or non-suicidal [5]. It is important to test similarities and differences, including in neural profile, between those with suicidal and non-suicidal self-harm to help us to resolve this debate. This will help us know whether to treat people with these behaviours differently in terms of risk management, treatment and advice on prognosis.

9.12.1 Approach to the Evidence

This section describes, and compares, biological findings (vs controls) in those with: (i) suicide attempts; (ii) suicidal ideation but not attempts; and (iii) non-suicidal self-injury. We begin by discussing brain imaging findings [6], listing brain areas with more important findings first. We group regions together within the ventral and dorsal prefrontal cortices in line with a novel model of suicidal thoughts and behaviours [6]. We then discuss findings from neuropsychology, neurochemistry and genetics. Given the fact that self-harm is seen across psychiatric diagnoses, and indeed in people with no mental illness [1], we do not limit the discussion to specific psychiatric diagnoses. We mainly discuss those studies where control groups have the same levels of mental illness as the self-harm group, thereby minimising confounding by mental illness.

9.12.2 Brain Imaging in Self-Harm and Suicidality

9.12.2.1 Suicide Attempts

The ventral prefrontal cortex comprises orbitofrontal, inferior frontal as well as ventromedial and ventrolateral prefrontal regions (Figure 9.12.1). These regions are particularly important in suicidality and modulation of suicidal thoughts [6]. There are multiple lines of evidence showing differences in the ventral prefrontal cortical structure and function between people with and without suicide attempts:

- lower grey and white matter volume in structural MRI
- greater activation during emotional processing and modulation, as well as memory processing, measured by functional MRI (fMRI)
- abnormalities of serotonin synthesis, transport and 5-HT1A receptors in people with high-lethality suicide attempts in positron emission tomography studies
- high levels of cytokine expression have been found in post-mortem studies [7].

The dorsal prefrontal cortex comprises regions within the medial and lateral prefrontal cortex (Figure 9.12.1). These regions are important in top-down control of suicidality and may play a key role in initiating suicidal

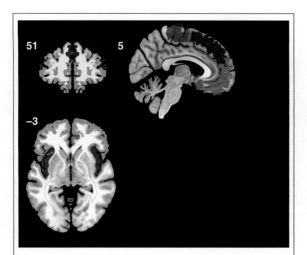

Figure 9.12.1 Dorsal prefrontal cortical (blue), ventral prefrontal cortical (green) and insular (red) regions of the brain (depicted at Montreal Neurological Institute (MNI) coordinates: $X = 5$, $Y = 51$ $Z = -3$, which are used to map locations in three dimensions in MNI space, a standard template of the brain, independent from individual differences in the size and overall shape of the brain) thought to be important in suicidal thoughts and behaviours.

behaviours and decision making [6]. Again, multiple studies have demonstrated differences in the dorsal prefrontal cortex between people with and without suicide attempts:

- reduced grey and white matter volume
- altered dorsal prefrontal cortex activation is seen in response to emotion processing, regulation and during cognitive control processing; notably, increased dorsal prefrontal cortex activation has been shown during higher-order cognitive control tasks in people with past suicide attempts compared to people with past suicidal ideation only
- regional cerebral blood flow and glucose metabolic rates are lower in people with past suicide attempts.

Together, it is thought that ventromedial and dorsomedial prefrontal cortical alterations may lead to situations where increased excessive negative thoughts (ventromedial prefrontal alterations) are not adequately inhibited or dampened (dorsal prefrontal cortical alterations) and may underlie critical risk situations that lead to suicidal attempts in vulnerable individuals [6]. In this model, insula and dorsal anterior cingulate cortices play an important role in switching between ventromedial and dorsal prefrontal cortical activity and may therefore be especially critical in suicidal attempts. In line with this idea, individuals with suicide attempts have smaller insular volume, and higher resting cerebral blood flow of the insula.

Alterations in the structure and function of other brain regions important for emotion and stress responses have also been reported. These results include findings of altered structure and/or function of the amygdala, hippocampus, putamen, temporal association cortex and cerebellum, as well as altered serotonin binding potential in these regions. However, so far, the results in these regions paint a rather mixed picture and require replication before any conclusions can be drawn. Future studies should include powerful designs (including higher numbers of participants) and take into account individual differences within groups, as impulsivity and aggression are both known to moderate neuroimaging findings in these brain regions.

9.12.2.2 Suicidal Ideation

In contrast to research on individuals with suicidal attempts, there has been much less research on the neural basis of suicidal ideation in individuals who have not attempted suicide [6], so findings here are even more preliminary. In these studies, suicidal ideation is associated with decreased ventral prefrontal cortical thickness and increased activation during cognitive control tasks. Crucially, there appears no difference between those with and without suicide attempts, suggesting that such alterations are related to suicidal ideation and not attempts. Altered functioning in the dorsal prefrontal cortex has also been reported during emotion processing and regulation in those with suicidal ideation. This includes lower dorsal prefrontal cortical activation during emotion processing (i.e. passive viewing of negative images), and greater dorsolateral prefrontal cortical activation during emotion regulation (i.e. regulation of responses to these images). Suicidal ideation is also associated with monoamine oxidase A density and neuroinflammation in the anterior cingulate cortex.

There has been even less research on other brain areas [6]. Suicidal ideation is associated with: altered putamen activation and functional connectivity; greater dorsal striatum responses during cognitive control [8]; increased superior temporal activation during error processing; reduced posterior cingulate cortex activation in self-referential processing; and decreased cerebellum activation while viewing negative emotional pictures. This suggests that a wide range of neural abnormalities across the brain underlie suicidal ideation.

Connectivity (as measured by correlated activation on fMRI) has been shown to be altered in individuals with suicidal ideation, including lower connectivity between the rostral anterior cingulate and orbitofrontal cortices, temporal pole and precuneus, and within the default-mode network; and greater connectivity between the amygdala and the parahippocampus, and the left ventral striatum and the dorsal anterior cingulate and prefrontal cortex. The amygdala and parahippocampus play an important role in emotional processing and memory, whereas the ventral striatum is central to many aspects related to reward, motivation and decision making. Stronger connectivity between these regions may underlie negative emotionality, possibly related to lower reward anticipation, which have both been observed in individuals suffering from suicidality. Of note, opposite findings have been reported in adults with suicide attempts compared

to those with suicidal ideation only: those with suicide attempts had reduced conflict-related dorsal anterior cingulate cortical connectivity with the dorsal ventrolateral prefrontal cortices, posterior cingulate cortex, parietal regions and temporal gyri, while those with suicidal ideation had increased conflict-related connectivity between the dorsal anterior cingulate cortex and precuneus (part of the default-mode network). Likewise, a separate study demonstrated regions with reduced connectivity to the dorsal anterior cingulate cortex to be different for the two groups: ventrolateral prefrontal cortex, orbitofrontal cortex, insula and striatum for suicidal ideation but dorsal prefrontal cortex and motor regions for suicide attempts. These findings are in line with the notion that there may be distinct neural mechanisms that underpin suicidal ideation and behaviours, and that alterations in both of these neural networks may lead to very high-risk states in vulnerable individuals.

9.12.2.3 Non-Suicidal Self-Injury

There has been less imaging research on individuals with non-suicidal self-injury only. Altered limbic activity during emotional processing has been reported; however, these results were no longer present when controlling for depressive symptoms, suggesting that depression and not non-suicidal self-injury underpins such altered functioning. Altered amygdala resting-state functional connectivity (with frontal areas, dorsal anterior cingulate cortex, supplementary motor area and occipital lobe) has also been reported in such cases. Finally, non-suicidal self-injury is associated with lower occipital and cerebellar emotion processing activation (to happy versus neutral faces).

9.12.3 Neuropsychology of Self-Harm and Suicidality

Individuals with suicidal and non-suicidal self-harm have poorer, more risky decision making. People with suicide attempts show high levels of cognitive and behavioural impulsivity on laboratory tasks. In contrast, while individuals with non-suicidal self-harm rate themselves as being more impulsive on questionnaire measures, almost all laboratory studies have failed to find an objective increase in impulsivity [9].

9.12.4 Neurochemistry of Self-Harm and Suicidality

Key neurochemical findings include:

- low levels of the neuroprotective brain-derived neurotrophic factor in people who have attempted suicide

- hypothalamic–pituitary–adrenal axis dysfunction (non-suppression of cortisol in the dexamethasone suppression test) in people who have attempted suicide

- evidence of inflammation, including raised C-reactive protein, erythrocyte sedimentation rate and interleukin 6 in people with suicidal thoughts

- abnormalities of the serotonin system, long known to be implicated in people who have made suicide attempts [10]

- low endogenous opiate levels have been found in people who have engaged in non-suicidal self-harm, a possible link with its addictive nature [11].

Recent studies on medication found clinically to improve suicidality/depression give further clues to the neurochemistry of self-harm. Lithium has roles is neuroprotection and neurotransmission throughout the brain, partly via inhibition of the glycogen synthase kinase 3 beta pathway [10]. It has long been known to improve suicidality in patients with affective disorder, independent of its effects on depression. It also improves grey matter volume in regions implicated in suicide (prefrontal and anterior cingulate cortices and the hippocampus) and improves impulsivity, decision making and aggression, all implicated in suicide attempts [10]. Based on its antidepressant effects, ketamine (a glutamate antagonist) has been trialed as an antisuicidal-thoughts agent, with positive results (independent of effects on depression) [12]; this suggests a role for the glutamatergic system in suicidal thoughts. Transcranial magnetic stimulation has been shown to reduce suicidality in young people, potentially through modulating GABAergic and glutamatergic imbalances [13].

9.12.5 Genetics of Self-Harm and Suicidality

Both non-suicidal self-harm and suicidal ideation are moderately heritable, with overlapping genetic influences responsible for a lot of the correlation between phenotypes [14]. There are no replicated findings of single genetic polymorphisms being associated with self-harm/suicidality. A polygenic risk score based on depression risk is associated with suicidal ideation, although that study did not find significant effects on non-suicidal self-harm or suicide attempts, and all effect sizes were very low (<0.25% of variance).

9.12.6 Limitations of the Literature

There are several important limitations in the literature reviewed. First, most studies on self-harm are cross-sectional [6]. Therefore, it is not possible to conclude whether the biological abnormalities themselves increase risk for self-harm, or are a consequence of the self-harm. This makes it impossible to state that such findings can help us in predicting who is at risk of future suicide attempts. However, one recent study demonstrated that participants with future suicide attempts had lower ventral and rostral prefrontal cortal grey matter volume and reduced connectivity in the dorsal prefrontal cortex and anterior limb of the internal capsule compared to participants without future suicide attempts, supporting a causal role [15]. Sample sizes are relatively small, which reduces the reliability of any findings reported in these studies. Most importantly, very few studies have included participants from all three groups under consideration (i.e. suicidal attempts, suicidal ideation and non-suicidal self-harm), and therefore it is very difficult to make conclusions comparing these groups.

Conclusions and Outstanding Questions

There has been a significant amount of research on individuals who have made suicide attempts [16]. In particular, multiple studies have demonstrated reduced grey matter volume and altered neural activation in both the ventromedial and dorsolateral prefrontal cortices. This is important and understandable given the important roles of these brain areas in, respectively, emotional responses (which may lead to suicidal thoughts) and behavioural control (which may lead to suicidal acts in response to such thoughts [6]). Abnormalities have also been found in multiple brain areas involved in emotion and behavioural regulation, including the amygdala, hippocampus, caudate, putamen, posterior cingulate cortex and cerebellum, and in connectivity across brain regions. Medication shown to improve fMRI response in these regions to 'hot'

9

cognitive tasks (i.e. emotion-influenced cognition, including response to emotional faces, regulation of response to emotional scenes and risky decision making) may be effective in reducing suicide attempts; and fMRI may be a useful biomarker of response in initial proof-of-concept studies. Of special usefulness may be medication that specifically works on neural pathways demonstrated to be different in those with suicidal ideation and suicidal acts. People who make suicide attempts have more risky decision making and greater impulsivity, and therefore medication which improves these may be effective.

Outstanding Questions

- Is there a pathophysiological distinction between suicidal and non-suicidal self-injury? Some clinical evidence suggests yes, but no adequately powered biological studies have compared these groups to date. Future studies need to compare individuals with

these two types of behaviour, to help to resolve the debate about this distinction.

- Non-specific increases in inflammation/neural excitation and reduced neuroprotection seem to be associated with suicidality and self-harm. Thus, medication that normalises these processes may be efficacious. Although lithium and ketamine do this, their side effects make their widespread use impractical. Might anti-inflammatory drugs (as currently being tested for depression) be effective for suicidality and self-harm?

- Studies have tended to take top-down approaches to suicidality and self-harm, using drugs like ketamine and lithium, initially tested due to antidepressant effects. Can we better target symptoms, with fewer side effects, using bottom-up pharmacological studies based on the specific neural/cognitive targets detailed above?

REFERENCES

1. Hawton K, Saunders KE, O'Connor RC. Self-harm and suicide in adolescents. *Lancet* 2012; 379(9834): 2373–2382.

2. Mars B, Heron J, Klonsky ED et al. Predictors of future suicide attempt among adolescents with suicidal thoughts or non-suicidal self-harm: a population-based birth cohort study. *Lancet Psychiatry* 2019; 6(4): 327–337.

3. O'Connor RC, Kirtley OJ. The integrated motivational–volitional model of suicidal behaviour. *Philos Trans R Soc London B* 2018; 373: 1754.

4. Ougrin D, Tranah T, Stahl D, Moran P, Asarnow JR. Therapeutic interventions for suicide attempts and self-harm in adolescents: systematic review and meta-analysis. *J Am Acad Child Adolesc Psychiatry* 2015 Feb; 54(2): 97–107.e2.

5. Wilkinson PO, Qiu T, Neufeld S, Jones PB, Goodyer IM. Sporadic and recurrent non-suicidal self-injury before age 14 and incident onset of psychiatric disorders by 17 years: prospective cohort study. *Br J Psychiatry* 2018; 212(4): 222–226.

6. Schmaal L, van Harmelen AL, Chatzi V et al. Imaging suicidal thoughts and behaviors: a comprehensive review of 2 decades of neuroimaging studies. *Mol Psychiatry* 2020; 25(2): 408–427.

7. Tonelli LH, Stiller J, Rujescu D et al. Elevated cytokine expression in the orbitofrontal cortex of victims of suicide. *Acta Psychiatr Scand* 2008; 117(3): 198–206.

8. Minzenberg MJ, Lesh TA, Niendam TA et al. Control-related frontal-striatal function is associated with past suicidal ideation and behavior in patients with recent-onset psychotic major mood disorders. *J Affect Disord* 2015; 188: 202–209.

9. Liu RT, Trout ZM, Hernandez EM, Cheek SM, Gerlus N. A behavioral and cognitive neuroscience perspective on impulsivity, suicide, and non-suicidal self-injury: meta-analysis and recommendations for future research. *Neurosci Biobehav Rev* 2017; 83: 440–450.

10. Malhi GS, Das P, Outhred T et al. Understanding suicide: focusing on its mechanisms through a lithium lens. *J Affect Disord* 2018; 241: 338–347.

11. Groschwitz RC, Plener PL. The neurobiology of non-suicidal self-injury (NSSI): a review. *Suicidol Online* 2012; 3: 24–32.

12. Ballard ED, Yarrington JS, Farmer CA et al. Characterizing the course of suicidal ideation response to ketamine. *J Affect Disord* 2018; 241: 86–93.

13. Croarkin PE, Nakonezny PA, Deng Z-D et al. High-frequency repetitive TMS for suicidal ideation in adolescents with depression. *J Affect Disord* 2018; 239: 282–290.

14. Maciejewski DF, Creemers HE, Lynskey MT et al. Overlapping genetic and environmental influences on nonsuicidal self-injury and suicidal ideation: different outcomes, same etiology? *JAMA Psychiatry* 2014; 71(6): 699–705.

15. Lippard ETC, Johnston JAY, Spencer L et al. Preliminary examination of gray and white matter structure and longitudinal structural changes in frontal systems associated with future suicide attempts in adolescents and young adults with mood disorders. *J Affect Disord* 2019; 245: 1139–1148.

16. Van Harmelen A-L, Schmaal L, Blumberg HP. Journal of Affective Disorders Special Issue on Suicide-Related Research: hopeful progress but much research urgently needed. *J Affect Disord* 2019; 251: 39–41.

9

Mai Wong and Ruaidhrí McCormack

9.13

Medically Unexplained Symptoms

OVERVIEW

Medically unexplained symptoms (MUS), commonly encountered in clinical practice, represent a complex set of symptoms and conditions. This chapter explores the definitions and concepts of MUS, the latest neuroscientific research and some important considerations regarding MUS investigation and treatment. More research needs to be done to fully understand the distress and functional impairment that MUS cause.

9.13.1 Definitions and Classification

In 1984, Oliver Sacks wrote about his recovery from a leg injury that was, in part, characterised by a disproportionate inability to control the limb (Sacks, 1984; Stone et al., 2012); reappraisal of his experience captures his perplexity, anxiety and self-evaluation while accepting that his persistent symptoms seemed to have a psychological cause.

Medically unexplained symptoms (MUS) is the umbrella term for symptoms that a patient ascribes (at least initially) to a physical cause, but which cannot be explained, in nature or degree, by structural or other specified organic pathology. MUS encompass a range of symptom-based disorders with complex and overlapping nosology, including somatoform disorders (ICD-10), bodily distress syndrome (ICD-11), somatic symptom disorder (DSM-5), dissociative/conversion disorders (ICD-10/11; DSM-5), persistent physical symptoms, and myriad specific diagnoses such as irritable bowel syndrome, fibromyalgia, non-cardiac chest pain, hyperventilation syndrome, multiple chemical sensitivity, etc. (according to the World Health Organization's (2010/2018) *International Classification of Diseases*, 10th/11th edition (ICD-10/11) and the American Psychiatric Association's (2013) *Diagnostic and Statistical Manual of Mental Disorders,* 5th ed. (DSM-5)). It is common for patients to present with complaints in various body systems and attend different specialists.

The complaints can be transient and short-lived, or become chronic and functionally impairing.

The heterogeneity in the nature and definitions of MUS creates a number of challenges. It impacts the quality and generalisability of the associated evidence base as researchers use different diagnostic terms to inform methods. Moreover, recruitment and research have tended to focus on specific system presentations. This makes it difficult to search the literature and hard to find any unifying neuroscientific or systems-based biological theories encompassing all MUS disorders. It also adds heuristic complexity, with each conceptual term giving more or less credence to neurobiological contributors while being variably used by different medical professionals. Patients get confused. As an example, one can explore and compare the terms 'somatoform pain disorder' and 'complex regional pain syndrome (CRPS)'.

The presence of these overlapping terms and their evolution likely relates to the fact that MUS present to every medical specialty, each with its own cultural outlook/terms and historical methods of diagnostic classification (e.g. 'somatoform disorder' is a psychiatric ICD diagnosis, while CRPS is often diagnosed by pain services; neurologists commonly use 'functional', while psychiatrists may use 'dissociative'). The clinical pathways of MUS patients lead them through multiple services, and this produces a documentation trail (and patient understanding) involving multiple terms. North's (2015) exploration of the historical and phenomenological considerations of classification provides further insight into some of these challenges, and definitions continue to evolve.

9.13.2 MUS and Neuroscience

Medically unexplained symptoms (MUS) may actually serve as a useful vehicle in integrating many of the latest neuroscience developments discussed elsewhere in this book. While the results of routine clinical tests are often normal, to paraphrase Sagan, the absence of evidence is not evidence of absence. The perception of physical symptoms inevitably involves pathophysiology to some degree, whether at a local system or neurological level. Any attempt to restrict the pathophysiological basis to neuroscience (or a body system) alone will be incomplete; irritable bowel syndrome, for example, is associated with a range of local gastrointestinal physiological changes not discussed here. This is particularly the case if the MUS constitute an 'overlay' on (i.e. are additional to) objective physical insult or injury.

Despite its critics, Engel's (1977, 1980) biopsychosocial model of health and illness continues to offer a putative scaffold to build our understanding of complex illnesses and their varied challenges. Particularly in MUS, there is a continual interplay between this triad of factors, both before and during illness development, and in the symptomatic phase alongside care relationships (Figure 9.13.1).

In the first instance, somatic syndromes have genetic associations – for example, Holliday et al. (2010) report associations between MUS and genes relevant to the serotoninergic system (*TPH2*, *HTR2A*) and the endocrine hypothalamic–pituitary–adrenal (HPA) axis (*SERPINA6*). Major histocompatibility complex/human leucocyte antigen (HLA) genes – classically associated with autoimmune diseases – have also been implicated in chronic pain, which is associated with the serotypes *HLA-B62* and *HLA-DQ8*. Ante/perinatal stressors and childhood traumas are known to result in epigenetic changes, which in turn affect the HPA axis, pain sensitivity and inflammatory cascades (e.g. see Zucchi et al., 2013). See Section 6.2 for more on the HPA axis.

There are structural and functional neuroanatomical changes in MUS; these may be a cause or consequence of illness. Voon et al. (2016) and Bègue et al. (2019) summarise the array of neuroanatomical changes in functional and somatic disorders. Figure 9.13.2 shows the brain areas

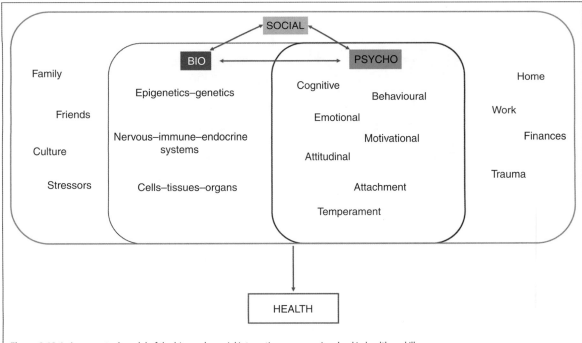

Figure 9.13.1 A conceptual model of the biopsychosocial interactive processes involved in health and illness.

Table 9.13.1 Neuroanatomical changes in functional neurological disorders (adapted from text in Voon, 2016)

Structural/functional neuroanatomical areas altered	Putative function
Perigenual anterior cingulate cortex/ventromedial prefrontal cortex, insula, amygdala	Emotional awareness, processing, regulation
Dorsolateral prefrontal cortex, dorsal anterior cingulate cortex, inferior frontal gyrus	Cognitive control
Temporoparietal junction, posterior cingulate cortex, precuneus	Self-referential processing
Supplementary motor area	Motor planning

affected, while Table 9.13.1 links some of these areas to putative cognitive or affective functions. The circuits between and through these areas are as relevant as the areas themselves, circuits governing functions such as attention, expectation, voluntariness and agency. Figure 9.13.2 gives a sense of the complexity seen in MUS neuroscience as individual areas are variably found to be increased or decreased in size in MUS depending on the presentation and/or the way the patients are grouped in the study.

There may be overarching links between these neuroanatomical changes, stress, adverse life events, post-traumatic stress disorder (PTSD) and MUS. The amygdala, anterior cingulate cortex, insula and orbitofrontal cortex are subject to stress-related neuroplasticity. The burden of adverse life events has been inversely correlated with left hippocampal volume, while PTSD has been inversely correlated with reduced perigenual/dorsal anterior cingulate cortex volume. Cingulo-insular, amygdalar and periaqueductal grey areas of the brain are proposed to form the 'salience network', a network which imbues interoceptive/visceral and nociceptive input with motivational, affective and threat-related meaning. Perez et al. (2019) draw interesting links between neuroanatomical changes in functional neurological disorder (FND) and PTSD subsequent to childhood sexual abuse, where the latter is more common in FND populations than the baseline, and childhood sexual abuse has also been linked with higher baseline cortisol and altered attentional processes (e.g. to angry faces).

The neurobiological relationship between chronic stress and chronic illness (in somatic/functional syndromes) is likely to be bidirectional and constitutes a vicious circle. Any characterisation of MUS as 'unreal' or an illegitimate use of health and social care, a stigma rooted in mind–body dualism, will aggravate chronic stress (e.g. see Drossman, 2016). The picture in MUS is nonetheless

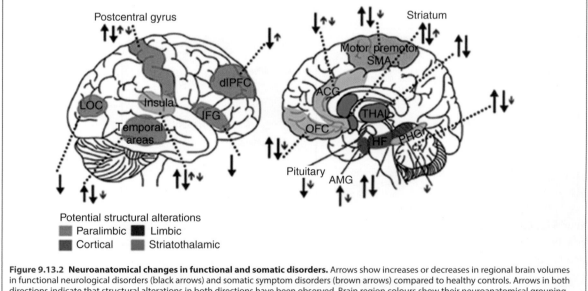

Figure 9.13.2 Neuroanatomical changes in functional and somatic disorders. Arrows show increases or decreases in regional brain volumes in functional neurological disorders (black arrows) and somatic symptom disorders (brown arrows) compared to healthy controls. Arrows in both directions indicate that structural alterations in both directions have been observed. Brain region colours show their neuroanatomical grouping. Abbreviations: ACG, anterior cingulate gyrus; AMG, amygdala; dlPFC, dorsolateral prefrontal cortex; HF, hippocampal formation; IFG, inferior frontal gyrus; LOC, lateral occipital cortex; OFC, orbitofrontal cortex; PHG, parahippocampal gyrus; SMA, supplementary motor area; THAL, thalamus. Reproduced from Bègue (2019).

complex, as inappropriate reliance on health and social care systems can itself form part of the pathology (see Subsection 9.13.3 below).

The autonomic nervous system – which includes the sympathetic system ('fight or flight'), the parasympathetic nervous system ('rest and digest') and the enteric (gut) nervous system – is a potential contributor to MUS. The autonomic nervous system is clearly linked with both emotional (particularly threat) responses and basic physiological functions outside conscious control (e.g. gastrointestinal peristalsis). MUS frequently manifests in organ systems with prominent autonomic nervous system control. The objective evidence for autonomic dysfunction is limited and often relies on measures of heart rate variability or respiratory sinus arrhythmia (i.e. the normal process where heart rate changes with inspiration and expiration), but Kolacz et al. (2018) provide a good introduction to polyvagal theory as it relates to gastrointestinal-system MUS. The vagus nerve is the major source of parasympathetic innervation to the body and there is interest in the use of vagus nerve stimulation for MUS given its use for epilepsy, primary headache disorders, bronchoconstriction, gastric motility disorders and depression and anxiety.

Many patients with MUS have comorbid depressive, anxiety or other mental disorders. Depressive and anxiety disorders are usually secondary, or at least they tend to appear subsequent to the MUS. Nonetheless, one must consider whether these disorders and MUS share common neurobiological pathways. MUS may be a physical variant of symptom expression in many mental disorders. Dissociative non-epileptic attacks are frequently seen in general hospital settings amongst patients with a primary diagnosis of personality disorder (see Harden et al., 2009).

9.13.3 MUS and Wider Considerations

In the absence of a comorbid anxiety or depressive disorder, the evidence for the use of drugs with antidepressant action in MUS is limited. This is particularly the case in conversion/dissociative disorders. Inferring MUS-related neuroscience from drug mechanisms is therefore unlikely to be helpful. Pharmacotherapy trials are more common in somatoform pain disorders (e.g. duloxetine, a serotonin and noradrenaline reuptake inhibitor; amitriptyline, a tricyclic antidepressant), possibly because earlier research

has shown greater benefit and/or because pharmacotherapy trials are common practice in pain medicine.

Repetitive transcranial magnetic stimulation (TMS) has been tried with some effect in studies of functional motor disorder, but is not in widespread clinical use. It remains unclear if its benefit is directly mediated through its effects on the cortex or indirectly by way of suggestion; the involuntary motor twitches that repetitive TMS generates may somehow restore a sense of agency or help in the behavioural process of regaining motor control (Garcin, 2017).

Excessive investigations for MUS, especially if invasive and repeated, can result in objective complications (e.g. adhesions or gastrointestinal bleeding/perforation with serial laparoscopies or gastrointestinal scopes) – these are cumulative on the symptom burden. Iatrogenic harm from physical treatments (including pharmacotherapy) adds another layer of pathology. Medication trials frequently lead to adverse effects, polypharmacy and dependence; patients with MUS often repeatedly present for medical input. Opioid analgesics, for example, have a range of neurobiological, endocrine and other adverse effects that may exacerbate MUS. Each medication needs to be monitored closely and prescribed only following careful (ideally specialist) individualised assessment.

Adaptive or maladaptive illness behaviour may complicate matters. For example, patients with chronic FND can develop contractures through disuse or lack of engagement with physiotherapists, and botulinum treatments may be required. Patients with somatoform pain may have oedema, vasomotor and trophic hair/nail/skin changes; these may be related to the underlying pathology or again partly related to limb disuse. Inappropriate demands for, and/or provision of, functional and social aids (e.g. wheelchairs, professional carers) can create dependent cycles where symptoms get worse, not better.

Such iatrogenic harm often stems from dysfunctional family and patient–professional dynamics; the care giver's 'wish to help' (perhaps alongside a perceived inability to do so) inadvertently becomes malign. Relationships and social contacts influence neurobiology, involving a range of neurotransmitters and neuroendocrine systems (e.g. oxytocin, serotonin, endogenous opioids, dopamine, cortisol), and activation of brain areas (e.g. dopaminergic reward regions such as the ventral striatum, ventral tegmental area, substantia nigra and ventromedial

9

prefrontal/orbitofrontal cortices) – see also Section 8.3 on attachment. Stahl (2017) also posits relationships as epigenetic events. Positive and negative interactions have neurobiological sequelae – supportive relationships with a psychotherapist and other relevant allied therapists (e.g. physiotherapy) are likely to be key variables in modulating and recovering from MUS.

Vrtička and Vuilleumier (2012) elaborate on this functional neurobiological model of social interaction. Relationships with prevailing health and social care systems are as relevant as human ones – if MUS manifest (even partly) as a physical proxy for psychological hurt or social disconnect, the way a system treats a patient is influential. Patients are often discharged from 'physical health services' as soon as MUS are diagnosed, and mental health services frequently lack the resources (and as a result, the experience) to assertively manage them.

Joint working with physical health professionals is often crucial to overcome the stigma associated with mental illness/health and the perception that professionals are rejecting of the patient's global experience. It can often be useful for multidisciplinary professionals to agree and streamline the language and MUS terms used when referring to a patient's symptoms; depending on their perception of psychological contributors, different terms having varying degrees of acceptability for each

individual patient. A cross-team agreement over MUS terms can reduce confusion and the patient's perception of stigma.

Conclusions and Outstanding Questions

In conclusion, MUS represent a complex set of disorders with multilayered interactions between the body, mind and environment interacting with neuro- and other biology. These interactions exist in a constant, dynamic alchemy and are a perpetual challenge for the patient and clinician alike – MUS are never as simple as they appear.

Outstanding Questions

- Do MUS have any unifying neurobiology?
- In what ways is the neurobiology of stress and trauma relevant to the aetiology and chronicity/severity of MUS?
- Can MUS classification systems be improved to facilitate higher-quality research?
- Can specific neuroanatomical circuits be consistently associated with specific MUS subtypes?
- Can understanding MUS neuroscience lead to effective treatments?
- How do therapeutic relationships affect neurobiology and modulate MUS?

REFERENCES

American Psychiatric Association. *Diagnostic and Statistical Manual of Mental Disorders*, 5th ed. (DSM-5). American Psychiatric Association, 2013.

Bègue, I., Adams, C., Stone, J., Perez, D. L. (2019). Structural alterations in functional neurological disorder and related conditions: a software and hardware problem? *Neuroimage Clin* 22: 101798.

Drossman, D. (2016). Functional gastrointestinal disorders: history, pathophysiology, clinical features, and Rome IV. *Gastroenterology* 150: 1262–1279.

Engel, G. (1977). The need for a new medical model: a challenge for biomedicine. *Science* 196(4286): 129–136.

Engel, G. (1980). The clinical application of the biopsychosocial model. *Am J Psychiatry* 137(5): 535–544.

Garcin, B., Mesrati, F., Husbch, C. et al. (2017). Impact of transcranial magnetic stimulation on functional movement disorders: cortical modulation or a behavioral effect? *Front Neurol* 8: 338.

Harden, C. L., Jovine, L., Burgut, F. T. et al. (2009). A comparison of personality disorder characteristics of patients with nonepileptic psychogenic pseudoseizures with those of patients with epilepsy. *Epilepsy Behav* 14(3): 481–483.

Holliday, K. L., Macfarlane, G. J., Nicholl, B. I. et al. (2010). Genetic variation in neuroendocrine genes associates with somatic symptoms in the general population: results from the EPIFUND study. *J Psychosom Res* 68(5): 469–474.

Kolacz, J., Porges, S. W. (2018). Chronic diffuse pain and functional gastrointestinal disorders after traumatic stress: pathophysiology through a polyvagal perspective. *Front Med* 5: 145.

North, C. (2015). The classification of hysteria and related disorders: historical and phenomenological considerations. *Behav Sci* 5: 496–517.

Perez, D. L., Matin, N., Barsky, A. et al. (2017). Cingulo-insular structural alterations associated with psychogenic symptoms, childhood abuse and PTSD in functional neurological disorders. *J Neurol Neurosurg Psychiatry* 88(6): 491–497.

Sacks, O. (1984). *A Leg to Stand On*. Harper & Row.

Stahl, S. (2017). Psychotherapy as an epigenetic 'drug': psychiatric therapeutics target symptoms linked to malfunctioning brain circuits with psychotherapy as well as with drugs. *J Clin Pharm Ther* 37: 249–253.

Stone, J., Perthen, J., Carson, A. J. (2012). 'A Leg to Stand On' by Oliver Sacks: a unique autobiographical account of functional paralysis. *J Neurol Neurosug Psychiatry* 83: 864–867.

Voon, V., Cavanna, A. E., Coburn, K. et al. (2016). Functional neuroanatomy and neurophysiology of functional neurological disorders (conversion disorder). *J Neuropsychiatry Clin Neurosci* 28(3): 168–190.

Vrtička, P., Vuilleumier P. (2012). Neuroscience of human social interactions and adult attachment style. *Front Human Neurosci* 6: 1–17.

World Health Organization (2010/2018). *International Classification of Diseases*, 10th/11th ed. (ICD-10/11). World Health Organization.

Zucchi, F. C. R., Yao, Y., Ward, I. D. et al. (2013) Maternal stress induces epigenetic signatures of psychiatric and neurological diseases in the offspring. *PloS One* 8(2): e56967.

9

National Neuroscience Curriculum Initiative online resources

Clinical Commentary: *What's All The Hysteria About? A Modern Perspective on Functional Neurological Disorders*

Elizabeth N. Madva, David A. Ross and Joseph J. Cooper

Clinical neuroscience conversations: *Functional Neurological Disorder*

Elizabeth Madva and Joseph J. Cooper

Colm Cunningham and
Mark A. Oldham

9.14 Delirium

OVERVIEW

Delirium presents with a clearly operationalised acute confusional state caused by an underlying neurophysiological disturbance. However, despite the tremendous public health significance of delirium, much of its underlying pathophysiology remains theoretical.

This section explores the neuroscience of delirium through the integration of fundamental neuroscience and clinical practice. Since delirium is a disorder defined by a clinical phenotype that may arise from multiple different biological underpinnings we use a conceptual model in which the psychiatric state, delirium, does not imply a specific biological explanation. Instead, this 'delirium disorder' model integrates distinct but synergistic contributors to delirium. The first element of this model is neurophysiological vulnerability to delirium, a portion of which appears to be remediable. The second element is the proximal physiological precipitant, and its interactions with baseline vulnerability, leading to the third element, brain pathophysiology, which will vary between different clinical settings. Once the pathophysiological disturbance crosses a certain domain-specific network threshold, the fourth element, a delirium-spectrum phenotype, manifests clinically. Together, these four elements can guide clinical approaches to patients with and at risk for delirium, and they also offer inroads for neuroscientific advance.

Delirium vulnerability involves physiological compromise at cellular or circuit levels, and the ways that physiological precipitants may interact with this underlying vulnerability appear to be heterogeneous. Delirium pathophysiology may involve multiple, variously overlapping disturbances including neurotransmitter-specific imbalance (e.g. dopamine, acetylcholine, glutamate or gamma-aminobutyric acid), acute impairment in brain energy metabolism (e.g. hypoperfusion, hypoxia, astrocytic dysfunction or impaired glucose utilisation) and/or acute neuroinflammation (e.g. cytokines, chemokine or immune cell activation). Ultimately, delirium occurs due to functional brain network disintegration.

9.14.1 What Is Delirium?

Delirium is characterised by an acute change in mental status attributable to physiological disruption. It is very common in acute medical and surgical populations, with a combined prevalence and incidence ranging from 10% to 50% among hospitalised older adults and up to 80% among ventilated patients in critical care [1]. Delirium predicts a host of adverse outcomes including longer stays in critical care and in hospital, greater healthcare costs, as well as increased risk of institutionalisation, subsequent dementia diagnosis and mortality [2]. Despite the tremendous public health burden delirium poses, its pathophysiology is poorly understood and remains largely theoretical [3].

9.14.2 The Concept of Delirium

In the 1980s, Lipowski introduced the unified concept of delirium [4], a model that has predominated among psychiatrists, geriatricians and intensivists since. However, the neurosciences have largely followed the tradition of Adams and Victor, who considered the hyperactive state of delirium tremens (also called alcohol withdrawal delirium) as the prototype of delirium, and used the concept of encephalopathy to describe other states of acute confusion [5]. Currently, the literatures on delirium and acute encephalopathy are highly segregated [5], suggesting that insights in each are likely overlooked by those who use the alternative term. Similarly, insights from fundamental neuroscience and animal model research are largely overlooked by clinical researchers.

Delirium is a disorder defined by a clinical phenotype that may arise from multiple pathophysiological pathways. The model 'delirium disorder' suggests a plurality of physiologically distinct states, which converge to cause critical brain network disruption: each clinical presentation is the result of a particular subset of physiological disturbances caused by the interaction of acute precipitants and a person's individual set of cognitive vulnerabilities [3]; see Figure 9.14.1.

9.14.2.1 Delirium Vulnerability

Each person has a unique pattern of delirium thresholds across multiple physiological domains. The inverse of delirium vulnerability is resilience or 'cognitive reserve'. Universal delirium risk factors include advanced age, cognitive impairment, frailty and multi-morbidity, though unique sets of risk factors vary based on patient population and clinical setting. The more severe the baseline risk is, the smaller the acute precipitant required to trigger an episode of delirium [6] (Figure 9.14.2). Evidence in humans and rodents reveals that

delirium risk increases in proportion to baseline cognitive impairment and associated neurodegeneration [7]. Neuroimaging and pathophysiological studies suggest that impaired connectivity in interhemispheric and fronto-thalamo-cerebellar networks and impairments in limbic and memory functions core pathophysiology predispose to delirium [8].

9.14.2.2 Acute Precipitants

The list of conditions that can precipitate delirium is practically innumerable (Table 9.14.1), but among them is the basic principle that if the acute insult or disturbance is severe enough (e.g. septic shock, central nervous system trauma), delirium can occur in any individual. In each patient, acute precipitants and baseline vulnerability interact to cause system failure [9].

9.14.2.3 Clinical Description of Delirium

In the *Diagnostic and Statistical Manual of Mental Disorders*, 5th edition (DSM-5) [10], delirium describes an acute change in mentation that tends to fluctuate. The cognitive phenotype is characterised by reduced ability to focus (aprosexia), sustain (hypoprosexia) or shift (perseveration) attention and reduced awareness of one's environment ('clouded sensorium' or qualitative 'confusion'). Delirium also requires a cognitive disturbance in addition to reduced attention, such as a memory deficit, disorientation, language disturbance, executive dysfunction or perceptual change. Delirium arousal may be specified as hyperactive, hypoactive or mixed level of activity.

The operationalised clinical phenotype of delirium allows for reliable detection, systematic screening and prompt identification. Dozens of delirium screening instruments are available to identify, characterise and evaluate the severity of delirium. Commonly used instruments include the family of Confusion Assessment Method instruments, the Delirium Rating Scale Revised 98 and the 'Arousal, Attention, Abbreviated Mental Test – 4, Acute change ('4AT')'. When selecting an instrument, clinicians should ensure that the instrument is valid in the population of interest.

9.14.3 Clinical Management of Delirium

The delirium disorder model suggests four treatment targets: (i) addressing a patient's unique pattern of

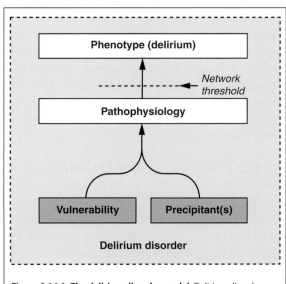

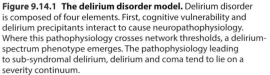

Figure 9.14.1 The delirium disorder model. Delirium disorder is composed of four elements. First, cognitive vulnerability and delirium precipitants interact to cause neuropathophysiology. Where this pathophysiology crosses network thresholds, a delirium-spectrum phenotype emerges. The pathophysiology leading to sub-syndromal delirium, delirium and coma tend to lie on a severity continuum.

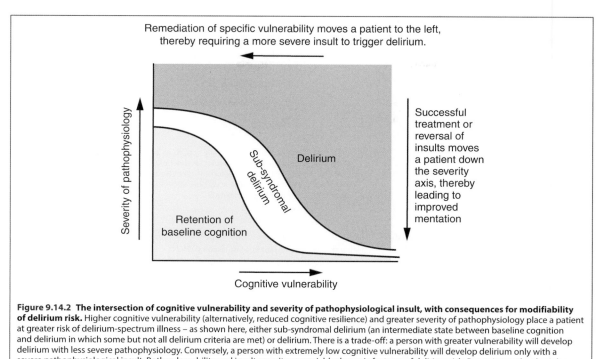

Remediation of specific vulnerability moves a patient to the left, thereby requiring a more severe insult to trigger delirium.

Severity of pathophysiology

Delirium

Sub-syndromal delirium

Retention of baseline cognition

Successful treatment or reversal of insults moves a patient down the severity axis, thereby leading to improved mentation

Cognitive vulnerability

Figure 9.14.2 The intersection of cognitive vulnerability and severity of pathophysiological insult, with consequences for modifiability of delirium risk. Higher cognitive vulnerability (alternatively, reduced cognitive resilience) and greater severity of pathophysiology place a patient at greater risk of delirium-spectrum illness – as shown here, either sub-syndromal delirium (an intermediate state between baseline cognition and delirium in which some but not all delirium criteria are met) or delirium. There is a trade-off: a person with greater vulnerability will develop delirium with less severe pathophysiology. Conversely, a person with extremely low cognitive vulnerability will develop delirium only with a severe pathophysiological insult. Both vulnerability and insult severity are variably dynamic features of delirium risk. Reversing pathophysiology will reduce the likelihood that a patient has delirium, as will remediation of pertinent factors of cognitive vulnerability (e.g. nutritional status or circadian rhythms). One expects this to have implications for both the prevention and treatment of delirium. That cognitive vulnerability has a theoretical lower limit would also suggest that remediating cognitive vulnerability stands to have a greater impact at higher levels of cognitive vulnerability. It is an important corollary of this theoretical model that treating specific neuropsychiatric symptoms of delirium might improve the phenotype without altering the core pathophysiology.

delirium vulnerability (alternatively conceived, factors that *promote cognitive* resilience or 'pro-cognitive' factors); (ii) the acute precipitants; (iii) the underlying pathophysiology; and (iv) the dangerous and distressing aspects of the delirium phenotype [11] ; see Table 9.14.2. The fact that delirium often persists for days or even weeks after an initial precipitant has resolved implies that it is inadequate to address precipitants alone. To the extent possible, one should differentiate between precipitants and any subsequent or arising pathophysiology.

Pro-cognitive factors are an essential aspect of addressing delirium vulnerability. These factors span both somatic and psychosocial domains, including functional brain connectivity, adequate cerebral perfusion, nutritional status, hydration, sleep–wake cycles, physical activity and cognitive/sensory stimulation. Subsumed under this category are multicomponent,

non-pharmacological interventions ('delirium bundles') that prevent some deliria in sufficiently at-risk populations [12]. Such interventions are thought to raise a patient's delirium threshold, for instance by reducing the likelihood of deficiency (e.g. enhancing cerebral perfusion prior to relative hypoxia or increasing nutritional stores for impending systemic expenditures) or supporting naturally restorative functions (e.g. sleep–wake), though such mechanisms remain theoretical. One also expects that targeted pharmacological and other biological interventions will prove to serve a similar pro-cognitive role as well. Supplementing psychosocial pro-cognitive factors with biological ones is likely to have the greatest benefits for those with baseline vulnerabilities.

Although mild cognitive impairment and dementia are major delirium risk factors, delirium is also associated with an increased risk of subsequent dementia [13, 14] and this

Table 9.14.1 Precipitants categorised by the mnemonic I WATCH DEATH

Precipitant	Subtypes	Potential pathophysiological mechanisms
Inflammation	Severe/systemic infection	Systemic effects (e.g. inflammation, reduced brain energy)
	Autoimmune	Specific neuronal activity changes plus systemic effects
Withdrawal	Alcohol/sedatives	Glutamatergic and adrenergic excess
Acute metabolic disturbance	Organ failure	Likely systemic effects with physiology based on organ (e.g. hepatic or uraemic encephalopathy)
	Electrolyte disturbance	Brain energy metabolism (e.g. low phosphate) or direct effect on network connectivity (e.g. sodium/oncotic pressure change)
Toxins	Medications	A variety of toxidromes possible, typically specific to a neurotransmitter (stimulants, dopamine, anticholinergics, acetylcholine), toxin (valproate-induced hyperammonaemia), direct physiological effect (sedative intoxication) or other specific syndromes (tacrolimus, posterior reversible encephalopathy syndrome; forms of antibiotic-associated encephalopathy)
	Drugs of abuse	A variety of toxidromes possible
	Poisons	A variety of toxidromes possible
Central nervous system	Paraictal (seizure-associated)	Likely due to network connectivity or specific neurotransmitters
	Structural change/lesions	Network connectivity, plus specific regional effects
	Demyelinating disease	Structural connectivity, plus specific regional effects
Hypoxia	Reduced delivery by blood	Reduced brain energy and other systemic effects
	Respiratory failure	
	Environmental	
Deficiency	B vitamins (e.g. B1, B3, B6)	Likely systemic effects, especially reduced brain energy
Endocrine	Hypoglycaemia	Reduced brain energy and likely other systemic effects
	Hyper-/hypothyroid	Likely systemic effects, especially reduced brain energy
Acute vascular	Perfusion-related (e.g. stroke, heart attack)	Brain-region specific, predominantly due to reduced brain energy
	Haemorrhage-related (e.g. subdural or subarachnoid)	May have mass-effect (i.e. direct effects on network connectivity) or cause vasospasm (i.e. subarachnoid haemorrhage)
Trauma	Numerous mechanisms	Likely systemic effects with specific effects on network connectivity due to diffuse axonal injury
Hematologic	Dyscrasias include thrombotic thrombocytopenia purpura, disseminated intravascular coagulation, haemolytic uraemic syndrome, hyperviscosity, transfusion reaction, etc.	Effects may be mediated by disruption in oxygen delivery (e.g. metabolic disruptions, haemolysis, reduced flow) or specific to the disease process (e.g. specific transfusion reaction)

association has led many to theorise that delirium may represent a preventable dementia risk factor. Specifically, delirium continues to be explored for its mechanistic links with Alzheimer's disease and related dementias [15]. In the largest analysis of delirium neuropathology to date, delirium in the last decade of life was associated with altered post-mortem brain pathology and with accelerated cognitive decline [16], which might suggest that delirium pathophysiology modifies the progression of pre-existing neuropathology in dementia. It bears noting, however, that not all delirium is likely to accelerate or inaugurate neuropathology, or to do so equally. That is, physiologically different causes of delirium are associated with different cognitive outcomes [17].

Understanding delirium pathophysiology will be the key to identifying interventions to treat the different physiologically distinct types of delirium (Figure 9.14.3). It is necessary to integrate basic neurobiology underpinning attention, arousal and cognition with insights from pharmacological routes to delirium, attempts to treat different deliria, and studies in healthy controls that illuminate key deliriogenic processes. Medication-induced deliria, in particular, provide insights into the neurophysiological basis for certain deliria: agents with highest risk of causing delirium include opioids, benzodiazepines and diphenhydramine (an antihistamine with anticholinergic properties) [18]. Currently, no medications are approved to prevent or treat delirium.

Table 9.14.2 An illustrative approach to addressing delirium

Clinical presentation	Addressing delirium vulnerability	Acute precipitant: intervention, where actionable	Addressing underlying pathophysiology*	Addressing behavioural and psychological features
29-year-old man with alcohol withdrawal delirium and autonomic instability	Nutritional status (thiamine repletion)	Abrupt removal of inhibitory tone: intervention targets resultant pathophysiology	Balance excitatory excess with GABAergic sedatives, gabapentin or valproic acid Reduce noradrenergic excess with alpha-2 agonists	Ensure safety of patient and others in view of hyperactivity
52-year-old man with alcoholic cirrhosis and active alcohol use disorder who develops hepatic encephalopathy when non-adherent with lactulose	Address nutritional deficiencies (especially B-complex), dehydration, disrupted sleep–wake cycles (non-pharmacological ± pharmacological), physical inanition (behavioural activation)	Non-adherence: variably remediable	Hyperammonaemia addressed with lactulose, rifaximin, or other interventions to eliminate ammonia	Ongoing monitoring for disruptive or dangerous behaviours and psychological distress
19-year-old woman who develops delirium with prominent psychosis due to anti-NMDA receptor antibody encephalitis, found to have ovarian teratoma	Limited vulnerability	Anti-NMDA receptor antibodies: corticosteroids, intravenous immunoglobulin, immunomodulators, ovarian teratoma resection	Glutamatergic over-activity (antiepileptics that augment GABA, benzodiazepines) and noradrenergic excess (clonidine, guanfacine)	Psychosis management chiefly by managing pathophysiology; consideration of antipsychotic should be balanced against risk for neuroleptic malignant syndrome in autoimmune encephalitis
65-year-old woman with accidental overdose of diphenhydramine	Address full range of physiological vulnerabilities using multicomponent interventions	Enteral medication ingestion: Gastrointestinal decontamination and supportive measures (as indicated)	Consider physostigmine for diagnostic clarification and to reverse anticholinergic toxidrome	Ongoing monitoring for disruptive or dangerous behaviours and psychological distress
79-year-old man with cerebrovascular disease and mild cognitive impairment admitted with hypoactive delirium due to urosepsis	Address full range of physiological vulnerabilities using multicomponent interventions (e.g. Hospital Elder Life Program)	Infection: antibiotics	Undefined: translational interventions needed to address effect of inflammation on the brain, brain metabolic deficiencies, circadian/sleep disruption	Target inanition with behavioural activation, frequent ambulation, bright lights during the day, consolidated sleep at night; consider stimulants/modafinil if marked inanition
67-year-old woman with pneumonia intubated for respiratory failure and with hyperactive delirium	Address full range of physiological vulnerabilities using multicomponent interventions (e.g. the intensive care unit liberation 'A-to-F' bundle)	Infection: antibiotics	Undefined: translational interventions needed to address effect of inflammation on the brain, brain metabolic deficiencies, circadian/sleep disruption	In addition to non-pharmacological approaches to restlessness or agitation, dexmedetomidine may be preferable to GABAergic sedatives or opioids; judicious use of haloperidol considered for acute concerns

* See reference [3] for further discussion of theorised translational interventions. Abbreviations: GABA, gamma-aminobutyric acid; NMDA, N-methyl-D-aspartate.

9.14.4 Underlying Pathophysiology: Specific Neurophysiological Accounts of Delirium

9.14.4.1 Dopamine: Delirium Phenotype and Antipsychotic Medications

As proof of concept, dopaminergic agents can cause delirium or isolated psychotic symptoms; however, according to current data there is limited evidence that dopamine plays any more than a minor role in most deliria. Most pharmacological approaches to delirium target its behavioural and psychological symptoms rather than any proven underlying physiology, and dopamine D2-blocking medications have long been used in delirium despite a lack of compelling evidence of dopaminergic excess in most deliria. This reflects a rational psychopharmacology approach since several of delirium's behavioural and psychological symptoms, when occurring in other conditions, are improved by medications with antipsychotic effects. Controlled clinical trials have broadly failed to conclude that such medications prevent or treat delirium [19, 20]; however, most of these studies have been conducted in heterogeneous deliria (e.g. critical care delirium). It is unlikely that modulating any single neurotransmitter system can address every physiologically distinct delirium. Antipsychotic drugs may be useful in managing agitation, delusions, hallucinations and emotional dysregulation during some deliria, but their use should be time-limited and restricted to managing severe or dangerous symptoms. Haloperidol has long been the 'drug of choice' in delirium because it exerts potent D2 blockade with no appreciable anticholinergic effect. The atypical agents quetiapine and olanzapine cause less D2 receptor blockade but have strong histamine (H1) and alpha-1-noradrenergic receptor antagonism and moderate anticholinergic activity. Limited evidence supports their use for delirium management.

9.14.4.2 Acetylcholine: Hypocholinergia and Anticholinergic Medications

There is some evidence for a hypocholinergic account of delirium: medications with anticholinergic effects can directly trigger delirium, particularly in older patients [21]. Delirium due to cholinergic antagonism has been observed in multiple clinical studies (e.g. amitriptyline and diphenhydramine), demonstrated experimentally in early psychiatric patient studies, induced with muscarinic acetylcholine receptor antagonists (atropine and scopolamine) in rodents, and illustrated via increased vulnerability of mice with basal forebrain cholinergic lesions. Direct disruption of the basal forebrain and pontine cholinergic systems produces delirium-like behavioural and EEG changes. However, evidence that cholinergic inhibition is sufficient to cause delirium does not imply that cholinergic dysfunction occurs in all deliria. One of the few clinical trials addressing this hypothesis found the cholinesterase inhibitor rivastigmine to be ineffective in treating critical care delirium [22]. Nevertheless, given that cholinergic dysfunction may underlie many deliria, particularly in older adults [21], and that cholinesterase inhibitors such as physostigmine can reverse anticholinergic toxicity, pro-cholinergic strategies deserve further investigation for delirium [23]. Whereas it is usually preferable to avoid psychotropic or other medications with significant anticholinergic activity (e.g. chlorpromazine, clozapine, tricyclic antidepressant medications, paroxetine, promethazine, diphenhydramine, procyclidine, hyoscine) in cognitively vulnerable adults, caution should be exercised when considering a change in psychotropic medications or psychotropic dosing during delirium (especially clozapine) as this risks psychiatric symptom relapse.

9.14.4.3 Glutamate, GABA and Excitatory–Inhibitory Balance

Some deliria reflect an excitatory–inhibitory imbalance. Several types of autoimmune encephalitis (e.g. antibodies to N-methyl-D-aspartate (NMDA) or gamma-aminobutyric acid (GABA) receptors) illustrate how dysregulated glutamate and GABA activity can cause delirium. Glutamatergic excess also occurs during alcohol withdrawal delirium (AWD) and – coupled with acute elevations in noradrenaline and dopamine and loss of GABAergic inhibitory control – leads to agitation, hallucinations, seizures and dysautonomia. Conversely, benzodiazepines enhance inhibitory tone and can cause delirium in a dose-dependent fashion [24]. Clearly, the excitatory–inhibitory balance is important given that benzodiazepines meaningfully counteract the excitatory state of AWD. Recently, there has been emerging use of gabapentin and valproic acid to mitigate glutamatergic excess and use of alpha-2 adrenoceptor agonists

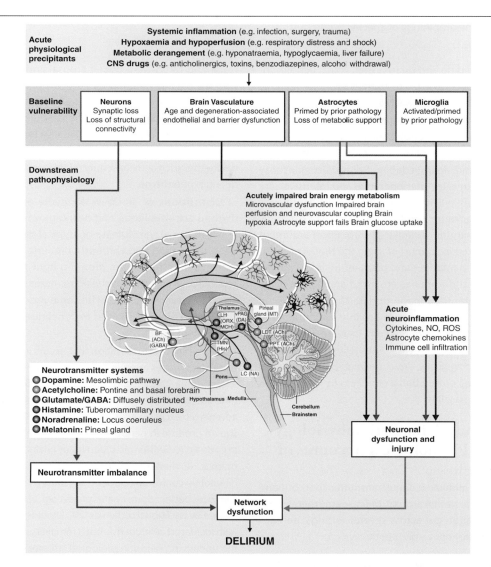

Figure 9.14.3 Acute physiological precipitants interact with baseline vulnerabilities to bring about downstream delirium pathophysiology. (View from top to bottom). A non-exhaustive list of acute physiological precipitants is shown here, but includes the major inflammatory, metabolic and neuropharmacological precipitants discussed in the text. These precipitants are superimposed on brains with variable degrees of underlying baseline vulnerability. These include changes to multiple cell populations arising from biological ageing and/or neurodegenerative disease, as shown. Such acute precipitants further disrupt brain networks already made vulnerable by changes in those populations. Neuronal network function is readily altered by multiple central nervous system acting drugs. Intuitively, if those networks/functions reliant on the neurotransmitters impacted by these drugs were already operating at diminished capacity, the acute neuropharmacological disruptions will impact those networks more severely. Distributed midbrain and brainstem nuclei include strong cholinergic, noradrenergic, dopaminergic and histaminergic drive from the tegmentum to the thalamus to activate cortical arousal and multiple monoaminergic nuclei that activate the cortex to modulate and integrate cortical activation, mediating appropriate levels of arousal. Widely distributed glutamatergic and GABAergic innervation, not shown here, will also have widespread effects on network activity. A number of medications including GABAergic sedatives, anaesthetics and anticholinergic drugs significantly alter arousal and are known to contribute to delirium. The vasculature may be vulnerable, at baseline, in two key ways: tissue perfusion and neurovascular coupling may be impaired in age-related pathology and leakiness of the blood–brain barrier may facilitate entry of toxins and inflammatory substances to the brain. Acute physiological disruptors such as respiratory distress and shock impose very marked constraints on the continued supply of oxygen and nutrients to the brain, with obvious consequences for neuronal network function. Microglia can be primed by existing pathology in the brain and further activated by acute inflammatory stimuli, secreting pro-inflammatory cytokines as well as reactive oxygen and nitrogen species into the surrounding brain tissue. The mediators produced during this amplified neuroinflammation can directly impact neuronal function but can also act directly on astrocytes. These astrocytes can also be primed during chronic brain pathology, becoming hypersensitive to acute inflammatory stimulation and secreting exaggerated levels of chemokines, which can drive recruitment of additional peripheral inflammatory cells to the brain. Activated astrocytes may also be impaired in their ability to support energy metabolism of neurons. All of these mechanisms (and others not shown) bring about neurotransmitter imbalance, neuronal dysfunction and injury and metabolic insufficiency, all of which may contribute to the most obvious proximate cause of delirium: impairment of network integration. Abbreviations: ACh, acetylcholine; BF, basal forebrain; CNS, central nervous system; DA, dopamine; GABA, gamma-aminobutyric acid; His, histamine; LC, locus coeruleus; LDT, laterodorsal tegmentum; LH, lateral hypothalamus; MCH, melanin-concentrating hormone; MT, melatonin; NA, noradrenaline; NO, nitric oxide; ORX, orexin; PPT, pedunculopontine tegmentum; ROS, reactive oxygen species; TMN, tuberomamillary nucleus; vPAG, ventral periaqueductal grey. Adapted by permission from Springer Nature: Saper et al. (2005) Hypothalamic regulation of sleep and circadian rhythms, vol 437; Nature 2005.

(dexmedetomidine and guanfacine), which act presynaptically (see Section 2.4.4) to counter the noradrenergic excess of alcohol withdrawal [25].

Benzodiazepines cause neuronal hyperpolarisation via positive allosteric modulation at the GABA-A receptor (see Section 2.4.3), leading to dose-dependent anxiolysis, amnesia and sleep/sedation. Benzodiazepines may be beneficial in select perioperative and intensive care settings or used judiciously to manage AWD, neuroleptic malignant syndrome, serotonin syndrome or catatonic features in delirium (a similar physiological argument has been offered in support of using the NMDA receptor antagonists amantadine and memantine in catatonia). However, benzodiazepines are listed among the Beers Criteria for Potentially Inappropriate Medication Use in Older Adults, and their use is broadly discouraged in patients with or at risk for delirium. Increased GABAergic tone reduces cortical network connectivity, consciousness and, hypothetically, drives delirium [26], particularly when structural or functional connectivity impairments are present at baseline.

9.14.5 Underlying Pathophysiology: Systemic Physiological Accounts of Delirium

In addition to individual neurotransmitter contributions, evidence suggests that arousal, brain energy metabolism and inflammation cut across several settings, perhaps representing key convergent pathways.

9.14.5.1 Arousal, Sleep–Wake Cycles and Circadian Rhythm

The fact that delirium presents with altered level of arousal strongly suggests alterations in the ascending reticular activating system – midbrain nuclei collectively controlling cortical arousal via thalamic activation (see Section 4.6). Alert wakefulness requires **tonic** (sustained) activation supported by cholinergic and histaminergic activity; transition to sleep involves **phasic** (transient) activation that causes thalamic synchronisation and an increase in delta activity, which is a characteristic EEG change during delirium.

The histaminergic tuberomamillary nuclei innervate cortical and limbic areas, supporting optimal arousal. There is a biologically plausible association between antihistamines and delirium risk since inhibition of

histamine can drive reduced arousal and is associated with hypoactive delirium [18]. Nevertheless, it remains unclear whether the anticholinergic effects of older antihistamines (e.g. diphenhydramine) account for the deliriogenic potential of such agents. It is also unclear whether antihistaminergic activity causes full syndromic delirium or whether such activity simply reinforces the hypoactive delirium phenotype.

Disruptions of sleep–wake cycle and circadian rhythms are ubiquitous, and delirium can feature states of pathological wakefulness or atypical sleep [27]. Both sleep-promoting and chronotherapeutic interventions (e.g. evening melatonin, morning light therapy, non-pharmacological approaches) are increasingly investigated to *prevent* delirium, with some promising results; however, analogous trials to *treat* delirium have shown inconsistent results [28].

The sympathetic activation that occurs in several types of delirium invites interventions to mitigate noradrenergic excess. Alpha-2 agonists including dexmedetomidine, clonidine and guanfacine are increasingly explored to combat adrenergic excess. Sedation with dexmedetomidine has shown promise in perioperative and critical care settings: in contrast to GABAergic sedatives or analgosedation with opioids, dexmedetomidine reduces arousal often without qualitative confusion ('clouded sensorium'). Also, the state it induces better approximates physiological sleep than that caused by traditional sedatives [29]. Opioids are associated with increased delirium risk, but it remains unclear whether the underlying neurophysiological stressor (causing pain) or the physiological effects of opioids drive delirium risk. Putative mechanisms of opioid-induced delirium include reduced arousal via mu antagonism, anticholinergic effects of metabolites (e.g. of meperidine and tramadol) or of 3-glucuronide metabolites (e.g. of morphine and hydromorphone) [30].

Whereas dysregulation of the hypothalamic–pituitary–adrenal axis has been studied as a contributor to delirium, the data remain inconclusive [9]. Supraphysiological doses of corticosteroids can cause mood elevation and psychosis in a dose-dependent fashion; however, steroid-induced delirium is rare. It is also possible that the effects of corticosteroids on sleep could play a role in a putative relationship with delirium, by reducing melatonin levels and altering brain sensitivity to GABA and glutamate [31].

9.14.5.2 Brain Energy Metabolism

The brain is energy demanding and requires adequate delivery of oxygen, glucose and other nutrients for higher-order functioning. In the 1959, Engel and Romano conceptualised delirium as a syndrome of 'cerebral insufficiency' occurring when the brain's energy requirements are inadequate [32]. In classic studies, they induced delirium experimentally in human volunteers: demonstrating that induced hypoxia (16,000 ft, ~50% in partial pressure of oxygen) and hypoglycaemia (44–49 mg/100 ml) caused EEG slowing, preceding reduced attention, awareness and comprehension.

Evidence supporting delirium as a state of energy insufficiency is growing: delirium is associated with impaired brain perfusion, reduced cerebral blood flow, low cerebral blood oxygenation, increased brain lactate and reduced brain glucose uptake (using fluorodeoxyglucose positron emission tomography imaging, see Section 3.1.5). Animal models demonstrate that sepsis triggers microcirculatory dysfunction preceding impaired brain oxygenation and loss of evoked potentials; that decreased glucose concentrations drive episodes of acute cognitive dysfunction; and that animals with existing neurodegeneration are highly susceptible to such perturbations [33]. The tricarboxylic acid (TCA), or Krebs, cycle is a key series of chemical reactions underlying aerobic metabolism. Thiamine is a crucial co-factor for TCA enzymes (pyruvate dehydrogenase, alpha-ketoglutarate dehydrogenase), and thiamine deficiency can cause delirium, presumably via impaired adenosine triphosphate (ATP) generation. Overall, the evidence reveals a temporal link between delirium and both brain hypoxia and impaired glucose metabolism, making metabolic insufficiency a plausible driver of delirium in inflammatory, infectious and metabolic scenarios. Although it is unclear whether this may underlie all deliria, there is a pressing need to test whether improving brain oxygenation and the availability and utilisation of glucose may benefit patients with delirium.

9.14.5.3 Inflammation

Peripheral inflammation – as occurs in bacterial and viral infections and after surgery or injury – is a well-appreciated delirium trigger. These types of insults share key inflammatory pathways including activation of Toll-like receptors on tissue macrophages and blood monocytes by pathogen- or damage-associated molecular patterns, leading to inflammatory mediator release (interleukin (IL) 1-beta, tumour necrosis factor alpha (TNFα), IL-6, IL-8, monocyte chemoattractant protein 1 and prostaglandins) at the site of insult [34]. Several of these mediators in blood or cerebrospinal fluid have been associated with delirium in multiple clinical settings.

There are many potential routes by which circulating inflammatory mediators can activate the brain to induce behavioural change: inflammatory mediators can act at receptors on neural afferents, the brain endothelium and circumventricular organs (areas with a more permeable blood–brain barrier than most of the brain) [35] but the precise mechanisms by which these mediators may drive delirium are poorly understood. Roles for microglial cells and infiltrating monocytes and mediators including IL-1β, TNFα and prostaglandin E2 in causing acute cognitive deficits have emerged from mouse models [34]. However, inflammatory mediators become elevated not only in patients experiencing delirium but in every case of sepsis, trauma and surgery. Therefore, prior brain vulnerabilities such as microglia and astrocyte priming by prior pathology, and underlying impairment of the blood–brain barrier and of neuronal network connectivity remain key determinants of whether peripheral inflammatory activation triggers delirium in any given patient. Inflammation can also drive hypercoagulation, leading to hypoxia, and can locally reprogram energy metabolism, thereby bridging inflammatory and energy insufficiency accounts of delirium.

9.14.5.4 Impaired Network Function and Delirium

Much of the preceding discussion concerns events relatively proximal to the precipitating factors. Downstream – that is, distal to precipitating factors – evidence suggests that different deliria converge on impairment of network connectivity. Diffusion tensor imaging studies show that decreased preoperative structural connectivity (i.e. disrupted structural connections between brain structures) predicts postoperative delirium [8]. Functional connectivity (i.e. the extent to which two or more connected regions show temporally coordinated increases and decreases in the functional MRI (fMRI) blood-oxygen-level-dependent signal) is a useful measure of which regions alter their coordinated activity during disruptions of normal function, and these

9

approaches are now being used to interrogate the alteration of consciousness that is central to delirium. During normal consciousness a key reciprocal relationship exists between the 'default-mode network' and the 'central executive network'. The former, involving the ventromedial prefrontal cortex and the posterior cingulate cortex, is active during resting-state fMRI. During more complex cognitive tasks and goal-directed behaviour brain activity switches to the central executive network, which involves the dorsolateral prefrontal cortex and posterior parietal cortex [36]. Functional MRI in mixed medical inpatients showed impaired functional connectivity between the intralaminar thalamic nuclei and both the cholinergic nucleus basalis and the dopaminergic ventral tegmental area, which recovered upon delirium resolution [37] . Moreover, using seed-based correlation with the posterior cingulate cortex as seed reference (i.e. testing how this region's activity correlates with activity in the rest of the brain), there was a correlation between posterior cingulate cortex and dorsolateral prefrontal cortex during delirium, contrasting with their anti-correlation in comparison subjects, suggesting that delirium is characterised by a reversal of the reciprocal relationship between the default-mode network and the central executive network. Frontoparietal connectivity is critical to sustained attention and, during delirium, frontal and parietal regions show decreased correlation. These changes were associated with increased slow-wave activity (delta and theta frequencies) in occipitoparietal and frontal cortices but delirium was present only when these slow-wave activity changes also occurred in more posterior areas. The transition to delirium was associated with a decrease in functional connectivity between frontal and posterior regions [38]. Systematic review suggests that impaired structural connectivity constitutes a significant risk factor for delirium but that functional network disintegration may be a key pathway to the delirium syndrome [39].

Conclusions and Outstanding Questions

Delirium is a very common and distressing condition whose prevalence is proportional to a person's baseline cognitive vulnerability and specific acute physiological insults. The literature does not support a singular physiological account of all deliria; rather, it suggests a variety of physiologically distinct conditions ultimately leading to network disruption. Thus a 'delirium disorder' model suggests physiologically distinguishable deliria: it traces the physiological rivulets that lead from the many potential precipitants to a convergent clinical phenotype. It appears increasingly unlikely that a singular intervention will prevent or treat the multiple physiological disruptions across deliria. Future research should define, characterise and evaluate specific physiological pathways rather than approach delirium as a singular clinical entity.

Outstanding Questions

- What extent of baseline delirium vulnerability is remediable, and how quickly can this vulnerability be reversed?
- Are there feasible, non-pathogenic physiological stress tests that may assess a patient's delirium risk?
- Can delirium be divided into discrete disturbances in neurophysiology, and what are these subtypes?
- What pharmacological interventions might prevent, reverse or manage physiologically discrete types of delirium?
- Which pathophysiological disturbances underlying delirium are neurotoxic?
- Does preventing delirium *ipso facto* reduce the risk of subsequent dementia?
- If so, how do different types of delirium pathophysiology interact with neural substrates to cause or accelerate neurodegenerative changes that lead to dementia?

REFERENCES

1. Inouye SK, Westendorp RG, Saczynski JS. Delirium in elderly people. *Lancet* 2014; 383(9920): 911–922.

2. Khachaturian AS, Hayden KM, Devlin JW et al. International drive to illuminate delirium: a developing public health blueprint for action. *Alzheimers Dement* 2020; 16(5): 711–725.

3. Oldham MA, Flaherty JH, Maldonado JR. Refining delirium: a transtheoretical model of delirium disorder with preliminary neurophysiologic subtypes. *Am J Geriatr Psychiatry* 2018; 26(9): 913–924.

4. Lipowski ZJ. *Delirium: Acute Brain Failure in Man*. Charles C. Thomas, 1980.

5. Slooter AJC, Otte WM, Devlin JW et al. Updated nomenclature of delirium and acute encephalopathy: statement of ten societies. *Intensive Care Med* 2020; 46(5): 1020–1022.

6. Inouye SK. Predisposing and precipitating factors for delirium in hospitalized older patients. *Dement Geriatr Cogn Disord* 1999; 10(5): 393–400.

7. Davis DHJ, Skelly DT, Murray C et al. Worsening cognitive impairment and neurodegenerative pathology progressively increase risk for delirium. *Am J Geriatr Psychiatry* 2015; 23(4): 403–415.

8. Cavallari M, Dai W, Guttmann CR et al. Neural substrates of vulnerability to postsurgical delirium as revealed by presurgical diffusion MRI. *Brain* 2016; 139(Pt 4): 1282–1294.

9. MacLullich AM, Ferguson KJ, Miller T, de Rooij SE, Cunningham C. Unravelling the pathophysiology of delirium: a focus on the role of aberrant stress responses. *J Psychosom Res* 2008; 65(3): 229–238.

10. American Psychiatric Association. *Diagnostic and Statistical Manual of Mental Disorders*, 5th ed. (DSM-5). American Psychiatric Association, 2013.

11. Oldham MA, Holloway RG. Delirium disorder: integrating delirium and acute encephalopathy. *Neurology* 2020; 95(4): 173–178.

12. Hshieh TT, Yang T, Gartaganis SL, Yue J, Inouye SK. Hospital elder life program: systematic review and meta-analysis of effectiveness. *Am J Geriatr Psychiatry* 2018; 26(10): 1015–1033.

13. Inouye SK, Marcantonio ER, Kosar CM et al. The short-term and long-term relationship between delirium and cognitive trajectory in older surgical patients. *Alzheimers Dement* 2016; 12(7): 766–775.

14. Richardson SJ, Davis DHJ, Stephan BCM et al. Recurrent delirium over 12 months predicts dementia: results of the Delirium and Cognitive Impact in Dementia (DECIDE) study. *Age Ageing* 2021; 50(3): 914–920.

15. Chan CK, Song Y, Greene R et al. Meta-analysis of ICU delirium biomarkers and their alignment with the NIA-AA Research Framework. *Am J Crit Care* 2021; 30(4): 312–319.

16. Davis DH, Muniz Terrera G, Keage H et al. Association of delirium with cognitive decline in late life: a neuropathologic study of 3 population-based cohort studies. *JAMA Psychiatry* 2017; 74(3): 244–251.

17. Girard TD, Thompson JL, Pandharipande PP et al. Clinical phenotypes of delirium during critical illness and severity of subsequent long-term cognitive impairment: a prospective cohort study. *Lancet Respir Med* 2018; 6(3): 213–222.

18. Clegg A, Young JB. Which medications to avoid in people at risk of delirium: a systematic review. *Age Ageing* 2011; 40(1): 23–9.

19. Oh ES, Needham DM, Nikooie R et al. Antipsychotics for preventing delirium in hospitalized adults: a systematic review. *Ann Intern Med* 2019; 171(7): 474–484.

20. Nikooie R, Neufeld KJ, Oh ES et al. Antipsychotics for treating delirium in hospitalized adults: a systematic review. *Ann Intern Med* 2019; 171(7): 485–495.

21. Hshieh TT, Fong TG, Marcantonio ER, Inouye SK. Cholinergic deficiency hypothesis in delirium: a synthesis of current evidence. *J Gerontol A* 2008; 63(7): 764–772.

9

22. van Eijk MM, Roes KC, Honing ML et al. Effect of rivastigmine as an adjunct to usual care with haloperidol on duration of delirium and mortality in critically ill patients: a multicentre, double-blind, placebo-controlled randomised trial. *Lancet* 2010; 376(9755): 1829–1837.

23. Field RH, Gossen A, Cunningham C. Prior pathology in the basal forebrain cholinergic system predisposes to inflammation-induced working memory deficits: reconciling inflammatory and cholinergic hypotheses of delirium. *J Neurosci* 2012; 32(18): 6288–6294.

24. Pandharipande P, Shintani A, Peterson J et al. Lorazepam is an independent risk factor for transitioning to delirium in intensive care unit patients. *Anesthesiology* 2006; 104(1): 21–26.

25. Maldonado JR. Novel algorithms for the prophylaxis and management of alcohol withdrawal syndromes: beyond benzodiazepines. *Crit Care Clin* 2017; 33(3): 559–599.

26. Sanders RD. Hypothesis for the pathophysiology of delirium: role of baseline brain network connectivity and changes in inhibitory tone. *Med Hypotheses* 2011; 77(1): 140–143.

27. Watson PL, Pandharipande P, Gehlbach BK et al. Atypical sleep in ventilated patients: empirical electroencephalography findings and the path toward revised ICU sleep scoring criteria. *Crit Care Med* 2013; 41(8): 1958–1967.

28. Lu Y, Li YW, Wang L et al. Promoting sleep and circadian health may prevent postoperative delirium: a systematic review and meta-analysis of randomized clinical trials. *Sleep Med Rev* 2019; 48: 101207.

29. Oldham M, Pisani MA. Sedation in critically ill patients. *Crit Care Clin* 2015; 31(3): 563–587.

30. Swart LM, van der Zanden V, Spies PE, de Rooij SE, van Munster BC. The comparative risk of delirium with different opioids: a systematic review. *Drugs Aging* 2017; 34(6): 437–443.

31. Cole JL. Steroid-induced sleep disturbance and delirium: a focused review for critically ill patients. *Fed Pract* 2020; 37(6): 260–267.

32. Engel GL, Romano J. Delirium, a syndrome of cerebral insufficiency. *J Chronic Dis* 1959; 9(3): 260–277.

33. Kealy J, Murray C, Griffin EW et al. Acute inflammation alters brain energy metabolism in mice and humans: role in suppressed spontaneous activity, impaired cognition, and delirium. *J Neurosci* 2020; 40(29): 5681–5696.

34. Wang P, Velagapudi R, Kong C et al. Neurovascular and immune mechanisms that regulate postoperative delirium superimposed on dementia. *Alzheimers Dement* 2020; 16(5): 734–749.

35. Dantzer R, O'Connor JC, Freund GG, Johnson RW, Kelley KW. From inflammation to sickness and depression: when the immune system subjugates the brain. *Nat Rev Neurosci* 2008; 9(1): 46–56.

36. Sridharan D, Levitin DJ, Menon V. A critical role for the right fronto-insular cortex in switching between central-executive and default-mode networks. *Proc Natl Acad Sci USA* 2008; 105(34): 12569–12574.

37. Choi SH, Lee H, Chung TS et al. Neural network functional connectivity during and after an episode of delirium. *Am J Psychiatry* 2012; 169(5): 498–507.

38. Tanabe S, Mohanty R, Lindroth H et al. Cohort study into the neural correlates of postoperative delirium: the role of connectivity and slow-wave activity. *Br J Anaesth* 2020; 125(1): 55–66.

39. van Montfort SJT, van Dellen E, Stam CJ et al. Brain network disintegration as a final common pathway for delirium: a systematic review and qualitative meta-analysis. *Neuroimage Clin* 2019; 23: 101809.

OVERVIEW

In this section, we describe psychiatric disorders in the perinatal period, with a focus on understanding the triggering of mood and psychotic disorders by childbirth (postpartum psychosis and postnatal depression). We define perinatal disorders and the perinatal period, and the issues around how these episodes of illness are dealt with in the current diagnostic classification systems – the World Health Organization's *International Classification of Diseases*, 11th edition (ICD-11) and the American Psychiatric Association's *Diagnostic and Statistical Manual of Mental Disorders*, 5th edition (DSM-5) [1, 2].

The mechanisms of the triggering of perinatal disorders remain poorly understood but there are a number of clear hypotheses that are being actively explored, namely hormonal, circadian rhythm disruption, immunological and genetic. We consider the evidence for each in turn. For example, hormonal changes which occur during pregnancy and the postpartum period are associated with the onset of psychiatric disorders at this time. Reproductive hormones (oestrogen and progesterone) increase significantly during pregnancy but decrease rapidly in the immediate postpartum. Vulnerable women may have an abnormal response to the normal physiological variation in the levels of these hormones. Changes in the hypothalamic–pituitary–adrenal (HPA) axis and thyroid axis may also be involved. First-onset postpartum autoimmune thyroid disorders often co-occur with postpartum mood disorders.

Pregnancy is also associated with a change in levels of inflammation and in immunological responses. Postpartum psychosis has been associated with T-cell and monocyte numbers, antineuronal autoantibodies and autoimmune encephalitis. Genetic factors may also contribute to the aetiology of perinatal disorders, and we review progress in identifying genetic markers in the age of genome-wide association studies and the use of polygenic risk scores. Finally, we outline what is known about potential imaging markers for perinatal illnesses.

9.15.1 Classification and Features of Perinatal Disorders

A wide variety of mental health disorders develop in relation to pregnancy and childbirth. Perinatal disorders can have major impacts on the mother, her new baby and her wider family. Understanding the neurobiological mechanisms of these disorders is important as it can provide clues to aetiology and influence the development of

novel treatment and prophylactic strategies, therefore reducing the potential negative impact of illness at this critical time.

The current classification systems do us no favours and vary in how they deal with episodes of perinatal mental illness. The *Diagnostic and Statistical Manual of Mental Disorders*, 5th edition (DSM-5) includes a specifier 'within 4 weeks of childbirth' and the *International Classification of*

Table 9.15.1 Severe mood disorders triggered by childbirth [3]

	Postnatal depression	**Postpartum psychosis**
Incidence per delivery	4–20%	0.1–0.3%
Typical onset after delivery	Within 6 months	First 2 weeks
Duration	Weeks to months	Weeks to months
Symptoms	Depressed mood, lack of pleasure, poor sleep/ appetite, suicidal thoughts, self-blame/guilt	Elated, irritable or depressed mood, lability of mood, confusion/perplexity, psychosis symptoms including delusions and hallucinations, rapidly changing clinical picture

Diseases, 11th edition (ICD-11) 'within about 6 weeks after delivery'. They both fail to distinguish between pregnancy and postpartum onsets, which might obscure important differences in aetiology. In this section, we focus on what is known about the triggering of mood disorders by pregnancy and childbirth, focusing on postnatal depression and postpartum psychosis (see Table 9.15.1 for definitions). We highlight key hypotheses, seminal studies and research approaches with the potential to increase our understanding of this topic.

Many psychiatric illnesses can present in pregnancy and the postpartum period, including anxiety disorders, obsessive–compulsive disorder, post-traumatic stress disorder (PTSD), schizophrenia and the focus of our section, postnatal depression and postpartum psychosis. Differences in illness definitions and study methodologies can explain the variations in reported epidemiology for postnatal depression and postpartum psychosis. For instance, in a recent systematic review of 58 studies [4], the incidence of postpartum depression in women without history of depression was found to be 12% [95% confidence interval (CI) 4%–20%] (ranging from 3.4% to 34% in different studies) and point-prevalence of 17% [95% CI 15%–20%] (ranging from 8% in Europe to 26% in the Middle East). Unlike postpartum psychosis, whether the incidence of depression peaks in the postpartum period is greatly debated [5]. A systematic review [6] found that the incidence of postpartum psychosis ranged between 0.1% and 0.3% of births across several countries; however, there were limited data, with only six studies reported.

It is clear, however, that childbirth is a potent trigger for severe mental illness. Population-based register studies [7–9] found that the first month after childbirth is associated with increased risk of psychiatric readmission, and women with a history of bipolar affective disorder are at particular risk of postpartum psychiatric readmissions.

The mechanisms behind this association, which are likely to involve a range of biopsychosocial factors, are still to be established. Psychological and social factors are clearly important for perinatal mental health in general, and postnatal depression in particular [5], but given the focus of this book on neurobiology we will limit ourselves to a discussion of biological factors (see Figure 9.15.1), which perhaps play a more important role in the aetiology of postpartum psychosis. We will consider four potential mechanisms: (i) hormonal; (ii) circadian rhythm disruption; (iii) immunological; and (iv) genetic.

9.15.2 Mechanisms of Triggering of Perinatal Disorders

9.15.2.1 Hormonal Factors

The dramatic rise in reproductive hormone levels (oestrogen and progesterone, specifically) through pregnancy, and their precipitous fall immediately postpartum at exactly the peak time of onset of psychiatric symptoms (see Figure 9.15.1), has led to the hypothesis that these hormones causally contribute to the onset of postpartum psychiatric disorders [11]. The literature, however, does not reveal consistent associations between the *levels* of reproductive hormones and symptoms [12]. It is, however, possible that women are differentially sensitive to the normal fluctuations associated with childbirth. In a seminal study by Bloch et al. of the role of gonadal steroid levels in postpartum mood disorders, the hormonal changes of pregnancy and parturition were simulated in euthymic women with and without a history of postpartum depression [11]. The study mimicked the supraphysiological gonadal steroid levels of pregnancy and withdrawal from these high levels by giving women a gonadotropin-releasing hormone agonist to induce hypogonadism, then administering supraphysiological doses of oestradiol and progesterone for 8 weeks, then withdrawing the oestradiol and progesterone. Five of the eight women with a history of postpartum depression (62.5%) and none of the eight women in the comparison group developed significant mood symptoms during the withdrawal period. These data support the involvement

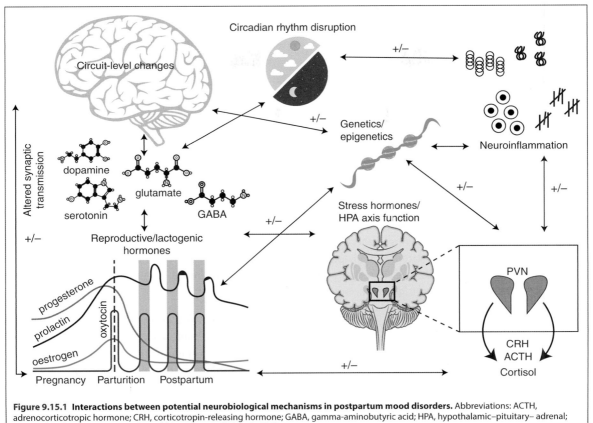

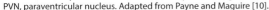

Figure 9.15.1 Interactions between potential neurobiological mechanisms in postpartum mood disorders. Abbreviations: ACTH, adrenocorticotropic hormone; CRH, corticotropin-releasing hormone; GABA, gamma-aminobutyric acid; HPA, hypothalamic–pituitary– adrenal; PVN, paraventricular nucleus. Adapted from Payne and Maguire [10].

of changes in the level of oestrogen and progesterone in postpartum depression, suggesting that women with a history of this disorder are differentially sensitive to the mood-destabilising effects of gonadal steroids. See Section 5.3 for more on the effects of sex hormones on the brain and symptoms.

The role of other hormonal systems has also been considered. The evidence is inconsistent for oxytocin: lower levels have been suggested to be predictive of postpartum depression, but the administration of oxytocin does not improve, and could actually worsen, depressive symptoms [10]. Levels of corticotropin-releasing hormone (CRH), adrenocorticotropic hormone (ACTH) and cortisol increase substantially during pregnancy and drop a few days following delivery, normalising at around 12 weeks postpartum – again corresponding to the period of high risk for mood disorders. There is little

evidence, however, linking hypothalamic–pituitary–adrenal (HPA) axis function to perinatal mood disorders over and above the known impact on mood episodes in general [13].

One potentially important recent lead comes from the development of a novel therapeutic approach to postpartum depression and points to the potential involvement of neurosteroids, metabolites of steroid hormones which have effects in the brain. Allopregnanolone, a metabolite of progesterone, is a positive allosteric modulator of gamma-aminobutyric acid (GABA) type A (GABA-A) receptors, which increases during pregnancy and decreases substantially after childbirth and has been implicated in postpartum depression. Brexanolone, a proprietary formulation of allopregnanolone (given by infusion), has demonstrated promise in phase 3 clinical trials and was recently approved in the United States as the first pharmacological therapy specifically indicated for postpartum depression [14].

9.15.2.2 Circadian Rhythm Disruption

Women experience changes in sleep quality and quantity in late pregnancy and following childbirth and there is a considerable body of evidence (outside of the perinatal context) showing that circadian rhythm disruption can trigger episodes of mood disorder, particularly mania. Although it has not been studied extensively, there is some evidence in support of the hypothesis that perinatal changes in sleep quality and quantity causally contribute to mood episodes. Subjective perinatal sleep disruption was associated with the development of postpartum depression [15] and night-time births and longer duration of labour were found to be associated with postpartum psychosis [16]. In addition, women with bipolar disorder who reported that sleep loss had triggered episodes of mania were more than twice as likely to have experienced postpartum psychosis, whereas having depressive episodes triggered by sleep loss was not associated with an increased rate of postpartum depression [17]. Notably, a number of neurotransmitters implicated in mood regulation, such as serotonin and dopamine, also influence sleep and circadian rhythms. Lithium, the gold-standard mood stabiliser, acts via the glycogen synthase kinase-3 beta, which is a regulator of the circadian clock.

9.15.2.3 Immunological Factors and Inflammation

Pregnancy and the postpartum period are a major immunological challenge and associated with significant immune alterations, and it is hypothesised that these changes may trigger mood disorders. During pregnancy, anti-inflammatory cytokines are elevated, whereas pro-inflammatory cytokines are downregulated. Childbirth abruptly shifts the immune system into a pro-inflammatory state, which lasts for several weeks. Oestradiol is known to regulate this change in immune function [18]. Some studies have found that postpartum depression is associated with lower T-cell number, increased interleukin (IL)-6, IL-1β, IL-8, tumour necrosis factor (TNF) and lower interferon (IFN) and IFN:IL-10 ratio. However, there have been conflicting reports on cytokines; for example, some studies did not find IL-6 [19] and TNF to be associated

with postpartum depression, but increased levels of TNF during pregnancy were associated with antecedent trauma [20].

A study examining the role of immune biomarkers found that women with postpartum psychosis did not display the expected pregnancy T-cell elevation and had monocytosis compared with postpartum women without symptoms [21]. A small number of women with postpartum psychosis, 2% (2/96), have been found to have potentially pathogenic antineuronal autoantibodies, consistent with an autoimmune encephalitis [22]. Further evidence supporting the immune hypothesis comes from first-onset postpartum autoimmune thyroid disorders often co-occurring with postpartum mood disorders, which may suggest overlapping aetiology [23]. New avenues of research on the influence of microbiota on the immune and stress systems perinatally are also being pursued [24].

9.15.2.4 Genetic Factors

There is an important genetic contribution to perinatal disorders, with evidence that perinatal depression is more heritable than non-perinatal depression (estimated heritabilities of 50% and 32%, respectively) [25]. The heritability of postpartum depression is estimated to be 40%, with one-third of the genetic variance being unique to perinatal depression and two-thirds shared with non-perinatal depression [25]. Family and linkage studies [26, 27] also suggest a genetic aetiology for postpartum psychosis. A number of linkage and candidate gene studies have been reported but have not yielded consistent results and perinatal sample sizes are not yet sufficient to power large-scale genome-wide approaches. However, large-scale collaborative efforts are underway to significantly increase the sample sizes for genome-wide approaches to both postpartum depression and postpartum psychosis.

Another potentially productive avenue of research is the study of peripheral blood gene expression profiles. MicroRNAs (miRNAs) are small, highly conserved non-coding RNA molecules involved in the regulation of gene expression, including immune activation. For instance, patients with postpartum psychosis showed altered expression of miR-146a and miR-212 in monocytes relative to healthy controls in one study [28].

9.15.3 Brain Imaging in Perinatal Disorders

Neuroimaging also has the potential to investigate women at high risk of perinatal disorders. Imaging studies in postpartum depression have found altered activity in the amygdala, prefrontal cortex, cingulate cortex and insula, but these findings are similar to studies of major depressive disorder in general [10]. Other studies show specific changes in relation to the peripartum period [29]. For instance, people with generalised anxiety and depression showed a hyperactive amygdala in response to emotional cues, while new mothers with depression and anxiety showed a decreased amygdala response to emotional cues (except those related to their infant [30]).

In postpartum psychosis there has only been one small imaging study conducted to date [31]. It found that women who developed a recent postpartum psychosis episode, compared with at-risk women who did not develop a postpartum psychosis episode, had a reduction in volume of parahippocampal gyrus, anterior cingulate cortex and postcentral gyrus, and these findings were similar to people with psychosis not related to childbirth. It also found that women at risk who do not develop postpartum psychosis episodes had larger volumes of superior and inferior frontal gyri when compared with healthy controls, suggesting a different cortical phenotype across the three groups. More research is clearly needed to establish if episodes in the perinatal period are neurobiologically distinct from those occurring at other times.

9.15.4 Future Directions

Compared with mood disorders in general, postpartum mood disorders may be a more homogeneous group. This allows for specific hypothesis to be tested and opens the potential to better understand not only postpartum disorders, but mood disorders in general. Despite this advantage, however, there are many potential reasons why our mechanistic understanding is limited. First, the heterogeneity of the conditions being studied. For instance, many people may be given a diagnosis of a postpartum psychosis based on the symptoms of the acute episode, but the aetiology and underlying diagnosis might be very different (e.g. bipolar disorder, schizophrenia or psychotic depression). Populations with postpartum depression may be even more heterogeneous, with an underlying diagnosis of recurrent depression, bipolar disorder or PTSD, for example. In some, episodes may be triggered by childbirth, but for others the timing may be purely coincidental.

Second, treatment studies for perinatal disorders have been limited to observational rather than interventional studies due to concerns about the impact of the treatment in pregnancy and breastfeeding – indeed, these are usual exclusion criteria for medication trials. The actions of drugs have often led to specific aetiological theories (e.g. dopaminergic theory of psychosis, serotonergic theory of depression) so the lack of treatments being developed for perinatal mental health disorders has perhaps hindered the research agenda. It is of note that the development of brexanolone described above has bucked this trend.

Third, potential biomarkers have mainly been limited to substances circulating in the blood, as other sources such as cerebrospinal fluid are more challenging to obtain, particularly in pregnancy and following childbirth. This is the reality for psychiatric research in general but may apply even more in the perinatal period.

Future directions of research into this field will need to investigate factors which specifically increase the risk of perinatal episodes over and above those that impact on the underlying condition. For example, in bipolar affective disorder, what is unique about the aetiology of the postpartum triggering of episodes – and how is this different to the aetiology of bipolar affective disorder in general? The paradigms described above which implicate specific perinatal changes in hormones, immune system, circadian rhythm and genetics are therefore avenues worth exploring further.

Conclusions and Outstanding Questions

Pregnancy and childbirth are associated with significant and large-scale biological changes. It is hypothesised that these are related to mechanisms triggering mood disorders and give clues to the aetiology of these conditions. The genetic, hormonal, circadian and immunological mechanisms described above are potentially highly interrelated. We are now, with the development of the research paradigms outlined above, as well as an increased awareness of the importance of perinatal mental illness, at the start of a revolution in our understanding. These scientific developments are a necessary step towards improving our understanding of the aetiology of these conditions and, it is hoped, towards better evidence-based treatment options for perinatal mood disorders.

Outstanding Questions

- What is the neurobiology of the triggering of mental illness by childbirth and does it vary across different diagnoses?

- Are perinatal episodes neurobiologically different from those occurring outside the perinatal period?

- Is the neurobiology of a first-onset postpartum psychosis different from severe perinatal episodes occurring in women with a history of bipolar affective disorder?

- How can further understanding of the aetiology of perinatal mental illness inform the classification of disorders?

- How can understanding the aetiology of perinatal mental illness lead to new therapeutic targets or more personalised approaches to the use of existing treatments?

REFERENCES

1. World Health Organization. *International Classification of Diseases*, 11th ed. (ICD-11). World Health Organization, 2018.

2. American Psychiatric Association. *Diagnostic and Statistical Manual of Mental Disorders*, 5th ed. (DSM-5). American Psychiatric Association, 2013.

3. Casanova Dias M, Jones I. Perinatal psychiatry. *Medicine* 2020; 48(12): 774–778.

4. Shorey S, Chee CYI, Ng ED et al. Prevalence and incidence of postpartum depression among healthy mothers: a systematic review and meta-analysis. *J Psychiatr Res* 2018; 104: 235–248.

5. Howard LM, Molyneaux E, Dennis CL et al. Non-psychotic mental disorders in the perinatal period. *Lancet* 2014; 384(9956): 1775–1788.

6. VanderKruik R, Barreix M, Chou D et al. The global prevalence of postpartum psychosis: a systematic review. *BMC Psychiatry* 2017; 17(1): 272.

7. Munk-Olsen T, Laursen TM, Pedersen CB, Mors O, Mortensen PB. New parents and mental disorders. *JAMA* 2006; 296(21): 2582.

8. Kendell RE, Chalmers JC, Platz C. Epidemiology of puerperal psychoses. *Br J Psychiatry* 1987; 150: 662–673.

9. Martin JL, McLean G, Martin D, Cantwell R, Smith DJ. Admission to psychiatric hospital for mental illnesses 2 years prechildbirth and postchildbirth in Scotland: a health informatics approach to assessing mother and child outcomes. *BMJ Open* 2017; 7(9): e016908.

10. Payne JL, Maguire J. Pathophysiological mechanisms implicated in postpartum depression. *Front Neuroendocrinol* 2019; 52: 165–180.

11. Bloch M. Effects of gonadal steroids in women with a history of postpartum depression. *Am J Psychiatry* 2000; 157(6): 924–930.

12. Schiller CE, Meltzer-Brody S, Rubinow DR. The role of reproductive hormones in postpartum depression. *CNS Spectr* 2019; 20: 48–59.

13. Meltzer-Brody S, Stuebe A, Dole N et al. Elevated corticotropin releasing hormone (CRH) during pregnancy and risk of postpartum depression (PPD). *J Clin Endocrinol Metab* 2011; 96(1): E40–E47.

14. Meltzer-Brody S, Colquhoun H, Riesenberg R et al. Brexanolone injection in post-partum depression: two multicentre, double-blind, randomised, placebo-controlled, phase 3 trials. *Lancet* 2018; 392(10152): 1058–1070.

15. Lawson A, Murphy KE, Sloan E, Uleryk E, Dalfen A. The relationship between sleep and postpartum mental disorders: a systematic review. *J Affect Disord* 2015; 176: 65–77.

16. Sharma V, Smith A, Khan M. The relationship between duration of labour, time of delivery, and puerperal psychosis. *J Affect Disord* 2004; 83(2–3): 215–220.

17. Lewis KJS, Di Florio A, Forty L et al. Mania triggered by sleep loss and risk of postpartum psychosis in women with bipolar disorder. *J Affect Disord* 2018; 225: 624–629.

18. Robinson DP, Klein SL. Pregnancy and pregnancy-associated hormones alter immune responses and disease pathogenesis. *Horm Behav* 2012; 62(3): 263–271.

19. Osborne LM, Monk C. Perinatal depression: the fourth inflammatory morbidity of pregnancy? Theory and literature review. *Psychoneuroendocrinology* 2013; 38(10): 1929–1952.

20. Blackmore ER, Moynihan JA, Rubinow DR et al. Psychiatric symptoms and proinflammatory cytokines in pregnancy. *Psychosom Med* 2011; 73(8): 656–663.

21. Bergink V, Burgerhout KM, Weigelt K et al. Immune system dysregulation in first-onset postpartum psychosis. *Biol Psychiatry* 2013; 73(10): 1000–1007.

9

22. Bergink V, Armangue T, Titulaer MJ et al. Autoimmune encephalitis in postpartum psychosis. *Am J Psychiatry* 2015; 172(9): 901–908.

23. Bergink V, Pop VJM, Nielsen PR et al. Comorbidity of autoimmune thyroid disorders and psychiatric disorders during the postpartum period: a Danish nationwide register-based cohort study. *Psychol Med* 2018; 48(08): 1291–1298.

24. Rackers HS, Thomas S, Williamson K, Posey R, Kimmel MC. Emerging literature in the microbiota–brain axis and perinatal mood and anxiety disorders. *Psychoneuroendocrinology* 2018; 95: 86–96.

25. Viktorin A, Meltzer-Brody S, Kuja-Halkola R et al. Heritability of perinatal depression and genetic overlap with nonperinatal depression. *Am J Psychiatry* 2016; 173(2): 158–165.

26. Jones I, Craddock N. Searching for the puerperal trigger: molecular genetic studies of bipolar affective puerperal psychosis. *Psychopharmacol Bull* 2007; 40(2): 115–128.

27. Jones I, Hamshere M, Nangle J-M et al. Bipolar affective puerperal psychosis: genome-wide significant evidence for linkage to chromosome 16. *Am J Psychiatry* 2007; 164(7): 1099–1104.

28. Weigelt K, Bergink V, Burgerhout KM et al. Down-regulation of inflammation-protective microRNAs 146a and 212 in monocytes of patients with postpartum psychosis. *Brain Behav Immun* 2013; 29: 147–155.

29. Pawluski JL, Lonstein JS, Fleming AS. The neurobiology of postpartum anxiety and depression. *Trends Neurosci* 2017; 40(2): 106–120.

30. Wonch KE, de Medeiros CB, Barrett JA et al. Postpartum depression and brain response to infants: differential amygdala response and connectivity. *Soc Neurosci* 2016; 11(6): 600–617.

31. Fusté M, Pauls A, Worker A et al. Brain structure in women at risk of postpartum psychosis: an MRI study. *Transl Psychiatry* 2017; 7(12): 1286.

National Neuroscience Curriculum Initiative online resources

Effects of Maternal Prenatal Stress: Mechanisms, Implications, and Novel Therapeutic Interventions

Amalia Londono Tobon, Andrea Diaz Stransky, David A. Ross and Hanna E. Stevens

This "stuff" is really cool: Tara Thompson-Felix, *"Crossing Barriers"* on pregancy and exosomes

Ute Stead

9.16   Sleep Disorders

OVERVIEW

Sleep disorders can be understood as conditions which affect either the quality, duration or timing of sleep, or present with unusual sleep-related behaviours. These are often associated with an impact on daytime functioning. In this section we look at the main groups of sleep disorders, followed by a review of the role of sleep in psychiatric conditions and the effect of psychotropic medication on sleep.

9.16.1 Classification of Sleep Disorders

Sleep disorders can be classified into the following groups: insomnia disorders, sleep-related breathing disorders, central disorders of hypersomnolence, circadian rhythm sleep–wake disorders, parasomnias, sleep-related movement disorders and other sleep disorders [1]. It is not uncommon for different sleep disorders to occur together.

9.16.1.1 Insomnia Disorder

Insomnia disorder is considered one of the most common sleep disorders, but prevalence rates vary widely, depending on methodology and criteria used. A survey in England found a 38.6% prevalence of insomnia symptoms, with 5.8% meeting the more stringent criteria for an insomnia disorder diagnosis [2]. Women are more frequently affected and this effect increases with older age [2, 3].

The diagnostic criteria for chronic insomnia disorder include difficulties initiating or maintaining sleep, or waking up earlier than desired. These are associated with either significant distress or impairment and have been occurring at least three times per week for 3 months. If the duration of symptoms is less than three months it is classified as short-term insomnia disorder [1]. There should be adequate opportunity for sleep and the sleep disturbance is not better explained by another disorder or substance misuse [1, 4]. The insomnia disorder may occur on its own, or it can be comorbid with other medical and psychiatric conditions. The previous classification as either 'primary' or 'secondary' has been abandoned in recent diagnostic manuals [5–7].

Insomnia can have a marked impact on quality of life [7]. It has been associated with adverse mental and physical health effects, including increased risk of depressive disorder [5–7] and suicide [6, 7], anxiety [5, 7], substance use [5], cardiovascular disorders [3, 6, 7] and type 2 diabetes [6, 7].

With regard to aetiology and pathophysiology, a range of cognitive–behavioural and neurobiological models have been proposed, pointing towards increased arousal as a core component [3, 5, 6]. This is supported by studies showing increased activity of the hypothalamic–pituitary–adrenal axis and the autonomic nervous system in insomnia [3, 5, 7]. On the neurobiological level, several mechanisms involved in regulating arousal and sleep (discussed in Section 5.2) are also considered to play a role in insomnia, with either an increased activity of the arousal systems, reduced activity of the sleep-promoting systems, or both [3]. The possibility of insomnia as a 'hybrid state' between wake and sleep, with different brain regions showing variations in sleep depth, has also been proposed [8]. Polysomnography studies have shown a reduction in slow-wave and rapid-eye-movement (REM) sleep and increased shifts between sleep stages, as well as more brief awakenings and micro-arousals, leading to increased fragmentation of sleep stages [3, 6]. The subjective perception of the sleep disturbance may be in excess of the polysomnographic findings and this is an area of ongoing research [6]. On the other hand, subgroups of objective short sleepers have been identified, suggesting different types of insomnia [3, 6].

Medication commonly used in insomnia either enhances sleep-promoting systems, such as GABAergic transmission and agonism at melatonin receptors, or inhibits neurotransmission in arousal systems [5, 7, 9]. Examples of the latter would be the sedating effect of H1 histamine antagonists ('antihistamines'), or hypocretin/orexin antagonists [5, 7, 9]. However, rather than medication, cognitive behavioural therapy for insomnia (CBT-I) is generally the recommended first-line treatment for insomnia [3, 6, 7]. One of the core components of the programme is sleep restriction, which aims to increase the homeostatic sleep drive (see Section 5.2). Other aspects include sleep education, sleep hygiene advice, stimulus control, relaxation and cognitive techniques [3, 6, 7].

9.16.1.2 Sleep-Related Breathing Disorders: Obstructive Sleep Apnoea

Obstructive sleep apnoea (OSA) is a common but underdiagnosed sleep-related breathing disorder [10, 11]. Features include loud snoring, observed apnoeas, choking or gasping in sleep, morning headaches and excessive daytime sleepiness [10, 12]. Male gender, increased age, obesity, enlarged neck circumference and certain craniofacial features are important risk factors [10, 12]. OSA has been associated with a decreased quality of life and a range of health conditions, such as cardiovascular, metabolic and mood disorders, with increased overall mortality [10, 12]. In addition, studies have indicated an increased risk of OSA in people with psychiatric disorders, especially depression and schizophrenia [10]. Recognition and subsequent treatment of OSA can improve mental and physical health outcomes, highlighting the importance of timely diagnosis [10, 12]. Screening tools, like the STOP-Bang Questionnaire, can be useful in this respect [11]. The underlying pathophysiological mechanism of OSA is complex. Repeated episodes of pharyngeal collapse during sleep result in partial or complete obstruction of the upper airway with reduced (hypopnoea) or complete (apnoea) cessation of airflow [5, 10, 13]. These obstructive events are associated with fluctuations in intrathoracic

pressure, intermittent hypoxia and brief arousals [12, 13]. They can occur numerous times overnight, often without the individual's awareness, resulting in significant fragmentation of sleep with daytime impairment of functioning [10, 12, 13].

9.16.1.3 Central Disorders of Hypersomnolence: Narcolepsy

Narcolepsy is a relatively rare neurological disorder, caused by loss of hypothalamic hypocretin/orexin neurons [5, 14]. This leads to instability of sleep–wake stages (see Section 5.2). Features include excessive daytime sleepiness, abnormal REM sleep (occurring at sleep onset or intruding into wakefulness), hypnagogic hallucinations, sleep paralysis, disturbed nocturnal sleep and cataplexy [5, 14]. Cataplexy is the sudden loss of muscle tone, usually triggered by strong emotions (e.g. laughter). It is specific to narcolepsy, but not mandatory for diagnosis [14]. Peak onset of symptoms is around 15 years of age, with a smaller peak between ages 30 and 40 years [14]. Autoimmune processes and genetic factors have been suggested as possible underlying causes of this disorder [5, 14].

9.16.1.4 Circadian Rhythm Sleep–Wake Disorders

Circadian rhythm sleep–wake disorders refer either to a disruption of the internal circadian timing mechanism, or to its misalignment with the 24-hour social and physical environment, such as that which occurs with shift work and jet lag [5].

9.16.1.5 Parasomnias

Parasomnias are sleep-related undesirable experiences or behaviours. They may occur at sleep onset, during sleep, between sleep stages or on arousal from sleep. Depending on the sleep stage affected, they are divided into non-rapid eye movement (NREM) and REM parasomnias [15, 16].

NREM parasomnias are associated with incomplete arousal from NREM sleep, usually deep (stage N3) sleep [15, 16]. They include confusional arousal, sleepwalking, sleep terrors, sexsomnias and sleep-related eating disorder [15, 16]. NREM parasomnias are very common in childhood, but the prevalence reduces to about 4% in adults [16].

REM parasomnias include nightmare disorder, recurrent isolated sleep paralysis and REM behaviour disorder (RBD) [15, 16]. In RBD, the usual muscle atonia during REM sleep is lost, allowing for dream enactment, often of violent dreams [15, 16]. RBD is associated with synucleinopathies (e.g. Parkinson's disease, dementia with Lewy bodies, multiple system atrophy) and may occur years before noticeable disease onset [15, 16]. RBD may also be associated with other neurological conditions, alcohol or hypnotic withdrawal, and with use of antidepressant medication [15, 16].

Complex sleep behaviours with reduced awareness and parasomnias such as sleepwalking have been reported with benzodiazepine and non-benzodiazepine hypnotic medication [17, 18].

9.16.1.6 Sleep-Related Movement Disorders

RESTLESS LEGS SYNDROME (WILLIS–EKBOM DISEASE)

Restless legs syndrome (RLS) is a neurological condition characterised by an irresistible urge to move the legs, usually accompanied by an unpleasant sensation. These features typically occur in the evening or at night, and when resting. Movement gives temporary relief [16, 19]. Prevalence rates have been estimated at between 3.9% and 14.3%, with increased rates in women and older age groups [16]. RLS has been found to be associated with depression [19]. Abnormal iron metabolism with reduced iron levels in the central nervous system and dopamine dysfunction (iron is a cofactor for dopamine production) have been suggested as pathophysiological factors in RLS [5, 16, 19]. The circadian fluctuation of dopamine might explain the onset of symptoms in the evening when dopamine levels are naturally low (see Section 5.2) [5].

PERIODIC LIMB MOVEMENT DISORDER

Periodic limb movement disorder (PLMD) refers to a condition with brief recurrent movements, usually of the lower limb during sleep, but that can also occur when awake [16]. Most patients with RLS experience PLMD, but not the other way round [5, 19]. It has been suggested that both conditions have a shared aetiology [16]. Several conditions have a strong association with RLS/PLMD, including iron deficiency, renal failure and pregnancy [5, 16].

RLS and PLMD may be induced or exacerbated by substances, including most antidepressant medications, lithium, dopamine antagonists (antipsychotic medication, antiemetics) and antihistamines [5, 17, 20].

9.16.2 The Role of Sleep in Psychiatric Disorders

Sleep disturbances in psychiatric disorders are common across diagnostic categories [21, 22]. They have traditionally been considered symptoms of these and are often part of diagnostic criteria [21, 22]. However, the relationship between mental health and sleep appears more complex. It has been proposed that sleep disturbances may be part of the mechanism underlying psychiatric disorders, and affect the onset and course of a range of psychiatric conditions [22–24].

For example, disturbed sleep:

- can lead to worse mental health outcomes, negatively affecting remission rates, treatment response and quality of life [21]
- has been shown to be a risk factor for suicidal thoughts and suicide in depressive disorder [6, 21]
- may precede the onset or relapse of a mental disorder (e.g. insomnia is a risk factor for depression, and disturbed sleep can be a prodrome of relapse in schizophrenia) [21–24]
- often persists during periods of remission and may be an indicator of likely recurrence [7, 21, 24].

There is a growing body of evidence showing that addressing sleep difficulties can have a positive effect on mental health outcomes, beyond improving sleep [22, 24]. This may also be the case for primary sleep disorders associated with increased risk of psychiatric disorders, such as insomnia and OSA [6, 7, 10, 11, 23, 25].

Looking at the relationship between mental health and sleep on a neurobiological level, the neurotransmitters and neural systems involved in the regulation of arousal and sleep also play an important role in psychiatric conditions (see Section 5.2.3) [22–24]. Interestingly, many of these systems are influenced by circadian rhythm and there is increasing awareness of the relationship between mental health and circadian factors [22, 23, 26]. As an example, abnormal serotonin function has long been implicated in mood and anxiety disorders, but serotonin is also involved in the regulation of the circadian system. It is thought to have a stabilising effect on the suprachiasmatic nucleus (the circadian 'master clock') and reduced serotonin input may be associated with a phase advance [22]. In addition, serotonin function is influenced by circadian factors, highlighting the reciprocal relationship between serotonin and the circadian system [22]. Supporting the idea of an aetiological interplay between circadian factors and psychiatric disorders, there is evidence for polymorphism of circadian-clock genes in mood disorders [5, 22, 26], attention deficit hyperactivity disorder [22] and schizophrenia/schizoaffective disorder [5, 22].

In addition to circadian changes, sleep studies in psychiatric conditions have shown disturbance of sleep continuity for most disorders and more specific changes in sleep architecture for some conditions [27]. The relationships between psychiatric conditions and specific sleep changes are summarised in Table 9.16.1. It is notable that some studies show conflicting results; confounding factors may include age, gender, comorbidities and use of medication [27]. Consequences of the observed sleep disturbances (e.g. reduced daylight exposure), social and behavioural changes, and environmental factors, may all further contribute to a destabilisation of the sleep–wake pattern [23, 28]. Psychotropic medication can also influence sleep, as we discuss in the next section.

9.16.3 Effects of Medication on Sleep

Medication can affect sleep in many ways, such as altering levels of sedation either by enhancing sleep-promoting systems, or inhibiting wake-promoting ones, and vice versa [20, 31]. Medication may also affect sleep architecture, in particular REM sleep (e.g. REM suppression by anticholinergic effects or serotonin (5-HT) reuptake inhibition) and slow-wave sleep (e.g. increased SWS with 5-HT2 antagonism) [20, 31, 32]. Medication that suppresses a particular stage of sleep may result in a rebound of that sleep stage on its discontinuation [32]. Disorders that interfere with sleep, such as restless legs syndrome, periodic limb movement disorder and obstructive sleep apnoea may be exacerbated by certain medications [5, 20, 31, 32].

Table 9.16.2 summarises the effects of a range of psychotropic medications on sleep. The table should be used only as a guide due to limited data, significant variability in methodology and potential confounding factors such as the populations studied, underlying conditions and comorbidities, and additional medication use.

Conclusions and Outstanding Questions

There is a complex, multidirectional relationship between sleep disorders, sleep in psychiatric conditions and the effects of psychotropic medication on sleep. Sleep disorders include a broad range of conditions which, if left untreated, can have a significant impact on physical and mental health. Conversely people with mental health conditions are more likely to develop sleep disorders which can affect the course and outcome of the illness. On a more detailed level, specific psychiatric conditions tend to show specific markers or changes in sleep patterns.

Sleep can also be impacted by psychotropic medication due to its action on neurochemical agents involved in sleep–wake regulation. Certain medications are known to exacerbate sleep disorders.

Having an understanding of the complex relationships between sleep, mental health and medication has the potential to improve outcomes in psychiatry and may even offer new treatment approaches.

Outstanding Questions

- In insomnia disorder, the subjective perception of reduced sleep may be in excess of the polysomnographic findings, with some people reporting complete absence of sleep, despite evidence to the contrary. How can this be explained?

- A broad range of medications are used as sleep aids, but many have significant adverse effects, become less effective with time or interfere with the natural sleep architecture. Can we develop effective hypnotics without these drawbacks?

- REM sleep changes have been observed in depression and many antidepressant medications suppress REM sleep. What is the role of REM sleep in depression? What is the significance of pharmacological suppression of REM sleep with regard to therapeutic response and long-term effects?

Table 9.16.1 Summary of sleep patterns associated with different psychiatric disorders [21, 24, 26–30]

	Subjective sleep–wake complaints	Circadian rhythm	Sleep continuity	REM sleep	Slow-wave sleep (SWS)/Sleep depth	Associations
Unipolar depression (features may vary with age and subtype)	Insomnia: • difficulties falling and staying asleep [21, 24, 26] • frequent night-time awakening [24] Non-refreshing sleep [24, 26] Daytime fatigue [26] Disturbing dreams [26] Hypersomnia [24]	Abnormal circadian rhythm of hormones and neurotransmitters (e.g. melatonin, cortisol) [26] Reduced melatonin release [26] Increased night-time body temperature [26] Melancholic type: • early morning wakening [24, 26] • diurnal mood variation [24] Phase changes: • possible phase advance (melancholic type, older adults) [26] • delayed sleep phase in youth, and bipolar affective disorder [26]	Decreased sleep continuity [24, 27]: • increased sleep onset latency • reduced sleep efficiency • increased sleep fragmentation • reduced total sleep time	Decreased REM sleep latency [21, 26] Increased REM sleep duration [21] (above REM sleep changes not confirmed in a recent study after controlling for comorbidities) [27] Increased REM density [27]	Reduced sleep depth [27] Decreased SWS (may persist in remission) [21, 24] Decreased ratio of SWS in the first relative to the second NREM period (fairly specific to depression) [24] (no reduction in SWS found in more recent meta-analysis) [27]	Bidirectional relationship with insomnia [21] Sleep disturbance predictive of onset/relapse of depressive episode [21, 24] Insomnia often persists in remission, leading to increased risk of relapse [24] Sleep disturbance risk factor for suicide [21] 'Eveningness' chronotype [26] Comorbidity with OSA [26]
Bipolar affective disorder (limited data)	Irregular sleeping pattern [29] Depressive episode: • hypersomnia or/and insomnia [21, 24, 29] Manic episode: • decreased need for sleep [21]	Short circadian period [26] Possible increased sensitivity of melatonin suppression to light [26] Variation in melatonin secretion: • manic episode: phase advanced [26] • depressive episode: phase delayed [26] Seasonal onset of manic episodes [26] Increased sensitivity to circadian shifts [29] Delayed sleep phase more common [26, 29] Link with polymorphism in circadian clock genes [26, 29]	Depressive episode: • similar to unipolar depression [29] Manic episode: • reduced sleep need, duration and efficiency [29]	Limited data Similar to unipolar depression, but increased REM fragmentation in depressive episode [26, 29]	Limited data [27]	Sleep disturbances may persist between episodes [29] Sleep loss predisposes to manic episodes [21] 'Eveningness' chronotype [26] High prevalence of insomnia [29]

	Subjective sleep–wake complaints	Circadian rhythm	Sleep continuity	REM sleep	Slow-wave sleep (SWS)/Sleep depth	Associations
Schizophrenia	Difficulties with sleep onset and maintenance [21] Reduced sleep quality [21] Excessive daytime sleepiness (possible medication effect) [30] Psychotic experiences (delusions and hallucinations) disturbing sleep [28, 30] Negative association with bed, due to past distressing experiences [28]	Circadian rhythm disturbance [21, 28] Tendency for sleep–wake reversal [21]	Disturbed sleep continuity: – Increased sleep latency [21, 30] – Decreased total sleep time [21, 30] – Decreased sleep efficiency [30] – Increased wake time overnight [21]	Previous findings of increased REM sleep latency [21, 30] not confirmed after controlling for comorbidities [27] No increased REM sleep pressure [27]	Decreased amount of slow-wave sleep [21] Reduced sleep depth [21, 27]	Sleep disturbance associated with prodrome and relapse [21, 30] Increased prevalence of insomnia, OSA and RLS/PLMD [21, 28, 30] Sleep disturbances linked to symptom severity [28, 30] Poor sleep environment and lack of daytime activities contributing factors [28] Sleep might be used as an escape from distressing experiences [28]
Generalised anxiety disorder (GAD) (limited data)	Difficulties falling and staying asleep [21]	Limited data	Increased sleep latency [21] Increased arousals and time awake after sleep onset [21]	No change in REM sleep latency or percentage [21]	Limited data Possible decreased slow wave sleep [21]	Insomnia may increase risk of GAD [21]

Notes: REM sleep latency: time between the onset of sleep and first REM sleep [27]. REM density: frequency of rapid eye movements during REM sleep [27]. REM pressure: shorter REM latency, increased REM density and duration of REM sleep [27]. Sleep efficiency: ratio of total sleep time to time in bed, expressed as percentage asleep while in bed [27]. Sleep onset latency: time from lights out to onset of sleep [27]. Abbreviations: NREM, non-rapid-eye-movement (sleep); OSA, obstructive sleep apnoea; REM, rapid-eye-movement (sleep); RLS, restless legs syndrome; PLMD, periodic limb movement disorder.

Table 9.16.2 The effects of psychotropic medication on sleep [5, 17, 20, 31–41]

Medication	Possible mode of action affecting sleep	Medications with antidepressant action				Other effects
		REM sleep	Slow-wave sleep (SWS)	Sleep continuity	RLS/PLMD	
Sedating tricyclic antidepressant medications (amitriptyline, trimipramine, clomipramine, doxepin) [17, 20,31–36]	Inhibition of 5-HT and NA uptake (except trimipramine) Antagonism at 5-HT2, HA (H1), m-ACh, alpha-1 adrenergic receptors Trimipramine: blocks 5-HT2 and D2 receptors	↓ REM sleep Clomipramine suppresses REM the most Doxepine suppresses REM relatively less Exception: ↔ Trimipramine	↑ SWS (variable effects, dependent on medication and population) ↔ Trimipramine	↑ sleep continuity Effects may reduce with time Variable effects between patients and volunteers	↑/↔? RLS/PLMD	Somnolence/daytime sedation Nightmares, vivid dreams May induce/exacerbate bruxism, REM sleep without atonia and RBD Doxepin is FDA (USA) approved for treatment of insomnia in very low doses (3–6 mg). Sleep promotion mainly due to antihistaminic effect Discontinuation effects may include insomnia, nightmares, REM rebound related excessive dreaming (similar effect for most antidepressants) Trimipramine: risk of tardive dyskinesia
Activating tricyclic antidepressant medications (desipramine, nortriptyline) [17, 20, 31–33, 35]	Inhibition of 5-HT and NA uptake (more selective for NA) Antagonism at m-ACh receptor	↓ REM sleep (milder effect for desipramine)	↑ SWS nortriptyline ↔ Desipramine	↓ sleep continuity Effects may reduce with time Variable effects between patients and healthy volunteers	↑/↔? RLS/PLMD	Insomnia Nightmares, vivid dreams May induce/exacerbate bruxism, REM sleep without atonia and RBD
SSRIs (fluoxetine most studied) [17, 20, 31–35]	Inhibition of 5-HT uptake	↓ REM (moderate effects)	↔ SWS (↓ fluoxetine)	↓ sleep continuity Less effect in depressed patients and reduces over time (except for fluoxetine)	↑ RLS/PLMD	Insomnia /daytime somnolence Nightmares May induce/ exacerbate bruxism, REM sleep without atonia and RBD REM sleep rebound after discontinuation
SNRIs (venlafaxine, duloxetine) [17, 20, 31–33, 35]	Inhibition of 5-HT and NA uptake	↓ REM (effect less in duloxetine)	↔ SWS (↔/↑ duloxetine)	↓ sleep continuity Effect less for duloxetine (dose dependent)	↑ RLS/PLMD (especially venlafaxine)	Nightmares, vivid dreams Insomnia/daytime somnolence May induce/exacerbate bruxism, REM sleep without atonia and RBD
SARIs (trazodone) [17, 20, 31–33, 35]	Antagonism at 5-HT2A, HA (H1), alpha-1-adrenergic receptors 5-HT reuptake inhibition	↔ REM	↑ SWS	↑ sleep continuity	↔? RLS/PLMD (less commonly associated)	↑↑ daytime somnolence More commonly used as hypnotic than as antidepressant (low dose, unlicensed use)
NaSSAs (mirtazapine) [17, 20, 31–33, 35]	Antagonism at 5-HT2, 5-HT3, HA (H1), alpha-1- and alpha-2-adrenergic receptors	↔ REM	↑ SWS	↑ sleep continuity	↑↑ RLS/PLMD	Nightmares, confusional states ↑↑ daytime somnolence ↑ sedation <30 mg (predominantly antihistaminergic effects at lower doses, at higher doses noradrenergic effects) Weight gain may enhance OSA

Table 9.16.2 (cont.)

Medications with antidepressant action

Medication	Possible mode of action affecting sleep	REM sleep	Slow-wave sleep (SWS)	Sleep continuity	RLS/PLMD	Other effects
NDRIs (bupropion) [17, 20, 31, 33, 35]	Inhibition of NA and DA uptake	↑/↔? REM	↓/↔? SWS	↓/↔? sleep continuity	↔/↑? RLS/PLMD	Insomnia Vivid dreams, nightmares
MAOIs [17, 20, 31, 33–35]	Inhibition of MAO	↓↓ REM (cases of complete REM suppression, less marked with reversible MAOI moclobemide)	↔/? SWS	↓ sleep continuity	↑ RLS/PLMD	Insomnia/ daytime sedation REM rebound on dose reduction and discontinuation (vivid dreams)
Agomelatine [20, 32, 33, 35]	Agonism at melatonergic MT1 and MT2 receptors Antagonism at 5-HT2C receptors	↔ REM	↔/↑ SWS (increase with repeated administration)	↑ sleep continuity	? RLS/PLMD	Improved subjective sleep

Medications with anxiolytic and hypnotic action

Medication	Possible mode of action affecting sleep	REM sleep	Slow-wave sleep (SWS)	Sleep continuity	RLS/PLMD	Other effects
Benzodiazepine receptor agonists: Benzodiazepines [5, 20, 32, 37]	GABA-A receptor modulator	↓/↔ REM	↓ SWS (increased effect at higher doses)	↑ sleep continuity	? RLS/PLMD	Somnolence Improved self-reported sleep Used for treatment of RLS/PLMD (not first line, unlicensed use)
Benzodiazepine receptor agonists: Non-benzodiazepines (zopiclone, zolpidem) [5, 17, 37, 38]	Binding at various subtypes of GABA-A receptor	↔/↓ REM (at clinical doses, may ↓ at increased doses)	↔ SWS (at clinical doses, may ↓ at increased doses)	↑ sleep continuity	? RLS/PLMD	Improved self-reported sleep. Possible association with parasomnias (sleepwalking, sleep-related eating disorder (zolpidem))
Buspirone [20, 32]	5-HT1A, 5-HT2 agonism, antagonism D2	↓/↔ REM	↔ SWS	↑ sleep continuity	? RLS/PLMD	

Table 9.16.2 (cont.)

		Medications with antipsychotic action				
Medication	Possible mode of action affecting sleep	REM sleep	Slow wave sleep (SWS)	Sleep continuity	RLS/ PLMD	Other effects
Typical antipsychotic medication (variable effects with different medication) [20, 31, 39]	Antagonist at DA, alpha-1-adrenergic, HA (H1), m-ACh (m1), 5-HT2 (low affinity) receptors	?/↓ REM (mild effect)	?/↑ SWS ↑ (haloperidol)	↑ sleep continuity	↑ RLS/PLMD	Somnolence/insomnia
Aripiprazole [20, 31, 39]	Partial DA (D2), 5-HT1A receptor agonist 5-HT2A, NA and HA (H1) antagonist	? REM	? SWS	? sleep continuity	↑ RLS/PLMD	Insomnia Less likely to cause daytime sedation
Clozapine [17, 20, 31, 39, 40]	Antagonism at DA (D1,2), 5-HT2, m-ACh, HA (H1), alpha-1 adrenergic receptors	↔ REM	↔↓/↑ SWS (variable findings)	↑ sleep continuity	↑ RLS/PLMD	High rate of daytime sedation Increased risk of weight gain (may increase risk of OSA)
Olanzapine [17, 20, 32, 39, 40]	Antagonism at HA (H1), 5-HT2A, DA (D 1,2), m-ACh (m1), alpha-1-adrenergic receptors	↔/↑ REM	↑ SWS	↑ sleep continuity	↑ RLS/PLMD	Insomnia /daytime sedation Increased risk of weight gain (may increase risk of OSA)
Quetiapine [20, 39, 40]	Antagonism at 5-HT2A, HA (H1), alpha-1-adrenergic, m-ACh (m1), DA (D2) receptors	↔/↓ REM	↔↓/↓ SWS	↔/↑ sleep continuity	↑ RLS/PLMD	Possible insomnia/daytime sedation (variable findings) Effects may vary between preparations (modified/ immediate release) and timing of administration
Risperidone [17, 20, 39, 40]	Antagonism at DA (D2), 5-HT2A, alpha-1-adrenergic receptors	↔/↓ REM	↑ SWS	↔/↑ sleep continuity	↑ RLS/PLMD	Possible insomnia/daytime sedation
Paliperidone (limited data) [17, 20, 36, 40]	Antagonism at DA (D2), 5-HT2A, alpha-1-adrenergic receptors	↑ REM	↑ SWS	↑ sleep continuity	↑ RLS/PLMD (likely, but limited data)	Possible insomnia Less daytime somnolence

9

Table 9.16.2 (cont.)

Medication	Possible mode of action affecting sleep	REM sleep	Slow wave sleep (SWS)	Sleep continuity	RLS/PLMD	Other effects
Lithium carbonate [5, 20, 32]	Not well understood	↓ REM	↑ SWS	Subjectively improved sleep	↑ RLS/PLMD	
Gabapentin [5, 19, 20, 32, 37]	Binds at alpha-2 delta subunit of voltage-gated calcium channels	↔/↑ REM	↑ SWS	↑ sleep continuity	↓ RLS/PLMD	Used as treatment for RLS/ PLMD (unlicensed use in UK)
Pregabalin [5, 19, 20, 32, 37]	Binds at alpha-2 delta subunit of voltage-gated calcium channels	↓/↔? REM	↑ SWS	↑ sleep continuity	↓ RLS/PLMD	Used as treatment for RLS/ PLMD (unlicensed use in UK)
Sodium oxybate (sodium salt of gamma-hydroxybutyrate (GHB)) [5, 32, 37, 41]	Agonist at GHB receptor, partial agonist at GABA-B receptors	Consolidates REM sleep in narcolepsy	↑ SWS	↑ sleep continuity	? RLS/PLMD	Licensed for narcolepsy with cataplexy (due to short half-life requires second nightly dose) Abuse potential due to euphoria inducing and growth-hormone promoting effects

Key: ↑, increased; ↓, decreased; ↑↓, variable effects/findings; ↔, no significant effect/limited effect; ↔?, equivocal findings; ?, unknown/insufficient data or information.

Abbreviations: ACh, acetylcholine; DA, dopamine; FDA, Food and Drug Administration (USA); GABA, gamma-aminobutyric acid; 5-HT, 5-hydroxytryptamine (serotonin); MAOI, monoamine oxidase inhibitor; NaSSA, noradrenaline and specific serotonin antagonist; NDRI, noradrenaline and dopamine reuptake inhibitor; NA, noradrenaline OSA, obstructive sleep apnoea; REM, rapid-eye-movement (sleep); RBD, REM behaviour disorder; RLS/ PLMD, restless legs syndrome/periodic limb movement disorder; SARI, serotonin antagonist and reuptake inhibitor; SNRI, serotonin–noradrenaline reuptake inhibitor; SSRI, selective serotonin reuptake inhibitor.

For references see online appendix; available at www.cambridge.org/CTNP.

REFERENCES

1. American Academy of Sleep Medicine. *International Classification of Sleep Disorders*, 3rd ed. American Academy of Sleep Medicine, 2014.

2. Calem M, Bisla J, Begum A et al. Increased prevalence of insomnia and changes in hypnotic use in England over 15 years: analysis of the 1993, 2000, and 2007 national psychiatric morbidity surveys. *Sleep* 2012; 35(3): 377–384.

3. Riemann D, Nissen C, Palagini L et al. The neurobiology, investigation, and treatment of chronic insomnia. *Lancet Neurol* 2015; 14: 547–558.

4. American Psychiatric Association. *Diagnostic and Statistical Manual of Mental Disorders*, 5th ed. (DSM-5). American Psychiatric Association, 2013.

5. Stahl SM, Morrissette DA. *Stahl's Illustrated Sleep and Wake Disorders*. Cambridge University Press, 2016.

6. Riemann D, Baglioni C, Bassetti C et al. European guideline for the diagnosis and treatment of insomnia. *J Sleep Res* 2017; 26: 675–700.

7. Wilson S, Anderson K, Baldwin D, Dijk D-J et al. British Association for Psychopharmacology consensus statement on evidence-based treatment of insomnia, parasomnias and circadian rhythm disorders: an update. *J Psychopharmacol* 2019; 33(8): 923–947.

8. Perlis ML, Ellis JG, DeMichele Kloss J, Riemann DW. Etiology and pathophysiology of insomnia. In Kryger M, Roth T, Dement WC (eds.), *Principles and Practice of Sleep Medicine*, 6th ed. Elsevier, 2017, pp. 769–784.

9. Krystal AD. New developments in insomnia medications of relevance to mental health disorders. *Psychiatr Clin North Am* 2015; 38(4):843–860.

10. Jokic R. Obstructive sleep apnoea. In Selsick H (ed.), *Sleep Disorders in Psychiatric Patients*. Springer-Verlag, 2018, pp. 213–238.

11. Chung F, Abdullah HR, Liao P. STOP-Bang Questionnaire. A practice approach to screen for obstructive sleep apnoea. *Chest* 2016; 149(3): 631–638.

12. Greenberg H, Lacticova V, Scharf SM. Obstructive sleep apnoea: clinical features, evaluation, and principles of management. In Kryger M, Roth T, Dement WC (eds.), *Principles and Practice of Sleep Medicine*, 6th ed. Elsevier, 2017, pp. 1110–1024.

13. Gottlieb DJ, Punjabi NM. Diagnosis and management of obstructive sleep apnoea: a review. *JAMA* 2020; 323(14): 1389–1400.

14. Perez-Carbonell L, Leschziner G. Clinical update on central hypersomnias. *J Thorac Dis* 2018; 10(Suppl 1): 112–123.

15. Fleetham JA, Fleming JA. Parasomnias. *CMAJ* 2014; 186(8): 273–280.

16. Breen DP, Hoegl B, Fasano A et al. Sleep-related motor and behavioural disorders: recent advances and new entities. *Mov Disord* 2018; 33(7): 1042–1055.

17. Doghramji K, Jangro WC. Adverse effects of psychotropic medications on sleep. *Psychiatr Clin North Am* 2016; 39: 487–502.

18. Kilduff TS, Mendelson WB. Hypnotic medications: mechanisms of action and pharmacological effects. In Kryger M, Roth T, Dement WC (eds.), *Principles and Practice of Sleep Medicine*, 6th ed. Elsevier, 2017, pp. 424–431.

19. Garcia-Borreguero D, Williams A-M. An update on restless legs syndrome ('Willis–Ekbom disease'): clinical features, pathogenesis and treatment. *Curr Opin Neurol* 2014; 27: 493–501.

20. Schweitzer PK, Randazzo AC. Drugs that disturb sleep and wakefulness. In Kryger M, Roth T, Dement WC (eds.), *Principles and Practice of Sleep Medicine*, 6th ed. Elsevier, 2017, pp. 480–498.

21. Krystal AD. Psychiatric disorders and sleep. *Neurol Clin* 2012; 30(4): 1389–1413.

22. Harvey AG, Murray G, Chandler RA, Soehner A. Sleep disturbance as transdiagnostic: consideration of neurobiological mechanisms. *Clin Psychol Rev* 2011; 31(2): 225–235.

23. Foster RG. Sleep, circadian rhythms and health. *Interface Focus* 2020; 10: 20190098.

24. Minkel JD, Krystal AD, Benca RM. Unipolar major depression. In Kryger M, Roth T, Dement WC (eds.), *Principles and Practice of Sleep Medicine*, 6th ed. Elsevier, 2017, pp. 1352–1362.

25. Freeman D, Sheaves B, Goodwin G, Yu L-M et al. The effects of improving sleep on mental health (OASIS): a randomised controlled trial with mediation analysis. *Lancet Psychiatry* 2017; 4: 749–758.

26. Hickie IB, Naismith SL, Robillard R et al. Manipulating the sleep–wake cycle and circadian rhythms to improve clinical management of major depression. *BMC Medicine*. 2013; 11(79): 1–27.

27. Baglioni C, Nanovska S, Regen W et al. Sleep and mental disorders: a meta-analysis of polysomnographic research. *Psychol Bull* 2016; 142(9): 969–990.

28. Waite F, Myers E, Harvey AG, Espie CA et al. Treating sleep problems in patients with schizophrenia. *Behav Cogn Psychother* 2016; 44: 273–287.

29. Harvey AG, Soehner AM, Buysse DJ. Bipolar disorder. In Kryger M, Roth T, Dement WC (eds.), *Principles and Practice of Sleep Medicine*, 6th ed. Elsevier, 2017, pp. 1363–1369.

30. Reeve S, Sheaves B, Freeman D. The role of sleep dysfunction in the occurrence of delusions and hallucinations: a systematic review. *Clin Psychol Rev* 2015; 42: 96–115.

31. Krystal AD. Antidepressant and antipsychotic drugs. *Sleep Med Clin* 2010; 5(4): 571–589.

32. Wilson S. Pharmacology of psychiatric drugs and their effects on sleep. In Selsick H (ed.), *Sleep Disorders in Psychiatric Patients*. Springer-Verlag, 2018, pp. 85–96.

33. Wichniak A, Wierzbicka A, Walecka M, Jernajczyk W. Effects of antidepressants on sleep. *Curr Psychiatry Rep* 2017; 19(63): 1–7.

34. Beitinger ME, Fulda S. Long-term effects of antidepressants on sleep. In Pandi-Perumal SR, Kramer M (eds.), *Sleep and Mental Illness*. Cambridge University Press, 2010, pp. 183–201.

35. Staner L, Staner C, Luthringer R. Antidepressant-induced alteration of sleep EEG. In: Pandi-Perumal SR, Kramer M (eds.), *Sleep and Mental Illness*. Cambridge University Press, 2010, pp. 202–221.

36. Van Gastel A. Drug-induced insomnia and excessive sleepiness. *Sleep Med Clin* 2018; 13: 147–159.

37. Roehrs T, Roth T. Drug-related sleep stage changes: functional significance and clinical relevance. *Sleep Med Clin* 2010; 5(4): 559–570.

38. Carlos K, Prado GF, Teixeira CDM et al. Benzodiazepines for restless legs syndrome. *Cochrane Database Syst Rev* 2017; 3: CD006939.

39. Krystal AD, Goforth HW, Roth T. Effects of antipsychotic medications on sleep in schizophrenia. *Int Clin Psychopharmacol* 2008; 23: 150–160.

40. Monti JM, Torterolo P, Pandi Perumal SR. The effects of second-generation antipsychotic drugs on sleep variables in healthy subjects and patients with schizophrenia. *Sleep Med Rev* 2017; 33: 51–57.

41. Joint Formulary Committee. *British National Formulary* (online). BMJ Group and Pharmaceutical Press. www.medicinescomplete.com.

<table>
<tr><td>**9.17**</td><td>**Eating Disorders**</td><td>Andreas Stengel and Sophie Scharner</td></tr>
</table>

OVERVIEW

Eating disorders are a group of heterogeneous mental disorders characterised by a distorted relationship to food and eating that often leads to abnormalities in body weight, including both extremes of the weight spectrum. In this section we focus on three disorders: anorexia nervosa, bulimia nervosa and binge eating disorder. Both anorexia nervosa and bulimia nervosa often have an early onset in adolescence or young adulthood and are much more common in females than in males, whereas binge eating disorder is nearly similarly prevalent in men and women (around 5%) and can start later in life [1]. Anorexia nervosa has the highest mortality rate (up to 20%) of any psychiatric disease and a prevalence around 1% in women [1]. Bulimia nervosa has a higher prevalence in women, around 2%, and occurs often undetected for longer periods [1]. Despite the huge impact that eating disorders can have on individuals and families, data on prevalence, frequency of specific symptoms and comorbidities are only sporadically available. The pathophysiology of these diseases is still only partially understood. There is still no specific pharmacological treatment available, which can be partially explained by the multifactorial origin of the diseases and the still insufficiently understood pathophysiology.

MRI has shown brain structural and functional changes associated with eating disorders. In structural MRI scans of anorexia nervosa patients, the most common finding is grey and white matter reduction, correlating with the extent of malnourishment and mostly reversible with recovery. In normal weight or overweight patients suffering from bulimia nervosa or binge eating disorder, there are usually more localised structural abnormalities (i.e. specific to particular brain regions). Most functional MRI (fMRI) studies of patients with anorexia nervosa focus on food, taste, physical appearance and social cognition, whereas studies on patients with bulimia nervosa and binge eating studies additionally focus on impulse inhibition and reward. The most common findings in anorexia nervosa are increased activation of the amygdala and altered activation of the cingulate cortex. In patients with bulimia nervosa and binge eating disorder, fMRI changes detected are often similar in both disorders: the most common findings are hypoactivity in the frontostriatal circuits and alterations in the insula, amygdala and frontal gyrus. In bulimia and binge eating disorder, there is generally a link between illness severity (measured as frequency of binge eating) and the extent of neural changes.

9.17.1 Anorexia Nervosa

The data and research related to anorexia nervosa are more comprehensive than for other eating disorders [2]. Clinically, anorexia nervosa is defined by the strong wish to lose or maintain body weight at abnormally low levels, usually by caloric restriction and hyperactivity [3]. Most patients suffer from a distorted body image [3] (see the diagnostic criteria in Table 9.17.1). Nine out of ten affected patients are women [1]. As far as it is understood, the pathophysiology of anorexia nervosa is multifactorial, with genetic susceptibility playing a role (genetics' impact on anorexia nervosa is not fully understood, but twin-based heritability estimates are at 50–60%) [4]. Evidence

Table 9.17.1 DSM-5 diagnostic criteria for anorexia nervosa

(A) Restriction of energy intake relative to requirements leading to a significantly low body weight in the context of age, sex, developmental trajectory and physical health. Significantly low weight is defined as a weight that is less than minimally normal or, for children and adolescents, less than that minimally expected.

(B) Intense fear of gaining weight or becoming fat, or persistent behaviour that interferes with weight gain, even though at a significantly low weight.

(C) Disturbance in the way in which one's body weight or shape is experienced, undue influence of body weight or shape on self-evaluation or persistent lack of recognition of the seriousness of the current low body weight.

From the *Diagnostic and Statistical Manual of Mental Disorders*, 5th edition DSM-5 [3].

from genome-wide association studies has identified genetic risk loci that correlate with risk loci for other psychiatric disorders, physical activity and metabolic (including glycaemic), lipid and anthropometric (body measurement) traits, supporting the idea that anorexia nervosa is a metabo-psychiatric disease [5]. We also know that psychosocial factors including personality, family structure and culture increase one's risk of suffering from anorexia nervosa [2]. The most frequent comorbidities are depression, obsessive–compulsive disorder and anxiety disorders [6]. Animal models have also been used to gain insight into pathophysiology. The most commonly used is a model called activity-based anorexia: in this model rodents have decreased access to food (only a few hours a day), but have a running wheel in their cage [7]. This leads to the rodents voluntarily exercising in the running wheel and, consequentially, losing body weight until they would starve to death [7]. Predisposing psychosocial and genetic factors are not mimicked in this model, but neuroendocrine changes including 'amenorrhoea' (the cessation of the oestrous cycle), changes in the activation of different brain nuclei and metabolic changes can be observed [8]. Since starvation is not 'voluntary', it is still not an ideal model for anorexia nervosa.

9.17.2 Biological Alterations in Anorexia Nervosa

There are many endocrine changes in patients with anorexia nervosa, including decreased leptin and insulin and increased ghrelin and cortisol [9] (see Section 5.1 for background on the regulation of appetite). So far, our understanding is that none of the endocrine changes are primary (i.e. they are a result of, rather than causative of, anorexia nervosa). Nonetheless, they have negative effects on the body (e.g. osteoporosis) and may lead to disease-self-perpetuating effects (vicious cycle) [9].

In structural MRI studies of patients with anorexia nervosa, the main finding is that grey matter volume and cortical thickness are lower in patients with anorexia nervosa [10]. These findings are temporary, as both lower volume and cortical thickness normalise with weight recovery. Animal studies suggest that this loss in volume is most likely derived from malnutrition and dehydration of astrocytes within the brain connective tissue [11]. These MRI findings are not disease-specific but rather weight-loss related, as patients with other diseases involving weight loss also suffer from a loss of grey matter volume and cortical thickness [10]. Additionally, the midbrain and the thalamus are often reduced in volume in anorexia nervosa patients [12]. This is interesting because the thalamus is a sensory relay station, critically involved in communication of incoming sensory information like taste and gustatory signals to the cerebral cortex, especially the frontal and insular regions, for further processing [13].

From functional MRI (fMRI) studies we know that the most important circuit involved in a patient's food-avoidance behaviour is the brain reward system [14]. This system processes an individual's motivation to eat by incorporating signals of hedonic pleasure from food intake and a specific food's perceived value [13] (Figure 9.17.1). Specifically, the circuitry includes:

- the insula, where the primary taste cortex is located
- the ventral striatum (consisting of the nucleus accumbens and the olfactory tubercle), which receives several dopaminergic and glutamatergic inputs from different sources and drives food approach
- the orbitofrontal cortex, which calculates the subjective value of a food
- the hypothalamus, which receives body signals on hunger and satiety and helps the higher-order decision making and food approach.

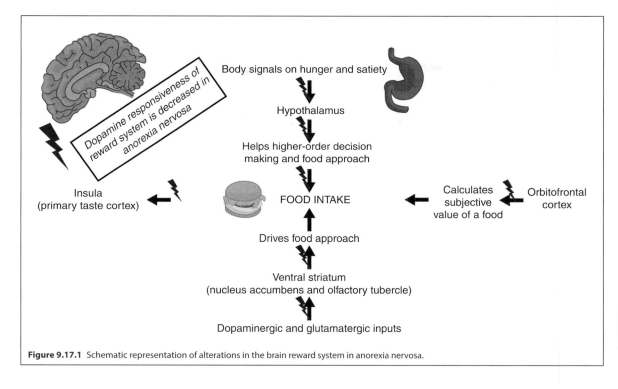

Figure 9.17.1 Schematic representation of alterations in the brain reward system in anorexia nervosa.

In anorexia nervosa, the dopamine responsiveness of the reward system is decreased [15]. Importantly, when considering pharmacological treatments for anorexia nervosa, the serotonin–dopamine receptor antagonist olanzapine has several metabolic side effects that might be beneficial [6] and has already shown potential in clinical trials. Another approach acknowledges that patients with anorexia nervosa often suffer from high anxiety levels that intensely interfere with a normal drive to eat [15]. Many patients with anorexia nervosa are prescribed a selective serotonin reuptake inhibitor (especially fluoxetine) to treat their comorbid mood disorder, anxiety disorder and obsessive–compulsive disorder, which sometimes also improves their eating behaviour [6].

Habit learning and striatal–frontal brain connectivity have also been shown to be altered in anorexia nervosa (Table 9.17.2), and these factors might play a role in the perpetuation of illness behaviour, an aspect of the disease that is difficult to overcome [2].

9.17.3 Bulimia Nervosa and Binge Eating Disorder

9.17.3.1 Bulimia Nervosa

Bulimia nervosa can go undiagnosed for years as patients maintain a normal body weight. Patients suffer from the wish to lose weight interjected with binge eating attacks in which they eat in a large amount of food in a short

Table 9.17.2 Key neurobiological and genetic changes in anorexia nervosa

Method	Finding
MRI	Grey matter volume, cortical thickness, midbrain and thalamus can all be reduced in size.
fMRI	Food avoidance behaviour originates from changes in brain reward system. Specifically, the dopamine responsiveness of the brain reward system is decreased.
	Perpetuation of illness behaviour might originate from altered striatal–frontal brain connectivity.
Genetic (genome-wide association studies)	Genetic risk for anorexia nervosa correlates with: genetic risk for other psychiatric disorders; physical activity; and metabolic (including glycaemic), lipid and anthropometric (body measurement) traits.

Table 9.17.3 DSM-5 diagnostic criteria for bulimia nervosa

(A) Recurrent episodes of binge eating. An episode of binge eating is characterised by BOTH of the following: 　(1) Eating in a discrete amount of time (e.g. within a 2-hour period) an amount of food that is definitely larger than what most individuals would eat in a similar period of time under similar circumstances. 　(2) Sense of lack of control over eating during an episode.
(B) Recurrent inappropriate compensatory behaviour in order to prevent weight gain, such as self-induced vomiting; misuse of laxatives, diuretics, or other medications; fasting; or excessive exercise.
(C) The binge eating and inappropriate compensatory behaviours both occur, on average, at least once a week for 3 months.
(D) Self-evaluation is unduly influenced by body shape and weight.
(E) The disturbance does not occur exclusively during episodes of anorexia nervosa.

From the *Diagnostic and Statistical Manual of Mental Disorders*, 5th edition DSM-5 [3].

amount of time [3]. These binge eating attacks are accompanied by a feeling of loss of control [3]. Patients try to prevent weight gain and engage in some kind of purging behaviour, such as self-induced vomiting, abuse of laxatives, diuretics (or other medication) or excessive exercise [3] (see also the diagnostic criteria in Table 9.17.3).

The first genome-wide association studies do not show overlap of the genetic risk variants for anorexia and bulimia nervosa, but more studies are necessary to be certain [16]. The most common psychiatric comorbidities in bulimia nervosa are depression and specific phobias (similar to anorexia nervosa). Other comorbidities include post-traumatic stress disorder (PTSD), attention deficit hyperactivity disorder and drug abuse disorder (the majority of cases being alcohol abuse disorder), which differs greatly from anorexia nervosa [17, 18]. Overall, trauma (PTSD) and impulse inhibition (drug abuse disorder) are more prevalent in bulimia nervosa than in anorexia nervosa [17, 18].

9.17.3.2 Binge Eating Disorder

Binge eating disorder is the most common of the three eating disorders, but it has the fewest data available. There are no genome-wide association studies on binge eating disorder to date. Patients with binge eating disorder have attacks of increased food intake in a short amount of time usually accompanied by a sense of lack of control [3]. Moreover, individuals suffering from binge eating disorder are in distress about the binging attacks and often feel ashamed [3] (see also the diagnostic criteria in Table 9.17.4). Patients with binge eating disorder have significantly more psychiatric comorbidities than obese patients without binge eating disorder. Again, the most common psychiatric diseases are depression and anxiety disorders; additional comorbidities include PTSD and trauma experiences, personality disorders (specifically borderline personality and avoidant personality disorder) and drug abuse [1].

Table 9.17.4 DSM-5 diagnostic criteria for binge eating disorder

(A) Recurrent episodes of binge eating. An episode of binge eating is characterised by both of the following: 　(1) Eating, in a discrete period of time (e.g. within any 2-hour period), an amount of food that is definitely larger than what most people would eat in a similar period of time under similar circumstances. 　(2) A sense of lack of control over eating during the episode (e.g. a feeling that one cannot stop eating or control what or how much one is eating).
(B) The binge eating episodes are associated with three (or more) of the following: 　(1) Eating much more rapidly than normal. 　(2) Eating until feeling uncomfortably full. 　(3) Eating large amounts of food when not feeling physically hungry. 　(4) >Eating alone because of feeling embarrassed by how much one is eating. 　(5) >Feeling disgusted with oneself, depressed or very guilty afterward.
(C) Marked distress regarding binge eating is present.
(D) The binge eating occurs, on average, at least once a week for 3 months.

From the *Diagnostic and Statistical Manual of Mental Disorders*, 5th edition DSM-5 [3].

9.17.4 Biological Alterations in Bulimia Nervosa and Binge Eating Disorder

Many studies combine bulimia nervosa and binge eating disorder patients and there are many shared findings [19]. Compared to unaffected individuals, patients with these disorders show diminished attentional capacity and learning early on in a task [19]. In tests of inhibitory control (how well an individual can suppress inappropriate or unwanted actions), patients with binge eating disorder and bulimia nervosa show general impairments in inhibitory control compared to healthy controls [20]. Patients with bulimia nervosa specifically show altered choice behaviour when tested for the degree of preference for immediate over delayed rewards, preferring more often the immediate reward compared to controls [21].

In structural MRI studies, patients with bulimia nervosa and binge eating disorder show increased grey matter volume in the medial orbitofrontal cortex, which is part of the brain reward system and is implicated in representing the hedonic value of food stimuli [13, 22]. Patients suffering from bulimia nervosa also show decreased inferior frontal grey matter [23] and reduced volume of the caudate nucleus (part of the frontostriatal circuit) [24].

Functional MRI studies of bulimia nervosa and binge eating disorder show hypoactivity in frontostriatal circuits and aberrant responses in the insula, amygdala, middle frontal gyrus and occipital cortex to a range of different stimuli or tasks [19]. The frontostriatal system has a central role in controlling goal-directed thoughts and behaviours, including inhibitory control and reward processing [13] – see also Section 5.15. Illness severity, which is defined as the frequency of binge eating or purging episodes, is related to greater neural changes as measured by fMRI [19]. The urge to binge eat seems to be mediated by a hyperactivity of the orbitofrontal cortex and the anterior cingulate cortex and hypoactivity of executive control networks, especially an impaired inhibitory control from the lateral prefrontal circuits [25]. It is notable that alterations in the corticostriatal circuits, with changes in the function of the prefrontal, insular and orbitofrontal cortices, as well as the striatum, are similar to those seen in studies of people with substance abuse [18, 26]. There are no animal models for bulimia nervosa and

Table 9.17.5 Key neurobiological changes in bulimia nervosa and binge eating disorder

Method	Finding
MRI	Bulimia nervosa and binge eating disorder: • increased grey matter volumes in the medial orbitofrontal cortex Bulimia nervosa: • volume reduction of the inferior frontal grey matter and the caudate nucleus
fMRI	Bulimia nervosa and binge eating disorder: • urge to binge eat might be mediated by a hyperactivity of the orbitofrontal cortex and the anterior cingulate cortex and a hypoactivity of the lateral prefrontal circuits • aberrant responses to a range of different stimuli or tasks were shown in the insula, amygdala, middle frontal gyrus and occipital cortex

binge eating disorder available. The key neurobiological changes in bulimia nervosa and binge eating disorder are summarised in Table 9.17.5.

Conclusions and Outstanding Questions

The eating disorders have high prevalence and mortality rates, but their pathophysiology is still only partially understood. In fMRI studies, the most common findings in anorexia nervosa are increased activation of the amygdala and altered activation of the cingulate cortex. The most common findings in patients with bulimia nervosa and binge eating disorder are hypoactivity in the frontostriatal circuits and alterations in the insula, amygdala and frontal gyrus.

Outstanding Questions

• Which of the neurocognitive changes are causes and which are consequences of the symptoms of the eating disorder?

• Given that eating disorders most likely have a multifactorial genesis, to what extent are eating disorders caused by psychosocial or genetic factors or physiological self-perpetuating processes?

• Can we identify new pharmaceutical treatments for eating disorders?

• What exactly do the different comorbidities for anorexia nervosa and bulimia nervosa imply for the neurobiology and maybe even pathogenesis of these eating disorders?

REFERENCES

1. Keski-Rahkonen A, Mustelin L. Epidemiology of eating disorders in Europe: prevalence, incidence, comorbidity, course, consequences, and risk factors. *Curr Opin Psychiatry* 2016; 29(6): 340–345.

2. Frank GKW, Shott ME, DeGuzman MC. Recent advances in understanding anorexia nervosa. *F1000Res* 2019; 8: F1000 Faculty Rev-504.

3. American Psychiatric Association. *Diagnostic and Statistical Manual of Mental Disorders*, 5th ed. (DSM-5). American Psychiatric Association, 2013.

4. Yilmaz Z, Hardaway JA, Bulik CM. Genetics and epigenetics of eating disorders. *Adv Genomics Genet* 2015; 5: 131–150.

5. Watson HJ, Yilmaz Z, Thornton LM et al. Genome-wide association study identifies eight risk loci and implicates metabo-psychiatric origins for anorexia nervosa. *Nat Genet* 2019; 51(8): 1207–1214.

6. Brockmeyer T, Friederich HC, Schmidt U. Advances in the treatment of anorexia nervosa: a review of established and emerging interventions. *Psychol Med* 2018; 48(8): 1228–1256.

7. Schalla MA, Stengel A. Activity based anorexia as an animal model for anorexia nervosa: a systematic review. *Front Nutr* 2019; 6: 69.

8. Scharner S, Prinz P, Goebel-Stengel M et al. Activity-based anorexia reduces body weight without inducing a separate food intake microstructure or activity phenotype in female rats mediation via an activation of distinct brain nuclei. *Front Neurosci* 2016; 10: 475.

9. Misra M, Klibanski A. Endocrine consequences of anorexia nervosa. *Lancet Diabetes Endocrinol* 2014; 2(7): 581–592.

10. Bernardoni F, King JA, Geisler D et al. Weight restoration therapy rapidly reverses cortical thinning in anorexia nervosa: a longitudinal study. *Neuroimage* 2016; 130: 214–222.

11. Frintrop L, Liesbrock J, Paulukat L et al. Reduced astrocyte density underlying brain volume reduction in activity-based anorexia rats. *World J Biol Psychiatry* 2018; 19(3): 225–235.

12. Miles AE, Voineskos AN, French L, Kaplan AS. Subcortical volume and cortical surface architecture in women with acute and remitted anorexia nervosa: an exploratory neuroimaging study. *J Psychiatr Res* 2018; 102: 179–185.

13. Duane Haines GAM. *Fundamental Neuroscience for Basic and Clinical Applications*, 5th ed. Elsevier, 2017.

14. Jiang T, Soussignan R, Carrier E, Royet JP. Dysfunction of the mesolimbic circuit to food odors in women with anorexia and bulimia nervosa: a fMRI study. *Front Hum Neurosci* 2019; 13: 117.

15. Monteleone AM, Castellini G, Volpe U et al. Neuroendocrinology and brain imaging of reward in eating disorders: a possible key to the treatment of anorexia nervosa and bulimia nervosa. *Prog Neuropsychopharmacol Biol Psychiatry* 2018; 80(Pt B): 132–142.

16. Hinney A, Friedel S, Remschmidt H, Hebebrand J. Genetic risk factors in eating disorders. *Am J Pharmacogenomics* 2004; 4(4): 209–223.

17. Patel RS, Olten B, Patel P, Shah K, Mansuri Z. Hospitalization outcomes and comorbidities of bulimia nervosa: a nationwide inpatient study. *Cureus* 2018; 10(5): e2583.

18. Munn-Chernoff MA, Johnson EC, Chou YL et al. Shared genetic risk between eating disorder- and substance-use-related phenotypes: evidence from genome-wide association studies. *Addict Biol* 2020; 26(1): e12880.

19. Donnelly B, Touyz S, Hay P et al. Neuroimaging in bulimia nervosa and binge eating disorder: a systematic review. *J Eat Disord* 2018; 6: 3.

20. Skunde M, Walther S, Simon JJ et al. Neural signature of behavioural inhibition in women with bulimia nervosa. *J Psychiatry Neurosci* 2016; 41(5): E69–E78.

21. Kekic M, Bartholdy S, Cheng J et al. Increased temporal discounting in bulimia nervosa. *Int J Eat Disord* 2016; 49(12): 1077–1081.

22. Frank GK, Shott ME, Riederer J, Pryor TL. Altered structural and effective connectivity in anorexia and bulimia nervosa in circuits that regulate energy and reward homeostasis. *Transl Psychiatry* 2016; 6(11): e932.

23. Westwater ML, Seidlitz J, Diederen KMJ, Fischer S, Thompson JC. Associations between cortical thickness, structural connectivity and severity of dimensional bulimia nervosa symptomatology. *Psychiatry Res Neuroimaging* 2018; 271: 118–125.

24. Coutinho J, Ramos AF, Maia L et al. Volumetric alterations in the nucleus accumbens and caudate nucleus in bulimia nervosa: a structural magnetic resonance imaging study. *Int J Eat Disord* 2015; 48(2): 206–214.

25. Seitz J, Hueck M, Dahmen B et al. Attention network dysfunction in bulimia nervosa: an fMRI study. *PLoS One* 2016; 11(9): e0161329.

26. Kessler RM, Hutson PH, Herman BK, Potenza MN. The neurobiological basis of binge-eating disorder. *Neurosci Biobehav Rev* 2016; 63: 223–238.

National Neuroscience Curriculum Initiative online resources

Expert video: *Carrie McAdams on Eating Disorders*

9

9.18	Epilepsy and Seizures	Manny Bagary

OVERVIEW

This section begins with a definition of epilepsy and the different types of seizure. Next, I describe epileptogenesis, the process leading to a hyperexcitable neuronal network which is predisposed to seizures. I consider the biological mechanisms thought to contribute to this, at the ion-channel, cell and network level, followed by a description of how investigations including EEG, MRI and genetic testing contribute to the understanding and management of epilepsy in individual patients. Finally, I discuss the neuropsychiatric symptoms associated with epilepsy, and the range of factors that may contribute to these.

9.18.1 Key Definitions and Types of Seizure

9.18.1.1 What Is Epilepsy?

Epilepsy is a disorder of the brain characterised by an enduring predisposition to generate unprovoked epileptic seizures and by the neurobiological, cognitive, psychological and social consequences of this condition. In the UK, incidence is estimated to be 50 per 100,000 per year and the prevalence of active epilepsy is estimated to be 5–10 cases per 1,000 [1]. The International League Against Epilepsy (ILAE) provided an operational definition of epilepsy in 2014 (Table 9.18.1) [2].

Table 9.18.1 ILAE operational definition of epilepsy [2]

Epilepsy is a disease of the brain defined by any of the following conditions:

(1) A least two unprovoked (or reflex) seizures occurring more than 24 hours apart.
(2) One unprovoked (or reflex) seizure and a probability of further seizures similar to the general recurrence risk (at least 60%) after two unprovoked seizures, occurring over the next 10 years.
(3) Diagnosis of an epilepsy syndrome.

Epilepsy is considered to be resolved for individuals who had an age-dependent epilepsy syndrome but are now past the applicable age or those who have remained seizure free for the last 10 years, with no seizure medicines for the last 5 years.

9.18.1.2 What Is a Seizure?

An epileptic seizure is a transient occurrence of signs and/or symptoms due to abnormal excessive or synchronous neuronal activity in the brain [3]. The effects of a seizure depend on which part of the brain is affected. Seizures typically last seconds or minutes but can be prolonged and continuous as in status epilepticus.

9.18.1.3 What Are the Different Seizure Types?

For clarity of nomenclature, a revised operational classification of seizure types was suggested by the ILAE in 2017, replacing previous nomenclature such as partial or complex partial seizures. Seizures are now classified as focal onset (with retained or impaired awareness), generalised onset or unknown onset, with subcategories of motor and non-motor features [4]; see Table 9.18.2.

9.18.1.4 What Is Epileptogenesis?

Epileptogenesis is the sequence of events that change a normal neuronal network into a hyperexcitable network predisposed to spontaneous, recurrent seizures. These changes may take several years and include the selective loss of inhibitory interneurons or the excitatory

Table 9.18.2 ILAE operational classification of seizure types[a]

Focal onset	Generalised onset	Unknown onset
Aware or impaired awareness		

Motor onset:
  automatisms
  atonic[b] (i.e. limp)
  clonic (i.e. rhythmic jerking)
  epileptic spasms[b] (i.e. trunk flexion)
  hyperkinetic (e.g thrashing/pedalling)
  myoclonic (i.e. arrhythmic jerking)
  tonic (i.e. extension or flexion postures)
	Motor:
	  tonic–clonic
	  clonic
	  tonic
	  myoclonic
	  myoclonic–tonic–clonic
	  myoclonic–atonic
	  atonic[b]
	  epileptic spasm[b]
		Motor:
		  tonic–clonic
		  epileptic spasms

Non-motor onset:
  autonomic (e.g. flushing, sweating, piloerection)
  behaviour arrest
  cognitive
  emotional
  sensory
	Non-motor (absence):
	  typical
	  atypical
	  myoclonic
	  eyelid myoclonia
		Non-motor:
		  behaviour arrest

Focal to bilateral tonic–clonic		Unclassified: inadequate information to place in other categories

[a] Adapted from [4]. [b] Focal or generalised, with or without alteration of awareness.

interneurons driving them. Additionally, sprouting of axonal collaterals can lead to self-reinforcing circuits of activity-dependent disinhibition. At present we do not have treatments which are antiepileptogenic.

9.18.2 Why Do Seizures Happen?

The hyperexcitable state associated with seizures can be considered at the level of ions, membranes, cells, circuits/synapses and large-scale neuronal networks.

The basic mechanism of neuronal excitability is the action potential, which is dependent on the movements of ions across the neuronal cell membrane, causing depolarisation. Ions implicated in ictogenesis – that is, the activity-dependent transition from the interictal (between seizures) state to a seizure – include sodium, potassium, calcium and chloride [5]. Action potentials induce membrane depolarisation, which propagates along axons to induce neurotransmitter release at the axon terminal. Neurotransmitter vesicle fusion with the presynaptic membrane requires coordination of proteins subserving docking, priming and fusion, in addition to calcium entry and neurotransmitter and vesicle recycling [6]. Mutations in presynaptic proteins

have been demonstrated to be associated with epilepsy [7, 8]. Postsynaptic mechanisms relevant to increased network activity include neurotransmitter reuptake, receptor desensitisation, receptor membrane trafficking and post-translational modifications of receptor subunits affecting transmitter affinity and channel gating [9].

At a network level, neuronal circuits with abnormal feedback due to cortical dysgenesis (abnormal cortical development), abnormalities in neuronal migration, over-activation of the mammalian target of rapamycin (mTOR) cell-signalling pathway or the compensatory rewiring following brain injury may lead to unnecessary neuronal connectivity and predispose to seizures.

Glutamate is the major excitatory neurotransmitter. Enhanced activation of postsynaptic glutamate receptors (ionotropic and metabotropic) is proconvulsant. Antagonists of N-methyl-D-aspartate (NMDA) and alpha-amino-3-hydroxy-5-methyl-4-isoxazole-propionic acid (AMPA) receptors are anticonvulsant. Gamma-aminobutyric acid (GABA) is the major inhibitory neurotransmitter and has two main receptor subtypes. GABA-A receptors are postsynaptic. Chloride ion influx hyperpolarises the membrane and inhibits action potentials.

GABA-A receptor agonists, such as barbiturates and benzodiazepines, suppress seizure activity.

A hyperexcitable state can occur from an alteration of intra- or extracellular ion concentration, increased excitatory synaptic neurotransmission, decreased inhibitory neurotransmission and summation leading to an excitatory postsynaptic potential (EPSP), which is a depolarisation in the membrane of a postsynaptic neuron. Temporal summation occurs when one presynaptic neuron repeatedly releases neurotransmitters over a period of time to cause an EPSP whereas spatial summation occurs when multiple presynaptic neurons release neurotransmitters synchronously to cause an EPSP.

Proposed mechanisms of neuronal synchronisation during seizures include:

- chemical synaptic interactions involving synaptic neurotransmitter release
- electrical coupling via gap junctions which directly connect adjacent cells, allowing molecules, ions and electrical impulses to directly pass through a regulated gate between cells
- ephaptic interactions whereby coupling of adjacent nerve fibres is a result of local electric fields
- activity-dependent interactions between neurons due to seizure-associated changes in transmembrane ion concentration gradients (Na^+, K^+, Cl^-, Ca^{2+}, H^+ and HCO_3^-), which may alter hyperexcitability in neuronal networks.

However, the precise mechanisms underlying the sudden episodic transition from normal activity or interictal spikes to seizures in hyperexcitable epileptic networks remain largely unexplained.

9.18.3 What Investigations Do We Use?

EEG was invented by the German psychiatrist, Hans Berger, in 1929 (see Section 3.1.4 for the basics of EEG). Electrical activity recorded by scalp electrodes mostly reflects a summation of excitatory and inhibitory postsynaptic potentials in apical dendrites of pyramidal neurons in superficial cortical layers that have the same relative orientation and polarity. EEG does not measure action potentials which are too short to be recorded. Many cells are synchronously activated. The summation of the dipoles (i.e. positive and negative charges) created at each of thousands of neurons creates an electrical

potential detectable at the scalp (see Figure 9.18.1). Each electrode can detect synchronous activity generated by approximately 6 cm^2 of cortex at gyral surfaces. The cortex in sulci generally does not contribute to the EEG potentials because the cortical dipoles generated in this location cancel each other out.

The cortical generators of the many normal and abnormal cortical activities recorded in the EEG are still largely unknown. Spatial sampling of the cortex in routine scalp EEG is incomplete, as significant amounts of cortex, particularly in basal and mesial (midline) areas of the hemispheres, are not covered by standard electrode placement. High-frequency oscillations are outside the conventional bandwidth of clinical EEG and include gamma oscillations (30–80 Hz), ripples (80–200 Hz) and fast ripples (200–500 Hz). Intracranial depth-electrode EEG recordings of fast ripples are closely correlated with the local epileptogenicity of the brain tissue.

The incidence of epileptiform discharge in routine EEG is 0.5% in healthy adults with no declared history of seizures, and 2–4% in healthy children and non-epileptic patients referred to hospital EEG clinics. The incidence increases to 10–30% in cerebral pathologies such as tumour or prior head injury (without seizures), requiring considerable care to establish a diagnosis. Sleep-EEG, ambulatory EEG or video-telemetry (simultaneous video and EEG) can be helpful to increase yield and capture the EEG correlate of an habitual paroxysmal event [10].

Brain MRI is the most useful imaging investigation, and is particularly indicated in those with epilepsy onset before the age of 2 years or in adulthood, likely focal onset based on history, or if seizures continue in spite of first-line medication [1]. See Section 3.1.5 for background on three-dimensional brain imaging in general. Epilepsy protocol MRI at 1.5 T or 3.0 T involves a set of MRI sequences including T1, T2, FLAIR and DWI sequences, which collectively improve the sensitivity and specificity of identifying relevant structural abnormalities such as hippocampal sclerosis and focal cortical dysplasia. Advanced imaging such as PET, SPECT (SISCOM; subtraction ictal single-photon emission CT coregistered to MRI), functional MRI or magnetoencephalography can also be helpful in MRI-negative drug-resistant focal epilepsy to determine an implantation strategy for stereo-EEG – a minimally invasive procedure with an array of intracranial depth electrodes inserted into the brain to identify the

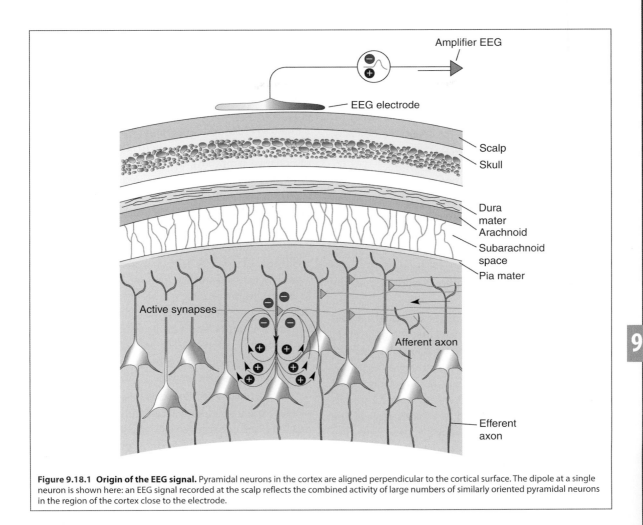

Figure 9.18.1 Origin of the EEG signal. Pyramidal neurons in the cortex are aligned perpendicular to the cortical surface. The dipole at a single neuron is shown here: an EEG signal recorded at the scalp reflects the combined activity of large numbers of similarly oriented pyramidal neurons in the region of the cortex close to the electrode.

epileptogenic zone and enable surgical planning of the limits of a potential resection.

A cognitive assessment can help to delineate deficits in relation to other investigations, particularly language and memory.

Genetic studies can be helpful. The main genetic variants associated with epilepsy are single-nucleotide polymorphisms (each polymorphism represents a difference in a single nucleotide), insertions, deletions and structural variation such as microdeletions/microduplications or chromosomal monosomy/trisomy (see Chapter 7).

The genes most likely to be related to epilepsy have diverse biological functions, including coding for ion-channel subunits, transcription factors and a vitamin B6 metabolism enzyme. Generalised epilepsies have

a stronger heritable component than focal epilepsies, although fewer single genes have been implicated in generalised epilepsies.

Genes most likely to be related to epilepsy include [11]:

- Ion-channel genes (*SCN1A*, *SCN2A*, *SCN3A*, *GABRA2*, *KCNN2*, *KCNAB1* and *GRIK1*)
- the transcription factors *ZEB2*, *STAT4* and *BCL11A*
- the histone modification gene *BRD7*
- the synaptic transmission gene *STX1B*
- the pyridoxine (vitamin B6) metabolism gene *PNPO*
- the *FANCL* gene, implicated in Fanconi anaemia and certain cancers
- the *PCDH7* gene, which codes for a membrane protein thought to function in cell–cell recognition

- the acetyl co-A transporter-1 protein gene *SLC33A1*
- the connexin gene *GJA1*, a component of gap junctions.

Clinically, the highest yield for genetic testing is ~5% for chromosome microarray analysis and 20–50% for sequencing via panel testing or exome analysis for epilepsy, with dysmorphic features, intellectual disability, autism and cognitive regression [12] .

9.18.4 Beyond Seizures: Neuropsychiatric Comorbidity

Epilepsy is associated with neurological (stroke, dementia, migraine) and neuropsychiatric (depression, psychosis, anxiety) comorbidities. Beyond seizure freedom, neuropsychiatric comorbidity (see Figure 9.18.2) and anticonvulsant adverse events are important treatable determinants of quality of life.

Epidemiological studies have demonstrated a higher prevalence of psychiatric disorders preceding the onset of seizure disorders, suggesting a bidirectional relationship [13, 14]. The prevalence of depression is doubled in epilepsy compared with the general population and a similar prevalence is seen in other neurological disorders such as multiple sclerosis and Parkinson's disease. The prevalence of psychosis in epilepsy is approximately five times higher than in the general population [15]. Postictal psychosis develops within a week of a cluster seizures and is often characterised by a lucid interval (i.e. a temporary improvement) over 12–72 hours. This is often followed by delirium or delusions (e.g. paranoid, non-paranoid, delusional, misidentifications) or hallucinations (e.g. auditory, visual, somatosensory, olfactory) in clear consciousness [16]. Postictal psychosis duration is between 1 day and 3 months [17]. In contrast, interictal psychosis is temporally unrelated to seizures. There is a relative absence of negative symptoms, with better premorbid as well as long-term functioning compared to schizophrenia. Nevertheless, cautious use of maintenance antipsychotic medications is usually required, with attention to their propensity to lower the seizure threshold.

Forced normalisation was described by Landolt in 1958 in patients with epilepsy in whom the emergence of neuropsychiatric symptoms followed treatment resulting in the EEG becoming more normal or entirely normal. This observation suggests a reciprocal relationship between seizure frequency and neuropsychiatric symptoms. Possible explanations include antiepileptic medication toxicity or exposing a latent neuropsychiatric disorder with improved seizure control.

The risk of completed suicide following diagnosis of epilepsy is increased, with a standardised mortality ratio of 3.5–10, and is associated with depression, anxiety and psychosis at higher rates than most other chronic conditions [18, 19].

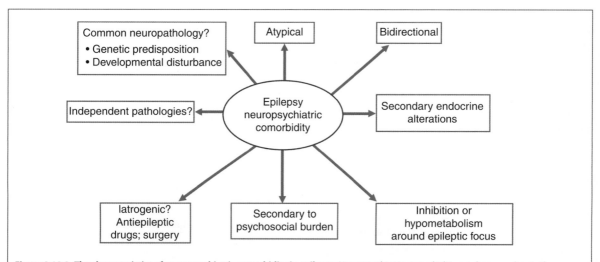

Figure 9.18.2 The characteristics of neuropsychiatric comorbidity in epilepsy. Neuropsychiatric comorbidity may be secondary to the psychosocial burden of epilepsy; it may reflect common (e.g. genetic or developmental) neuropathology; it may be secondary to antiepileptic drugs; it may reflect the neurophysiological or endocrine effects of the seizures themselves; or it may be an independent pathology. There are bidirectional interactions between epileptic and psychiatric symptoms.

Although not fully understood, the shared mechanisms of epilepsy and mental health comorbidity may include aberrant serotonergic, GABAergic and glutamatergic neurotransmitter systems. Disturbances in opioid signalling have been implicated in mood disorders and suicidality, with phasic postictal changes of opioid receptor availability also reported in temporal lobe epilepsy [20].

Recent evidence suggests some postictal behavioural impairments may be related to a severe prolonged hypoperfusion/hypoxia. The relationship of this cyclooxygenase-2-dependent mechanism to neuropsychiatric symptoms remains to be established [21].

Both temporal lobe epilepsy and schizophrenia are associated with aberrant hippocampal excitatory synaptic transmission [22]. Both epilepsy and depression are reported to be associated with an abnormal hypothalamic–pituitary–adrenal axis causing excessive glucocorticoid signalling, with downstream effects on neurotransmitters like serotonin, and producing excessive cell loss and atrophy in limbic brain regions. The role played by mechanisms of neuroinflammation may also be relevant. Pro-inflammatory cytokines such as interleukin 1 beta (IL-1β) are reported to be proconvulsant through a reduction in glutamate uptake by glial cells [23] and *IL1B* gene polymorphisms (rs16944, rs114643) have been found to predict a lack of response to selective serotonin reuptake inhibitors [24].

Genetic predisposition is likely to contribute to the increased vulnerability to psychosis in epilepsy. 22q11.2 deletion syndrome (DiGeorge or velocardiofacial syndrome) has a variable phenotype but is associated with seizures, psychosis and mood disorder. Mutations in the leucine-rich glioma inactivated 1 (*LGI1*) gene (10q22–24) cause autosomal-dominant partial (focal) epilepsy with auditory features, ranging from unformed sounds such as buzzing, ringing or clicking; distortions such as volume changes or muffling; and complex sounds such as a specific radio jingle or singer.

Conclusions and Outstanding Questions

While our understanding of the neurobiology of epilepsy has increased, and there are multiple anticonvulsants which can control or prevent seizures, there are at present no anti-epileptogenic treatments, that is, treatments which target the underlying pathological process leading to the development of neuronal hyperexcitability. Beyond seizure control, neuropsychiatric comorbidity is a key determinant of quality of life in this patient group. If we are to improve treatment approaches, we require a better understanding of the underlying biology of these symptoms, and better tools to determine the factors contributing to neuropsychiatric symptoms in a given patient.

Outstanding Questions

- What is the pathophysiological basis of idiopathic epilepsy?
- What triggers the sudden transition between interictal spiking and the generation of seizure activity in hyperexcitable epileptic neuronal networks?
- Why is there a delay (36–48-hour lucid period) between seizures and the onset of postictal psychiatric symptoms?

REFERENCES

1. National Institute for Health and Care Excellence. Epilepsies: diagnosis and management. Clinical guideline. NICE, 2012.

2. Fisher RS, Acevedo C, Arzimanoglou A et al. A practical clinical definition of epilepsy. *Epilepsia* 2014: 55(4): 475–482.

3. Fisher RS, van Emde Boas W, Blume W et al. Epileptic seizures and epilepsy: definitions proposed by the International League Against Epilepsy (ILAE) and the International Bureau for Epilepsy (IBE). *Epilepsia* 2005; 46: 470–472.

4. Fisher RS, Cross H, French JA. Operational classification of seizure types by the International League Against Epilepsy: Position Paper of the ILAE Commission for Classification and Terminology. *Epilepsia* 2017: 58(4): 522–530.

5. Staley K. Molecular mechanisms of epilepsy. *Nat Neurosci* 2015; 18(3): 367–372.

6. Kaeser PS, Regehr WG. Molecular mechanisms for synchronous, asynchronous, and spontaneous neurotransmitter release. *Annu Rev Physiol* 2014; 76: 333–363.

7. Rajakulendran S, Kaski D, Hanna MG. Neuronal P/Q-type calcium channel dysfunction in inherited disorders of the CNS. *Nat Rev Neurol*; 2012; 8(2): 86–96.

8. Lazarevic V, Pothula S, Andres-Alonso M, Fejtova A. Molecular mechanisms driving homeostatic plasticity of neurotransmitter release. *Front Cell Neurosci* 2013; 7: 244.

9. Staley K. Molecular mechanisms of epilepsy. *Nat Neurosci* 2015; 18(3): 367–372.

10. Smith SJ. EEG in the diagnosis, classification, and management of patients with epilepsy. *J Neurol Neurosurg Psychiatry* 2005; 76(Suppl II): ii2–ii7.

11. Abou-Khalil B, Auce P et al. The International League Against Epilepsy Consortium on Complex Epilepsies. Genome-wide mega-analysis identifies 16 loci and highlights diverse biological mechanisms in the common epilepsies. *Nat Commun* 2018; 9: 5269.

12. Poduri A. When should genetic testing be performed in epilepsy patients? *Epilepsy Curr* 2017; 17(1): 16–22.

13. Chang YT, Chen PC, Tsai IJ et al. Bidirectional relation between schizophrenia and epilepsy: a population-based retrospective cohort study. *Epilepsia* 2011; 52: 2036–2042

14. Hesdorffer DC, Ishihara L, Mynepalli L et al. Epilepsy, suicidality, and psychiatric disorders: a bidirectional association. *Ann Neurol* 2012; 72: 184–191.

15. Clancy MJ, Clarke MC, Connor DJ, Cannon M, Cotter DR. The prevalence of psychosis in epilepsy: a systematic review and meta-analysis. *BMC Psychiatry* 2014; 14: 75.

16. Logsdail S, Toone B. Post-ictal psychoses: a clinical and phenomenological description. *Br J Psychiatry* 1988; 152: 246–252.

17. Trimble M, Kanner A, Schmitz B. Postictal psychosis. *Epilepsy Behav* 2010; 19: 159–161.

18. Christensen J, Vestergaard M, Sidenius P, Agerbo E. Epilepsy and risk of suicide: a population-based case–control study. *Lancet Neurol* 2007; 6: 693–698.

19. Lönnqvist JK. Psychiatric aspects of suicide. In Hawton K, van Heeringen K (eds.), *The International Handbook of Suicide and Attempted Suicide*. John Wiley & Sons, 2000, pp. 107–120.

20. Hammers A, Asselin MC, Hinz R et al. Upregulation of opioid receptor binding following spontaneous epileptic seizures. *Brain* 2007; 130: 1009–1016.

21. Farrell JS, Colangeli R, Wolff MD et al. Postictal hypoperfusion/hypoxia provides the foundation for a unified theory of seizure-induced brain abnormalities and behavioral dysfunction. *Epilepsia* 2017; 58(9): 1493–1501.

22. Nakahara S, Adachi M, Ito H et al. Hippocampal pathophysiology: commonality shared by temporal lobe epilepsy and psychiatric disorders. *Neurosci J* 2018: 4852359.

23. Hu S, Sheng WS, Ehrlich LC, Peterson PK, Chao CC. Cytokine effects on glutamate uptake by human astrocytes. *Neuroimmunomodulation* 2000; 7: 153–159.

24. Baune BT, Dannlowski U, Domschke K et al. The interleukin-1b (IL1B) gene is associated with failure to achieve remission and impaired emotion processing in major depression. *Biol Psychiatry* 2010; 67: 543–549.

9

<table>
<tr><td>**9.19**</td><td>**Electroconvulsive Therapy**</td><td>**George Kirov and Pascal Sienaert**</td></tr>
</table>

George Kirov and Pascal Sienaert

OVERVIEW

Electroconvulsive therapy (ECT) remains the most effective treatment for severe or treatment-resistant depression, especially for those presenting with psychotic or catatonic features (Kirov et al., 2021). It might exert its effects via different biological mechanisms that remain to be fully understood.

9.19.1 Effectiveness of Electroconvulsive Therapy

Electroconvulsive therapy (ECT) was first developed in Rome in 1938 by Ugo Cerletti and Lucio Bini. It was first used to treat patients who suffered with schizophrenia, but it soon became clear that the best results were achieved in those suffering with severe depression. ECT works best for the most severely ill patients (Kellner et al., 2020): those with psychomotor retardation or psychotic symptoms, with remission rates up to 95% among the latter, provided they complete the ECT course (Petrides, 2001). Indeed, ECT is the most effective treatment for severe depression, with effect sizes in randomised controlled trials about twice as high as pharmacotherapy (UK ECT Review Group, 2003). One of the largest studies (253 patients) achieved 75% remission rate (defined as a final score of less than 10 points on the 24-item Hamilton Depression Rating Scale, recorded on two consecutive occasions), far in excess of any other treatment modality (Husain et al., 2004); see Figure 9.19.1. It is reserved as a second-line treatment in practice due to adverse effects in some patients (see below) and because of practical considerations.

9.19.2 Mechanism of Action

It is known that good quality seizures are required in order to achieve good therapeutic outcomes. ECT works by passing a brief-pulse repetitive electric current through the head of the patient, which elicits a grand mal seizure. The current produced by modern devices consists of brief pulses of between 0.25 and 1 milliseconds, at frequencies of 20–120 Hz. The amount of electric charge depends on individual differences in seizure threshold, which increases with age and in patients taking benzodiazepines or anticonvulsant medications. For best therapeutic effect, a seizure needs to be elicited with an electric charge that exceeds the seizure threshold by at least 30% when administered bilaterally, and 500% when administered unilaterally (Sackeim et al., 1993). Higher doses tend to be more effective but are also associated with worse postictal confusion and memory problems. Several modifications to ECT delivery have been introduced since 1938 and although they have minimised cognitive side effects, none has increased the efficacy of the treatment (Bailine, 2019).

ECT induces multiple changes in the brain. The antidepressant effect of ECT is probably not due to one single effect on brain function, but to several biological effects that work in concert to produce the unparalleled improvements in depression:

- **Neurotransmitter changes**. ECT-induced seizures result in enhancement of serotonergic neurotransmission and activation of the mesocorticolimbic dopamine system. Increases in gamma-aminobutyric acid (GABA), noradrenaline and glutamate have also been documented.

- **Neuroplasticity**. ECT is a potent inducer of hippocampal neuroplasticity, i.e. synaptogenesis and neurogenesis (Bouckaert et al., 2014; Rotheneichner

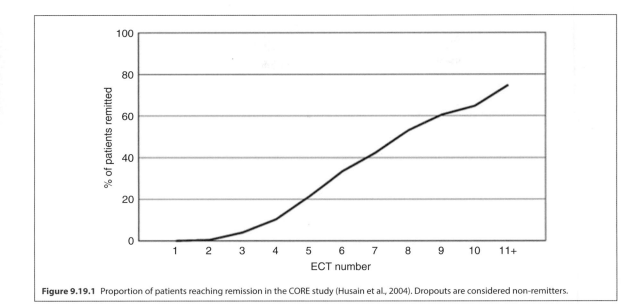

Figure 9.19.1 Proportion of patients reaching remission in the CORE study (Husain et al., 2004). Dropouts are considered non-remitters.

et al., 2014). Figure 9.19.2 shows increased cell proliferation in the dentate gyrus of the hippocampus of mice treated with electric shocks. In humans, rather than causing grey matter shrinkage, significant but transient increases in hippocampal volume have been consistently observed after ECT (Wilkinson et al., 2017). These do not correlate with clinical improvements, complicating the interpretation of these changes (Sartorius et al., 2019).

- **Functional connectivity.** An intuitive line of investigation is to test the possibility that ECT resets the functional connectivity in areas of the brain that have been affected by depression. Several neuronal networks have been shown to share increased resting-state connectivity to the dorsomedial prefrontal cortex in depression. This could account for the depressive ruminations, increased vigilance and emotional and autonomic dysregulation observed in depressed patients (Sheline et al., 2010). ECT was indeed found to reduce the excessive frontal functional cortical connectivity in depressed patients (Perrin et al., 2012). Other studies have reported conflicting data, showing reduced functional connectivity between the dorsomedial prefrontal cortex and the posterior cingulate cortex in depression, and restoration of this connectivity following ECT (Bai et al., 2019). A uniform pattern of changes in brain connectivity is unlikely to be present in all depressed

patients, therefore different mechanisms could be playing a role in different types of depression and in different individuals. Future research should focus on examining the changes in functional connectivity that are associated with remission during successful ECT. This could also answer more fundamental questions about the neurobiology of depression.

9.19.3 Cognitive Side Effects

There is no reported credible evidence that ECT causes brain damage as measured by histopathology. In fact, increases in hippocampal volume have been observed, as outlined above. Large studies using the Danish national registry data have shown that ECT does not increase the risk for dementia (Osler et al., 2018) or stroke (Rozing et al., 2018). Nevertheless, a substantial proportion of people undergoing ECT report varying degrees of both anterograde and retrograde memory problems. Anterograde amnesia is limited to a few days after an ECT course and results improve beyond baseline levels on follow-up (Semkovska and McLoughlin, 2010). Repeated courses of ECT do not lead to cumulative cognitive deficits (Kirov et al., 2016) and maintenance ECT does not result in worsening of memory problems (Bailine et al., 2019). Even patients with late-life depression do not, on average, show deleterious cognitive effects 6 months following an ECT course. There are, however, considerable differences at an

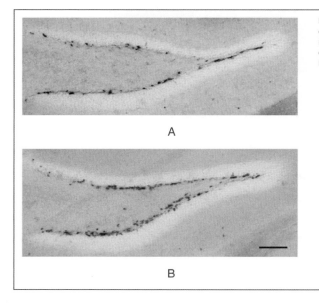

Figure 9.19.2 Bromodeoxyuridine-labelled cells in the dentate gyrus demonstrate increased cell proliferation after electric shocks in mice. **(A)** Image from a mouse in the sham group. **(B)** Image from the experimental electroconvulsive shock group. Image reproduced from Rotheneichner et al. (2014).

individual level. Most patients will tolerate the treatment course, some will experience a cognitive enhancement and a small group of patients can experience significant and more lasting cognitive side effects (Obbels et al., 2018).

Conclusions and Outstanding Questions

ECT is a highly effective treatment for some of the most severe psychiatric presentations. Despite that, it suffers with a poor image among the general public and its use is severely restricted in some countries. High-quality neuroscientific studies and more publicity are needed to raise the public profile of this treatment, and thus allow higher numbers of suitable patients to benefit from it.

Outstanding Questions

- How can we improve the image of ECT?
- Neuroimaging studies using the latest techniques should be able to answer better the question as to how ECT works. Could this potentially contribute towards personalised treatments for severe psychiatric disorders?

REFERENCES

Bai T, Wei Q, Zu M et al. (2019). Functional plasticity of the dorsomedial prefrontal cortex in depression reorganized by electroconvulsive therapy: validation in two independent samples. *Hum Brain Mapp* 40(2): 465–473.

Bailine SH, Sanghani SN, Petrides G (2019). Maintenance electroconvulsive therapy is not acute electroconvulsive therapy. *J ECT* 35(1): 1–2.

Bouckaert F, Sienaert P, Obbels J et al. (2014). ECT: its brain enabling effects. A review of electroconvulsive therapy-induced structural brain plasticity. *J ECT* 30(2): 143–151.

Husain MM, Rush AJ, Fink M et al. (2004). Speed of response and remission in major depressive disorder with acute electroconvulsive therapy (ECT): a Consortium for Research in ECT (CORE) report. *J Clin Psychiatry* 65(4): 485–491.

Kellner CH, Obbels J, Sienaert P (2020). When to consider electroconvulsive therapy (ECT). *Acta Psychiatr Scand* 141(4): 304–315.

Kirov G, Owen L, Ballard H et al. (2016). Evaluation of cumulative cognitive deficits from electroconvulsive therapy. *Br J Psychiatry* 208(3): 266–270.

Kirov G, Jauhar S, Sienaert P, Kellner CH, McLoughlin DM (2021). Electroconvulsive therapy for depression: 80 years of progress. *Br J Psychiatry* 219: 594–597.

Obbels J, Verwijk E, Vansteelandt K et al. (2018). Long-term neurocognitive functioning after electroconvulsive therapy in patients with late-life depression. *Acta Psychiatr Scand* 138: 223–231.

Osler M, Rozing MP, Christensen GT et al. (2018). Electroconvulsive therapy and risk of dementia in patients with affective disorders: a cohort study. *Lancet Psychiatry* 5(4): 348–356.

Perrin JS, Merz S, Bennet DM et al. (2012). Electroconvulsive therapy reduces frontal cortical connectivity in severe depressive disorder. *Proc Natl Acad Sci USA* 109: 5464–5468.

Petrides G, Fink M, Husain MM et al. (2001). ECT remission rates in psychotic versus nonpsychotic depressed patients: a report from CORE. *J ECT* 17(4): 244–253.

Rotheneichner P, Lange S, O'Sullivan A et al. (2014). Hippocampal neurogenesis and antidepressive therapy: shocking relations. *Neural Plast* 2014: 723915.

Rozing MP, Jorgensen MB, Osler M (2019). Electroconvulsive therapy and later stroke in patients with affective disorders. *Br J Psychiatry* 214(3):168–170.

Sackeim HA, Prudic J, Devanand DP et al. (1993). Effects of stimulus intensity and electrode placement on the efficacy and cognitive effects of electroconvulsive therapy. *N Engl J Med* 328(12): 839–846.

Sartorius A, Demirakca T, Böhringer A et al. (2019). Electroconvulsive therapy induced gray matter increase is not necessarily correlated with clinical data in depressed patients. *Brain Stimul* 12(2): 335–343.

Semkovska M, McLoughlin DM (2010). Objective cognitive performance associated with electroconvulsive therapy for depression: a systematic review and meta-analysis. *Biol Psychiatry* 68(6):5 68–77

Sheline YI, Price JL, Yan Z, Mintun MA (2010). Resting-state functional MRI in depression unmasks increased connectivity between networks via the dorsal nexus. *Proc Natl Acad Sci USA* 107: 11020– 11025.

UK ECT Review Group (2003). Efficacy and safety of electroconvulsive therapy in depressive disorders: a systematic review and meta-analysis. *Lancet* 361: 799–808.

Wilkinson ST, Sanacora G, Bloch MH (2017). Hippocampal volume changes following electroconvulsive therapy: a systematic review and meta-analysis. *Biol Psychiatry Cogn Neurosci Neuroimaging* 2: 327–335.

9

National Neuroscience Curriculum Initiative online resources

Expert video: *Sarah H. Lisanby on ECT*

Camilla L. Nord

9.20	**Brain Stimulation**

OVERVIEW

One of the best examples of translation from neuroscience to psychiatric treatment is brain stimulation, an array of techniques aimed at modulating the activity and/or plasticity of particular brain structures. Brain stimulation is not new: as far back as ancient Rome, the physician Scribonius Largus wrote of electrical stimulation to relieve migraine (although he employed a torpedo fish, a species of electric ray). Today, a number of invasive and non-invasive brain stimulation techniques show efficacy in treating psychiatric disorders. What these distinct approaches have in common is their ability to target specific neural regions more directly than traditional pharmacological or psychological approaches (see Figure 9.20.1). This capacity to influence the very circuits implicated in neuroscience studies has contributed to some transformative discoveries, but has faced key translational challenges, including response variability and inadequate placebos.

9.20.1 Non-Invasive Brain Stimulation

The two most common forms of non-invasive brain stimulation are **transcranial magnetic stimulation** (TMS) and **transcranial direct current stimulation** (tDCS). TMS uses brief, high-current pulses to induce a magnetic field, indirectly activating neurons, and causing an increase or decrease in brain activity in a localised target region [1]. There is substantial evidence that repetitive high-frequency TMS pulses over the left dorsolateral prefrontal cortex are effective for major depressive disorder [2], purportedly by restoring activity in this area of the prefrontal cortex, a commonly described source of aberrant activation in neuroimaging studies in depression (often, but not always, showing hypoactivation) [3]. More limited evidence suggests TMS might be helpful in other psychiatric conditions: targeting the ventromedial prefrontal cortex, for example, shows promise as a treatment for addiction disorders [4]. However, the precise mechanisms by which TMS might exert treatment effects in psychiatric disorders are still largely unknown.

tDCS is a mild electrical current that has a more diffuse effect than TMS (see Figure 9.20.1), evoking brain activation changes both locally and in anatomically connected but spatially distant regions [5]. At a neuronal level, anodal tDCS (using the positive electrode) increases the membrane potential of neurons towards depolarisation (rather than eliciting firing), and is also thought to induce longer-term effects via synaptic plasticity, along with more complex neuronal changes. tDCS has been suggested as a putative treatment for a variety of psychiatric disorders, particularly depression. Many trials show moderately large effects of five or more left dorsolateral prefrontal cortical tDCS sessions on depression symptoms [6], but there have also been notable null results [7]. Mirroring this, many neuroscience studies in healthy populations report improvements in short-term memory and other cognitive measures during or immediately after tDCS delivery [8], whilst other studies find broadly null effects [9] (though note that the analytical approach of the latter meta-analysis has been criticised). Despite this relatively mixed picture, experimental tDCS

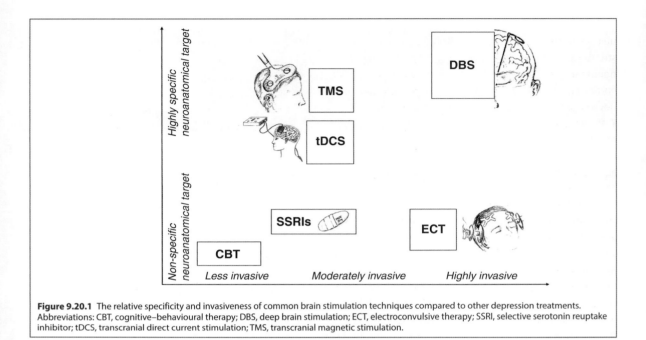

Figure 9.20.1 The relative specificity and invasiveness of common brain stimulation techniques compared to other depression treatments. Abbreviations: CBT, cognitive–behavioural therapy; DBS, deep brain stimulation; ECT, electroconvulsive therapy; SSRI, selective serotonin reuptake inhibitor; tDCS, transcranial direct current stimulation; TMS, transcranial magnetic stimulation.

studies have inspired a wealth of commercial ventures selling simple tDCS kits, and a dedicated public following among devotees of so-called 'neurohacking'.

Perhaps most notably from a neuroscience perspective, both TMS and tDCS have a limited depth of penetrance, with biological effects rapidly falling off with increasing depth. As such, non-invasive brain stimulation is often restricted to targeting superficial neural structures. This limits their ability to directly modulate activity in the deep cortical and subcortical regions that play a fundamental role in psychiatric disorders, such as the amygdala or striatum (although note indirect modulation of deep structure occurs [10], for example ventrolateral prefrontal cortex TMS evokes focal modulation of amygdala activation). In contrast, surgical brain simulation (and potentially some novel types of non-invasive brain stimulation such as focused ultrasound stimulation), has the capacity to directly target these deeper structures.

9.20.2 How Can We Target Deeper Structures?

The most well-known form of brain stimulation in psychiatry, other than electroconvulsive therapy (see Section 9.19), is **deep brain stimulation** (DBS). In open-label studies, DBS evokes profound short- and long-term improvements in patients with intractable depression [11]; DBS electrodes typically target the subgenual anterior cingulate cortex, ventral capsule or nucleus accumbens). However, randomised controlled trials (RCTs) have been inconclusive, potentially due to the importance of peri-surgical effects of the stimulation and/or inadequate parameter optimisation. More recently, exploration of new targets such as the medial forebrain bundle has been coupled with more innovative trial designs – such as intraoperative exploration of the psychotropic effects of stimulation to guide electrode placement [12]. In patients with intractable obsessive–compulsive disorder, DBS of the ventral capsule and the anteromedial subthalamic nucleus are both effective in treating the symptoms of this disorder [13] (see also Section 9.6.3). One of the most innovative DBS approaches is personalised closed-loop stimulation, where recordings from particular brain areas inform stimulation parameters in real time – an approach recently found to be effective in a single case study of a patient with treatment-resistant major depression [14]. However, a surgical approach like DBS is not intended to be a first-line treatment for any psychiatric disorder. To that end, DBS studies serve a dual purpose: they can also highlight novel targets which might be suitable for targeting with non-invasive brain stimulation.

The major technical hurdle for non-invasive brain stimulation is most techniques' inability to stimulate deeper structures with any degree of specificity (as stimulation necessarily passes through more superficial regions and often becomes more diffuse with depth). There are newer approaches that may change this, however. Deep TMS can penetrate several centimetres below the skull, modulating deep prefrontal targets such as the medial prefrontal cortex. In a recent double-blind trial, this approach significantly benefited patients with obsessive–compulsive disorder [15]. More recently, studies around the world have begun investigating a new noninvasive stimulation technique, focused ultrasound stimulation, which has the ability to modulate very deep structures with extreme precision [16]. While the majority of studies have been conducted in non-human animals, preliminary human work has shown potential for stimulation of deeper structures such as the insula [17], which has been implicated in a number of psychiatric disorders [18]. Clinical trials in psychiatric disorders are currently underway, although some safety and efficacy questions have yet to be answered.

9.20.3 Challenges for the Future of Brain Stimulation Research

9.20.3.1 Placebo Control

A major challenge across all forms of brain stimulation, both invasive and non-invasive, is adequate placebo control. This is a critical issue in DBS and TMS studies, which, respectively, have no or poor double-blind placebo stimulation options (ideally, the placebo would be some form of non-therapeutic stimulation indistinguishable from the intervention). Sham surgery, where an electrode is implanted but not stimulated, can be used as a control for DBS, and the lack of placebo stimulation does not typically prevent successful blinding of patients in DBS studies. However, TMS produces an intense, albeit short-lived sensation, which is difficult to replicate with sham stimulation: the lack of adequate placebo could certainly magnify the effects described in the literature. tDCS evokes milder sensations than TMS, and many tDCS studies show effective double-blind-controlled placebo stimulation, but at higher stimulation amplitudes people start to be able to differentiate between real and placebo stimulation [19].

9.20.3.2 Interindividual Variability and Mechanistic Insight

As with all other psychiatric treatments, response to brain stimulation interventions varies substantially between individuals. Myriad anatomical and physiological properties contribute to this variability. Interindividual variability makes replication challenging, contributing to some of the inconsistencies in the brain stimulation literature. To address this, researchers have begun to add mechanistic measures, such as brain activation, to trials and studies. For instance, in patients with addiction disorders, TMS was found to specifically modulate cue reactivity (brain activation while viewing disorder-specific cues); this procedure could localise individually specified target coordinates [4]. Mechanistic approaches might also identify responders and non-responders: in an RCT of tDCS combined with psychological therapy for depression, left dorsolateral prefrontal cortical activation measured with functional MRI predicted later response to tDCS in this region of the prefrontal cortex [7].

Conclusions and Outstanding Questions

The future of brain stimulation requires more refined ways to customise stimulation based on the particular disruptions found in an individual patient. This would require a degree of mechanistic insight into DBS, TMS and tDCS that it is only possible to develop following carefully controlled experimental studies and innovatively designed RCTs. Still, brain stimulation offers remarkable potential to develop novel psychiatric treatments based on insights from neuroscience.

Outstanding Questions

- What are the long- and short-term neural changes evoked by each type of brain stimulation?
- What is the optimal design for a DBS trial?
- How can we adjust TMS, tDCS and DBS parameters on an individual scale to improve patients' response to each intervention?
- Could focused ultrasound or another form of non-invasive brain stimulation safely and selectively target deeper structures in psychiatric disorders?

REFERENCES

1. Hallett M. Transcranial magnetic stimulation and the human brain. *Nature* 2000; 406: 147–150.

2. O'Reardon JP, Solvason HB, Janicak PG et al. Efficacy and safety of transcranial magnetic stimulation in the acute treatment of major depression: a multisite randomized controlled trial. *Biological Psychiatry* 2007; 62: 1208–1216.

3. Wang X-L, Du M-Y, Chen T-L et al. Neural correlates during working memory processing in major depressive disorder. *Progress in Neuro-Psychopharmacology and Biological Psychiatry* 2015; 56: 101–108.

4. Kearney-Ramos TE, Dowdle LT, Lench DH et al. Transdiagnostic effects of ventromedial prefrontal cortex transcranial magnetic stimulation on cue reactivity. *Biological Psychiatry: Cognitive Neuroscience and Neuroimaging* 2018; 3: 599–609.

5. Stagg CJ, Lin RL, Mezue M et al. Widespread modulation of cerebral perfusion induced during and after transcranial direct current stimulation applied to the left dorsolateral prefrontal cortex. *Journal of Neuroscience* 2013; 33: 11425–11431.

6. Brunoni AR, Moffa AH, Sampaoi-Junior B et al. Trial of electrical direct-current therapy versus escitalopram for depression. *New England Journal of Medicine* 2017; 376: 2523–2533.

7. Nord CL, Chamith Halahakoon D, Limbachya T et al. Neural predictors of treatment response to brain stimulation and psychological therapy in depression: a double-blind randomized controlled trial. *Neuropsychopharmacology* 2019; 44(9): 1613–1622.

8. Filmer HL, Mattingley JB, Dux PE. Modulating brain activity and behaviour with tDCS: rumours of its death have been greatly exaggerated. *Cortex* 2020; 123: 141–151.

9. Cooney Horvath J, Forte JD, Carter O. Quantitative review finds no evidence of cognitive effects in healthy populations from single-session transcranial direct current stimulation (tDCS). *Brain Stimulation* 2015 8(3): 535–550.

10. Sydnor VJ, Cieslak M, Duprat R et al. Cortical–subcortical structural connections support transcranial magnetic stimulation engagement of the amygdala. *Science Advances* 2022; 8(25): eabn5803.

11. Mayberg HS, Lozano AM, Voon V et al. Deep brain stimulation for treatment-resistant depression. *Neuron* 2005; 45: 651–660.

12. Coenen VA, Bewernick BH, Kayser S et al. Superolateral medial forebrain bundle deep brain stimulation in major depression: a gateway trial. *Neuropsychopharmacology* 2019; 44: 1224–1232.

13 Tyagi H, Apergis-Schoute AM, Akram H et al. A randomised trial directly comparing ventral capsule and anteromedial subthalamic nucleus stimulation in obsessive compulsive disorder: clinical and imaging evidence for dissociable effects. *Biological Psychiatry* 2019; 85(9): 726–734.

14. Scangos KW, Khambhati AN, Daly PM et al. Closed-loop neuromodulation in an individual with treatment-resistant depression. *Nature Medicine* 2021; 27(10): 1696–1700.

15. Carmi L, Tendler A, Bystritsky A et al. Efficacy and safety of deep transcranial magnetic stimulation for obsessive-compulsive disorder: a prospective multicenter randomized double-blind placebo-controlled trial. *American Journal of Psychiatry* 2019; 176(11): 931–938.

16. Folloni D, Verhagen L, Mars RB et al. Manipulation of subcortical and deep cortical activity in the primate brain using transcranial focused ultrasound stimulation. *Neuron* 2019; 101(6): 1109–1116.e5.

17. Legon W, Strohman A. Non-invasive neuromodulation of sub-regions of the human insula differentially affect pain processing and heart-rate variability. *bioRxiv* 2023; https://doi.org/10.1101/2023.05.05.539593.
18. Nord CL, Lawson RP, Dalgleish T. Disrupted dorsal mid-insula activation during interoception across psychiatric disorders. *American Journal of Psychiatry* 2021; 178(8): 761–770.
19. O'Connell NE, Cossar J, Marston L et al. Rethinking clinical trials of transcranial direct current stimulation: participant and assessor blinding is inadequate at intensities of 2mA. *PLoS One* 2012; 7(10): e47514.

National Neuroscience Curriculum Initiative online resources

What We've Got Here Is Failure to Communicate: Improving Interventional Psychiatry With Closed-Loop Stimulation

Katherine W. Scangos and David A. Ross

The Electrochemical Brain: Lessons From The Bell Jar and Interventional Psychiatry

Joseph J. Taylor, Hedy Kober and David A. Ross

What to say: The Electrochemical Brain: Lessons from The Bell Jar and Interventional Psychiatry

This "stuff" is really cool: Noah Philip, *"Current Reality"* on conditioning and direct current stimulation in PTSD

Jane Eisen

This "stuff" is really cool: Mahendra Bhati, *"Psychosurgery, Past & Future" on deep brain stimulation in psychiatry*

Expert video: *Flavio Frohlich on Mechanisms of Brain Stimulation*

Expert video: *Scott Aaronson on Vagus Nerve Stimulation*

10

Neurodegeneration

James B. Rowe and
Alexander G. Murley

10.1

A Neurodegenerative Cascade of Causality

James B. Rowe and
Alexander G. Murley

OVERVIEW

The burden of dementia on health and social and economic well-being is enormous, whether viewed in terms of the 40 million people living with dementia (predicted 75 million by 2030) or the trillion-dollar cost per annum (predicted $2 trillion by 2030) [1]. In many parts of the world, mental health services provide the backbone to dementia diagnosis and management. The sections in this chapter focus on neurodegenerative disorders although several non-degenerative causes of dementia are considered alongside. Neurodegenerative disorders commonly present with changes in personality and behaviour that lead to referral for psychiatric assessment. Other common psychiatric disorders can mimic dementia, or complicate its management.

Guidance on specific investigative protocols and treatment options are available elsewhere (e.g. www.nice.org.uk) and will differ between countries. Here, we review the principles of neurodegeneration and the advances in understanding their aetiology that are changing the approach to diagnosis and shaping new strategies for prevention and treatment. We refer to the disabling loss of cognitive functions as dementia (as in Alzheimer's dementia or frontotemporal dementia), while the term 'disease' refers to the associated neuropathology. This distinction is important to bear in mind when considering pre-symptomatic and prodromal clinical states in which there is disease activity but not yet dementia.

We emphasise the commonalities across neurodegenerative diseases. These include convergent mechanisms of disease; the concept and use of biomarkers; evolving concepts of disease that encompass prodromal states and pre-symptomatic stages, as well as domain-based approaches; the impact of genetic versus environmental influences; and the challenges of comorbidity.

There is no direct link between the genetic and molecular foundations of neurodegeneration and the syndromes we observe as clinicians. There is instead a complex cascade of causes and effects, illustrated in

Figure 10.1.1, applicable with variation to Alzheimer's disease, Parkinson's disease, frontotemporal dementias, Huntington's disease, progressive supranuclear palsy, corticobasal degeneration and others.

10.1.1 Genetics

The cascade begins with genetic and environmental factors. Monogenic causes of dementia are uncommon. Less than 5% of cases are attributable to single mutations for Alzheimer's disease (e.g. *PSEN1*, *PSEN2*, *APP* genes), Parkinson's disease and dementia with Lewy bodies (e.g. *LRRK2*, *SNCA*, *VPS35* genes). Monogenic cases are often identified by young onset or atypical features and family history. For behavioural variant frontotemporal dementia ~30% is autosomal dominant (e.g. *C9orf72*, *MAPT* and *GRN* genes), and Huntington's disease is defined by its CAG expansions in the Huntingtin (*HTT*) gene.

The discovery of genes often begins with classical syndromes, but clinical–genetic correlations often dissipate. As illustrated in Figure 10.1.2, even coarse clinical categories do not remain true to the genes that were first associated with them [2]. A practical consequence for clinicians is the need to adopt panel-based gene tests (i.e. testing multiple genes simultaneously). There can

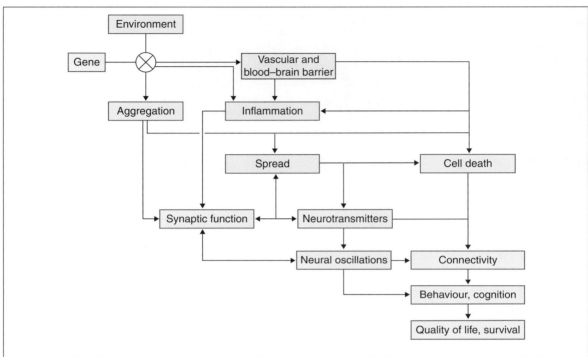

Figure 10.1.1 The pathogenesis of neurodegenerative dementias is represented by a cascade of events. The details vary between Alzheimer's disease, Parkinson's disease and dementia with Lewy bodies, frontotemporal dementias etc. in terms of which gene, which protein, which regions of cellular vulnerability to death and which symptoms arise. But there is extensive overlap and convergence between diseases. Each element of the cascade is associated with a set of biomarkers and potential for transdiagnostic assays and interventions.

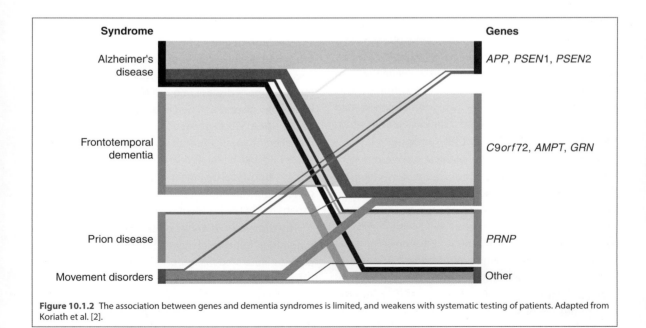

Figure 10.1.2 The association between genes and dementia syndromes is limited, and weakens with systematic testing of patients. Adapted from Koriath et al. [2].

be clinical clues to the gene (e.g. marked asymmetric atrophy on structural brain imaging is associated with granulin precursor (*GRN*) gene mutations) but these are not reliable for individual diagnosis and management.

The problem with genetics is exacerbated by pleiotropy: a specific mutation may cause multiple syndromes. For example, *C9orf72* hexanucleatide expansions may cause frontotemporal dementia, motor neuron disease, ataxia, chorea, parkinsonism or aphasia, alone or in combination. Presenilin-1 (*PSEN1*) gene mutations cause amnestic Alzheimer's type dementia, but also frontotemporal dementia and/or parkinsonism. Pleiotropy may arise from genetic moderators. For example, transmembrane protein 106B (*TMEM106B*) variants protect carriers of *GRN* and *C9orf72* mutations from symptom onset and brain atrophy [3], while a leucine-rich repeat kinase 2 (*LRRK2*) variant modifies survival in progressive supranuclear palsy [4]. The discovery of such protective variants requires detailed phenotyping in large genotyping studies.

There are common risk alleles for neurodegeneration. For example, mutations and polymorphism of the glucocerebrosidase (*GBA*) gene are found in 5–10% of dementia with Lewy bodies and Parkinson's disease, with younger onset, faster progression and increased dementia [5, 6]. However, 90% of carriers do not develop either disease. Polymorphisms in the apolipoprotein E (*APOE*) gene also modulate cognition, brain structure and function. The ε4 allele is associated with a two to three times increased risk of dementia. More than half of patients with Alzheimer's disease carry an ε4 allele. But so does a quarter of the healthy population, and ε4 cannot be considered a causal mutation. Note that the proposed early-life advantage of APOE-ε4 (known as antagonistic pleiotropy) has not been substantiated [7].

Rather than focus on single gene causes, polygenic risk scores sum the effect of multiple genes which, although weak in their individual effects, collectively confer substantial risk of disease. Polygenic risk scores are increasingly sophisticated and accurate in predicting Alzheimer's disease in clinical and neuropathological studies [8, 9]. Polygenic risk is also observed for frontotemporal dementia [10], including loci common to risk of Alzheimer's disease and Parkinson's disease. The genes affected by the variants composing the polygenic score highlight the complexity of the aetiological cascade, including inflammation.

10.1.2 Inflammation

The last decade has provided compelling evidence for neuroinflammation in multiple neurodegenerative disorders. For example, genome-wide association studies identify genes for inflammatory and immunological pathways with Alzheimer's disease, Parkinson's disease and dementia with Lewy bodies, frontotemporal dementias, Huntington's disease and progressive supranuclear palsy [10–15]. Each of these disorders has been associated with elevated markers of inflammation in blood or cerebrospinal fluid samples ante mortem, or microglial activation on post-mortem brain histology (i.e. staining and microscopy).

Positron emission tomography (PET; see Section 3.1.5) studies, using ligands that bind to activated microglia and/or astrocytes, consistently show elevated neuroinflammation in Alzheimer's disease, Parkinson's disease with and without dementia, frontotemporal dementias, Huntington's disease, progressive supranuclear palsy, corticobasal degeneration and prion disease [16–19].

The emerging evidence of direct synaptotoxicity of activated microglia [20] suggests that neuroinflammation is harmful, not simply a response to other neuronal injury or epiphenomenal. Neuroinflammation occurs many years before symptom onset [21]; and predicts the future rate of cognitive decline [22]. The influence of neuroinflammation may also provide a link between delirium in response to systemic infection and its exacerbation of dementia (see Section 9.14 for more on inflammation in delirium). The challenge now is to develop immunotherapeutic strategies that target detrimental neuroinflammation without leaving patients prone to systemic infections.

10.1.3 Prion-Like Disease Progression

Neurodegenerative diseases are dynamic but their rate-limiting step remains controversial. This is critical, as to slow the rate-limiting step would slow the overall course of disease. There are preclinical (animal) models of neurodegenerative diseases which recapitulate many of the disease processes and pathological features of human dementias. However, the large scale and long lifespan of humans, and the genetic and immunological differences across species, mean that rate-limiting steps may differ

10

between species, and between different diseases, even if homologous processes occur in each of the principal degenerative dementias and their respective preclinical models.

One candidate is the aggregation of misfolded proteins. Abnormal protein aggregates are found in Alzheimer's disease (including beta-amyloid and 3R- and 4R-tau), Parkinson's disease (alpha-synuclein), frontotemporal dementias (3R- or 4R-tau or TAR DNA-binding protein 43 (TDP-43)), Huntington's disease (huntingtin), progressive supranuclear palsy and corticobasal degeneration (4R-tau) and prion disease (prion protein). 3R- and 4R-tau are isoforms (alternative versions) of the microtubule-associated protein derived from the microtubule-associated protein tau (*MAPT*) gene that differ by having three (3R) or four repeats (4R) of the microtubule-binding domain. The amplification of protein aggregates is associated with (i) chemical modification (e.g. phosphorylation) that affects conformation and adhesion; (ii) templating onto existing 'seed' molecules, in a chain reaction; and (iii) reduced clearance by neuronal autophagy (the homeostatic removal of unnecessary or dysfunctional cellular components). There is evidence for these processes in preclinical models, and also clinical studies, with drug development in progress against each [23].

However, a second critical process for disease progression is the spread of these aggregates through the brain. The spread of misfolded proteins in monomeric or oligomeric forms preserves the molecular strains that have distinct ultrastructure and pathogenicity [24, 25]. The spread follows the pathways of brain connectivity rather than anatomical proximity. Trans-synaptic transfer of pathological tau has multiple potential mechanisms, which vary according to the aggregation and conformation of the disease-specific protein [26, 27]. Clinical trials to reduce cell-to-cell transfer of tau species are underway in several neurodegenerative diseases.

For Alzheimer's disease, there has been much discussion as to whether beta-amyloid or tau is the more important. Beta-amyloid plaques are a prerequisite for Alzheimer's disease, while amyloid oligomers are toxic to neurons and their synapses, and the disease can arise from mutations affecting the amyloid precursor protein, or the enzymes that cleave it [28]. However, for people with symptomatic Alzheimer's disease, the degree and location of the amyloid load is at best weakly related to the syndrome severity and phenotype [29]. Moreover, clearance of even a high percentage of amyloid by diverse anti-amyloid therapies does not improve prognosis for symptomatic patients [30]. In contrast, the degree of tauopathy has been closely linked to disease severity [31], and the location of tauopathy is strongly linked to clinical phenotype (e.g. amnestic versus logopenic versus posterior cortical atrophy variants) [32]. However, mutations affecting tau lead to frontotemporal lobar degeneration rather than Alzheimer's disease pathology. Rather than dispute the primacy of amyloid or tau, it is better to recognise that they are both toxic, and indeed synergistic in their neuronal toxicity and pro-inflammatory effects [33]. The efficacy of future treatment strategies may therefore depend on the stage of disease, or combination therapies.

It has been suggested that all neurodegenerative dementias are 'prion-like' [23]. The term prion refers to proteins that acquire abnormal conformations and as a result become self-propagating. This was characterised initially in the classic prion diseases, like Creutzfeldt–Jakob disease and kuru, in which there was also evidence of transmissibility within species by ingestion or surgical inoculation. Later, cross-species transmission from ingestion of animal prion protein in the 1990s led to the new variant Creutzfeldt–Jakob disease outbreak. However, sporadic late-onset neurodegenerative disease might arise from an initial stochastic formation of proteins with prion-like properties: once initiated, there follows amplification and spread as above.

However, the phrase prion-like can cause confusion. There are critical differences between classic prion diseases and the common dementias. The prion-like properties of protein tau do not mean that common neurodegenerative tauopathies are transmissible like classical prion diseases; nor that, in the clinical context, reference to prion disease is helpful for the majority of patients with common dementias.

10.2 **Prodromal Disease and Mild Cognitive Impairment**

James B. Rowe and
Alexander G. Murley

The dichotomy of dementia diagnosis (healthy adult versus patient) conflicts with the gradually progressive nature of neurodegeneration. There may be a memorable first event – such as a fall, or getting lost – but usually symptoms emerge against an individual's normal ability and behaviour. In other words, they start **mild**.

The term 'mild cognitive impairment' (MCI) refers to the presence of subjective complaint (i.e. symptoms) corroborated by formal tests, over and above age-related norms, but with minimal impact on functioning. The concept of MCI is well established in the context of prodromal Alzheimer's disease, typically with isolated memory deficits [34, 35]. MCI should be used as a positive diagnosis, in the presence of measurable changes in at least one cognitive domain. It should not be used when there are subjective cognitive symptoms without objective deficit. And it should not be used to shy from discussion of Alzheimer's disease by name or instead of acknowledging uncertainty about a clinical diagnosis of Alzheimer's disease.

There are several problems with the term MCI. First, it is not specific: only a proportion of people with MCI have an underlying neurodegenerative pathology. In response, research and clinical practice increasingly adopt the use of biomarkers of Alzheimer's disease pathology, in conjunction with the clinical diagnosis of MCI. High tau and low beta-amyloid levels in cerebrospinal fluid, or increased amyloid on brain PET, or elevated levels of specific forms of phosphorylated tau in blood (pTau181, pTau217), are excellent indicators of the presence of underlying Alzheimer's disease neuropathology.

Second, there is no clear distinction between MCI and Alzheimer-related dementia, defined by the presence of functional impairment. Only a fraction of people with MCI progress to dementia: approximately 10% per year, although the figure varies widely according to clinical context. To recognise Alzheimer's disease early, with confidence, would aid clinical management and clinical trials.

The National Institute of Neurological and Communicative Diseases and Stroke–Alzheimer's Disease and Related Disorders Association (NINCDS–ADRDA) criteria (used to diagnose Alzheimer's disease) originally required only clinical and neuropsychological evidence of dysfunction for a diagnosis of probable Alzheimer's disease. They have been revised to incorporate cerebrospinal fluid or PET biomarkers [36]. To be positive for biomarkers of Alzheimer pathology greatly increases the likelihood of dementia, as do certain cognitive impairments. For example, deficits in allocentric spatial processing (i.e. the locations of objects relative to each other, independent of viewpoint) and paired-associates learning (i.e. encoding and retrieving newly formed associations between pairs of stimuli) are especially relevant [37, 38]. Cerebrospinal fluid biomarkers are standard in clinical practice, indicating the presence of Alzheimer's disease [39]. The amyloid-beta 1-42 peptide is reduced with Alzheimer's (and dementia with Lewy bodies, in the 40% of cases where there is dual pathology) while total tau and phosphorylated tau are elevated. Sensitivity and specificity (versus healthy controls) are typically in the region of 80–85%. However, the interpretation of such results depends on the clinical context because of the prior likelihood of a person having Alzheimer's pathology. At age 60 years, the prior probability of a healthy person having Alzheimer's disease is very low, so a positive biomarker greatly changes the posterior (after test) probability of having the disease. But, at 85 years, the prior probability of a healthy person having latent Alzheimer's disease pathology is ~30%, and a 'positive' biomarker test is less informative, and may divert attention away from other causes of symptoms. In the secondary-care memory-clinic setting, cerebrospinal fluid biomarkers are useful to diagnose Alzheimer's disease (versus non-Alzheimer's disease) if young cases are selected [40], but a positive test result becomes progressively less informative as age increases above 70. These tests may soon be superseded by blood-based biomarkers including Alzheimer-specific forms of phosphorylated tau.

Biomarker-positive MCI is often interpreted as evidence that Alzheimer's disease pathology is the cause of symptoms. This may be the case, especially for younger patients for whom the prior probability of Alzheimer's disease pathology is low. But, by the age of 80 years, a third of otherwise healthy adults (without memory symptoms) are positive for Alzheimer's disease biomarkers, reflecting latent (asymptomatic) pathology [41]. The biomarker status is not in that case sufficient to attribute symptoms to Alzheimer's disease pathology (at least not in isolation). Such variation in the positive predictive value for a test according to the prevalence of a disease is not unique to dementia biomarkers, but its consequences must not be overlooked in memory assessment services.

A third problem is that thresholds may vary between clinical practice, observational studies and clinical trials. For example, to prevent people without Alzheimer's disease pathology entering clinical trials, a high threshold on biomarkers is preferred, and this will exclude some people with Alzheimer's disease. In clinic, a lower threshold may be used, lowering the false-negative rate but increasing the false-positive rate, reflecting a balance of probability. Such thresholding issues are inevitable where diagnostic dichotomies are imposed on continuous variables. But for patients, the consequence can be confusion and distress.

The impact of the concept of MCI on Alzheimer's disease clinical practice and research fuelled efforts to define analogous states for other disorders. MIC is common in Parkinson's disease, and associated with dementia [42]. However, there is significant heterogeneity in the cognitive domains affected. Parkinson's disease MIC impairment is more heterogeneous that Alzheimer's disease MIC. The common patterns of early mild deficits (e.g. executive dysfunction) are not a *forme fruste* of the dementia phenotype (e.g. visuospatial and amnestic impairment). In this respect, the relationship between those with Parkinson's disease-associated MCI and those with Parkinson's disease and dementia differs from that between those who have Alzheimer's disease with MCI and Alzheimer's disease with dementia.

It is even more of a challenge to identify sensitive and specific criteria for 'frontotemporal dementia with MCI' or 'frontotemporal dementia with mild **behavioural** impairment', especially with the extent of pleiotropy discussed above. Apathy may develop subtly, years before the onset of disease is recognised [43], and resemble common psychiatric disorders like depression, or reactive stress to mid-life events. However, clinical trials for prevention and disease modification urgently require research criteria for these conditions. These are under development by international consortia allied to the Frontotemporal Dementia Prevention Initiative.

James B. Rowe and Alexander G. Murley

10.3 Preclinical Stages of Neurodegenerative Disease

The advent of biomarkers highlighted the pre-symptomatic stage of neurodegenerative disease, among apparently healthy adults with normal cognition (Figure 10.3.1A). This preclinical stage comes before the period of mild early symptoms and signs, which is called the prodromal phase. With genetic aetiology, one can study healthy pre-symptomatic adult mutation carriers many years before symptoms. This is underway through international collaborations such as the Dominantly Inherited Alzheimer Network, the Genetic Frontotemporal Dementia Initiative and Parkinson's Progression Markers Initiative genetic cohort. These international collaborations have much in common, with large cohorts (500–1,500) of patients and healthy first-degree relatives; followed longitudinally with 'deep phenotyping' of multiple blood, cerebrospinal fluid and imaging biomarkers and neuropsychological evaluation. Multimodal PET imaging, neurophysiology, eye-tracking, wearables and other phenotyping tools augment core protocols.

Despite differences between the diseases, they all have measurable consequences of the neurodegeneration many years before symptom onset; and there is a cascade of biomarkers that serve to detect and quantify the progression of pathology. The cascade of biomarkers (Figure 10.3.1B) is to be distinguished from the cascade of pathological processes (Figure 10.1.1), since the signal-to-noise and dynamic range of biomarkers will determine when they become clinically useful to detect the emergence of neuropathological and clinical features (Figure 10.3.1C).

Where genetics and family history allow prediction of age of onset, the genetic initiatives supplement longitudinal designs to assess very early changes in biological and functional aspects of disease. For example, autosomal-dominant Alzheimer's disease mutation carriers have elevated cortical amyloid levels 15 years before estimated onset of symptoms (Figure 10.3.1C),

hypometabolism 10 years before onset and atrophy 5 years before. Longitudinal data suggest an acceleration of atrophy around the time of symptom onset [44, 45]. Similarly, volumetric reductions in frontal and temporal brain regions emerge 10–15 years before the expected onset of frontotemporal dementia [46]. Reduced brain perfusion and increased neuroinflammation emerge many years before symptom onset. In Huntington's disease, accelerated atrophy – especially of the caudate nuclei – is underway more than 10 years from expected onset [47].

Where disorders lack a frequent genetic cause, alternative strategies are required to systematically interrogate pre-symptomatic states. For example, the UK Biobank recruited around 500,000 healthy adults in middle age, with baseline genotyping, cognitive measures, health and lifestyle assessment. They have been followed systematically with recall testing, and electronic health record surveillance augmented by MRI in a subset. A decade on, there are many cases of common sporadic neurodegeneration (several thousand cases of Alzheimer's disease and Parkinson's disease to date, rising rapidly each year). The next few years will see rapid expansion of insights from the UK Biobank, as the cohort ages and, with it, manifests their previously latent neurodegenerative disease.

Atrophy on MRI is a late effect of neurodegeneration – the graveyard of cortical pathology. It is non-specific with respect to the cellular and biochemical processes. These can be quantified from constituents of body fluids. Neurofilament light protein (NFL) is an index of large-fibre axonal degeneration, reliably measured in cerebrospinal fluid and more recently in blood. It is elevated in Alzheimer's disease, frontotemporal dementia, Huntington's disease and progressive supranuclear palsy. What it lacks in diagnostic specificity, it makes up for in its ability to detect pre-symptomatic degeneration, and its potential as a **proximity marker** when those

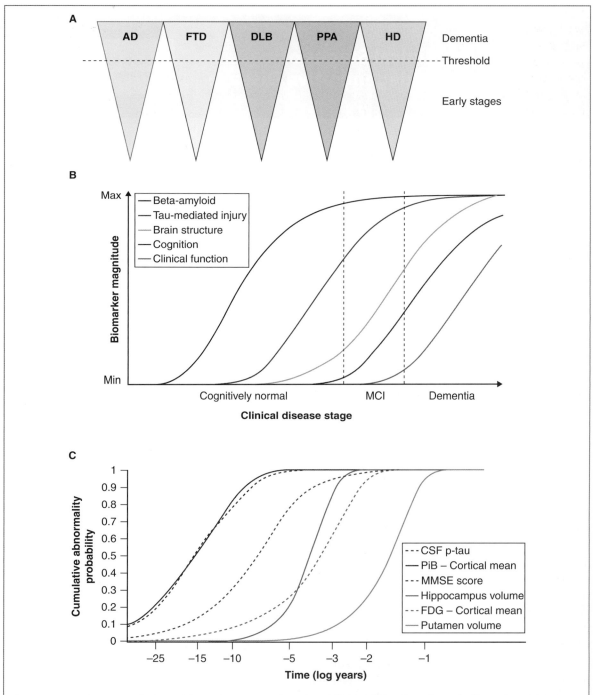

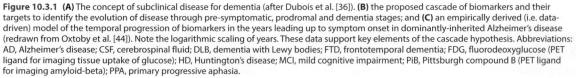

Figure 10.3.1 (A) The concept of subclinical disease for dementia (after Dubois et al. [36]). **(B)** the proposed cascade of biomarkers and their targets to identify the evolution of disease through pre-symptomatic, prodromal and dementia stages; and **(C)** an empirically derived (i.e. data-driven) model of the temporal progression of biomarkers in the years leading up to symptom onset in dominantly-inherited Alzheimer's disease (redrawn from Oxtoby et al. [44]). Note the logarithmic scaling of years. These data support key elements of the cascade hypothesis. Abbreviations: AD, Alzheimer's disease; CSF, cerebrospinal fluid; DLB, dementia with Lewy bodies; FTD, frontotemporal dementia; FDG, fluorodeoxyglucose (PET ligand for imaging tissue uptake of glucose); HD, Huntington's disease; MCI, mild cognitive impairment; PiB, Pittsburgh compound B (PET ligand for imaging amyloid-beta); PPA, primary progressive aphasia.

at risk of dementia approach symptom onset (i.e. to reveal how close a patient is to developing disease). In Huntington's disease, for example, NFL rises through the pre-symptomatic approach to onset, and does so faster in proportion to the number of CAG repeats in the *HTT* gene (see Figure 10.3.2) [48]. NFL is elevated in progressive supranuclear palsy and corticobasal syndrome, providing around 90% diagnostic accuracy versus controls [49]. In frontotemporal dementia, although NFL levels vary markedly between individuals, an increase in NFL

heralds the imminent onset of symptoms. The changes in NFL are not disease-specific, but partially reflect the rate of neurodegeneration, which is highest in amyotrophic lateral sclerosis, intermediate in frontotemporal dementia, Huntington's disease and progressive supranuclear palsy, but overlapping with normal ranges in Parkinson's disease and dementia with Lewy bodies.

Cerebrospinal fluid and blood biomarkers are increasing their sensitivity and range. For example, neuroinflammation is reflected in markers such as the chitinase-3-like

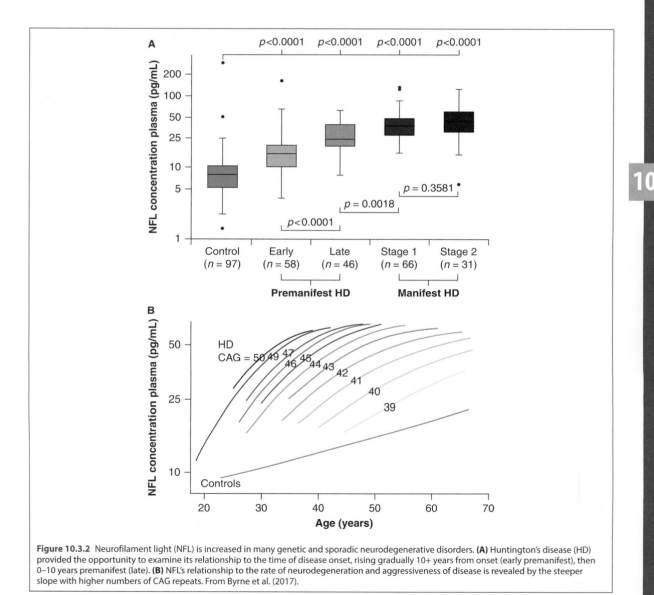

Figure 10.3.2 Neurofilament light (NFL) is increased in many genetic and sporadic neurodegenerative disorders. **(A)** Huntington's disease (HD) provided the opportunity to examine its relationship to the time of disease onset, rising gradually 10+ years from onset (early premanifest), then 0–10 years premanifest (late). **(B)** NFL's relationship to the rate of neurodegeneration and aggressiveness of disease is revealed by the steeper slope with higher numbers of CAG repeats. From Byrne et al. (2017).

protein 1 ('YKL-40') and triggering receptor expressed in myeloid cells 2 (TREM2) proteins, which correlate with PET indices of inflammation [50]. Synaptic degeneration is identified early in preclinical models and people with Alzheimer's disease pathology in terms of presynaptic (synaptosomal-associated protein 25 (SNAP25), growth-associated protein 43 (GAP43)) and postsynaptic (neurogranin (NRGN)) proteins [51].

The recognition of pre-symptomatic, prodromal, MCI and dementia states in a spectrum of disease is widely accepted. But, in addition to this spectrum of temporal progression, there is a spectrum of phenotypes that has received less attention but which is equally important if clinical trials are to be effective and inclusive, with results that generalise to benefit the widest possible patient population.

**James B. Rowe and
Alexander G. Murley**

10.4 Spectra, Domains and Dimensions of Neurodegenerative Disease

The syndromes caused by Alzheimer's disease pathology, dementia with Lewy bodies, frontotemporal lobar degeneration and progressive supranuclear palsy pathology are each diverse. For example, Alzheimer's disease commonly presents with amnesia (and hippocampal atrophy), but it can also present with visuospatial deficits (posterior cortical atrophy), logopenic progressive aphasia (temporoparietal atrophy), corticobasal syndrome (parkinsonism, dystonia, apraxia and higher cognitive deficits) or a behavioural/dysexecutive syndrome [52]. The pathology of alpha-synuclein-containing Lewy bodies can present with motor parkinsonism (clinical Parkinson's disease), dementia (clinical dementia with Lewy bodies) or autonomic and sleep disturbance. Even specific gene mutations causing frontotemporal dementia (e.g. *C9orf72*, *GRN* or *MAPT*) can present with behavioural change, progressive aphasia or parkinsonism, alone or in combination [40, 53]. With time, patients progress to a less differentiated dementia affecting multiple domains. For a discussion of language in neurodegenerative disease, see Subsection 5.17.4. For memory in neurodegenerative disease see Subsection 5.14.3.

Such heterogeneity of phenotypes is a challenge and an opportunity. The opportunity lies in the potential to extend the benefits of a disease-modifying drug identified in one phenotype of a given pathology, to the other phenotypes. Care is needed to ensure the risk–benefit assessment is favourable in other phenotypes which may have differential trajectories [49]. There is also the opportunity to identify the mechanistic determinants of phenotypic variance, whether genetic (e.g. *TMEM106B*, *LRRK2* above) or environmental [54]. Modifiers of clinical phenotype might be enhanced, opening new therapeutic strategies to avert disease.

The challenge lies in the inevitable failure of categorical diagnostic systems, and the failure of clinical trials that do not pertain to the relevant aspect of disease. For example,

several strategies to counteract the effect of *GRN* mutations are ready for clinical trials. Such treatments might even be used pre-symptomatically, so as to prevent frontotemporal dementia. But how should a trialist measure the efficacy of a compound, if the mutation can cause aphasia and/or parkinsonism and/or personality change? Can these domains of illness be captured in a single scale?

Instead, we propose a dimensional approach to disease. This has been standard practice in psychiatric research for many years, formalised in the National Institute for Mental Health Research Domains Criteria (RDoC) initiative. It is time for a 'neurological RDoC', to examine the origins of clinical phenotypes, and to identify the intermediate phenotypes that express convergence of causal mechanisms and foundations for treatable symptoms.

The dimensions of clinical phenotypes can then be interrogated with enhanced statistical power across diagnostic groups, and in relation to severity rather than arbitrary categorisation. The genetic, molecular, cellular, pharmacological, physiological and connectomic basis of the dimensions can then be characterised. It is not a search for diagnostic biomarkers, but a data-driven framework to understand brain–behaviour disorder. For example, consider the heterogeneity of syndromes caused by frontotemporal lobar degeneration [55]. Patients can be placed in diagnostic categories, under current criteria, but these diagnostic groups are confluent rather than distinct in symptomatology. The dimensional approach can be understood by the analogy of a continuous colour space rather than discrete colours (recall, the colours of a rainbow are a cultural artefact, not physics), illustrated in Figure 10.4.1. To treat a problem like impulsivity, one can then identify the causes of impulsivity, address the underlying mechanism and treat the impulsive patient regardless of their diagnostic label. Conversely, if a patient does not express a given dimension, do not treat it, even if others with the same diagnosis are affected.

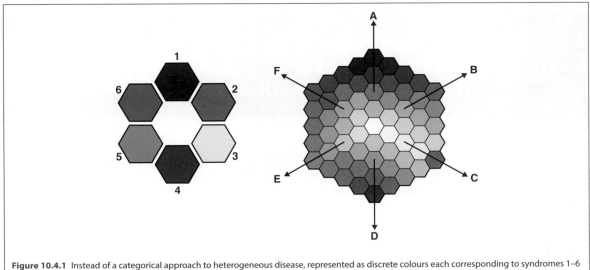

Figure 10.4.1 Instead of a categorical approach to heterogeneous disease, represented as discrete colours each corresponding to syndromes 1–6 (left), diseases can be represented by orthogonal dimensions A–F (right). An individual patient might lie anywhere in the continuous dimensional space. For example, if 1–6 were the syndromes caused by frontotemporal dementia (behavioural variant, semantic variant, logopenic variant, progressive supranuclear palsy, corticobasal syndrome), the dimensions A–F might correspond approximately to impulsivity, semantics, logopenia, agrammatism, apraxia/dystonia and gaze palsy/falls. Patients with mixed syndromes lie within intermediate colours, e.g. progressive supranuclear palsy with corticobasal syndrome, or corticobasal syndrome with non-fluent agrammatism [55].

10.5 Reserve, Resilience and Resistance to Neurodegeneration

James B. Rowe and Alexander G. Murley

We have seen that there is a long period of neurodegeneration in the absence of symptoms. This asymptomatic period highlights the issues of functional reserve, resilience and tolerance – that function (cognition, activities and roles etc.) can be maintained despite pathology (molecular pathology, neuroinflammation, synaptic loss, atrophy).

A temporal dissociation between pathology onset and symptoms onset may be the result of reserve. Higher reserve refers to a greater starting capacity in a system, such as more neurons or synapses. This capacity is gradually used up, until a functional threshold is crossed when a critical proportion is degenerated. Reserve may also be considered in terms of cognitive systems, in the way that neural resources are used to mediate cognitive processes.

Resilience refers to the capacity of a dynamic system to withstand neurodegeneration (or other injury). It may result from the inherent organisation of a neurocognitive system. For example, cognitive functions that depend on a distributed network are more likely to survive random lesions to the network. However, some of what is referred to currently as resilience may be reduced injury to the brain by lesions that are associated with comorbid diseases and risk factors, rather than resilience of the brain to the effects of injury and degeneration.

In families affected by genetic forms of frontotemporal dementia, atrophy clearly emerges more than a decade before expected symptom onset [46]. However, the efficiency of information transfer in large-scale brain networks is maintained, until around the time of symptom onset, after which there is a precipitate decline in proportion to clinical disease severity [56]. One interpretation is that symptoms are held off for as long as the neurocognitive system can compensate for cell loss in such a way as to maintain functional connectivity. These compensatory mechanisms are eventually overwhelmed. To harness the potential of such mechanisms will require formal models of compensation [57].

Resilience and reserve are not synonymous. Reserve speaks to capacity in a neurocognitive system, while resilience speaks to adaptability and compensation. Parallel systems, such as bilateral language representations, may provide both reserve and resilience. Education, occupation and lifestyle factors are often used as proxies for cognitive reserve, but they may also confer resilience. The differentiation between resilience and reserve is made difficult by recruitment biases into research cohorts (typically towards higher health, wealth and education and lower comorbidity), and the paucity of long-term phenotyping with consistent methodology.

Cellular mechanisms can also determine the functional consequences of pathology. For example, the burden of aggregated misfolded protein tau has been closely associated with the phenotype and severity of Alzheimer's disease [29]. However, in preclinical models at least, cells can be induced to resist the effects of high levels of aggregated misfolded tau [58]. The causes of reserve, resilience and resistance provide immediate routes to reduce the risk and burden of dementia, particularly through modification of environmental risk factors, which we turn to in the next section.

We have seen that the diagnostic and prognostic relevance of biomarkers changes with age, and that as people reach their 90s, the presence of Alzheimer's disease pathology becomes less predictive of cognitive impairment. This apparent age-related dissociation between pathology and symptoms has several possible causes. There may be cohort differences between those who are young now versus those who were young in the past; or bias towards more benign forms of pathology in later life; with slower replication rates for misfolded proteins that can be mitigated by autophagy; or a change in corollary pathogenic processes like inflammation. There is also the dissociation between the less toxic plaques/tangles seen on microscopy and the more toxic oligomeric misfolded proteins that are not visible. Age would be expected to increase the number of chronic aggregates of amyloid and tau that are seen on light microscopy (or measured by PET scans), even without changing the toxicity of invisible oligomers. Such an effect would lead to apparent resilience to the disease, as measured by aggregate burden.

<table>
<tr><td>**10.6**</td><td>**Environmental Causes of Neurodegenerative Disease**</td><td>**James B. Rowe and Alexander G. Murley**</td></tr>
</table>

In the seminal report of the Lancet Commission on dementia [54] the identification of contributory risk factors, their effect size and their modifiabilty, led to a startling conclusion: as much as 40% of dementia could be prevented by immediate application of known interventions. Not by a novel disease-modifying treatment but a systematic approach to resolve and reduce risk factors across the lifespan. Early-life education; mid-life obesity, hypertension and hearing loss; and later life exercise, smoking, social isolation, diabetes, depression and pollution contribute to this potential for dementia prevention.

Some of the environmentally modifiable risk factors may have genetic influences, such as obesity, hearing loss and hypertension. But the key message is the modifiability of the risk by environmental measures – calling on collaboration across political, healthcare, educational and social services to promote and support individuals' engagement with dementia prevention. Many of the preventive measures operate at a national policy level, or require access to services that may not be available in many areas. It is important therefore that the optimism around the potential for dementia prevention is not re-cast to imply blame on those that have developed dementia.

There are two other lines of inquiry that support the importance of modifiable environmental factors.

First, twin studies of neurodegeneration indicate high heritability of late-life Alzheimer's disease at 50–60% [59], but the twin discordance suggests that environmental factors influence the start of beta-amyloid and tau aggregation [60]. Second, some neurodegenerative diseases have in effect died out. For example, the prion disease kuru, which reached epidemic levels during the 1950s and 1960s among the Fore people in the Eastern Highlands of Papua New Guinea, has not been seen for over a decade. A second example is the amyotrophic lateral sclerosis–parkinsonism–dementia complex of Guam (Lytico–bodig disease). In 1950 it was the leading cause of death in Chamorro adults, but has now all but disappeared. These examples, albeit rare and with the potential for gene–environment interactions, confirm that environmental changes can, in principle, eradicate neurodegenerative disease.

There are other well-known and common environmental contributors to dementia, like alcohol, HIV and traumatic brain injury. Alcohol misuse is a common cause of cognitive decline. It is injurious by multiple mechanisms, including direct chronic neurotoxicity, interactions with vitamin B1 depletion in Wernicke–Korsakoff syndrome, increased risk of head trauma and neglect of beneficial lifestyle and healthcare measures. This brings us to the complex issue of comorbidity.

10.7 Comorbidity and Dual Pathology in Neurodegenerative Disorders

James B. Rowe and
Alexander G. Murley

Descriptions of the aetiology of neurodegenerative disorders often focus on their specific molecular and genetic basis of archetypical phenotypes. Clinical trials usually focus on unequivocal and unconfounded cases, through strict inclusion and exclusion criteria. This is understandable in terms of clarity of didactic teaching, and clinical trial efficiency. However, comorbidity is the norm, not the exception. The Cognitive Function and Ageing Study monitored dementia, mild cognitive impairment and major comorbidities (anaemia, Parkinson's disease, breathing difficulties, angina, hypertension, diabetes mellitus, peripheral vascular disease, transient ischaemic attack, stroke or heart attack). With a mean age of 74 years, over half of participants reported comorbidities, and 12% had three or more [61].

Comorbidity may alter the performance of diagnostic tests; modify the phenotype; and worsen prognosis, through biological interactions or by undermining optimal care. Comorbidity may change the safety of medication. And the dementia may undermine good care and engagement in health maintenance activities to mitigate the comorbid condition. For example, diabetes and Alzheimer's disease are mutually detrimental. Comorbidity does not necessarily arise from shared genetic correlations; for example Alzheimer's disease and stroke may have separate genetic risks and a high prevalence of 'mixed' vascular disease and Alzheimer's disease [62].

In addition to systemic comorbidities, many people have dual cerebral pathologies. Cerebrovascular disease, including small vessel disease and stroke, is especially common. With cerebral amyloid angiopathy (a condition in which amyloid protein is deposited in the walls of brain blood vessels), even a single microhaemorrhage identified by MRI worsens the prognosis of Alzheimer's disease. Small vessel disease, associated with hypertension and

diabetes, is frequently seen on MRI as white matter hyperintensities, whose extent correlates with cognitive impairment in neurodegenerative disorders. Interestingly, vascular and inflammatory contributions to dementia are related [63, 64]. A systematic approach to these interactions may facilitate risk reduction and new treatment strategies.

Dual pathology also includes dual degenerative processes. For example, in dementia with Lewy bodies around 40% of people have comorbid Alzheimer's disease pathology at post-mortem or ante-mortem biomarker studies [65], often in conjunction with vascular white matter lesions. This is twice the prevalence that would be expected by chance in view of age-related norms. Dual pathology is common with frontotemporal lobar degeneration, including around 8% with dementia with Lewy bodies ≥ Braak stage IV [66]. Among patients with primary frontotemporal lobar degeneration as the cause of a phenotype for which frontotemporal dementia had been considered as a diagnosis, 54% had some Alzheimer's disease neuropathology, though at low levels in most cases; 16% had cerebrovascular disease, 11% dementia with Lewy bodies, 39% limbic argyrophilic grain disease and 8% had incidental or contributing TDP-43 proteinopathy. Where the clinical diagnostic confidence of frontotemporal dementia was low, a third had pathological Alzheimer's disease but copathologies were common including dementia with Lewy bodies 33%, cerebrovascular disease 13%, argyrophilic grain disease 50% and TDP-43 in 22% of cases [67]. Limbic-predominant age-related TDP-43 encephalopathy (LATE) is a less-well-known neuropathology of later life, with TDP-43 proteinopathy, affecting medial temporal lobe structures, leading to amnesia. It is likely to be a major contributor to non-Alzheimer's disease dementia in the older population. The genetic associations of LATE (*GRN*,

TMEM106B, *ABCC9*, *KCNMB2* and *APOE*) suggest shared pathogenic mechanisms with both frontotemporal lobar degeneration and Alzheimer's disease, including dysregulation of inflammatory pathways, as a reminder of the commonalities in the cascade of events leading to the many neurodegenerative disorders.

Conclusions and Outstanding Questions

We began with the burden of dementia, and complexity of the cascade of events from genetics, through inflammation and prion-like propagation of disease, ending on the complexity of comorbidity and dual pathology. We have seen how each of the neurodegenerative disorders presents a spectrum over time – from long asymptomatic stages, through prodromal symptoms, and on to dementia – and a spectrum of clinical syndromes, even with the same genetics and neuropathology. To end the chapter, and the book, we can be optimistic that it is already plausible to prevent 40% of the burden of dementia, and that the cascade of causality in Figure 10.1.1 presents a wealth of opportunities to treat and prevent the remainder. Indeed, there are approximately 150 agents currently in clinical trials as disease-modifying treatments for

Alzheimer's disease alone [68], with rapid innovations and increasing clinical trials for the non-Alzheimer's dementias. We can be optimistic about the eventual success of new treatments, and your input will be key to this success.

Outstanding Questions

- How do we design clinical trials to show the ability of interventions to prevent dementia in dementia gene mutation carriers?
- How can we exploit the differences between individuals with the 'same disease' to identify and exploit the intrinsic modifying mechanisms?
- How do we work across professional boundaries to deliver the 40% reduction indicated as already feasible by the Lancet Commission?
- Our individual personality, language, social context and autobiographical experience shape the expression of neurodegenerative dementias – how can this human dimension inform the model of neurodegeneration so as to improve individual care?
- Will genetics or clinical phenotyping be a more effective means to precision medicine?
- Why do some older adults manage to carry a lot of neuropathology without dementia?

10

REFERENCES FOR CHAPTER 10

1. Alzheimer's Disease International. World Alzheimer Report. The global impact of dementia: an analysis of prevalence, incidence, cost and trends. 2015. www.alz.co.uk/worldreport2015.

2. Koriath, C. et al. Predictors for a dementia gene mutation based on gene-panel next-generation sequencing of a large dementia referral series. *Mol Psychiatry* 2020; 25(12): 3399–3412.

3. Nicholson, A. M., R. Rademakers. What we know about *TMEM106B* in neurodegeneration. *Acta Neuropathol* 2016; 132(5): 639–651.

4. Jabbari, E. et al. Genetic determinants of survival in progressive supranuclear palsy: a genome-wide association study. *Lancet Neurol* 2021; 20(2): 107–116.

5. Maple-Grodem, J. et al. Association of *GBA* genotype with motor and functional decline in patients with newly diagnosed Parkinson disease. *Neurology* 2021; 96(7): e1036–e1044.

6. Winder-Rhodes, S. E. et al. Glucocerebrosidase mutations influence the natural history of Parkinson's disease in a community-based incident cohort. *Brain* 2013; 136(Pt 2): 392–399.

7. Henson, R. N. et al. Effect of apolipoprotein E polymorphism on cognition and brain in the Cambridge Centre for Ageing and Neuroscience cohort. *Brain Neurosci Adv* 2020; 4: 2398212820961704.

8. Escott-Price, V. et al. Polygenic risk score analysis of pathologically confirmed Alzheimer disease. *Ann Neurol* 2017; 82(2): 311–314.

9. Escott-Price, V. et al. Common polygenic variation enhances risk prediction for Alzheimer's disease. *Brain* 2015; 138(Pt 12): 3673–3684.

10. Ferrari, R. et al. Genetic architecture of sporadic frontotemporal dementia and overlap with Alzheimer's and Parkinson's diseases. *J Neurol Neurosurg Psychiatry* 2017; 88(2): 152–164.

11. Chia, R. et al. Genome sequencing analysis identifies new loci associated with Lewy body dementia and provides insights into its genetic architecture. *Nat Genet* 2021; 53(3): 294–303.

12. Ittner, L. M. et al. Dendritic function of tau mediates amyloid-beta toxicity in Alzheimer's disease mouse models. *Cell* 2010; 142(3): 387–397.

13. Dewan, R. et al. Pathogenic huntingtin repeat expansions in patients with frontotemporal dementia and amyotrophic lateral sclerosis. *Neuron* 2021; 109(3): 448–460e4.

14. Kunkle, B. W. et al. Genetic meta-analysis of diagnosed Alzheimer's disease identifies new risk loci and implicates Aβ, tau, immunity and lipid processing. *Nat Genet* 2019; 51(3): 414–430.

15. Hoglinger, G. U. et al. Identification of common variants influencing risk of the tauopathy progressive supranuclear palsy. *Nat Genet* 2011; 43(7): 699–705.

16. Passamonti, L. et al. ^{18}F-AV-1451 positron emission tomography in Alzheimer's disease and progressive supranuclear palsy. *Brain* 2017; 140(3): 781–791.

17. Bevan-Jones, W. R. et al. Neuroinflammation and protein aggregation co-localize across the frontotemporal dementia spectrum. *Brain* 2020; 143(3): 1010–1026.

18. Surendranathan, A. et al. Early microglial activation and peripheral inflammation in dementia with Lewy bodies. *Brain* 2018; 141(12): 3415–3427.

19. Tai, Y. F. et al. Microglial activation in presymptomatic Huntington's disease gene carriers. *Brain* 2007; 130(Pt 7): 1759–1766.

20. Hong, S. et al. Complement and microglia mediate early synapse loss in Alzheimer mouse models. *Science* 2016; 352(6286): 712–716.

21. Bevan-Jones, W. R. et al. *In vivo* evidence for pre-symptomatic neuroinflammation in a *MAPT* mutation carrier. *Ann Clin Transl Neurol* 2019; 6(2): 373–378.

22. Malpetti, M. et al. Microglial activation and tau burden predict cognitive decline in Alzheimer's disease. *Brain* 2020; 143(5): 1588–1602.

23. Prusiner, S. B. Biology and genetics of prions causing neurodegeneration. *Annu Rev Genet* 2013; 47: 601–623.

24. Ahmed, Z. et al. A novel *in vivo* model of tau propagation with rapid and progressive neurofibrillary tangle pathology: the pattern of spread is determined by connectivity, not proximity. *Acta Neuropathol* 2014; 127(5): 667–683.

25. Uemura, N. et al. Cell-to-cell transmission of tau and alpha-synuclein. *Trends Mol Med* 2020; 26(10): 936–952.

26. De La-Rocque, S. et al. Knockin' on heaven's door: molecular mechanisms of neuronal tau uptake. *J Neurochem* 2021; 156(5): 563–588.

27. Gibbons, G. S., V. M. Y. Lee, J. Q. Trojanowski. Mechanisms of cell-to-cell transmission of pathological tau: a review. *JAMA Neurol* 2019; 76(1): 101–108.

28. Selkoe, D. J., J. Hardy. The amyloid hypothesis of Alzheimer's disease at 25 years. *EMBO Mol Med* 2016; 8(6): 595–608.

29. Ossenkoppele, R. et al. Tau PET patterns mirror clinical and neuroanatomical variability in Alzheimer's disease. *Brain* 2016; 139(Pt 5): 1551–1567.

30. Lu, L. et al. Anti-Aβ agents for mild to moderate Alzheimer's disease: systematic review and meta-analysis. *J Neurol Neurosurg Psychiatry* 2020; 91(12): 1316–1324.

31. Murray, M. E. et al. Clinicopathologic and ^{11}C-Pittsburgh compound B implications of Thal amyloid phase across the Alzheimer's disease spectrum. *Brain* 2015; 138(Pt 5): 1370–1381.

32. Ossenkoppele, R. et al. Distinct tau PET patterns in atrophy-defined subtypes of Alzheimer's disease. *Alzheimers Dement* 2020; 16(2): 335–344.

33. Nisbet, R. M. et al. Tau aggregation and its interplay with amyloid-beta. *Acta Neuropathol* 2015; 129(2): 207–220.

34. Petersen, R. C. et al. Aging, memory, and mild cognitive impairment. *Int Psychogeriatr* 1997; 9 (Suppl 1): 65–69.

35. Albert, M. S. et al. The diagnosis of mild cognitive impairment due to Alzheimer's disease: recommendations from the National Institute on Aging–Alzheimer's Association workgroups on diagnostic guidelines for Alzheimer's disease. *Alzheimers Dement* 2011; 7(3): 270–279.

36. Dubois, B. et al. Research criteria for the diagnosis of Alzheimer's disease: revising the NINCDS–ADRDA criteria. *Lancet Neurol* 2007; 6(8): 734–746.

37. Ritchie, K. et al. Allocentric and egocentric spatial processing in middle-aged adults at high risk of late-onset Alzheimer's disease: the PREVENT dementia study. *J Alzheimers Dis* 2018; 65(3): 885–896.

38. Barnett, J. H. et al. The Paired Associates Learning (PAL) Test: 30 years of CANTAB translational neuroscience from laboratory to bedside in dementia research. *Curr Top Behav Neurosci* 2016; 28: 449–474.

39. Paterson, R. W. et al. Cerebrospinal fluid in the differential diagnosis of Alzheimer's disease: clinical utility of an extended panel of biomarkers in a specialist cognitive clinic. *Alzheimers Res Ther* 2018; 10(1): 32.

40. Boelaarts, L., J. F. M. de Jonghe, P. Scheltens. Diagnostic impact of CSF biomarkers in a local hospital memory clinic revisited. *Dement Geriatr Cogn Disord* 2020; 49(1): 2–7.

41. Toledo, J. B. et al. Alzheimer's disease cerebrospinal fluid biomarker in cognitively normal subjects. *Brain* 2015; 138(Pt 9): 2701–2715.

42. Goldman, J. G. et al. Evolution of diagnostic criteria and assessments for Parkinson's disease mild cognitive impairment. *Mov Disord* 2018; 33(4): 503–510.

43. Malpetti, M. et al. Apathy in presymptomatic genetic frontotemporal dementia predicts cognitive decline and is driven by structural brain changes. *Alzheimers Dement* 2021; 17(6): 969–983.

10

44. Oxtoby, N. P. et al. Data-driven models of dominantly-inherited Alzheimer's disease progression. *Brain* 2018; 141(5): 1529–1544.

45. Benzinger, T. L. et al. Regional variability of imaging biomarkers in autosomal dominant Alzheimer's disease. *Proc Natl Acad Sci USA* 2013 110(47): E4502–E4509.

46. Rohrer, J. D. et al. Presymptomatic cognitive and neuroanatomical changes in genetic frontotemporal dementia in the Genetic Frontotemporal dementia Initiative (GENFI) study: a cross-sectional analysis. *Lancet Neurol* 2015; 14(3): 253–262.

47. Tabrizi, S. J. et al. Biological and clinical manifestations of Huntington's disease in the longitudinal TRACK-HD study: cross-sectional analysis of baseline data. *Lancet Neurol* 2009; 8(9): 791–801.

48. Byrne, L. M. et al. Neurofilament light protein in blood as a potential biomarker of neurodegeneration in Huntington's disease: a retrospective cohort analysis. *Lancet Neurol* 2017; 16(8): 601–609.

49. Jabbari, E. et al. Diagnosis across the spectrum of progressive supranuclear palsy and corticobasal syndrome. *JAMA Neurol* 2020; 77(3): 377–387.

50. Toppala, S. et al. Association of early beta-amyloid accumulation and neuroinflammation measured with [(11)C]PBR28 in elderly individuals without dementia. *Neurology* 2021; 96(12): e1608–e1619.

51. Pereira, J. B. et al. Untangling the association of amyloid-beta and tau with synaptic and axonal loss in Alzheimer's disease. *Brain* 2021; 144(1): 310–324.

52. Galton, C. J. et al. Atypical and typical presentations of Alzheimer's disease: a clinical, neuropsychological, neuroimaging and pathological study of 13 cases. *Brain* 2000; 123 (Pt 3): 484–498.

53. Rowe, J. B. Parkinsonism in frontotemporal dementias. *Int Rev Neurobiol* 2019; 149: 249–275.

54. Livingston, G. et al. Dementia prevention, intervention, and care: 2020 report of the Lancet Commission. *Lancet* 2020; 396(10248): 413–446.

55. Murley, A. G. et al. Redefining the multidimensional clinical phenotypes of frontotemporal lobar degeneration syndromes. *Brain* 2020; 143(5): 1555–1571.

56. Rittman, T. et al. Functional network resilience to pathology in presymptomatic genetic frontotemporal dementia. *Neurobiol Aging* 2019; 77: 169–177.

57. Gregory, S. et al. Testing a longitudinal compensation model in premanifest Huntington's disease. *Brain* 2018; 141(7): 2156–2166.

58. Radford, H. et al. PERK inhibition prevents tau-mediated neurodegeneration in a mouse model of frontotemporal dementia. *Acta Neuropathol* 2015; 130(5): 633–642.

59. Pedersen, N. L. et al. How heritable is Alzheimer's disease late in life? Findings from Swedish twins. *Ann Neurol* 2004; 55(2): 180–185.

60. Konijnenberg, E. et al. The onset of preclinical Alzheimer's disease in monozygotic twins. *Ann Neurol* 2021; 89(5): 987–1000.

61. Stephan, B. C. et al. Occurrence of medical co-morbidity in mild cognitive impairment: implications for generalisation of MCI research. *Age Ageing* 2011; 40(4): 501–507.

62. Anttila, V. et al. Analysis of shared heritability in common disorders of the brain. *Science* 2018; 360(6395): eaap8757.

63. Low, A. et al. Inflammation and cerebral small vessel disease: a systematic review. *Ageing Res Rev* 2019; 53: 100916.

64. Horsburgh, K. et al. Small vessels, dementia and chronic diseases: molecular mechanisms and pathophysiology. *Clin Sci (Lond)* 2018; 132(8): 851–868.

65. Jansen, W. J. et al. Prevalence of cerebral amyloid pathology in persons without dementia: a meta-analysis. *JAMA* 2015; 313(19): 1924–1938.

66. Forrest, S. L. et al. Coexisting Lewy body disease and clinical parkinsonism in frontotemporal lobar degeneration. *Neurology* 2019; 92(21): e2472–e2482.

67. Perry, D. C. et al. Clinicopathological correlations in behavioural variant frontotemporal dementia. *Brain* 2017; 140(12): 3329–3345.

68. Cummings, J. et al. Alzheimer's disease drug development pipeline: 2022. *Alzheimers Dement* 2022; 8(1): e12295.

National Neuroscience Curriculum Initiative online resources

Metabolism and Memory: Obesity, Diabetes, and Dementia

Daniel Shalev and Melissa R. Arbuckle

Amyloid: From Starch to Finish

Hannah L. Krystal, David A. Ross and Adam P. Mecca

Clinical neuroscience conversations: *Neurobiology of Alzheimer's Disease*

Adam P. Mecca

10

National Neuroscience Curriculum Initiative online resources

So Happy Together: The Storied Marriage Between Mitochondria and the Mind

Ruth F. Mccann and David A. Ross

This "stuff" is really cool: Noah Philip, *"Placebo Effect"*

This "stuff" is really cool: Roel Mocking, *"Forget Everything"* on fatty acids and psychiatric disorders

This "stuff" is really cool: Youngsun Cho, *"Precision Medicine"*

Expert video: *Jon Kar Zubieta on The Placebo Effect*

Index

Index

Index

Index

Index

Index

Index

Index

Index